Drug Delivery
An Integrated Clinical and Engineering Approach

Drug Delivery
An Integrated Clinical and Engineering Approach

Edited by
Yitzhak Rosen
Pablo Gurman
Noel M. Elman

CRC Press
Taylor & Francis Group
Boca Raton London New York

CRC Press is an imprint of the
Taylor & Francis Group, an **informa** business

CRC Press
Taylor & Francis Group
6000 Broken Sound Parkway NW, Suite 300
Boca Raton, FL 33487-2742

First issued in paperback 2019

ISBN-13: 978-1-4665-6594-4 (hbk)
ISBN-13: 978-0-367-86765-2 (pbk)

Visit the Taylor & Francis Web site at
http://www.taylorandfrancis.com

and the CRC Press Web site at
http://www.crcpress.com

Contents

Foreword

This book is a comprehensive overview in the much needed area of drug delivery. It addresses a critical unmet need, the approach of integrating the clinical and engineering disciplines for drug delivery optimization and advancement. This integration is a must, requires a patient-oriented approach, and is a key foundation in drug delivery development.

Furthermore, the book focuses on important advances and discusses how an integrated approach was used for these advances. It consists of 21 chapters, starting with a thorough introduction to drug delivery and pharmacokinetics, followed by diverse clinical examples of this integration. The book discusses the following areas and their advances: oral and intrathecal drug delivery; insulin delivery and artificial pancreas; micro- and nanotechnology for drug delivery, including applications of micro- and nanotechnology in vaccines; inflammatory diseases; airway diseases and the use of nanoparticles as tracking systems; biomaterial-based delivery systems, including chitosan and microsponges; gene delivery, cancer drug delivery with a focus on stem cells; cardiac drug delivery; intravitreal drug delivery; and drug delivery in obstetrics and gynecology as well as an important chapter on FDA regulation of drug delivery systems.

As an experienced clinician and discoverer of a new autoimmune syndrome (ASIA Syndrome), developer of novel therapeutics, publisher of numerous papers and books, and editor in chief of two journals on autoimmunity (*Autoimmunity Reviews* IF-7.95 and *Journal of Autoimmunity* IF 8.4), it is my hope that all clinicians and engineers involved in advancing drug delivery will find in this book a useful resource. Therefore, I give this book the highest recommendation.

Yehuda Shoenfeld, MD, FRCP, MaACR
Head of Zabludowicz Center for Autoimmune Diseases
Sheba Medical Center, Affiliated with Tel Aviv University

Acknowledgments

We, as editors, take this opportunity to acknowledge all the contributors, editorial staff, family, and friends for greatly assisting us in making this important book publication a reality.

Editors

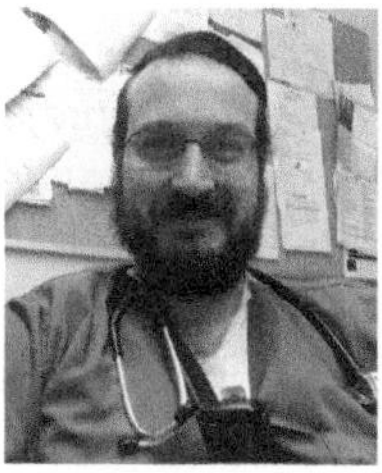

Yitzhak Rosen, MD, is a graduate of the Tel Aviv University of Medicine. He completed an internal medicine residency at Coney Island Hospital and is currently a fellow at the Cardiovascular Division of SUNY Downstate Medical Center in Brooklyn, New York. He has worked as a research scientist at the Institute for Soldier Nanotechnologies, Massachusetts Institute of Technology (MIT). He is also the president and CEO of Superior NanoBioSystems LLC, a biomedical company. He has served in the Israel Defense Forces (IDF) as a medical officer and physician in militarily active areas. He completed a medical internship at the Rabin Medical Center and has worked at the Oncology Institutes of both the Rabin and the Sheba Medical Centers in Israel. He has invented a microfluidic chip platform, funded by the Defense Advanced Research Projects Agency (DARPA), for effecting extremely rapid blood typing and cross-matching for mass casualties in collaboration with the MEMS and Nanotechnology Exchange. In addition, he is the inventor of several medical ultrasound technologies.

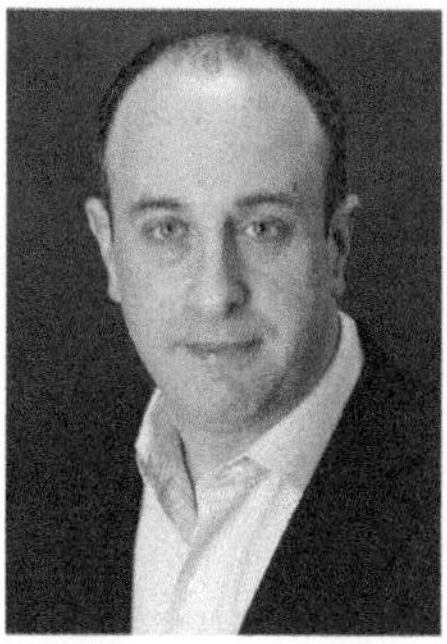

Pablo Gurman, MD, earned his MD degree from Buenos Aires University School of Medicine in 2002, where he worked at the Pharmacology Department for 10 years. He is currently the chief medical officer at GearJump Technologies, a biotechnology company dedicated to developing innovative solutions to public health problems. Prior to this appointment, he was a research scientist at the Materials Science and Engineering Department at the University of Texas-Dallas, as well as a research collaborator at Dr. Elman's group at the Institute for Soldiers Nanotechnologies at the Massachusetts Institute of Technology (MIT). Dr. Gurman was a visiting scientist at Argonne National Laboratory, where he worked under the artificial retina program.

Gurman's primary research interests involve micro- and nanotechnology for medical diagnostics and therapeutics, controlled release technologies, and biomaterials.

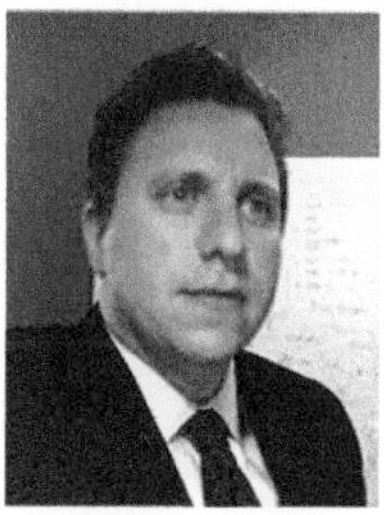

Noel M. Elman, PhD, is the CEO and founder of GearJump Technologies, LLC, a company dedicated to development of biotechnological solutions for public health applications. Dr. Elman is also a lecturer in technology and innovation at the Buenos Aires Institute of Technology. He worked at Draper Laboratory, an MIT-affiliated DoD-supported R&D center, where he was an appointed distinguished member of the technical staff. Prior to this appointment, he was a research scientist and principal investigator at the Institute for Soldier Nanotechnologies at MIT, leading a translational research group focused on developing technologies for biotech, biomed, and public health applications. In addition, he was appointed an Innovation Fellow at Massachusetts General Hospital. Dr. Elman's research focus is on rapid translation from idea conceptualization to experimental realization. He earned his bachelor's and master's degrees in electrical engineering at Cornell University, and his PhD degree in electrical engineering at Tel Aviv University. He performed postdoctoral studies at MIT, investigating several micro- and nanodevices for therapeutics and diagnostics.

Contributors

Lissa Nurrul Abdullah
Cancer Science Institute of Singapore
National University of Singapore
Singapore

Sharifa Al-Zahrani
School of Pharmacy
Queen's University
Belfast, United Kingdom

José L. Arias
Department of Pharmacy and Pharmaceutical Technology
Faculty of Pharmacy
University of Granada
Campus Universitario de Cartuja s/n
Granada, Spain

Shimon Ben-Shabat
Department of Clinical Pharmacology
School of Pharmacy
Faculty of Health Sciences
Ben-Gurion University of the Negev
Beer-Sheva, Israel

Luis Bruno Blanch
Medicinal Chemistry
Department of Biological Sciences
School of Sciences
National University of La Plata (UNLP)
La Plata, Argentina

María J. Blanco-Prieto
Department of Pharmacy and Pharmaceutical Technology
School of Pharmacy
University of Navarra
Pamplona, Spain

Maximiliano L. Cacicedo
Nanobiomaterials Laboratory
Institute of Applied Biotechnology (CINDEFI, UNLP-CONICET-CCT La Plata)
Department of Chemistry
School of Sciences
Universidad Nacional de La Plata
La Plata, Argentina

Guillermo R. Castro
Nanobiomaterials Laboratory
Institute of Applied Biotechnology (CINDEFI, UNLP-CONICET-CCT La Plata)
Department of Chemistry
School of Sciences
National University of La Plata
La Plata, Argentina

SriKrishna Chandran
University Hospitals of Cleveland
Cleveland, Ohio

Mohini Chaurasia
Amity Institute of Pharmacy
Amity University
Lucknow, India

Manish K. Chourasia
Pharmaceutics Division
CSIR-Central Drug Research Institute
Lucknow, India

Edward Kai-Hua Chow
Department of Pharmacology
Yong Loo Lin School of Medicine
and
Cancer Science Institute of Singapore
National University of Singapore
Singapore

Ana Costa
CESPU
Instituto de Investigação e Formação Avançada em Ciências e Tecnologias da Saúde
Department of Pharmaceutical Sciences
Gandra-PRD, Portugal

Arik Dahan
Department of Clinical Pharmacology
School of Pharmacy
Faculty of Health Sciences
Ben-Gurion University of the Negev
Beer-Sheva, Israel

Jonathan Daich
Superior NanoBioSystems LLC

Eyal Dassau
Harvard John A. Paulson School of Engineering and Applied Sciences
Harvard University
Cambridge, Massachusetts

Simón Pascual-Gil de Gómez
Department of Pharmacy and Pharmaceutical Technology
School of Pharmacy
University of Navarra
Pamplona, Spain

Paula Díaz-Herráez
Department of Pharmacy and Pharmaceutical Technology
School of Pharmacy
University of Navarra
Pamplona, Spain

Ryan F. Donnelly
School of Pharmacy
Queen's University
Belfast, United Kingdom

Mazen M. El-Hammadi
Department of Pharmacy and Pharmaceutical Technology
Faculty of Pharmacy
University of Granada
Campus Universitario de Cartuja s/n
Granada, Spain

and

Department of Pharmaceutics and Pharmaceutical Technology
Faculty of Pharmacy
Damascus University
Damascus, Syria

Noel M. Elman
GearJump Technologies, LLC
Brookline, Massachusetts

Steven J. Fallows
School of Pharmacy
Queen's University
Belfast, United Kingdom

Pedro Fonte
CESPU
Instituto de Investigação e Formação Avançada em Ciências e Tecnologias da Saúde
Department of Pharmaceutical Sciences
Gandra-PRD, Portugal

and

REQUIMTE
Department of Chemistry
University of Porto
Porto, Portugal

Elisa Garbayo
Department of Pharmacy and Pharmaceutical Technology
School of Pharmacy
University of Navarra
Pamplona, Spain

Julie Gehl
Department of Oncology
C*EDGE (Center for Experimental Drug and Gene Electrotransfer)
Copenhagen University Hospital
Herlev, Denmark

Pablo Gurman
Gur&Gor LLC
Revere, Massachusetts

Yael Hants
Department of Obstetrics and Gynecology
Hadassah–Hebrew University Medical Center, Ein Kerem
Jerusalem, Israel

Sarit Helman
Department of Obstetrics and Gynecology
Shaare Zedek Medical Center
Jerusalem, Israel

Mark Ihnen
Kentucky Eye Care
Louisville, Kentucky

Germán A. Islan
Nanobiomaterials Laboratory
Institute of Applied Biotechnology (CINDEFI, UNLP-CONICET-CCT La Plata)
Department of Chemistry
School of Sciences
Universidad Nacional de La Plata
La Plata, Argentina

Sanjay K. Jain
Pharmaceutics Research Project Laboratory
Department of Pharmaceutics
Dr. Hari Singh Gour University
Sagar, Madhya Pradesh, India

Ridhima Juneja
Department of Chemistry
University of Delhi
Delhi, India

Stephen Kuperberg
SUNY Downstate Medical Center
Department of Critical Care and Pulmonary Medicine
Brooklyn, New York

Jennifer Lane
Drexel University College of Medicine
Philadelphia, Pennsylvania

Maelíosa T. C. McCrudden
School of Pharmacy
Queen's University
Belfast, United Kingdom

Ellis Meng
Department of Biomedical Engineering
Ming Hsieh Department of Electrical Engineering
University of Southern California
Los Angeles, California

Vivek K. Pawar
Pharmaceutics Division
CSIR-Central Drug Research Institute
Lucknow, India

Mahyar Pourriahi
SUNY Downstate Medical Center
Department of Medicine
Brooklyn, New York

Felipe Prósper
Hematology, Cardiology and Cell Therapy
Clínica Universidad de Navarra and Foundation for Applied Medical Research
University of Navarra
Pamplona, Spain

Masturah Bte Mohd Abdul Rashid
Department of Pharmacology
Yong Loo Lin School of Medicine
National University of Singapore
Singapore

Aaron Richler
Brookdale University Hospital
Brooklyn, New York

Yitzhak Rosen
SUNY Downstate Medical Center
Department of Medicine, Cardiovascular Division
Brooklyn, New York

and

Superior NanoBioSystems LLC
New Jersey

Indrajit Roy
Department of Chemistry
University of Delhi
Delhi, India

Omar Saleh
Department of Ophthalmology
Jordan University of Science and Technology
Irbid, Jordan

Bruno Sarmento
CESPU
Instituto de Investigação e Formação Avançada em Ciências e Tecnologias da Saúde
Department of Pharmaceutical Sciences
Gandra-PRD, Portugal

and

INEB
Institute of Biomedical Engineering
University of Porto
Porto, Portugal

Shlomit Schaal
Department of Ophthalmology and Visual Sciences
University of Massachusetts Medical School
Worcester, Massachusetts

Komal Sethi
Department of Chemistry
University of Delhi
Delhi, India

Roya Sheybani
Department of Biomedical Engineering
University of Southern California
Los Angeles, California

Satish Shilpi
Pharmaceutics Research Project Laboratory
Department of Pharmaceutical Sciences
Dr. Hari Singh Gour University
Sagar, Madhya Pradesh, India

and

Department of Pharmaceutics
Ravishankar College of Pharmacy
Bhopal, Madhya Pradesh, India

Joseph Shivers
Columbia University College of Physicians and Surgeons
New York, New York

David Shveiky
Department of Obstetrics and Gynecology
Hadassah–Hebrew University Medical Center, Ein Kerem
Jerusalem, Israel

Teresa Simón-Yarza
Department of Pharmacy and Pharmaceutical Technology
School of Pharmacy
University of Navarra
Pamplona, Spain

Yuvraj Singh
Pharmaceutics Division
CSIR-Central Drug Research Institute
Lucknow, India

Sandra Soares
CESPU
Instituto de Investigação e Formação Avançada em Ciências e Tecnologias da Saúde
Department of Pharmaceutical Sciences
Gandra-PRD, Portugal

Rishabh Srivastava
Department of Pharmaceutics
Rajiv Academy for Pharmacy
Mathura, India

Alan Talevi
Biopharmacy
Department of Biological Sciences
School of Sciences
National University of La Plata (UNLP)
CCT La Plata CONICET
La Plata, Argentina

Tan Boon Toh
Cancer Science Institute of Singapore
National University of Singapore
Singapore

Neeraj Vij
Department of Pediatric Respiratory Science
The Johns Hopkins University School of Medicine
Baltimore, Maryland

and

College of Medicine
Central Michigan University
Mt Pleasant, Michigan

Matthew Wright
Nanosight Ltd.
Wiltshire, United Kingdom

Howard Zisser
Dept. of Chemical Engineering
University of California, Santa Barbara
Santa Barbara, California

1 An Introduction to Key Concepts in Drug Delivery

Stephen Kuperberg, Mahyar Pourriahi, Jonathan Daich, Aaron Richler, Pablo Gurman, Noel M. Elman, and Yitzhak Rosen

CONTENTS

OVERVIEW

Drug delivery is a broad and active area of research involving a multidisciplinary approach whose integrative aim is to assist in reaching the optimization of drug efficacy by effective delivery of the active drug component to its target tissue while minimizing toxicity. The purpose of this chapter in particular and the book as a whole is to address clinical and engineering integration approaches for drug delivery systems. The clinical aspect involves understanding the unmet need and the clinical implications involved. It also requires understanding the individual clinical and biological differences of patients. Moreover, generating clinical and biological data is critical for drug delivery as this data can delineate the optimized pathway for a particular drug and its delivery system. In addition, pathophysiology of disease can affect drug delivery; for example, inflammation may greatly alter the disposition of a medication, thereby modifying its efficacy, such as drug penetration to a particular tissue [1–3]. The engineering aspect, on the other hand, involves either the manipulation of the physicochemical properties of the active ingredient or formulation (pharmaceutical engineering) or the fabrication of devices based on mechanical engineering principles in order to achieve a desired pharmacokinetic–pharmacodynamics profile of the active principle (drug delivery devices).

Integration of clinical and engineering principles involves a constant interaction between these two disciplines, and therefore, this book is intended for both the drug delivery engineer and the clinician. This chapter briefly discusses the rudimentary foundations of pharmacology that must be considered when designing drug delivery systems and provides clinical examples where drug delivery systems are playing a critical role. In addition, a brief description of novel approaches in drug delivery will be described to illustrate the fast development of this field.

DRUG DELIVERY: ROUTES OF ADMINISTRATION

There are numerous routes of drug delivery with enteral and parenteral being the most common. Enteral routes of drug administration can include oral, sublingual, or rectal. Parenteral routes include injections, such as intravenous, intramuscular, and subcutaneous. The routes of drug administration influence the pharmacokinetics of the drug. This includes the bioavailability, the rate of onset, peak effect, and duration of action of the drug [1].

Oral Route

A drug that is given through the oral route must first go through what is known as the *first-pass effect* or *first-pass metabolism.* In the first-pass effect, the drug is first partially metabolized in the gut wall; then it enters the portal venous system into the liver where it is further metabolized before reaching the systemic circulation and receptor target sites. The first-pass effect alters the bioavailability of the drug before it reaches its receptor target sites. This explains why different routes for the same drug require different doses for the same drug to have the same efficacy [1,2].

The oral route is the most commonly preferred route for drug administration. Other routes are considered when problematic circumstances arise in which the oral route cannot be used. These include the following:

1. When the patient has nausea or vomiting and cannot tolerate oral medication
2. When the patient is unconscious and/or has limited swallowing ability
3. When the drug is inactivated by digestive enzymes or acidic gastric fluid or metabolized by gastrointestinal (GI) flora
4. When there is overall poor drug absorption occurring due to an edematous GI tract that is seen in fluid overload states [1,2]

Sublingual Route

With the sublingual route, the drug avoids the first-pass effect and thus avoids alteration in its bioavailability by being absorbed directly into the systemic vascular system. This allows a very rapid delivery of the active compound, such as sublingual nitroglycerin for cardiac chest pain [1,2].

Rectal Route

Drugs administered by the rectal route have a bioavailability of approximately 50%, and even this approximation may greatly vary due to the intricate venous drainage system of the rectum. The superior portion of the rectum has veins draining into the liver whereas the distal portion of the rectum has veins draining straight into the vena cava, thus bypassing the first-pass effect [1,2].

Parenteral Routes

Parenteral routes include intravenous, intramuscular, and subcutaneous. Their key advantages include administration to unconscious patients and to patients with poor enteral absorption. These routes provide a quick onset of action and 100% bioavailability; therefore, no dose adjustment is required. Their disadvantage is the need for trained personnel, a short duration of action, risk of infection, and dermal irritation [1,2].

Miscellaneous Routes

The inhalation route is used for respiratory diseases, such as asthma and COPD. Intranasal and intrathecal routes are used for a drugs whose target site is the brain but which are unable to penetrate the blood–brain barrier. Topical routes are used for local effect on areas of skin. Intradermal routes are used for sustained release of a drug, for example, pain management drugs, such as the fentanyl patch. Liposomes, biodegradable microspheres, and various polymer conjugates are also typical components that can be used for sustained delivery. The ocular route is utilized as well; for example, beta blocker eye drops are commonly used for the management of elevated intraocular pressure, and these drops can actually even affect the heart rate as they can reach other targets outside their local use. Target delivery involves delivering the drug to a targeted tissue while overcoming many of the host's biological barriers. This may be done using a combination of encapsulating nanoparticles and monoclonal antibodies [3].

Drug Elimination

Drug elimination occurs by embolization by the liver as discussed previously. Drugs are also eliminated in the kidneys where they get filtered into the urine. Some drugs get eliminated through other means, such as from the lungs, but the liver and kidney are the most common organs responsible for drug metabolism and excretion [1,2].

KEY CONCEPTS IN PHARMACODYNAMICS

A *receptor* is any cell component that when it interacts with a *ligand* (a drug or an organic molecule) will bring about a biological effect. Receptors are mostly made up of proteins, but they differ from each other based on their unique biological effects. Thus, the receptor determines the biological effect not the ligand that binds it [1,2].

The majority of drugs are designed to either stimulate or inhibit receptors. A drug that stimulates is called an *agonist*, and a drug that inhibits is called an *antagonist*. A drug that antagonizes a receptor prevents natural agonists from binding and thus prevents a downstream biological effect [1,2].

As the concentration of an agonist increases in the systemic circulation, the more receptors are bounded and the greater the biological effect. The relationship between a drug's concentration and its biological effect can be plotted as effect versus drug concentration, which will resemble a hyperbolic curve. Increase in drug concentration initially has a linear response curve and then plateaus as maximal effect is reached no matter what the drug concentration is. This plateau occurs due to all the receptors becoming saturated. *Efficacy* refers to the effect of the drug. The more effect, the more efficacious the drug. *Potency* refers to the drug concentration required for the effect to happen. The lower the concentration of a drug needed for the effect to occur, the more potent the drug [1,2].

Therapeutic Window

Drugs require a certain minimum concentration to have a desired effect. This is called the *minimum effective dose*. However, drugs can also have undesired effects that occur if the concentration gets too high. The *minimum toxic dose* is the minimum dose of a drug that will cause an undesired effect. The *therapeutic window* is the dosage range between minimum effective dose and minimum toxic dose. Drugs with a small therapeutic window must be cautiously administered and have frequent concentration monitoring to avoid toxic doses [1,2].

DRUG DELIVERY SYSTEMS: PHARMACEUTICAL SYSTEMS VERSUS DRUG DELIVERY DEVICES

A drug delivery system can be defined as a formulation or a device that facilitates the introduction of a therapeutic substance into the body with the objectives of improving its efficacy and safety. This can be done by controlling the rate, time, and place of release of the drug in the body [4]. Drug delivery formulations refer to the application of pharmaceutical principles to modify the active principle or its excipients to improve drug pharmacokinetics, pharmacodynamics, or both. Improved efficacy (pharmacodynamics) can be achieved by improving the interaction of the drug with its target (cell receptors), and rate, time, and place of released can be improved, for example, through the use of microscale and nanoscale carriers, such as liposomes, nanocapsules, magnetic nanoparticles, dendrimers, and other type of transporters.

Drug delivery devices, on the other hand, encompasses a wide range of systems that differ in their complexity, form factor, mechanical components, and materials. Drug delivery devices range from pumps designed to control the rate at which a drug is administered or released to the bloodstream and iontophoretic transdermal patches that increase the permeability of the skin to improve drug absorption to simple syringes or polymeric tubes to allow the passage of the drug from a reservoir to the circulatory system (catheters).

DRUG DELIVERY SYSTEMS: CLINICAL APPLICATIONS

Diabetes and Insulin Delivery Systems

Technology has added greatly to the treatment of diabetes. For years, patients with diabetes were dependent only on subcutaneous, intravenous, and intramuscular preparations of insulin. These have been burdensome and painful methods for patients who have become accustomed to sticking themselves with needles for glucose management.

Technosphere insulin, marketed as Affrenza®, is a new product that has brought much hope for a painless and convenient insulin regimen. Patients can now use this preparation as they would any other short-acting insulin by combining it with their basal insulin [5,6]. Affrenza works by combining human insulin with a small carrier, fumaryl diketopiperazine (FDKP), which consists of crystallized microparticles two microns in size. Once the particles are inhaled and inside alveoli, the FDKP and insulin are rapidly absorbed with FDKP mostly excreted by the kidney while the insulin is rapidly distributed in the bloodstream. Studies have shown that it reaches a peak blood level in less than 15 minutes [5–7].

FDA approval was based on two phase 3 trial studies: AFFINITY 1 and AFFFINITY 2. The AFFINITY 2 trial was a randomized, double-blind, placebo-controlled study with insulin-naïve T2DM patients that showed glycemic efficacy when compared to a placebo inhaler as the TI group showed both larger reductions in HA1c and a larger percentage of patients that achieved goal HA1c <7%. In the AFFINITY 1 trial, patients with T1DM were given a regimen of inhaled insulin (TI) with basal insulin Glargine or Aspart (short-acting insulin) with Glargine. Results showed mean decreases in HA1c that were significantly more in the subcutaneous insulin group compared to the TI group with a noninferiority margin of 0.19% [8]. In a meta-analysis of more than 12 studies of patients with T1DM or T2DM, results showed that the decrease from baseline HA1c was greater with subcutaneous insulin versus inhaled, which had an absolute mean of reduction in HA1c of 0.55% in the subcutaneous group (pittas). A study by Rosenstock et al. compared TI to Aspart with similar and noninferior decreases in HA1c, the parameter that is used by clinicians to determine 3-month cumulative glucose levels [9].

Besides common side effects of hypoglycemia and throat pain/irritation cough (25%–35% of patients), studies have shown significant side effects, such as increased incidence of bronchospasm in patients with chronic lung disease. In addition, further long-term study will be required due to its association with increased incidence of lung cancer as post-marketing studies have shown to have a fourfold increased risk of primary lung cancers [7].

Cancer and Antineoplastic Drug Delivery Systems

Most of the known cancers at the present time are treated partially or entirely with chemotherapy agents. Unfortunately, the problem with using chemotherapy agents is the indiscriminate action of drugs to all cells, which forces decreased dosing, which results in low concentrations of the drug available for treatment of cancerous cells. Various recent nanotechnological advances have been made.

Ideally, the most effective drug delivery system would be to provide a biodegradable nontoxic carrier that would have a structure that would enhance uptake and bioavailability for the delivery of the therapeutic treatment of tumor cells.

Silk fibrin is a fibrinous protein made by silkworms that has been showing much success in various trials. For years, silk protein has been used in biotechnology for biofilms, nanofibers, nanoparticles, and three-dimensional porous scaffolds [10]. Besides it being biodegradable, it has been shown to have cell-adhesive, anti-inflammatory, low immunogenicity, and non-thrombogenic properties [11].

SF was first used to deliver emodin, a tyrosine kinase inhibitor, in patients who had developed resistance to traditional chemotherapy drugs [12]. More recently, curcumin, a highly potent anticancer agent used against pancreatic cancer, cervical colorectal cancer, and multiple myeloma, was studied in vivo after encapsulation with SF protein. Gupta et al. found that after encapsulating the compound with SF it provided higher efficacy against breast cancer cells due to curcumin's known activity against Her2 and NF-kB pathways [13]. In a similar manner to how viruses and prion diseases gain entry into cells by using an amyloid-like antiparallel beta sheet structure of proteins for adhesion and subsequent penetration by endocytosis, the SF-coated curcumin microparticles have a similar beta sheet structure, which, when combined, forms a barrel-like structure, and when subsequently exposed to cilia of cancer cells, endocytosis occurs and cell death follows within 1 hour [11].

Another promising delivery system is the use of folate as an augmentation to the SF carrier, which enhances the specificity of the carrier. Folate, which is a requirement in DNA synthesis, is highly needed in the hyperactive DNA-synthesizing cancer cells. By attaching folate to a SF carrier carrying a specific drug, specificity is enhanced, and in addition, drug toxicity is decreased by increasing site-specificity by targeting the highly active cells, which subsequently lowers the needed doses of chemotherapeutic agents. Subia et al. attached folate to SF protein loaded with doxorubicin in vivo against breast cancer cells [14].

Technological advances such as these continue. Silk protein, due to its bioavailability and nontoxic properties, shows great promise to the field of drug delivery and for much broader applications for future health care [15].

Epilepsy and Benzodiazepines Drug Delivery Systems

Benzodiazepines, made up of a benzene ring fused with a diazepam ring, are psychoactive drugs that enhance the effects of gamma-aminobutyric acid by binding to the benzodiazepine receptor, resulting in anxiolytic, hypnotic, sedative, anticonvulsant, and muscle relaxant effects [16–19]. Their wide utilization and varied formulation make this drug a prime example for the clinical setting of a drug delivery mechanism. Around 1%–2% of all emergency department visits are due to seizures. While most are self-limited, approximately 6% of seizure visits are prolonged convulsions or rapidly recurrent convulsions without recovery of consciousness (status epilepticus), which is a true emergency [16–19]. While the utilization of primary anticonvulsants can terminate these episodes, emergent cases require an escalation to benzodiazepines to achieve seizure cessation [3,16–19].

Emergent treatment of status epilepticus is required to help prevent systemic pathology. While most emergency departments use parenteral (intravenous, intramuscular) administration of benzodiazepines to terminate the seizure, this is a difficult task outside of the hospital setting. Parenteral administration provides an immediate release of benzodiazepine (lipid-soluble substance) that crosses the blood–brain barrier and helps terminate the seizures [2]. It is due to this immediate effect that parenteral therapy remains a gold standard. Outside of the hospital setting or in an actively seizing patient, this method is much less ideal due to the inability to achieve an intravenous line or delay in giving therapy. Thus, other methods are used to deliver this antiepileptic drug [16–19]. For example, a diazepam autoinjector was developed, allowing the administration of diazepam in the prehospital setting. The autoinjector does not require an IV line and is easy for medical practitioners to administer during a seizure episode. Moreover, patients could also carry these autoinjectors with them, and should a seizure episode occur, these devices allow to a relative or any person to use it by following easy-to-follow instructions [20].

Enteral administration of benzodiazepine can be used in these cases. The suppository form of these drugs can be inserted rectally, where the drug is absorbed due to the high vascularity of the rectum. The drug absorption is more erratic using this method and can result in a low blood concentration or delayed response [2]. Buccal formulations, mostly used with children in Europe, also exist, which is applied on the inside of the cheeks. The buccal membrane is similarly heavily vascularized [3]. Fast-dissolving tablets have also been suggested for the out-of-hospital setting, which would act similarly to sublingual nitroglycerine that dissolves rapidly and is absorbed by the sublingual vasculature [4]. Regular tablets would not be beneficial in this situation due to the inability of the patient to swallow and the delayed response of the drug due to the first-pass metabolism [2,16–19].

OTHER EXAMPLES OF DRUG DELIVERY SYSTEMS

Many other drug delivery system approaches also exist. For example, intrathecal pumps and injections have been used to deliver drugs to the cerebrospinal fluid. Many drugs have poor absorption in the brain due to the blood–brain barrier, and this mechanism serves as a way to circumvent this barrier. Imipenem, a beta-lactam antibiotic, has three times higher levels, lasting four times longer in the brain as opposed to conventional intravenous therapy. Its bactericidal effects are not dose-dependent but rather time-dependent; therefore, intrathecal administration can play a big role in meningitis or brain abscess therapy [21].

NOVEL APPROACHES IN DRUG DELIVERY

Gene Delivery: DNA and RNA as Payloads for Drug Delivery

New concepts of drug delivery have emerged, leading to new opportunities for delivery not only of chemical compounds and small molecules, but for delivery of genes through DNA or RNA or, more recently, silent RNA (RNAi). In DNA and RNA delivery, a sequence codifying for a therapeutic protein is delivered to the cell. The genetic material will be integrated in the host genome and further transcribed to RNA, which will ultimately lead to gene expression to a protein product. This is the basis for what is known as gene therapy. In contrast, in RNAi delivery, the genetic material in the form of an RNA sequence quenches the expression of a defect protein by combining with the complementary sequence of RNA of the host, preventing the expression of this RNA sequence. There many different ways in which genes can be delivered to cells, including viral and nonviral methods.

Cell Delivery

Recently, it became possible to deliver genetically engineered cells as a therapeutic modality for a variety of clinical conditions. Genetic engineering of cells involves the modification of a cell product to express a desired therapeutic protein. These modified cells are then injected into the patient, allowing the production of a protein product in vivo. Further encapsulation of cells in special capsules prevents the implanted cells from being rejected by the immune system once implanted in the human body.

A product based on encapsulated genetically engineered cells for the treatment of ocular disorders of the posterior chamber was recently developed and is now undergoing clinical trials [22].

NOVEL TARGETS IN DRUG DELIVERY: CANCER STEM CELL DELIVERY

With the discovery of stem cells (cells capable of self-renewal and differentiation into many different cell types) within tumors, often responsible for cancer relapse, the idea of selective elimination of cancer stem cell populations has generated great interest as a potential cancer therapy. In one modality, a chemotherapeutic drug encapsulated in a nanoparticle expressing a particular ligand on its surface is selectively uptaken by the tumor based on the enhanced and permeability retention effect (EPR) due to increased permeability of the vessels supplying the tumor, allowing extravasation of the delivery product. Some of the issues that make cancer stem cell delivery a challenge include chemo resistance of stem cells to the therapeutic agent by the expression of enzymes capable of detoxification of the chemotherapeutic drug and the expression of drug transporters across the cell membrane that extrude the therapeutic drug out of the cell.

Novel Delivery Modalities Based on the Carrier: Micro and Nanosystems

Microtechnology encompasses the manipulation of matter at the microscale (1–100 microns) while nanotechnology encompasses techniques that deal with objects in the 1–100 nm range. The use of microtechnology in medicine originated in the 1990s with the development of the first pressure sensors for cardiovascular applications. With the continuous evolution of MEMS, toward the 2000s, the concept of MEMS drug delivery systems emerged, and by 2012, the first human clinical trial with an implantable microchip was demonstrated [23,24]. MEMS key advantages include active control, which allows tailoring of delivery time, rate, and volume at any time after the device has been implanted; small form factor, allowing minimally invasive procedures; improved biological performance; improved overall performance due to increased functionality in a small space; multiple pharmacotherapies in a single device; low cost; high reproducibility (similar payload across a batch of devices); lower power consumption; and high reliability because many of these devices do not contain mobile parts, thus decreasing the chances of failure, which paved the way for a wide number of clinical applications, including delivery of vasopressin for the emergency setting (hemorrhagic shock), delivery of PTH for osteoporosis, delivery of anticancer agents for the treatment of glioblastoma, and transdermal delivery of vaccines among others.

Nanotechnology is revolutionizing the field of drug delivery due to the nanoscale size of delivery carriers or active ingredients (nanopharmaceuticals), which results in increased surface-to-volume ratio, leading to increased solubility and rate of adsorption and increased permeability through vessel walls, allowing the active principle to penetrate biological barriers (e.g., blood–brain barrier, blood–retinal barrier). Nanopharmaceuticals have already reached the market, and many others are in the pipeline [25].

SUMMARY

Drug delivery represents an interdisciplinary field that brings together engineering principles and medical knowledge in order to overcome pharmacological issues arising from lack of efficacy or unacceptable toxicity of current pharmacotherapies. Understanding the clinical data (patient differences in clinical response to specific drugs, pathophysiology of different clinical states) can assist in optimizing drug delivery systems by understanding the biological microenvironment affecting pharmacokinetics (drug absorption, drug metabolism, and drug elimination) and drug pharmacodynamics (drug receptor interaction, downstream cell signaling pathways) while engineering principles can assist in the design and development of new devices and pharmaceutical formulations based on the data provided by the medical practitioner.

This book covers some of these general topics while at the same time introducing the reader to novel concepts in the drug delivery field. Chapter 2 provides a comprehensive description of pharmacokinetics. Chapters 3 through 5, and 11 provide illustrative examples of pharmaceutical engineering to improve drug pharmacokinetics, including the use of biomaterials. Chapter 6 describes the role of drug delivery devices for the management of diabetic patients through the development of an artificial pancreas. The incorporation of micro- and nanotechnology for drug delivery systems is covered in Chapters 7 through 10, 14, and 18. The importance of specific routes of administration to overcome biological barriers to address some serious medical conditions is described in Chapter 15 (Intrathecal Drug Delivery). Specific medical conditions that can benefit from drug delivery systems can be found in Chapter 13 (Infectious Disease Drug Delivery), Chapter 17 (Cardiac Drug Delivery), Chapter 19 (Intravitreal Drug Delivery), and Chapter 20 (Drug Delivery Obstetrics and Gynecology). Novel approaches in drug delivery are covered in Chapter 12 (Gene Delivery by Electroporation) and Chapter 16 (Cancer Stem Cell Drug Delivery). Last but not least, Chapter 21 covers the regulatory aspects of drug delivery systems.

In summary, successful drug delivery involves a multidisciplinary and integrated engineering and clinical approach. This book is therefore a useful resource for the medical practitioner and the engineer interested in drug delivery systems and the technologies currently available and others being investigated to address unmet clinical needs in a variety of medical fields.

REFERENCES

1. Brunton, L., Chabner, B., Knollmann, B. 2011. *Goodman and Gilman's: The Pharmacological Basis of Therapeutics*, 12th ed. New York. McGraw-Hill Education/Medical.
2. Kasper, D., Fauci, A., Hauser, S., Longo, D., Jameson, J., Loscalzo, J. 2015. *Harrison's Principles of Internal Medicine*, 19th ed. New York. McGraw-Hill Education/Medical.
3. Anselmo, A., Mitragotri, S. 2014. An overview of clinical and commercial impact of drug delivery systems. *J Control Release* 190: 1–674.
4. Jain, K. K. 2008. Drug delivery systems: An overview. *Methods Mol Biol.* 437: 1–50.
5. Pittas, A. G. et al. Efficacy, safety, and patient acceptability of Technosphere inhaled insulin for people with diabetes: A systematic review and meta-analysis. *Lancet Diabetes Endocrinol.* 3 (11): 886–894.
6. Rendell, M. 2014. Technosphere inhaled insulin (Afrezza). *Drugs Today.* 50 (12): 813–827.
7. Klonoff, D. C. 2014. Afrezza inhaled insulin: The fastest-acting FDA-approved insulin on the market has favorable properties. *J Diabetes Sci Technol.* 18 (6): 1071–1073.
8. Goldberg, T., Wong, E. 2015. Afrezza (insulin human) inhalation powder: A new inhaled insulin for the management of type-1 or type-2 diabetes mellitus. *P&T.* 40 (11): 735–741.

9. Rosenstock, J., Lorber, D. L., Gnudi, L. et al. 2010. Prandial inhaled insulin plus insulin glargine versus twice daily biaspart insulin for type 2 diabetes: A multicentre randomized trial. *Lancet*. 375: 2244–2253.
10. Numata, K., Kaplan, D. L. 2010. Silk-based delivery systems of bioactive molecules. *Adv Drug Deliv Rev*. 62 (15): 1497–1508.
11. Mathur, A. B., Gupta, V. 2010. Silk fibroin-derived nanoparticles for biomedical applications. *Nanomedicine*. 5 (5): 807–820.
12. Cheema, S. K., Gobin, A. S., Rhea, R., Lopez-Berestein, G., Newman, R. A., Mathur, A. B. 2007. Silk fibroin mediated delivery of liposomal emodin to breast cancer cells. *Int J Pharm*. 341 (1–2): 221–229.
13. Gupta, V., Aseh, A., Ríos, C. N., Aggarwal, B. B., Mathur, A. B. 2009. Fabrication and characterization of silk fibroin-derived curcumin nanoparticles for cancer therapy. *Int J Nanomedicine*. 4: 115–122.
14. Subia, B., Chandra, S. 2014. Folate conjugated silk fibroin nanocarriers for targeted drug delivery. *Integr Biol (Camb)*. 6 (2): 203–214.
15. Zhao, Z., Li, Y., Xie, M.-B. 2015. Silk Fibroin-Based Nanoparticles for Drug Delivery. *Int J Mol Sci*. 16 (3): 4880–4903.
16. McMullan, J., Sasson, C., Pancioli, A. 2010. Midazolam versus diazepam for the treatment of status epilepticus in children and young adults: A meta-analysis. *Acad Emerg Med*. 17 (6): 575–582.
17. Sirven, J., Waterhouse, E. 2003. Management of status epilepticus. *Am Fam Physician*. 68 (3): 469–476.
18. Anderson, M. 2013. Buccal midazolam for pediatric convulsive seizures: Efficacy, safety, and patient acceptability. *Patient Prefer Adherence*. 7: 27–34.
19. Peeters, E. 2010. Treatment of epileptic seizures as medical emergencies: A prospective analysis of a decision tree for nonmedically trained staff. *Seizure*. 9 (7): 473–479.
20. Meridian technologies. URL:http://www.meridianmeds.com/products/diazepam.
21. Wang, Y., Qiu, L., Dong, J. et al. 2013. Comparison of the pharmacokinetics of imipenem after intravenous and intrathecal administration in rabbits. *Eur Rev Med Pharmacol Sci*. 17 (6): 711–719.
22. Neurotech website. URL:http://www.neurotechusa.com/ect-platform.html.
23. Santini, J. T., Jr., Cima, M. J., Langer, R. 1999. A controlled-release microchip. *Nature*. 28; 397 (6717): 335–338.
24. Farra, R., Sheppard, N. F., Jr., McCabe, L., Neer, R. M., Anderson, J. M., Santini, J. T., Jr., Cima, M. J., Langer, R. 2012. First-in-human testing of a wirelessly controlled drug delivery microchip. *Sci Transl Med*. 22; 4 (122): 122ra21.
25. Weissig, V., Pettinger, T. K., Murdock, N. 2014. Nanopharmaceuticals (part 1): Products on the market. *Int J Nanomedicine*. 9: 4357–4373.

2 An Introduction to Pharmacokinetics

From Conventional to Advanced Systemic Drug Delivery Systems

Alan Talevi, Luis Bruno Blanch, and Guillermo R. Castro

CONTENTS

AN OVERVIEW OF SOME GENERAL ASPECTS OF CONVENTIONAL DRUG DELIVERY SYSTEMS

In order to comprehend the peculiarities of advanced drug delivery (nano)system pharmacokinetics, we should first briefly discuss some general aspects of conventional drug delivery systems. This chapter focuses on systemic medications, that is, pharmaceutical systems meant to deliver the active ingredient(s) to systemic circulation from which it is transported by the blood to its molecular target at a given site of action. We define conventional systemic drug delivery systems as pharmaceutical vehicles intended to release the active ingredient at a certain place with a certain kinetic so that the *free* drug eventually reaches systemic circulation from which it will eventually distribute to other tissues.

An important principle to establish pharmacokinetic/pharmacodynamic relationships is the free drug hypothesis [1]. Such hypothesis states that, under certain conditions, (a) the free drug concentrations at both sides of a given biological barrier are the same at the stationary state and (b) the free drug concentration in the biophase (i.e., the vicinity of the molecular target) determines the intensity of the pharmacological effect. The first part of the hypothesis, of enormous pharmacokinetic value, is verified whenever the stationary state is achieved provided that the drug transport across the biological membrane only involves passive diffusion. Additionally, the drug molecules are not only in the free state within the body, but also a fraction of them is often found interacting nonspecifically with plasma proteins or body tissues. However, in the case of conventional drug delivery systems, it is important to keep in mind that a drug molecule must be free in the site of absorption media before absorption can proceed, no matter if it is verified through passive or active processes. In other words, drug release from the vehicle is a necessary condition for absorption to take place if conventional drug delivery systems are considered. A corollary of this fact is that conventional drug delivery systems can only modulate, in a direct way, drug release and absorption processes while they have little direct influence on drug disposition (distribution and elimination processes).

Another relevant aspect of conventional drug delivery systems is nonspecific drug distribution in the body. Putting it into simple words, the entire body is potentially exposed to the drug molecules so that some—relatively few—drug molecules reach their site of action, which is often confined to a very limited region of the organism. Therefore, large doses of the active ingredient are administered just to compensate for this untargeted distribution, which brings about a number of potential adverse, off-site effects. The fact is that drug levels in the blood (or more precisely, in plasma) can be used as a tracer for drug concentration at the site of action (in the background of a conventional drug delivery system aimed at systemic delivery, there is a direct relationship between the plasma drug level and the drug concentration at the biophase) and thus provide a valid measure of bioavailability. This explains why most pharmacokinetic studies rely on analysis of plasma drug concentration–time curves. This is fortunate because assessment of drug levels directly at the biophase would imply extremely invasive approaches (fluid sampling from a given organ).

DRUG ABSORPTION, DISTRIBUTION, AND ELIMINATION

It is convenient to briefly discuss the definition of these three processes that will frequently appear in the chapter. Essentially, these terms refer to mass transfer processes. Drug absorption denotes the transfer of drug mass units from the site of administration to systemic circulation, that is, arterial blood. Although absorption usually encompasses transport across a number of serial biological barriers, frequently the transfer rate across one of such barriers becomes the rate-limiting step of the global process. Except for the enteral, the administration site and preferred absorption site are generally the same or anatomically immediate. In the enteral route, the dosage form is administered orally, and the preferred absorption site is usually the small intestine, due to its special absorptive adaptations (crypts, villi, and microvilli). This does not mean that for certain enterically delivered drugs absorption cannot start or conclude in other regions of the gastrointestinal site. However, the anatomical distance between the administration and absorption sites occasionally impacts the absorption lag time and thus the time to reach effective drug levels at the target.

Drug distribution refers to the drug transfer from systemic circulation to other tissues and backward. It may be significantly impacted by nonspecific, reversible interaction with plasma proteins and tissue components.

Elimination denotes the transfer of a drug from the organism to the environment. Frequently, during the elimination process, drugs are converted into derivatives that are more easily removed or excreted (see next section).

DRUG CLEARANCE: METABOLISM AND EXCRETION

Chemical compounds found within an organism can be generally classified into two fundamental categories [2]. The first category encompasses physiological compounds, or endobiotics, which are chemicals having essential biological functions, such as water, nutrients, and micronutrients and also endogenous molecules with physiological functions. Naturally, physiological compounds are expected to be present within a living organism. On the other hand are *xenobiotics*, which (as denoted by the *xeno-* prefix) refer to foreign compounds, which enter the body but have no essential physiological functions (even though they frequently modify body functions) or to physiological elements that are present at un-physiologically high levels after uptake from an external source. Examples of xenobiotics include environmental pollutants and food additives, such as colorants, artificial sweeteners, and preservatives. In most cases, drugs can be clearly conceived as xenobiotics. Because, as foreign entities, xenobiotics are potentially toxic, organisms have developed a number of protective strategies that either prevent their uptake or promote their removal. These evolutionary strategies can be basically divided into three approaches: (a) preventing the entry of the xenobiotic to the body or to sensitive organs (i.e., the brain) through selective barriers, (b) physical elimination (i.e., excretion) of the xenobiotic, and (c) chemical elimination (or biotransformation or xenobiotic metabolism). The major excretion routes of drugs in humans are urinary and hepato-biliary excretion. Drugs are renally excreted through two processes: glomerular filtration and tubular secretion [3,4]. The extent of the former depends on the molecular weight and charge of the drug and on whether the drug is bound too strongly to plasma proteins (for the majority of excreted medications, the drug excretion is limited to unbound drug in plasma). Since filtration is size-dependent, we will see later that advanced drug delivery nanosystems may be used to reduce excretion by considering the size threshold for glomerular filtration. Tubular secretion relies on a concerted system of membrane active transporters.

These two processes are counteracted by tubular reabsorption, which is primarily a passive process thus favored for lipophilic unionized drugs (and thus, highly dependent on urine pH). In fact, the general object of biotransformation reactions is to convert xenobiotics to more polar derivatives (metabolites) in order to promote their excretion (renal or biliar) by minimizing the reabsorption processes [5]. Even though every cell in the body retains some level of drug-metabolizing capability, the major organ where drug metabolism occurs is the liver, which expresses particularly high levels of drug-metabolizing enzymes. Other important drug-metabolizing organs include the gut, kidneys, and lungs [5,6].

Xenobiotic biotransformation typically includes a number of parallel and/or sequential reactions that configure the metabolic pathway of a given drug. Back in the 1940s, R. T. Williams coined the classification of xenobiotic metabolism into phase I and phase II reactions, which reflects the fact that frequently a phase I reaction exposes or introduces a reactive functional group to a parent molecule, and subsequently, a phase II reaction conjugates such active metabolite mostly with polar species that drastically increase polarity (and thus excretion) and/or terminate bioactivity. The order is, however, not strict: Phase II reactions may occur without or before phase I [2,7]. Phase I reactions are also known as *functionalization reactions* and include redox reactions and hydrolysis. Cytochrome P450 is responsible for most xenobiotic oxidations, which constitute the bulk of phase I metabolism. Phase II reactions are also termed *conjugation reactions* and conjugate their substrates to a number of moieties that include glucuronic acid, glutathione, sulfate, amino acids, and others. Phase I products usually retain some level of activity (in some cases, they even have more activity than the parent molecules or are highly toxic) while Phase II products tend to be inactive and innocuous. Both phase I and phase II reactions are catalyzed by metabolic enzymes; thus, substrates of such enzymes should be in their free form for biotransformation to proceed. This is usually the case for conventional drug delivery systems but not necessarily for advanced ones. It should also be highlighted that large molecules are not cleared via the same mechanisms as small molecules [3].

A practical way to express the ability of the whole body or a given organ to remove drug from plasma is *plasma clearance* (*Cl*) [8]. When considering the overall ability of the body to eliminate (either chemically or physically) a certain drug, it is termed body or total or systemic clearance, expressed as drug elimination rate (*Re*) and it is calculated as the overall elimination rate scaled by the corresponding plasma concentration:

$$Cl = \frac{Re}{Cp}, \tag{2.1}$$

where *Cp* is the drug concentration in plasma. It is interesting to note, however, that plasma clearance is often defined as the volume of plasma cleared from the drug per unit of time. The more accurate definition would regard it as the volume of plasma that contains the amount of drug that is eliminated per time unit. Considering drug elimination as a first-order process, all the saturable systems that take part in drug elimination are far from being saturated. Also, if the Michaelis kinetic model applies, drug concentrations are much smaller than the Michaelis constants of the saturable processes involved, and the previous expression can be rewritten as follows:

$$Cl = \frac{kA(t)}{Cp(t)}, \tag{2.2}$$

where K is the elimination rate constant, and *A(t)* is the total amount of drug in the body at a given moment *t*. Bear in mind that within the one-compartment pharmacokinetic model *A(t)* equals the volume of distribution V multiplied by *Cp(t)* (see the section devoted to the one-compartment open model) then

$$Cl = kV, \tag{2.3}$$

which demonstrates an interesting aspect of *Cl* whenever linear kinetics are considered: While the rate of elimination and *Cp(t)* are time-dependent (and thus assume instantaneous values), *Cl* is constant (since V and k are constants) and therefore a true pharmacokinetic parameter. The total plasma clearance is the sum of organ clearances (the contribution of each organ to the elimination processes). Generally, clearance by organs other than the kidneys and the liver is negligible. While urinary clearance is associated with the compound appearing in urine, it is important to note that renal clearance may involve both biotransformation and excretion of a given substance and thus is not necessarily equivalent to urinary clearance [9]. Hepatic clearance includes drug loss due to metabolization in the liver and secretion into the bile.

PRESYSTEMIC METABOLISM

The term *presystemic metabolism* (or *first-pass metabolism* or simply *presystemic effect*) denotes the loss of a drug via biotransformation prior to reaching general, systemic circulation (i.e., before reaching the aorta). Strictly speaking, it includes any extraction of drug prior to general circulation. Therefore, presystemic metabolism may occur in several organs, depending on the administration route: the gut, the liver, the lungs, or even the skin (for the transdermal route). However, the extent of first-pass metabolism in other organs is often negligible compared to that of the liver and the gut. What is more, no matter if a drug is administered enterally or parenterally into venous circulation, it has to pass through the lungs before entering general circulation so that the lung first-pass effect will tend to cancel out any bioavailability calculation [10]. Thus, presystemic metabolism is usually used as a synonym for the intestinal (including gut lumen, gut wall, and bacterial metabolism) and hepatic first-pass effect, and it is generally accepted that the presystemic effect is relevant for the oral and, to a lesser degree, rectal administration routes [11] and bypassed by all the others. Biotransformation of drug molecules that reach an organ through arterial blood (e.g., blood that reaches the liver through the hepatic artery) is termed systemic metabolism.

THE ONE-COMPARTMENT OPEN MODEL

Pharmacokinetics is the study of absorption, distribution, and elimination from a quantitative point of view by studying the time course of drug concentration profiles in readily accessible body fluids, such as plasma, urine, or saliva, leading to understanding, interpretation, and prediction of concentration–time profiles [12]. Pharmacokinetic analysis can be used to design a dosage regimen and, occasionally, to optimize a drug delivery system. There are a number of pharmacokinetic models that can be used for such purposes, from classical compartmental models to the more complex physiologically based models and noncompartmental analysis. Classical compartmental models depict the body as one or more compartments with no anatomical meaning. Each such abstract compartment is considered kinetically homogeneous. The typical output of these model is $Cp(t)$, and each empirical compartment is represented by an exponential term. Although useful for data description and interpolation, classical compartmental models usually behave poorly at extrapolation: Because their parameters do not have a physiological interpretation, it is difficult to predict how they change when the underlying physiology changes [13]. In other words, sometimes it is difficult to adapt classical compartmental models to pathological or physiological conditions that modify drug disposition.

Here we briefly review the simplest of the classical compartmental models: the one-compartment open model. The model is illustrated in Figure 2.1.

According to the model, a given quantity of drug (the drug dose D) is administered to the body. A fraction of such dose (the bioavailable fraction F) reaches systemic circulation unaltered. The model makes two important assumptions. First, the model is represented by a single compartment assuming that plasma and tissue drug levels reach equilibrium instantaneously (instantaneous distribution). Although this is of course not true, it is a reasonable approximation provided all tissues that receive significant levels of drug approach equilibrium with plasma in a small time period compared to the elimination half-life. As a corollary, the relationship between the total amount of drug within the body A and Cp is a constant, the apparent volume of distribution V. Second, elimination is considered a first-order process (the rate of elimination is proportional to A). Linear elimination is also a realistic assumption in most therapeutic situations because drug concentrations are often much less than the

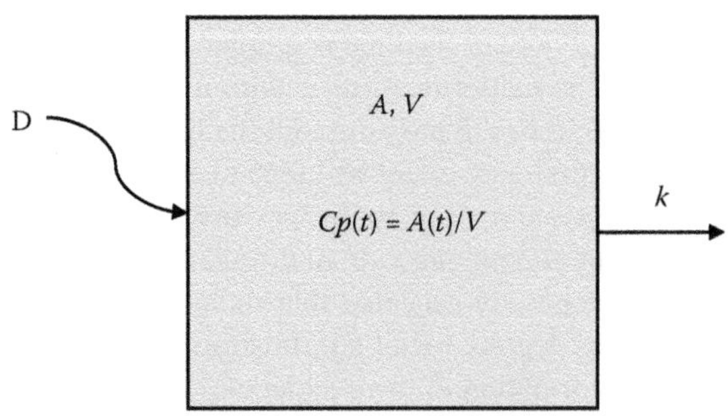

FIGURE 2.1 Scheme of the one-compartment open model.

Km value of enzymes and transporters involved in elimination. In contrast, absorption kinetics depends on the chosen route of administration and the delivery system. The simpler cases are instantaneous absorption (a reasonable assumption for bolus IV injection), zero-order absorption (useful to model drug levels when a drug enters systemic circulation at a constant rate, e.g., IV perfusion and sustained-release dosage forms), and first-order absorption (when a drug enters systemic circulation at a rate that is proportional to the amount of drug remaining to be absorbed at the site of absorption, a sensible approximation for extravascular administration of immediate-release dosage forms).

For instantaneous absorption, since the whole dose enters systemic circulation at time zero, the mass balance for a single dose is simply the following:

$$\frac{dA}{dt} = -kA. \tag{2.4}$$

After solving the differential equation and integrating between zero and a given time t (since A at time zero equals the dose) we obtain the following:

$$A = De^{-kt}. \tag{2.5}$$

Taking the natural logarithm of both sides of the previous expression provides the log-linear form

$$\ln A = \ln D - kt. \tag{2.6}$$

These expressions can be easily turned into plasma concentrations versus time relationships by dividing both sides of Equation 2.5 by the apparent volume of distribution:

$$Cp = \frac{A}{V} = C_0 e^{-kt} \tag{2.7}$$

and then

$$\ln Cp = \ln C_0 - kt, \tag{2.8}$$

where C_0 represents the initial plasma level, obtained by dividing the dose D by V (remember that the one-compartment model assumes instantaneous distribution throughout the whole compartment). Note that k is expressed in time^{-1} units (e.g., h^{-1}). Figure 2.2a shows the concentration–time curve for a bolus IV injection. Figure 2.2b illustrates the log-linear transformation. If the log transformation did not produce a line, then the one-compartment model would not be appropriate to describe the drug pharmacokinetics, and generally, more complex models (e.g., multicompartment ones) should be applied.

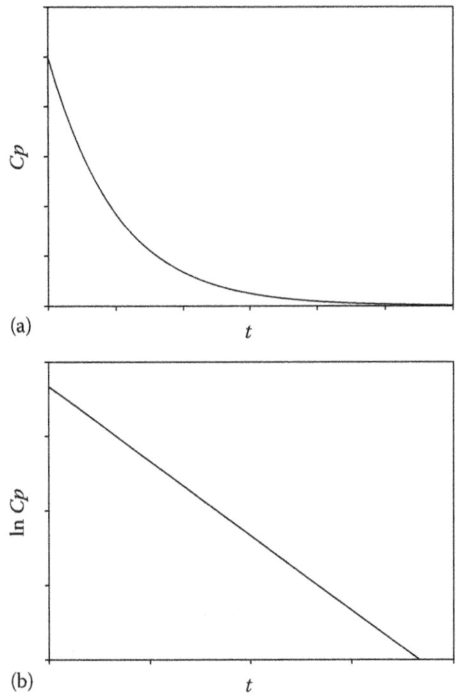

FIGURE 2.2 (a) Plasma concentration–time curve for a drug that follows the one-compartment model, considering instantaneous absorption. (b) Log-linear transformation of the plasma concentration–time curve for a drug that follows the one-compartment model, considering instantaneous absorption.

Due to the linear kinetics assumption, elimination half-life (the time that the body requires to eliminate half of any given drug amount) is constant and can be easily deduced from Equation 2.6 as the following:

$$t_{1/2,\text{elim}} = \frac{\ln 2}{k}. \tag{2.9}$$

Zero-order absorption is typically used for continuous IV infusion. In the case of zero-order absorption and as long as infusion continues at a constant rate, the mass balance equation assumes the following form:

$$\frac{dA}{dt} = k_0 - kA, \tag{2.10}$$

where k_0 is the steady flow rate at which the drug is delivered into systemic circulation. It is expressed in mass units divided by time units (e.g., mg h^{-1}). Solving

Equation 2.10 provides the subsequent relationship of the amount of drug in the body as a function of time:

$$A = \frac{k_0}{k}(1 - e^{-kt}) \tag{2.11}$$

and dividing the amount of drug in the body by the volume of distribution,

$$Cp = \frac{k_0}{kV}(1 - e^{-kt}). \tag{2.12}$$

The reader may remember that kV is no other thing than the total body clearance as stated in Equation 2.3. The concentration–time curve then shows an exponential rise to a maximum (Figure 2.3). When large times are considered, e^{-kt} tends to zero. The factor $(1 - e^{-kt})$ approaches 1 as time grows, and Cp approaches the so-called steady-state plasma concentration, Cp_{ss}, which is the following:

$$Cp = \frac{k_0}{kV}. \tag{2.13}$$

There are a couple of points that should be highlighted from the previous analysis. First, a simple way to estimate total clearance for a given drug is to infuse it via IV and assess drug levels at steady state because infusion rate is known by the experimentalist. Second, the steady-state drug level depends only on the infusion rate and the body clearance. Of them, only the infusion rate can be easily and predictably modified in a clinical scenario.

A pertinent question in a clinical setting is how long it takes to achieve steady-state drug levels. We will call such time t_{ss} (time to reach steady state). Since the curve presented in Figure 2.3 approaches Cp_{ss} asymptotically, the formal (and clinically

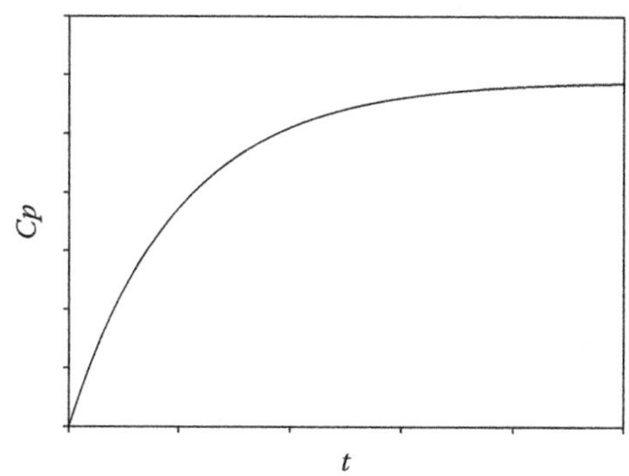

FIGURE 2.3 Plasma concentration–time profile for a drug that follows the one-compartment model, considering zero-order absorption.

irrelevant) answer to the question would be that steady state is achieved when time approaches infinity. A more practical way to answer the question is to compute the time needed to approach steady state to a certain (reasonable) degree. Let us compute, for instance, the required time to achieve 99% of the steady-state level.

$$0.99\,Cp = \frac{k_0}{kV}(1 - e^{-kt_{ss}}). \tag{2.14}$$

From Equation 2.13, the previous expression is equivalent to the following:

$$0.99 = (1 - e^{-kt_{ss}}), \tag{2.15}$$

which, after some algebraic manipulation and replacing k by ln $2/t_{1/2,\mathrm{elim}}$ from Equation 2.9 provides the following solution:

$$-\frac{\ln 0.01}{\ln 2} t_{1/2} = 6.64 t_{1/2} = t_{ss}. \tag{2.16}$$

Equation 2.16 shows that it takes almost seven elimination half-lives to reach 99% of steady-state drug levels. Interestingly, t_{ss} depends only on the elimination rate constant k. By increasing the infusion rate, one might increase drug levels at steady state, but the time required to reach steady state will not be affected.

It is relevant to note that the infusion time needed to reach steady state might be too long for those drugs with large $t_{1/2,\mathrm{elim}}$ while some therapeutic settings demand achieving effective concentrations in an urgent manner. At this point, it is useful to briefly discuss the *superposition principle* [14]. It states that the plasma concentrations after multiple doses of a drug (e.g., a drug administered by two or more different delivery methods) is equal to the sum of concentrations that would have resulted from each dose being given individually. The principle is valid as long as all elimination processes follow linear kinetics for the considered drug levels. Under these circumstances, the single-dose models described in this chapter can be coupled to predict concentrations in a multiple dosing scenario. Now we apply the superposition principle to immediately reach the steady state for an IV infusion shown in Equation 2.13. Imagine that, at the same instant that IV infusion starts at k_o perfusion rate, an IV bolus of k_o/k mass units is injected. After the superposition principle, the plasma concentration at any time (while the infusion continues) is given by the contribution of both delivery methods:

$$Cp = Cp,\ bolus + Cp,\ infusion = \frac{k_0}{k\ V} e^{-kt} + \frac{k_0}{k\ V}(1 - e^{-kt}). \tag{2.17}$$

As observed in Figure 2.4, as long as the infusion goes on, the total Cp in this therapeutic setting will be none other than $\frac{k_0}{kV}$, the drug level in the steady state for

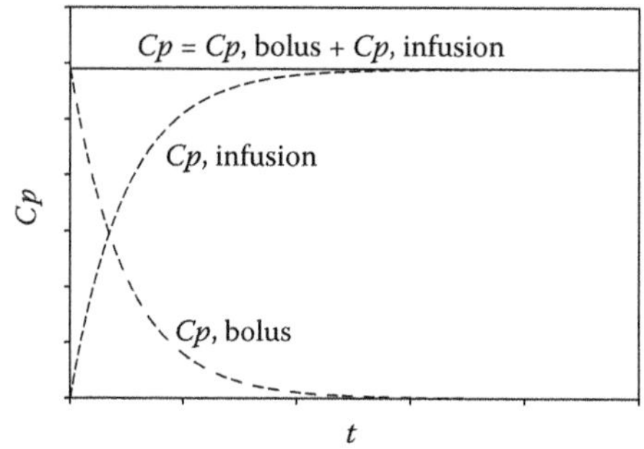

FIGURE 2.4 Plasma concentrations for drug delivery by both bolus IV injection and IV infusion for a general where the bolus IV dose has been designed to be a loading dose for the infusion.

an IV infusion. Such an IV bolus of k_o/k delivered at the beginning of an IV infusion administration is called a *loading dose*. Whenever infusion is interrupted, only the elimination process remains, and the mass balance equation reduces to Equation 2.4; that is, the concentration–time curve will be mathematically described by a simple exponential decay.

Finally, we should consider the mass balance for first-order absorption.

$$\frac{dA}{dt} = K_a F D e^{-k_a t} - kA. \tag{2.18}$$

Solving the differential equation and dividing by V we arrive at

$$Cp = \frac{FD}{V}\left(\frac{k_a}{k_a - k}\right)(e^{-kt} - e^{-k_a t}), \tag{2.19}$$

where k_a stands for the absorption rate constant, which is usually much larger than k (otherwise, flip-flop kinetics are observed [15]). Figure 2.5 shows the concentration–time curve for a drug dosage that follows first-order absorption.

The most common drug therapy interventions consist of administering a given dose of the drug at regular intervals (usually 4, 6, 8, 12, or 24 hours to help treatment adherence). Although it falls beyond the scope of this chapter, by following the superposition principle and coupling multiple single-dose equations, it can be easily demonstrated that, after a number of doses, a steady state is reached (essentially, the remaining drug levels from previous doses have to be taken into account in the calculations). During steady state, plasma drug levels fluctuate between approximately fixed steady-state maximum ($Cp_{max,ss}$) and minimum ($Cp_{min,ss}$) concentrations (in contrast, steady-state levels are constant in the case of IV infusion). Figures 2.6 and 2.7 illustrate the evolution of plasma levels for multiple-dose IV and extravascular. The time between successive doses or the *dosing interval* is denoted as τ (*tau*).

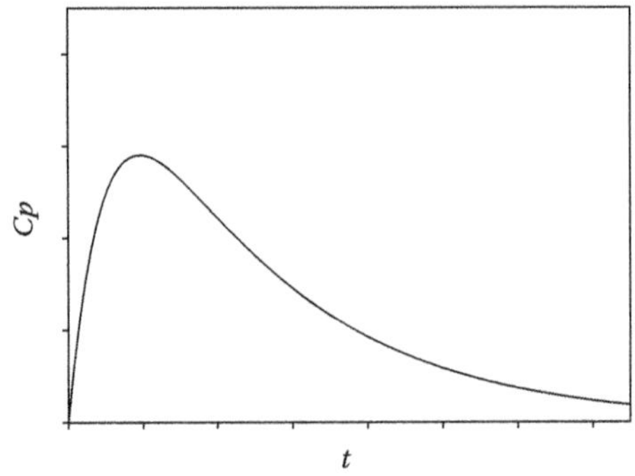

FIGURE 2.5 Plasma concentrations for drug delivery with first-order absorption (typically observed for immediate release extravascular delivery systems).

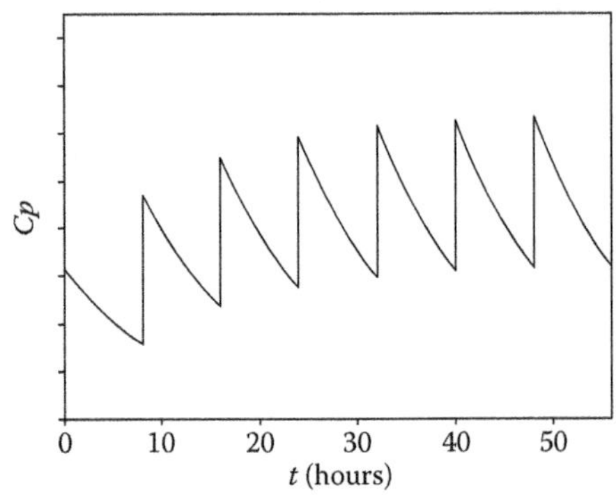

FIGURE 2.6 Concentration–time profile for multiple IV bolus administered at regular intervals (in this example, 8 hours).

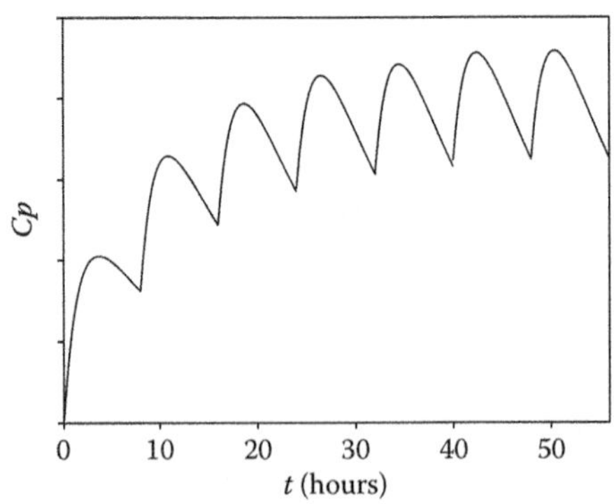

FIGURE 2.7 Concentration–time profile for extravascular multiple doses delivered at regular intervals (in this example, *tau* equals 8 hours).

Ideally, $Cpss,_{max}$ and $Cpss,_{min}$ should remain within the therapeutic window in order to achieve effective concentrations without toxic reactions. Because during steady state the mean rate of drug entry into the body equals the mean rate of drug elimination (so that net drug level remains the same):

$$\frac{FD}{\tau} = kVCp_{ave,ss} = ClCp_{ave,ss}. \tag{2.20}$$

Equation 2.20 is helpful to design a dosing regimen to achieve a given average steady-state drug concentration $Cp_{ave,ss}$, which generally is a priori set around the middle of the therapeutic range. It is important to realize that, theoretically, infinite D/τ relationships can provide the same average steady-state levels. There are, however, some constraints that must be considered. First, the larger the chosen dose, the larger the fluctuation of drug concentrations around $Cp_{ave,ss}$, which implies a larger probability that the drug concentration goes out of the therapeutic range during treatment. Second, the possible doses that can be selected depend on the available dosage units. Third, as has been already underlined, only a limited number of possible *taus* are usually chosen in a clinical setting to assure a comfortable dosing schedule and promote treatment adherence.

ADMINISTRATION ROUTES: ADVANTAGES AND LIMITATIONS RELATED TO CONVENTIONAL DELIVERY SYSTEMS

We present a short discussion of the most important routes of administration for systemic medications along with examples of particularly important therapies administered through each of them. Routes majorly used for topical purposes or very infrequent routes have not been considered.

Oral Route: Enteral, Sublingual, and Buccal

The oral route (*per os*, po) includes all the delivery systems taken through the mouth. It is by far the most widely used route of administration. Different considerations, however, should be taken into account depending on which place absorption of the drug is meant to take place. Most drugs are intended to be dissolved and absorbed within the stomach and/or the gut (enteral administration). In some cases, however, the drug is expected to dissolve within the mouth and absorbed either sublingually (systemic delivery through the mucosal membranes lining the floor of the mouth) or bucally (through the mucosal membranes lining the cheek) [16,17].

Enteral administration is the most natural, convenient, and generally the safest administration route. Since the drug accesses systemic circulation in a slow manner, side effects linked to exposure to high drug levels tend to be reduced. It is a highly versatile route (the active ingredient may be delivered through a very wide spectrum of dosage forms, for example, pharmaceutical solutions, soft and hard capsules, suspensions, tablets) and economic, compared to other parenteral routes [16,18]. There are, however, certain disadvantages that preclude the general use of the enteral route for systemic medications. It is the route associated to higher variability in patient response (due to a diversity of factors, such as irregular drug absorption, constitutional gut makeup, and presence and nature of food constituents at time of drug ingestion, among others). It presents a slow onset of action (in fact, the second slowest after transdermal delivery). Typical onset of action is 30 to 90 minutes after drug intake, which is inconvenient in an emergency situation. Some drugs produce adverse effects on the gastrointestinal mucosa (irritation, bleeding, vomiting, nausea). For example, nonsteroidal anti-inflammatory agents, such as aspirin or diclofenac, present irritating and ulcerative action with occasional serious complications, such as bleeding [19]. A major limitation of enteral administration is the low oral bioavailability of many drugs, owing to inactivation of the drug by acid reaction in the stomach and/or by gastrointestinal enzymes (e.g., hydrolytic enzymes), presystemic metabolism, and poor penetration of the intestinal membrane. For instance, poor aqueous solubility, affinity for drug efflux transporters, and presystemic biotransformation by cytochrome P-450 metabolic enzymes limit oral bioavailability and preclude the oral administration of taxanes [20]. Another class of drugs that present limited bioavailability *po* are peptide and protein drugs [21–23]. Many factors act as major barriers in the successful delivery of intact protein/peptide: poor permeability through the intestinal mucosa due to high molecular weight and poor lipophilicity; denaturation in the extreme acidic gastric medium; and digestion by gastric, pancreatic, and intestinal proteases. A very illustrative example of such a challenge is insulin, which is currently administered through the subcutaneous route with a series of inherent disadvantages (see the subcutaneous route subsection) [24]. A final limitation of the enteral route is that the patient must be conscious or be cooperative to deliver the drug.

The sublingual and buccal routes solve some of the limitations of the enteral route, retaining many of its advantages [25]. The oral cavity is well vascularized, and the blood vessels drain directly into the jugular vein, avoiding the first-pass effect and hydrolysis in the gastrointestinal tract. Interestingly, the cellular turnover in the buccal region is about 4–14 days, which allows the use of mucoadhesive devices for controlled-release applications (a strategy that has proven difficult to implement in the stomach due to its fast turnover). Finally, the microenvironment in the oral cavity can be easily and transiently modified with minimal side effects (e.g., to improve drug absorption). Some disadvantages linked to these routes are the small absorptive area, the continuous secretion of saliva that leads to drug dilution and removes the drug from the absorption site, and the risk of swallowing and/or choking by involuntarily swallowing the delivery system. Although the bad taste and odor of some drugs pose a general problem to the oral route, it is especially problematic for buccal or sublingual delivery systems because the residence time of the drug in the mouth increases compared to the enteral route. Classical examples of drugs delivered through these routes are nitroglycerine, nicotine, and fentanyl formulations. Available dosage forms include lozenges, sprays, chewing gum, bioadhesive tablets, effervescent tables, and thin films (thin strips). In the last years, the buccal and sublingual routes have attracted increasing attention as delivery routes for vaccines and immunotherapeutic treatment of allergies [26] (Figure 2.8).

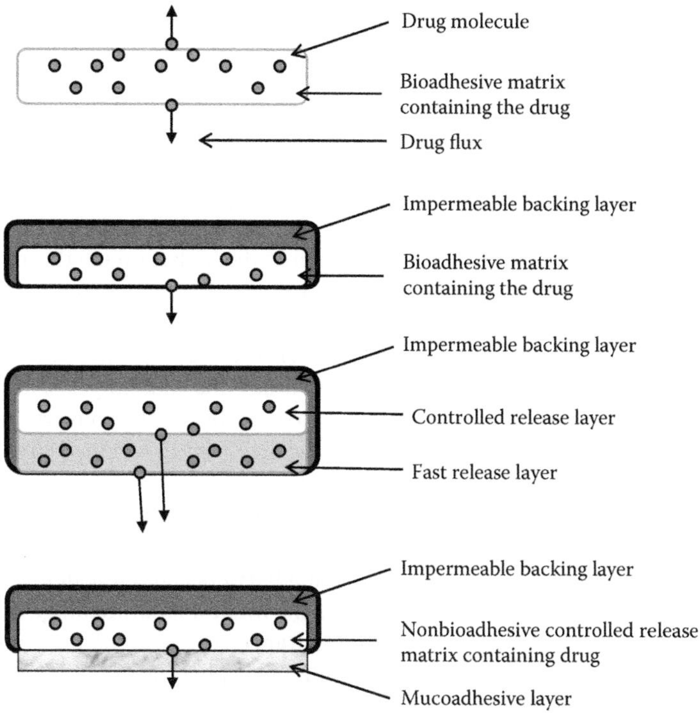

FIGURE 2.8 Schematic representation of some adhesive buccal drug delivery systems. (Reproduced from Paderni et al., Oral local drug delivery and new perspectives in oral drug formulation. *Oral Surg. Oral Med. O.*, 2013, under permission of Elsevier.)

Rectal Route

Drug rectal administration for systemic effects is infrequent. The main advantage of this route is that it avoids the gastric aggressive environment and (at least partially) the hepatic first-pass effect. Whether rectal administration bypasses presystemic metabolism completely or partially depends on the localization of the suppository: Although the lower and middle part of the rectum are drained, in that order, by the inferior and middle rectal veins, which are directly connected to systemic circulation, the upper rectum is drained by the superior rectal vein, a tributary of the portal system. This route may be used to treat unconscious patients when access to the intravenous route is difficult (or IV dosage forms cannot be formulated due to solubility issues) or when the intramuscular route is not well accepted. There are significant differences between countries in terms of acceptability of enemas and suppositories by patients. Moreover, the quantity of drug absorbed through the rectum is usually quite erratic and unpredictable. The pharmaceutical formulation plays a major role in rectal absorption. Occasionally, rectal administration of drugs for systemic delivery proves cathartic. Rectal diazepam has been used for decades to control repetitive or prolonged seizures in children (*status epilepticus*, cluster of seizures) with approved rectal gel preparations [27].

Parenteral Route

Although etymologically the term *parenteral* would comprise all the nonenteral routes, it is generally used for those routes of administration in which drug is given through an injection. Among these, intravenous, intramuscular, and subcutaneous are the most commonly used. Two general drawbacks of the parenteral route is that, on the one hand, it requires trained professionals to perform drug administration, and on the other, strict sterility requirements make the dosage forms much more expensive. Furthermore, once the drug has entered the body through this route, it is very difficult to remove the drug in case of severe toxic reactions to the drug (e.g., idiosyncratic reactions or accidental overdose). Last, it is a poorly tolerated route for many patients. The parenteral route, however, is the chosen delivery way in an emergency context due to the associated fast drug bioavailability and thus rapid onset. A comparison of the typical relative bioavailability of parenteral routes is presented in Figure 2.9 (the figure is only qualitative, and the relative bioavailability depends on a number of factors, including the drug, the dosage, and others; for instance, in specific cases, the subcutaneous route may be faster than the intramuscular one).

The intravenous route presents no absorption barriers and thus can be generally considered the administration route linked to the highest bioavailability. Since the whole dose accesses circulation almost simultaneously, it is highly probable to observe adverse reactions if, due to interindividual pharmacokinetic variability, the drug levels exceed the upper limit of the (individual) therapeutic window for a given patient. An important requisite for intravenous medications is that they must not interfere with blood circulation. This implies that neither suspensions nor emulsions can be administered IV to avoid the risk of emboli. Thus, only aqueous solutions are allowed through this route. It is also important that the drug maintains in solution after injection. The previous considerations pose a major technical issue, particularly when developing a dosage form for bolus IV injection. In that case, the dose has to be dissolved in a very small volume (often around 5 ml). What

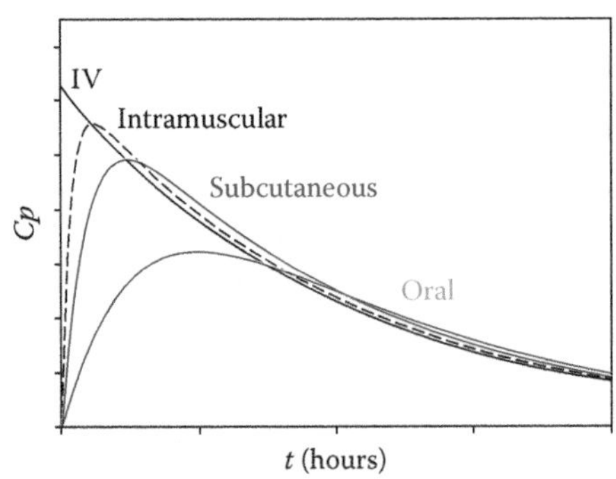

FIGURE 2.9 General concentration time–profiles for IV, intramuscular, and subcutaneous routes, compared to oral administration. F was arbitrarily considered equal to 1 for the parenteral routes and to 0.85 for the oral route.

is more, there is only a limited spectrum of cosolvents to help dissolve the drug, and many of them have intrinsic toxicity. The traditional formulations of taxanes (Figure 2.10) constitute a good example of this issue because their clinical applications have been limited by their poor aqueous solubility. The first approved paclitaxel formulation uses a 1:1 mixture of Cremophor EL® and ethanol to increase the solubility of the intravenously administered drug [28]. However, Cremophor EL may have serious adverse side effects, including severe hypersensitivity reactions, neurotoxicity, nephrotoxicity, and hypotensive vasodilatation [29,30]. Similar issues have been observed with the available docetaxel preparation, which is a concentrated injectable solution containing the drug in a vehicle composed of polysorbate 80 diluted with dehydrated ethyl alcohol in water. Several toxic side effects have resulted from the administration of these formulations [31]. For these reasons, it is recommended that patients treated with these formulations of taxanes are premedicated with oral corticosteroids to reduce the incidence and severity of adverse reactions to the vehicle. All in all, the intravenous route may be the only option when poor permeability forbids other routes. For example, the antibiotic vancomycin (Figure 2.11) must be given IV for systemic therapy since, due to its hydrophilic nature and high molecular weight, it partitions poorly across the gastrointestinal mucosa. Moreover, due to its short half-life, it is often injected twice a day or through continuous infusion [32].

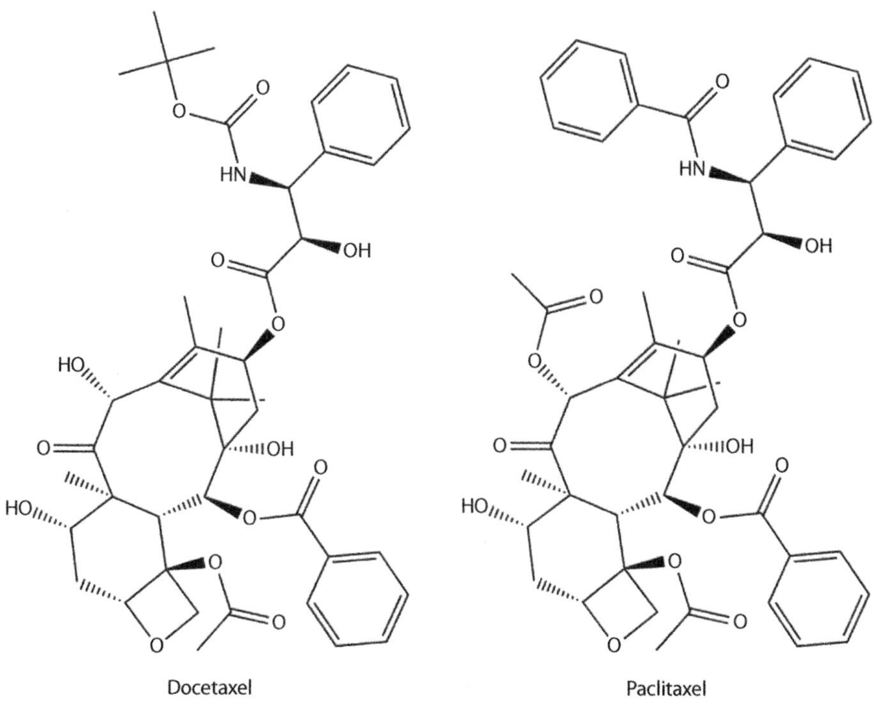

FIGURE 2.10 Due to their poor aqueous solubility IV delivered taxanes have to be dissolved in cosolvents that produce safety issues.

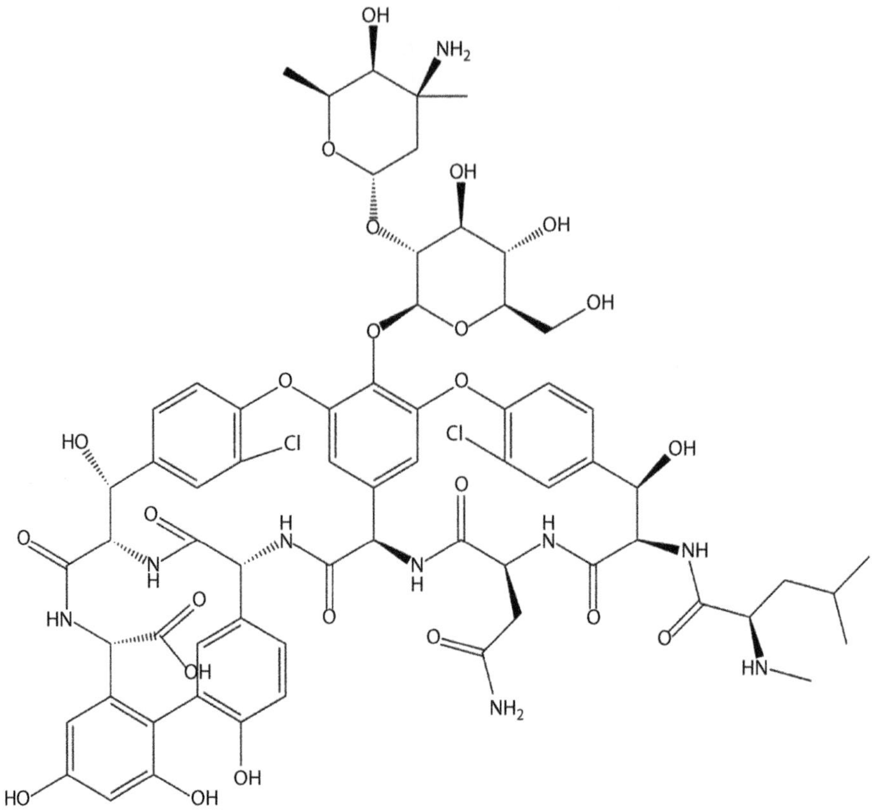

Vancomycin

FIGURE 2.11 The high hydrophilicity and molecular weight of vancomycin demand IV administration.

Intramuscular injections are performed deep into skeletal muscles, typically the deltoid, gluteal, or lumbar muscles. Both aqueous and oleaginous solutions and dispersions might be used with rapid effects or depot activity, which makes this route more versatile than the intravenous one. Nevertheless, it should be noted that oleaginous intramuscular formulations are especially painful, owing to local necrosis, irritation, and inflammatory reactions [33].

Long-lasting intramuscular depot preparations of antipsychotic drugs constitute a nice example of the applicability of such systems [34]. Basically, a prodrug is formulated by binding an alcohol radical from the parent compound to a long-chain fatty acid, forming an ester (Figure 2.12).

The slow partitioning of the prodrug out of the oily vehicle limits the rate at which ubiquitous tissue esterases can release the active ingredient from the prodrug. The intramuscular depot injections are administered at intervals of 1 to 4 weeks, facilitating treatment compliance in psychotic patients known to be noncompliant with oral medication. In general, the length of the fatty acids is inversely related to the rate of

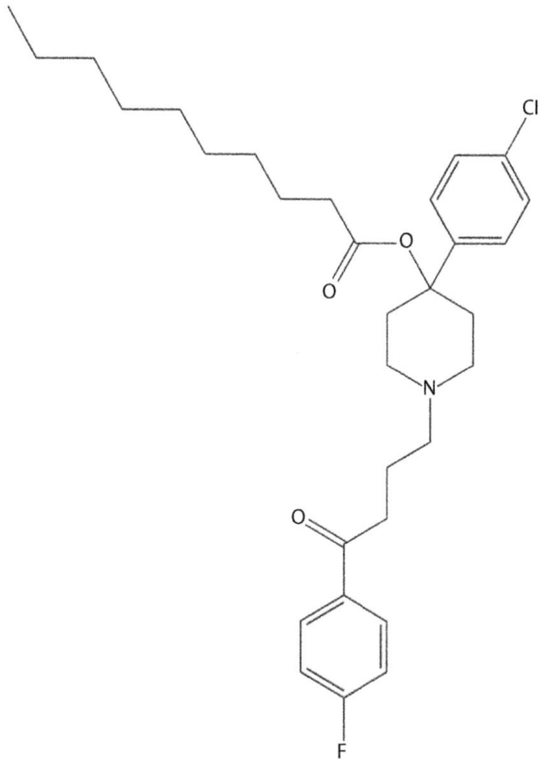

Haloperidol decanoate

FIGURE 2.12 A prodrug of haloperidol used for intramuscular depot systems.

release of the prodrug from the oily depot. Of course, the nature of the oily vehicle also plays a role in the process of drug absorption. Another alternative to control the rate of absorption is the delivery of slowly soluble salt forms.

And last, the subcutaneous route admits either the injection of a drug as a suspension or solution or, alternatively, the implantation of a device for long-term drug release. An important aspect of this route is that it allows self-administration in emergency situations. The maximum amount of volume that can be administered through intermittent subcutaneous injections is around 2–3 ml; thus, drugs administered by this route must be either potent in small concentrations or very soluble. Absorptions are faster and more predictable than in the case of enteral medication although the vascularity of the subcutaneous tissue is less than that of muscle for which absorption is generally slower than in the intramuscular route. Vasodilators can be used to improve drug absorption while vasoconstrictor agents have the opposite effect. The main disadvantage of this route is its inconvenience: Irritating drugs or very viscous suspensions may produce abscesses or necrosis and may be painful to the patient. Heparin and insulin are the most important drugs routinely administered subcutaneously. Multiple injections present a number of drawbacks, however, such as local pain, risk of hyperinsulinemia, and insulin lipohypertrophy, for which rotation of the injection site is recommended. Clinical trials have showed that a significant proportion of diabetic patients fail to achieve lasting glycemic control owing to noncompliance, and psychological barriers associated with multiple daily injections (like needle anxiety) have been described [35]. Some studies indicate insulin pumps (continuous subcutaneous insulin infusion) have a positive impact on patients' quality of life [36,37]. Alternatively, insulin glargine (an engineered insulin analogue that after injection forms microcrystals/microprecipitates that slowly release insulin) provides 18–26 hour control over glycemia with a more physiological insulin profile.

Transdermal Route

Transdermic (percutaneous) therapeutic systems are sustained-release delivery systems aiming to provide stable plasma drug levels (Figure 2.13). To access systemic circulation, a drug applied onto the skin must be released from its vehicle, partition into the stratum corneum, and diffuse through the epidermis and the dermis to reach capillaries.

Percutaneous absorption is influenced by multiple factors, among them drug physicochemical properties, such as drug concentration; surface area to which the delivery system is applied; vehicle composition; hydration of the skin; thickness of the skin; and amount of time permitted in contact with the skin. Preferentially, nonionic, lipophilic molecules of low molecular weight are absorbed quickly through this route. Traditional delivery systems applied onto the skin, such as ointments, creams,

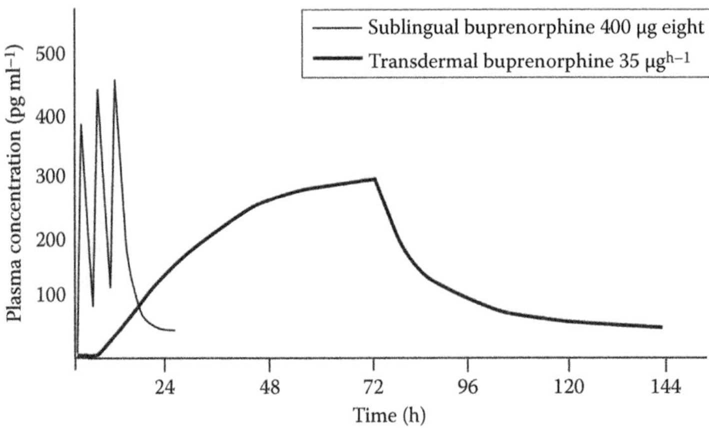

FIGURE 2.13 Comparison of sublingual and transdermal buprenorphine administration. Note that transdermal delivery provides a fluctuation-free concentration–time profile that resembles IV continuous infusion. (Reproduced from L. Margetts, R. Sawyer, *Crit. Care Pain*. 7, 171–176, 2007, under permission of Oxford University Press.)

lotions, and pastes, are nowadays reserved for topical purposes, which are out of the scope of this chapter. For percutaneous absorption, the chosen delivery systems today are adhesive patches, which are fundamentally of two types: those that allow the skin itself to control the rate of absorption (or matrix system or monolithic) in which the drug is incorporated into a polymer matrix from which it is continuously released to the skin (Figure 2.14) and those that control the rate of drug delivery by including a rate-limiting membrane between the drug reservoir (usually a solution or gel) and the skin (reservoir system) (Figure 2.15). Reservoir patches give tighter control of the delivery rate but can have an initial burst release and, if the membrane is damaged, include a risk of accidental overdose, which is much less probable with the matrix systems [38]. It should be underlined that, due to the slow absorption process, there is a delay between the patch application and the development of the effective plasma concentration. The time to achieve steady-state concentrations depends on the drug and may sometimes be achieved only after several patch applications. After that, drug levels will be maintained as long the patches are applied. The percutaneous route is highly accepted and promotes treatment adherence due to elimination of multiple dosing schedules. Naturally, it bypasses hepatic first-pass metabolism (although some drugs may be metabolized in the skin itself) and—since it produces almost constant drug levels—it tends to present no side effects. Nevertheless, the diffusion barrier posed by the skin is the major obstacle of this route, which is only feasible for potent drugs because only low-plasma drug levels are usually achieved.

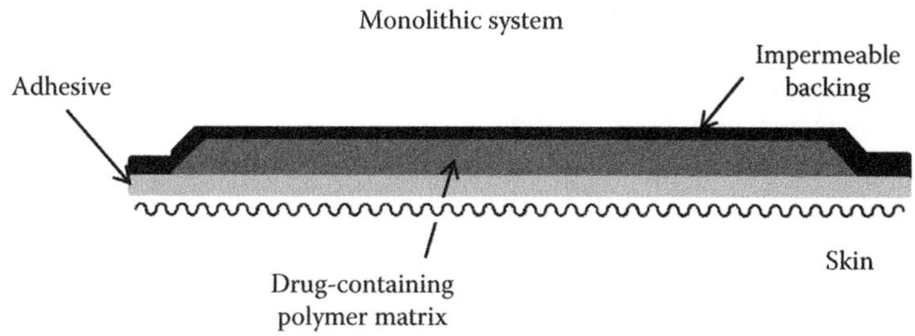

FIGURE 2.14 Matrix-type transdermal patch.

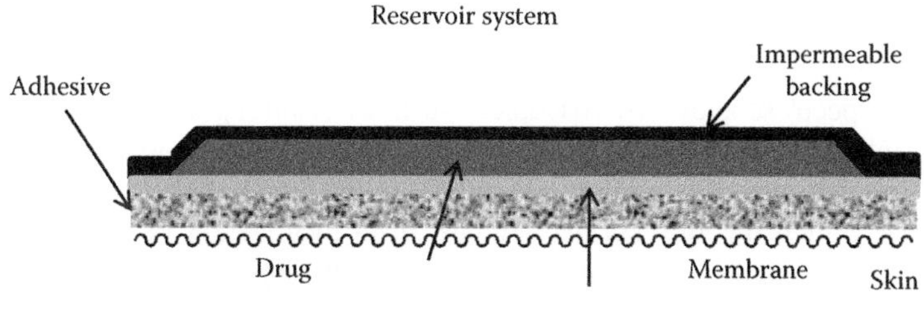

FIGURE 2.15 Reservoir-type transdermal patch.

The route is not practicable for irritating or sensitizing drugs. In order to help drug transfer, a number of strategies have been developed from chemical permeation enhancers (e.g., ethanol, propylene glycol, organic acids) to physical methods (iontophoresis, ultrasound, heat, microneedles).

Advanced Drug Delivery (Micro and Nano) Systems

Micro- and nanodevices present a number of features that have spawned a complete new therapeutic paradigm when they are used as drug delivery devices. Taking into account the definition of nanostructures made by the National Science Foundation, a nanomaterial is an object with at least one dimension between 1 and 100 nm. However, this definition, made only from the physical point of view, does not make sense from the physiological point of view because, for example, nano-objects of 200 nm or less are able to go inside the cells. Also, for instance, many studies demonstrated that particles with a diameter of millimeters are considered excellent drug carriers for sustainable drug delivery. Based on the experimental data, micro- and nanocarriers were analyzed in the same group.

The main advantages of using nanocarriers as drug delivery carriers can be considered as the following:

1. Well-defined control of the interaction between the nanocarrier and the drug.
2. Precise sustained release of the drug in specific targets.
3. Increase drug therapeutic efficiency.
4. Reduction of drug dispersion along the body.
5. Access to interstitial areas of tissues and/or ability to surpass biological barriers (e.g., blood–brain barrier).
6. Reduction of undesirable drug side effects.
7. Nanodevices composed of multicargo "smart" depots with specific drug release profiles based on targets.
8. Specific targeting of the drug by structural modification of the carrier appended with molecules required by pathological cells or tissues. Typical examples are the high requirements of folic acid and/or "biological" iron by tumor cells but also the use of specific antibodies to decorate the carrier surface.

The use of nanoobjects as drug delivery devices implies intensive and extensive preliminary studies of the relationship between the drug and the cargo. Most of the studies involved the use of many combined techniques, such as advanced microscopies and spectroscopies. Microscopies, such as scanning electron microscopy (SEM), transmission electron microscopy (TEM), confocal microscopy, fluorescent microscopy, and atomic force microscopy (AFM), are common tools in system characterization, which involves surface studies, drug localization in the carrier, and properties of the carrier (pore diameter, homogeneity, dispersion, etc.). Also, highly sensitive synchrotron and/or bench spectroscopies, such as FTIR, RAMAN, and fluorescence, among other techniques are providing powerful tools for the characterization of the functional groups involved in the interaction between the drug molecules and the carrier components. In this way, a fine-tuning of the nanocarriers can made based on the specific properties of the drug, allowing the control and modification of the interactions between the drug and the carrier. The main tailoring involves the changes in specific functional groups, like hydroxyl and/or carboxyl residues, to enhance the hydrophilic interactions by chemical and/or enzymatic approaches. Similarly, the attachment of nonpolar groups (e.g., aromatic motifs) using similar methodologies increases the interaction between hydrophobic groups of the carrier and the drug molecule (e.g., poorly soluble drugs under physiological conditions).

Nanosystems and Solubility and Absorption Issues

It has been already discussed that several drugs (e.g., taxanes) cannot be administered enterally due to their poor solubility, and others (e.g., proteins and peptide drugs, gene therapies, and small drug therapies such as vancomycin) present limited oral bioavailability due to their lack of stability within the gastrointestinal tract and permeability issues. When administered within a nanosystem, a drug might well reach systemic circulation in a non-free state. In other words, drug release from the vehicle may occur *after* drug absorption. For the first time in history, a pharmaceutical delivery system might influence drug distribution and elimination processes in a direct manner. Therefore, encapsulation within a micro- or nanocarrier with tailored physicochemical properties might serve to overcome the drug's intrinsic characteristics that impair its pharmacokinetic profile. Figure 2.16 shows different

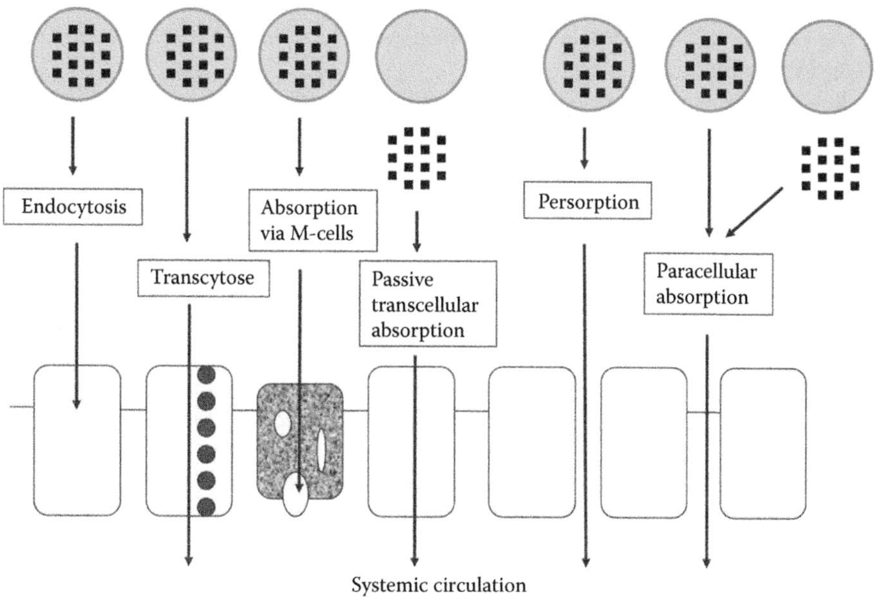

FIGURE 2.16 Different mechanisms through which micro- and nanocarriers might enhance drug uptake. (Reproduced from A. Bernkop-Schnürch, *Eur. J. Pharm. Sci.*, 49, 272–277, 2013, under permission of Elsevier.)

routes through which a nanocarrier might enhance drug uptake and improve systemic bioavailability [39,40]. As illustrated there, the drug–nanocarrier complex can reach systemic circulation through trancytosis and the paracellular route. In the case of oral delivery, they can reach the lymphoid system via M-cells (a quite unexplored absorption route that some authors suggest might be the predominant particle uptake route). Alternatively, systems that release their payload when they are in intimate contact with the absorption membrane have also been conceived: A comparatively steeper concentration gradient on the mucosa (the driving force of passive diffusion) would be achieved this way. The efficacy of this strategy could be improved by adhesive systems and/or by incorporating mucolytic enzymes to the particles. Furthermore, colloidal drug carriers might also conceal drugs from biochemical barriers to permeability, such as multidrug efflux transporters from the ABC superfamily.

For example, Manjunath and Venkateswarlu [41] formulate clozapine (an antipsychotic drug with oral bioavailability below 30% due to significant first-pass hepatic metabolism) as solid–lipid nanoparticles in order to favor intestinal lymphatic transport and evade portal circulation. A remarkable 91.8% relative bioavailability (compared to intravenous administration) and a significant increase in the mean residence time were achieved. Similarly, Feng et al. developed poly(lactic-co-glycolic acid) (PLGA) nanoparticles, poly(lactide)-vitamin E TPGS (PLA-TPGS) nanoparticles, and PLA-TPGS montmorillonite (PLA-TPGS/MMT) nanoparticles to accomplish efficient oral delivery of docetaxel, avoiding first-pass extraction and Pgp efflux transport [42]. The authors compared the bioavailability of the nanoparticulated systems (in rats) to that of intravenous administration. The oral bioavailability of the PLA-TPGS nanoparticle formulation achieved a remarkable 91.3% compared to intravenous administration.

Regarding the use of nanocarriers to circumvent efflux pumps, many examples can be cited. The poorly soluble Pgp-substrate propanolol was conjugated to a PAMAM three-generation dendrimer to enhance the transport of propranolol across Caco-2 cells. This PAMAM–propranolol prodrug was shown to bypass the efflux system [43]. In a related study, prodrugs between the smaller and less toxic one-generation PAMAM dendrimer and the water-insoluble Pgp substrate terfenadine were synthesized using succinic acid or succinyl-diethylene glycol as linkers. All of the PAMAM–terfenadine prodrugs were more hydrophilic than the parent drug [44]. An increase in the apparent permeability coefficient of terfenadine in both apical-to-basolateral and basolateral-to-apical directions was observed with the apparent permeability being larger in the apical-to-basolateral direction. Similar results were obtained with paclitaxel- and doxorubicin-loaded nanolipid carriers [45], which showed 34.3- and 6.4-fold reversal powers (compared to solutions of the same drugs) when tested on different multidrug-resistant cell lines.

Nanosystems and Biodistribution

The source for biophase bioavailability can be the systemic bioavailability following common routes of administration (described previously) or—directly—the site-specific biophase bioavailability for the formulations capable of cellular internalization in the body location where the drug and its molecular target will interact. As commented at the beginning of this chapter, the rationale of using nanosystems for targeting is based on the fact that nanocarriers will be able to deliver a concentrated dose of a drug in the vicinity of the targets and thus reduce the drug exposure to healthy tissues [46]. Drug targeting can be achieved by taking advantage of the distinct pathophysiological features of diseased tissues. Targeting strategies include passive targeting, active targeting, stimuli-responsive distribution, and more recently, synergic combinations of the previous through multifunctional nanosystems (Figure 2.17) [47,48]. Briefly, passive targeting exploits the irregular, leaky blood vessels and the lack of functional lymphatic drainage in tumor tissue to preferentially locate the drug carrier complex in the cancerous cells (enhanced permeability and retention effect, EPR). A similar approach can be conceived for the treatment of other conditions in which vascular permeability is increased (e.g., inflammation). Active targeting is achieved by conjugating targeting ligands (antibodies, sugars, peptides, vitamins) that selectively bind to receptors, which are upregulated in the target tissue. Stimuli-responsive distribution takes advantage of specific environmental signals (such as pH changes, reductive environment, magnetic fields, and others) to locate and release the drug. This is also known as triggered targeting or smart systems. Targeted delivery systems are

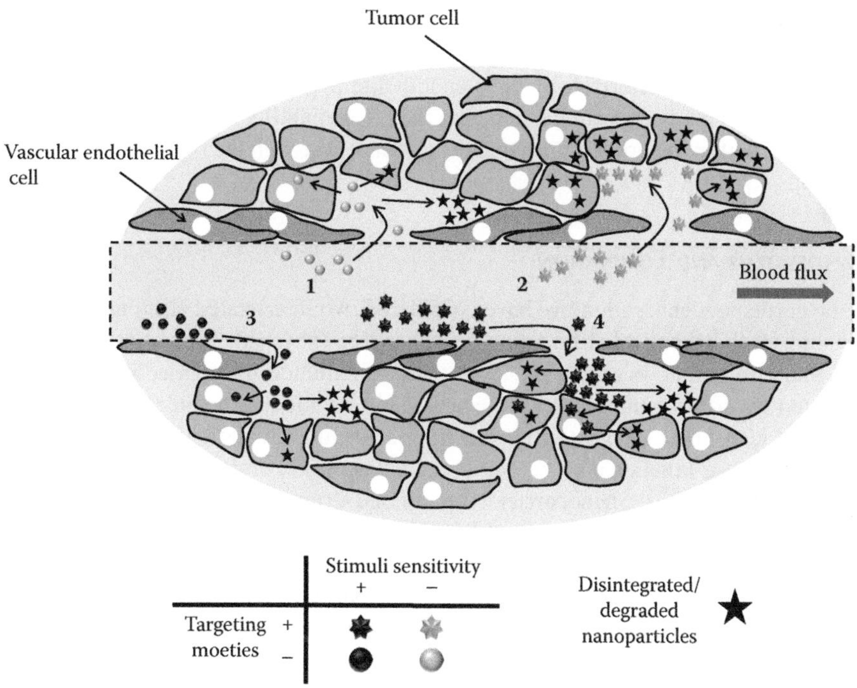

FIGURE 2.17 Different simple or combined targeting strategies, applied in this case to tumor targeting. (Reproduced from S. Kim, J.-H. Kim, O. Jeon, I. C. Kwon, K. Park, *Eur. J. Pharm. Biopharm.*, 71, 420–430, 2009, under permission of Elsevier.)

currently going beyond tissue or cellular targeting, achieving even subcellular targeting (engineered nanoparticle subcellular interactions) with great promise in the field of gene delivery and organelle-specific diseases [49].

An example of synergistic combinations is presented in work of Khoee et al. [50], who developed a pH-sensitive polymeric NP targeted with folate groups and loaded with the anticancer drug quercetin. The formulation is produced by radical polymerization of three monomers: methacrylated poly(lactic-co-glycolic acid) (mPLGA) as a lipophilic domain, acrylated methoxy poly(ethylene glycol) (aMPEG) as a hydrophilic domain and N-2-[(tertbutoxycarbonyl) amino] ethyl methacrylamide (Boc-AEMA) as a pH-responsive segment, followed by the removal of the protecting amine group (Boc) and the conjugation of the resulting copolymer with activated folic acid. Finally, the drug—which is poorly soluble in water—is loaded into the NP by a nanoprecipitation method. In vitro release experiments showed that quercetin release from the NP was pH-dependent and much faster at pH 5.8 than pH 7.4. The results indicated a conformational change in AEMA chains from a compacted shape to an expanded one with a decrease in the pH values. In the expanded conformation, the drug can diffuse out from the NP more easily than in a compact form. The folate group is expected to increase the specificity in the delivery of the encapsulate by the pH-sensitive NP. Other similar examples (among many others) include magnetic NP targeted with folate [51], biotin-conjugated pH-responsive polymeric micelles [52], and pH and redox dual-responsive nanoparticles functionalized with cRGD peptide [53].

Colloidal systems may also be applied to improve the bioavailabilty of a drug in some tissues characterized by poor endothelial permeability. Particularly, much effort has been made regarding enhancing the bioavailability of central nervous system agents within the brain, improving drug transfer through the blood–brain barrier [54–56].

Nanosystems and Elimination

In the correspondent section, we have considered two interrelated elimination ways: metabolism (biochemical elimination) and excretion (physical elimination). We have also underlined that, occasionally, excretion is facilitated through active transport mediated by efflux pumps. As has been already mentioned, nanodelivery systems may well keep their integrity after reaching systemic circulation. Simultaneously, the drug release kinetics may be engineered. Therefore, entrapment or encapsulation of a drug within a nanocarrier with defined drug release kinetics or stimuli-responsive drug release may be used to prolong the retention time in blood. Many reports agree that particles with a hydrodynamic diameter below 5.5–6 nm are rapidly excreted into urine [57–59]. Therefore, nanoparticles with diameters above that threshold would tend to increase drug half-life due to reduced renal filtration. What is more, since the basement membrane of glomerulus is mainly composed of glycosaminoglycans, negatively charged polysaccharides, it also exhibits permselectivity toward charged macromolecules [57]. Positively charged macromolecules are then filtered more effectively than anionic macromolecules. On the other hand, interactions between the drug and efflux transporters or metabolic enzymes are impeded as long as the drug is encapsulated within the nanocarrier. This may explain, for instance, why the elimination half-life of docetaxel is dramatically expanded from 4.5 hours (intravenous administration of free docetaxel) to an astonishing half-life of more than 118 hours (oral administration within a nanocarrier) in the already mentioned work from Feng et al. [42]. Note that in the background of this new therapeutic paradigm, the elimination half-life does not necessarily reflect the intrinsic elimination half-life of the drug (the ability of the body to remove free drug), but the sum of the parallel elimination of free drug and drug entrapped in colloidal systems, which represents an unprecedented situation until the nano era.

While nanocarriers of adequate size can escape glomerular filtration, a major obstacle to achieving long blood circulation time is the uptake by the reticulo-endothelial system (the mononuclear phagocyte system, a part of the immune system composed primarily by monocytes and macrophages and located mainly in the lymph nodes, the spleen, and the liver), which is capable of engulfing not only microorganisms, but also foreign particles (among them nanocarriers). The clearance of nanoparticles after intravenous administration can occur within 5 minutes [60]. It has long been recognized that surface properties and size are the major determinants of clearance and distribution of colloidal particles [61]. Ancient Egyptians knew that ink colloidal particles could be stabilized by adding natural polymers. Similarly, surface attachment of surfactants and natural or synthetic polymers can be used to increase the blood circulation time. Unmodified nanoparticles rapidly adsorb plasma proteins (mainly opsonins) and as a consequence are promptly removed from the bloodstream by the reticulo-endothelial system. Coating the nanoparticles with hydrophilic polymers or surfactants provides an aqueous shield around the nanoparticle, thus decreasing the extent of opsonization and the subsequent recognition by the mononunclear phagocyte system. Poly(ethyleneglycol) (PEG)-grafted nanocarriers (also known as stealth nanoparticles) have been extensively used for this purpose. What is more, it has been observed that PEGylation can also improve brain uptake [62]. The effect of particle size on in vivo distribution has also been studied [63], suggesting that particle sizes below 100 nm tend to increase circulation lifetime. However, a number of limitations to the use of PEG have also been described [64]. Several reports indicate that upon subsequent administrations of PEGylated systems, an immune response could be elicited, leading to rapid blood clearance and undesirable side effects that hamper their clinical utility; this immune response includes the production of anti-PEG antibodies and is commonly known as the accelerated blood clearance phenomenon [65–67]. There are indications that such phenomenon depends on the nature and content of the nanocarriers [67,68]. Interestingly, the accelerated blood clearance can be abrogated pharmacologically [69]. The level of induction of the immune response strongly depends on the time interval between doses. PEG also hinders the cellular uptake of the colloidal entities [64]. This later issue can be possibly overcome by the development of cleavable, stimuli responsive PEG-derivatized nanoparticles [70–71]. Alternatively, uncoated nanoparticles might be used for lymphatic targeting or Kupffer cell targeting.

Another point to take into account is the characteristics and properties of the nanocarriers related to physiology of the patient. Some nano-objects were found to be toxic, such as quantum dots, dendrimers, and also metallic and metal oxide nanoparticles, and with the exceptions of specific and particular cases cannot be used as carriers for drug delivery. Additionally, the behavior of the nanocarrier is related to the environment, and under physiological conditions, for example, in the bloodstream, it is difficult to believe that the nanocarrier could not interact with some biomolecules, modifying many properties, such as rheological, and also their distribution along the body, degradation, elimination, and so on.

In summary, the main clearance mechanism for drugs entrapped within nanocarriers are not the traditional drug elimination mechanisms acting on free drug released from conventional drug delivery systems (i.e., renal elimination of the parenteral drug or its metabolites); instead, the immune response arises as the major clearance determinant and thus limiting factor to long circulating nanodelivery systems.

In Vivo Monitoring

It has previously been discussed that, once distribution has been completed, the plasma drug levels will present a direct relationship with the drug levels in other tissues. In fact, if the free drug hypothesis applies, the free drug concentration at steady state will be the same at both sides of any biomembrane permeable to the drug. Therefore, biophase bioavailability is often studied indirectly through systemic bioavailability. Such approximation is reasonable for conventional drug delivery systems with non-targeted distribution. But what about advanced targeted nanosystems? Intuitively, the relationship between drug levels in plasma and drug levels in the biophase can be much more evasive or dubious. However, nanotechnology itself offers some solutions that may completely change the nature of pharmacokinetic studies through noninvasive in vivo monitoring of vehicle distribution and drug delivery. For instance, quantum dots (fluorescent semiconductor nanocrystals) feature small size and versatile surface chemistry, allowing their incorporation within virtually any nano drug delivery device with minimal effect on overall characteristics, and offer superb optical properties for real-time monitoring [72], making it possible to understand the biological fate of a drug in great detail. QDs, however, often contain cadmium, which is highly toxic in its soluble form. Gold nanoparticles and fluorophore-doped silica nanoparticles are examples of alternative luminescent nanosystems, which might prove more biocompatible, as well as magnetic nanoparticles [73,74]. Note, however, that these systems are inorganic in nature (and nonbiodegradable), which arouses safety concerns. For instance, a study on the in vivo toxicity on rodents of gold nanoparticles showed that administration of 8 mg/kg/week of 8- to 37-nm particles produced, from day 14, severe side effects, such as camel-like backs and crooked spines [75]. Histological examination revealed various degrees of abnormality in the liver, lung, and spleen of gold nanoparticle–treated mice. The median survival time was also significantly reduced. We are still missing standardized procedures and coordinated research programs that allow us to reach general conclusions on the biosafety of nanosystems [76,77]. Since the biodistribution and toxicology of nanoparticles strongly depend on a multiplicity of factors, such as dose, size, and shape, it has been pointed out that nanotoxicological studies without careful characterization of the physicochemical properties of the studied systems is not meaningful [77]. Evaluation of the final fate of the nanoparticles and their effect on protein and gene expression levels are critical issues that to the moment have been scarcely, insufficiently investigated [77,78]. Ultrasound-enhanced drug delivery is a yet unexplored option to inorganic nanoparticle-based monitoring: Because echogenic behavior may be achieved with biodegradable materials, real-time monitoring of the drug delivery process may be accomplished, minimizing potential safety issues [79].

CONCLUSIONS

Throughout this chapter, the basic pharmacokinetic considerations regarding conventional systemic drug delivery systems, including the free drug hypothesis; the notion of nonspecific distribution; definitions of absorption, distribution, and elimination processes; the basic equations of the one-compartment open model; and the more common routes of drug administration, together with their advantages and disadvantages, were overviewed. In the last section, we envision a whole change in the field of biopharmacy and pharmacokinetics due to the ongoing introduction of advanced, nano delivery systems. Such drug vehicles have brought us near to our dreamed of, ideal drug delivery vector, owing to unprecedented possibilities including targeted distribution and in vivo monitoring of drug release. Additionally, the opportunity of systemic delivery of nanocarrier–drug conjugates enables a complete modification of a drug biopharmaceutic profile, providing solutions to solubility, stability, and permeability issues. Consequently, more convenient delivery routes can be explored for problematic therapeutics (peptides, genes, anticancer agents), expanding their clinical utility.

REFERENCES

1. Smith, D. A.; Di, L.; Kerns, E. H. The effect of plasma protein binding on *in vivo* efficacy: Misconceptions in drug discovery. *Nat. Rev. Drug. Discov.* 2010, 9, 929–939.
2. Testa, B.; Krämer, S. D. The biochemistry of drug metabolism—And introduction. Part 1. Principles and overview. *Chem. Biodivers.* 2006, 3, 1053–1101.
3. Taft, D. R. Drug excretion. In *Pharmacology. Principles and Practice.* Hacker, M.; Bachmann, K.; Messer, W. (eds), Academic Press, 2009.
4. Wilkinson, J. N.; Moppett, I. K.; Hardman, J. G. Modes of drug elimination. *Anaesth. Intens. Care* 2008, 9, 362–365.
5. Bachmann, K. Drug metabolism. In *Pharmacology. Principles and Practice.* Hacker, M.; Bachmann, K.; Messer, W. (eds), Academic Press, 2009.
6. Jennen, D. G. J.; Gaj, S.; Giesbertz, P. J.; van Delft, J. H. M.; Evelo, C. T.; Kleinjans, J. C. S. Biotransformation pathway maps in WikiPathways enable direct visualization of drug metabolism related expression changes. *Drug Discov. Today* 2010, 15, 851–858.
7. King, R. S. Biotransformations in drug metabolism. In *Drug Metabolism Handbook. Concepts and Applications.* Nassar, A. F.; Hollenberg, P. F.; Scatina J. (eds), John Wiley & Sons, 2009.
8. Toutain, P. L.; Bousquet-Mélou, A. Plasma clearance. *J. Vet. Pharmacol. Therap.* 2004, 27, 415–425.
9. Lohr, J. W.; Willsky, G. R.; Acara, M. A. Renal drug metabolism. *Pharmacol. Rev.* 1998, 50, 107–141.
10. Welling, P. G. Factors influencing absorption and bioavailability after enteral administration. In *Pharmacokinetics. Processes, Mathematics and Applications.* American Chemical Society, 1997.

11. van Hoogdalem, E. J.; de Boer, A. G.; Breimer, D. D. Pharmacokinetics of rectal drug administration, part I. *Clin. Pharmacokinet.* 1991, 21, 11–26.
12. Dhillon, S.; Gill, K. Basic pharmacokinetics. In *Clinical Pharmacokinetics*. Dhillon, S.; Kostrsewski, A. (eds), Pharmaceutical Press, 2006.
13. Aarons, L. Physiologically based pharmacokinetic modelling: A sound mechanistic basis is needed. *Br. J. Clin. Pharmacol.* 2005, 60, 581–583.
14. Byers, J. P.; Sarver, J. G. Pharmacokinetic modeling. In *Pharmacology. Principles and Practice*. Hacker, M.; Bachmann, K.; Messer, W. (eds), Academic Press, 2009.
15. Yánez, J. A.; Remsberg, C. M.; Sayre, C. L.; Forrest, M. L.; Davies, N. M. Flip-flop pharmacokinetics—Delivering a reversal of disposition: Challenges and opportunities during drug development. *Ther. Deliv.* 2011, 2, 643–672.
16. Alexander, K. Dosage forms and their routes of administration. In *Pharmacology. Principles and Practice*. Hacker, M.; Bachmann, K.; Messer, W. (eds), Academic Press, 2009.
17. Shojaei, A. H. Buccal mucosa as a route for systemic drug delivery: A review. *J. Pharm. Pharmaceut. Sci.* 1998, 1, 15–30.
18. Verma, P.; Thakur, A. S.; Deshmukh, K.; Jha, A. K.; Verma, S. Routes of drug administration. *Int. J. Pharm. Stud. Res.* 2010, 1, 54–49.
19. Lanas, A. A review of the gastrointestinal safety data—A gastroenterologist's perspective. *Rheumatology* 2010, 48, ii3–ii10.
20. Jibodh, R. A.; Lagas, J. S.; Nuijen, B.; Beijnen, J. H.; Schellens, J. H. Taxanes: Old drugs, new oral formulations. *Eur. J. Pharmacol.* 2013. Published ahead of print. doi: 10.1016/j.ejphar.2013.02.058.
21. Parka, K.; Kwon, I. C.; Park, K. Oral protein delivery: Current status and future prospect. *React. Func. Polym.* 2011, 71, 280–287.
22. Morishita, M.; Peppas, N. A. Is the oral route possible for peptide and protein drug delivery? *Drug Discov. Today* 2006, 11, 905–910.
23. Gupta, S.; Arushi, J.; Chakraborty, M.; Sahni, J.; Ali, J.; Dang, S. Oral delivery of therapeutic proteins and peptides: A review on recent developments. *Drug Deliv.* 2013, 20, 237–246.
24. Kinesh, V. P.; Neelam, D. P.; Punit, B. P.; Bhavesh, S. B.; Pragna, K. S. Novel approaches for oral delivery of insulin and current status of oral insulin products. *Int. J. Pharm. Sci. Nanotechnol.* 2010, 3, 1057–1064.
25. Pather, S. I.; Rathbone, M. J.; Senel, S. Current status and the future of buccal drug delivery systems. *Expert. Opin. Drug. Deliver.* 2008, 5, 531–542.
26. Senel, S.; Rathbone, M. J.; Cansiz, M.; Pather, I. Recent developments in buccal and sublingual delivery systems. *Expert. Opin. Drug. Deliver.* 2012, 9, 615–628.
27. Anderson, G. D.; Saneto, R. P. Current oral and non-oral routes of antiepileptic drug delivery. *Adv. Drug Deliv. Rev.* 2012, 64, 911–918.
28. Tarr, B. D.; Yalkowsky, S. H. A new parenteral vehicle for the administration of some poorly water soluble anti-cancer drugs. *J. Parenter. Sci. Technol.* 1987, 41, 31–33.
29. ten Tije, A. J.; Verweij J.; Loos W. J.; Sparreboom A. Pharmacological effects of formulation vehicles: Implications for cancer chemotherapy. *Clin. Pharmacokinet.* 2003, 42, 665–685.
30. Gelderblom, H.; Verweij, J.; Nooter, K.; Sparreboom, A. Cremophor EL: The drawbacks and advantages of vehicle selection for drug formulation. *Eur. J Cancer.* 2001, 37, 1590–1588.
31. Hennenfent, K. L.; Govindan, R. Novel formulations of taxanes: A review. Old wine in a new bottle? *Ann. Oncol.* 2006, 17, 735–749.
32. Van Bambeke, F. Glycopeptides and glycodepsipeptides in clinical development: A comparative review of their antibacterial spectrum, pharmacokinetics and clinical efficacy. *Curr. Opin. Invest. Drugs* 2006, 7, 740–749.

33. Sartorius, G.; Fennell, C.; Spasevska, S.; Turner, L.; Conway, A. J.; Handelsman, D. J. Factors influencing time course of pain after depot oil intramuscular injection of testosterone undecanoate. *Asian J. Androl.* 2010, 12, 227–233.
34. Cocoman. A.; Murray, J. Intramuscular injections: A review of the best practice for mental health nurses. *J. Psychiatr. Ment. Health Nurs.* 2008, 15, 424–434.
35. Korytkowski, M. When oral agents fail: Practical barriers to starting insulin. *Int. J. Obesity* 2002, 26, S18–S24.
36. Lichtenberger-Geslin, L.; Boudailliez, B.; Braun, K.; Bach, V.; Mercier, A.; Bony-Trifunovic, H. Does insulin pump therapy improve quality of life and satisfaction in children and adolescents with type 1 diabetes? *Arch. Pediatr.* 2013, 20, 248–256.
37. Kesavadev, J.; Balakrishnan, S.; Ahammed, S.; Jothydev, S. Reduction of glycosylated hemoglobin following 6 months of continuous subcutaneous insulin infusion in an Indian population with type 2 diabetes. *Diabetes Technol. Ther.* 11, 517–521.
38. Margetts, L.; Sawyer, R. Transdermal drug delivery: Principles and opioid therapy. *Contin. Educ. Anaesth. Crit. Care Pain.* 2007, 7, 171–176.
39. Bernkop-Schnürch, A. Nanocarrier systems for oral delivery: Do we really need them? *Eur. J. Pharm. Sci.* 2013, 49, 272–277.
40. Bakhru, S. H.; Furtado, S.; Morello, P.; Mathiowitz, E. Oral delivery of proteins by biodegradable nanoparticles. *Adv. Drug Deliv. Rev.* 2013, 65, 811–821.
41. Manjunath, K.; Venkateswarlu, V. Pharmacokinetics, tissue distribution and bioavailability of clozapine solid lipid nanoparticles after intravenous and intraduodenal administration. *J. Control. Release* 2005, 107, 215–228.
42. Feng, S. S.; Mei, L.; Anitha, P.; Gan, C. W.; Zhou W. Y. Poly(lactide)–vitamin E derivative/montmorillonite nanoparticle formulations for the oral delivery of docetaxel. *Biomaterials* 2009, 30, 3297–3306.
43. D'Emanuele, A.; Jeyprasesphant, R.; Penny, J.; Attwood, D. The use of a dendrimer-propranolol prodrug to bypass efflux transporters and enhance oral bioavailability. *J. Control. Release* 2004, 95, 447–453.
44. Najlah, M.; Freeman, S.; Attwood, D.; D'Emanuele, A. Synthesis and assessment of first generation polyamidoamine dendrimer prodrugs to enhance the celular permeability of P-gp substrates. *Bioconjugate Chem.* 2007, 18, 937–946.
45. Zhang, X. G.; Miao, J.; Dai, Y. Q.; Du, Y. Z.; Yuan, H.; Hu, F. Q. Reversal activity of nanostructured lipid carriers loading cytotoxic drug in multi-drug resistant cancer cells. *Int. J. Pharm.* 2008, 361, 239–244.
46. Leucuta, S. E. Systemic and biophase bioavailability and pharmacokinetics of nanoparticulate drug delivery systems. *Curr. Drug Deliv.* 2013, 10, 208–240.
47. Bellera, C.; Gantner, M. E.; Ruiz, M. E.; Talevi, A. Recent advances on nanotechnology applications to cancer drug therapy. *J. Cancer Res. Update* 2013, 2, 151–185.
48. Kim, S.; Kim, J.-H.; Jeon, O.; Kwon, I. C.; Park, K. Engineered polymers for advanced drug delivery. *Eur. J. Pharm. Biopharm.* 2009, 71, 420–430.
49. Huang, J. G.; Leshuk, T.; Gu, F. X. Emerging nanomaterials for targeting subcellular organelles. *Nano Today* 2011, 6, 478–492.
50. Khoee, S.; Rahmatolahzadeh, R. Synthesis and characterization of pH-responsive and folated nanoparticles based on self-assembled brush-like PLGA/PEG/AEMA copolymer with targeted cancer therapy properties: A comprehensive kinetic study. *Eur. J. Med. Chem.* 2012, 50, 416–427.
51. Sahu, S. K.; Maiti, S.; Pramanik, A.; Ghosh, S. K.; Pramanik P. Controlling the thickness of polymeric shell on magnetic nanoparticles loaded with doxorubicin for targeted delivery and MRI contrast agent. *Carbohydr. Polym.* 2012, 87, 2593–2604.
52. Kim, J. H.; Li, Y.; Kim, M. S.; Kang, S. W.; Jeong, J. H.; Lee, D. S. Synthesis and evaluation of biotin-conjugated pH-responsive polymeric micelles as drug carriers. *Int. J. Pharm.* 2012, 427, 435–442.

53. Remant-Bahadur, K. C. R.; Thapa, B.; Xu, P. pH and redox dual responsive nanoparticle for nuclear targeted drug delivery. *Mol. Pharm.* 2012, 9, 2719–2729.
54. Pinzon-Daza, M. L.; Campia, I.; Kopecka, J.; Garzon, R.; Ghigo, D.; Rigant, C. Nanoparticle- and liposome-carried drugs: New strategies for active targeting and drug delivery across blood–brain barrier. *Curr. Drug. Metab.* 2013, 14, 625–640.
55. Vlieghe, P.; Khrestchatisky, M. Medicinal chemistry based approaches and nanotechnology-based systems to improve CNS drug targeting and delivery. *Med. Res. Rev.* 2013, 33, 457–516.
56. Kreuter, J. Nanoparticulate systems for brain delivery of drugs. *Adv. Drug. Deliv. Rev.* 2012, 64, 213–222.
57. Yamashita, F.; Hashida, M. Pharmacokinetic considerations for targeted drug delivery. *Adv. Drug Deliv. Rev.* 2013, 65, 139–147.
58. Longmire, M.; Choyke, P. L.; Kobayashi, H. Clearance properties of nano-sized particles and molecules as imaging agents: Considerations and caveats. *Nanomedicine (Lond)* 2008, 3, 703–717.
59. Choi, H. S.; Liu, W.; Liu, F.; Nasr, K.; Misra, P.; Bawendi, M. G.; Frangioni, J. V. Design considerations for tumour-targeted nanoparticles. *Nat. Nanotechnol.* 2010, 5, 42–47.
60. Wohlfart, S.; Gelperina, S.; Kreuter, J. J. Transport of drugs across the blood–brain barrier by nanoparticles. *J. Control. Release* 2012, 161, 264–273.
61. Storm, G.; Belliot, S. O.; Daemenb, T.; Lasic, D. D. Surface modification of nanoparticles to oppose uptake by the mononuclear phagocyte system. *Adv. Drug Deliv. Rev.* 1995, 17, 31–48.
62. Zara, G. P.; Cavalli, R.; Bargoni, A.; Fundaro, A.; Vighetto, D.; Gasco, M. R. Intravenous administration to rabbits of non-stealth and stealth doxorubicin-loaded solid lipid nanoparticles at increasing concentrations of stealth agent: Pharmacokinetics and distribution of doxorubicin in brain and other tissues. *J. Drug Target.* 2002, 10, 327–335.
63. Yadav, K. S.; Chuttani, K.; Mishra, A. K.; Sawant, K. K. Effect of size on the biodistribution and blood clearance of etoposide-loaded PLGA. *PDA J. Pharm. Sci. Technol.* 2011, 65, 131–139.
64. Gomes Da Silva, L. C.; Fonseca, N. A.; Moura, V.; De Lima, P.; Simoes, S.; Moreira. Nanotechnological platforms for siRNA delivery in cancer therapy: Paradigms and challenges. *J. Accounts Chem. Res.* 2012, 45, 1163–1171.
65. Zhao, Y.; Wang, C.; Wang, L.; Yang, Q.; Tang, W.; She, Z.; Deng, Y. A frustrating problem: Accelerated blood clearance of PEGylated solid lipid nanoparticles following subcutaneous injection in rats. *Eur. J. Pharm. Biopharm.* 2012, 81, 506–513.
66. Ishida, T.; Kiwada, H. Anti-polyethyleneglycol antibody response to PEGylated substances. *Biol. Pharm. Bull.* 2013, 36, 889–891.
67. Saadati, R.; Dadashzadeh, S.; Abbasian, Z.; Soleimanjahi, H. Accelerated blood clearance of PEGylated PLGA nanoparticles following repeated injections: Effects of polymer dose, PEG coating, and encapsulated anticancer drug. *Biol. Pharm. Bull.* 2013, 36, 889–891.
68. Shiraishi, K.; Yokoyama, M. Polymeric micelles possessing polyethyleneglycol as outer shell and their unique behaviors in accelerated blood clearance phenomenon. *Biol. Pharm. Bull.* 2013, 36, 878–882.
69. Nagao, A.; Abu Lilaa, A. S.; Ishida, T.; Kiwada, H. Abrogation of the accelerated blood clearance phenomenon by SOXL regimen: Promise for clinical application. *Int. J. Pharm.* 2013, 441, 395–401.
70. Nie, Y.; Gunther, M.; Gu, Z.; Wagner, E. Pyridylhydrazone-based PEGylation for pH-reversible lipopolyplex shielding. *Biomaterial* 2011, 32, 858–869.
71. Matsumoto, S.; Christie, R. J.; Nishiyama, N.; Miyata, K.; Ishii, A.; Oba, M.; Koyama, H.; Yamasaki, Y.; Kataoka, K. Environment-responsive block copolymer micelles with a disulfide cross-linked core for enhanced siRNA delivery. *Biomacromolecules* 2009, 10, 119–127.

72. Probst, E. E.; Zrazhenskiv, P.; Bagalkot, V.; Gao, X. Quantum dots as a platform for nanoparticle drug delivery vehicle design. *Adv. Drug. Deliv. Rev.* 2013, 65, 703–718.
73. Probst, J.; Dembski, S.; Milde, M.; Rupp. S. Luminescent nanoparticles and their use for in vitro and in vivo diagnostics. *Expert Rev. Mol. Diagn.* 2012, 12, 49–64.
74. Ho, D.; Sun, X.; Sun, S. Monodisperse magnetic nanoparticles for theranostic applications. *Acc. Chem. Res.* 2011, 44, 875–882.
75. Chen, Y. S.; Hung, Y. C.; Liau, I.; Huang, G. S. Assessment of the in vivo toxicity of gold nanoparticles. *Nanoscale Res. Lett.* 2009, 4, 858–864.
76. Khlebtsov, N. G.; Dykman, L. A. Biodistribution and toxicity of gold nanoparticles. *Nanotechnol. Russia* 2011, 6, 17–42.
77. Fadeel, B.; García-Bennett, A. E. Better safe than sorry: Understanding the toxicological properties of inorganic nanoparticles manufactured for biomedical applications. *Adv. Drug Deliv. Rev.* 2010, 62, 362–374.
78. Colombo, M.; Carregal-Romero, S.; Casula, M. F.; Guriérrez, M.; Morales, P.; Böhm, I. B.; Heverhagen, J. T.; Propseri, D.; Parak, W. J. Biological applications of magnetic nanoparticles. *Chem. Soc. Rev.* 2012, 41, 4306–4334.
79. Mo, S.; Coussios, C.-C.; Sevmour, L.; Carlisle, R. Ultrasound-enhanced drug delivery for cancer. *Expert Opin. Drug. Deliv.* 2012, 9, 1525–1538.

3 Transporter- and Enzyme-Targeted Prodrugs for Improved Oral Drug Delivery

Arik Dahan and Shimon Ben-Shabat

CONTENTS

INTRODUCTION

Prodrugs are bioreversible derivatives of drug molecules designed to overcome pharmaceutical, pharmacokinetic, or pharmacodynamic barriers such as low oral absorption, lack of site-specificity, insufficient chemical stability, poor solubility, toxicity, unacceptable taste/odor, etc. The prodrug approach becomes more and more popular and successful; to date, around 10% of all the world's marketed medications are prodrugs, 20% of all small molecular medicines approved between 2000 and 2008 were prodrugs, and when focusing on 2008 approved drugs, it emerges that over 30% of them were prodrugs (Huttunen et al., 2011; Stella, 2010).

During the past decade, the pharmaceutical sciences have undergone a molecular revolution; no longer relying on empirical fitting based on plasma levels, the modern absorption, distribution, metabolism, and excretion (ADME) research considers molecular/cellular factors, for example, membrane influx/efflux transporters and cellular protein expression and distribution. This molecular revolution had a great impact on the field of drug design and delivery in general and the utilization of the prodrug approach in particular as is highlighted in this chapter.

Increasing the intestinal absorption following oral administration is the most frequent rationale for prodrug design. To improve oral absorption, a classic prodrug approach can be adopted to mask charged/polar moieties and enhance drug lipophilicity and passive diffusion. This may be achieved by various carboxylic acid esters, which release the active carboxylic acid after hydrolysis (Beaumont et al., 2003).

In recent years, the understanding of membrane transporters has promoted a novel "targeted-prodrug" approach utilizing carrier-mediated transport to increase intestinal permeability (Dahan et al., 2012; Han and Amidon, 2000). Certainly, this type of approach requires substantial knowledge of the molecular and function characteristics of these membrane transporters.

Prodrugs must be converted to the active parent drug to exert the therapeutic effect. This activation process is not necessary specific; however, a good understanding of the possible activating enzymes will help the rational design of successful prodrugs. By considering enzyme–substrate specificity, it is possible to overcome poor site-specificity, leading to the desired higher efficacy accompanied by lower toxicity.

In this chapter, we present the concepts of a modern (vs. traditional) biopharmaceutical approach to orally administered prodrugs. We discuss the new opportunities that the continuous advancement in related fields, for example, molecular and computational biology, brings to the field of oral drug delivery via prodrug.

TARGETING TRANSPORTERS IN PRODRUG DESIGN

The classical approach for prodrug design uses the nonspecific strategy of covalently modifying the drug of interest by attaching hydrophilic functionalities (e.g., phosphate) to increase the solubility in the aqueous GI milieu (Amidon et al., 1980; Fleisher et al., 1996; Stella and Nti-Addae, 2007), or lipophilic moieties (e.g., ester) to increase the passive permeability through the GI wall (Bernard, 2009; Ettmayer et al., 2004; Rautio et al., 2008). On the other hand, the molecular revolution enabled more sophisticated strategies in prodrug design to emerge in which promoieties are covalently attached to the molecule of interest to selectively target certain membrane transporters and enzymes. This modern strategy offers a remarkable potential for improving drug bioavailability and selectivity of poorly absorbed drug molecules (Han and Amidon, 2000; Majumdar et al., 2004).

The recent advances in biochemistry and molecular biology have delivered a lot of information on the function and expression of transporters and enzymes. Many transporters are expressed on the intestinal enterocytes that may be selectively targeted. These include the organic anion transporter (OAT) family (Tamai, 2012), the organic cation transporter (OCT) family (Jonker and Schinkel, 2004; Koepsell et al., 2007), the sodium-dependent bile acid transporter (ASBT) family (Balakrishnan and Polli, 2006), the sodium-dependent glucose transporter (SGLT) family (Cao et al., 2006), the monocarboxylate transporter (MCT) family (Tsuji, 1999; Varma et al., 2010), the amino acid transporter PAT1 (Anderson et al., 2004; Thwaites and Anderson, 2011), the amino acid transporter $ATB^{0,+}$ (Ganapathy and Ganapathy, 2005; Hatanaka et al., 2004), the folate transporter (PCFT) (Qiu et al., 2006; Zhao et al., 2011), and the oligopeptide transporter (PEPT1) (Bai and Amidon, 1992; Brandsch et al., 2008; Kikuchi et al., 2009; Lee et al., 1999). These transporters have been extensively characterized and have been shown to play important roles in the absorption of certain nutrients and drugs (Giacomini et al., 2010; Martinez and Amidon, 2002; Mizuno et al., 2003; Shugarts and Benet, 2009). Since significant information is available on the substrate specificity of these transporters, drug moieties could be chemically modified to enhance their oral absorption via targeting intestinal transporters. Of all the intestinal transporters, PEPT1 has captured the greatest attention as a drug transport pathway, mainly due to wide distribution throughout the entire small intestine, broad substrate specificity, and high capacity. PEPT1 is characterized as a high-capacity, low-affinity transporter, predominantly expressed in the small intestine, and accepts dipeptides, tripeptides, and peptidomimetic drugs, such as β-lactam antibiotics and ACE inhibitors (Jappar et al., 2011; Kikuchi et al., 2009). Thus, PEPT1 targeted prodrugs may be a most promising strategy for oral drug delivery.

Zanamivir and oseltamivir are the two FDA-approved neuraminidase inhibitors for the treatment of influenza infection. Oseltamivir (Tamiflu®) is a carboxylic acid ester that may represent a successful example for the "traditional" approach for prodrug design. The very low oral bioavailability (>5%) of oseltamivir carboxylate increased to approximately 80% for oseltamivir in humans (Aoki and Doucette, 2001). While incidences of resistance against oseltamivir have been reported in the literature (Le et al., 2005), there are no such reports with zanamivir to date. However, the polar nature of zanamivir results in very low oral bioavailability (~2%) for this clinically important compound (Cass et al., 1999). A modern prodrug approach was taken in trying to improve zanamivir's absorption following oral administration, targeting PEPT1 for carrier-mediated transport (Varghese Gupta et al., 2011). For this purpose, a series of acyloxy ester prodrugs of zanamivir conjugated with amino acids were synthesized and characterized for chemical stability, membrane transport, and enzymatic activation. In comparison to zanamivir, the L-valyl prodrug of zanamivir showed a threefold higher uptake by PEPT1 overexpressing cells, indicating recognition between the prodrug and the transporter. Subsequent intestinal permeability studies of zanamivir's L-valyl and other amino acid prodrugs compared to the parent drug in Caco-2 transepithelial experiments and in the rat jejunal perfusion model confirmed that this mechanistic targeted prodrug strategy significantly improves the intestinal epithelial cell permeability of zanamivir (Figure 3.1) (Varghese Gupta et al., 2011). Since no oral delivery route of zanamivir currently exists (Miller et al., 2010), despite the high clinical importance of this drug in fighting the common seasonal flu as well as the recent H1N1 global pandemic (Dawood et al., 2009), this work demonstrates that the modern approach for prodrug design has the potential to provide the high oral bioavailability necessary for oral zanamivir therapy and hence to enable new treatment options.

Since amino acid ester prodrugs have been found to be substrates for PEPT1, a variety of amino acid, dipeptide, and tripeptide prodrugs have been investigated for their suitability as substrates for PEPT1. These include the anticancer agent floxuridine (Landowski et al., 2005; Tsume et al., 2011; Tsume et al., 2008); the antiviral agents acyclovir, gancyclovir, and zidovudine (Han et al., 1998; Li et al., 2008); the anticancer agents melphalan (Mittal et al., 2005) and gemcitabine (Song et al., 2005); the antihypotensive agent midodrine (Tsuda et al., 2006); the antiosteoporotic agent alendronate (Ezra et al., 2000), and others. These studies have assured that mono amino acid and dipeptide ester prodrugs generally provide enhanced PEPT1-mediated transport and, as a result, improved oral absorption and bioavailability.

An additional study that successfully utilizes the transporter-mediated absorption approach by targeting PEPT1 was recently published (Gupta, 2013 #113). In this study,

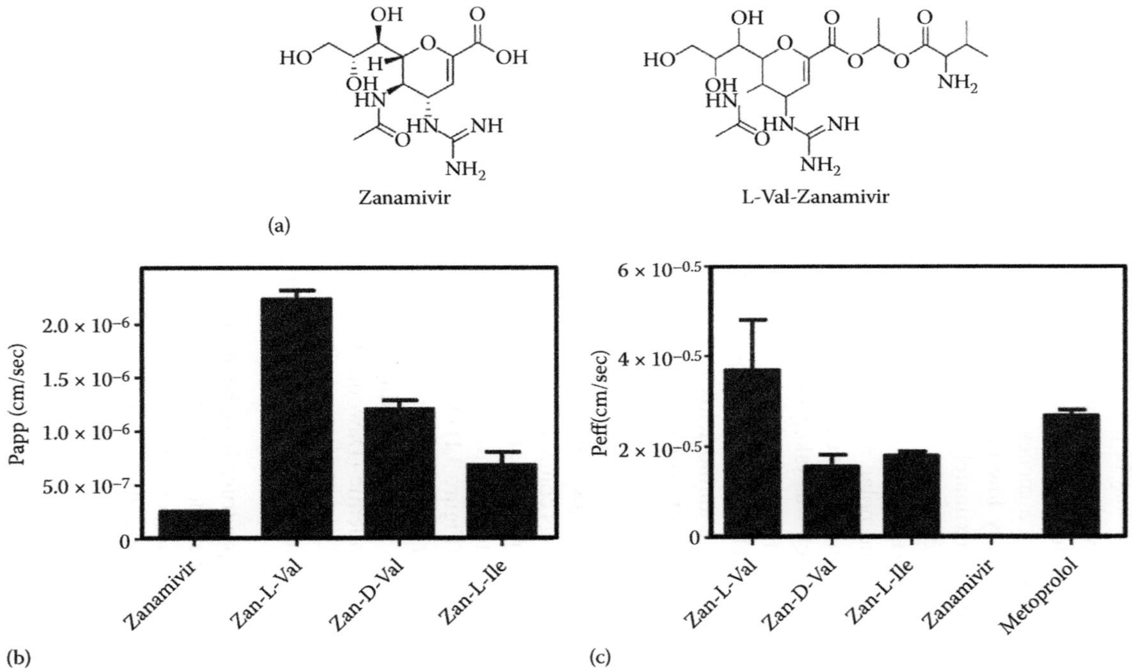

FIGURE 3.1 Molecular structure of zanamivir and its L-valyl prodrug (a), and the permeability of zanamivir and its amino acid prodrug across Caco-2 monolayers (b), and in the single-pass rat jejunal perfusion method (c). (Reproduced from Varghese Gupta, S., Gupta, D., Sun, J., Dahan, A., Tsume, Y., Hilfinger, J., Lee, K.-D., Amidon, G. L., *Molecular Pharmaceutics*, 8, 2358–2367, 2011, with permission.)

the highly active polar antiviral agent, guanidine oseltamivir carboxylate, which represents very low oral bioavailability (4%), was investigated. In order to improve the insufficient oral bioavailability of guanidine oseltamivir, a series of acyloxy(alkyl) ester prodrugs conjugated with amino acids were synthesized and characterized for chemical stability, membrane transport, and enzymatic activation. The intestinal permeability of the amino acid prodrugs were compared with that of the parent drug in Caco-2 cell monolayers and also in the rat jejunal perfusion model, showing a two- to fivefold increase in permeability. The amino acid prodrug showed a 30-fold increase in affinity for PEPT1 compared to the parent drug and a three- to sixfold higher affinity for PEPT1 compared to valacyclovir, a well-known PEPT1 substrate, indicating high recognition between the prodrugs and the transporter. The most promising antiviral derivative for oral delivery was found to be the guanidine oseltamivir carboxylate-I-Val. The systemic oral bioavailability of this compound in mice was found to be 28% under fed conditions and 48% under fasted conditions while the parent drug exhibited bioavailability of only 5% under both fed and fasted state (Figure 3.2) (Gupta, 2013).

Targeting of monocarboxylate transporter type 1 (MCT1) has also been shown to result in enhanced intestinal prodrug/drug absorption. MCT1, a low-affinity, high-capacity transporter that transports unbranched aliphatic monocarboxylates, is widely expressed along the entire intestinal tract (Halestrap and Meredith, 2004). XP13512 is a carbamate prodrug of the GABA analogue gabapentin; since gabapentin suffers from many poor pharmacokinetic properties, including high variability, saturable absorption and lack of dose proportionality, an efficient prodrug may allow significantly better drug-like properties. It has been shown that following oral administration of XP13512 the systemic bioavailability of gabapentin was dramatically increased in preclinical (Cundy et al., 2004a) and clinical (Cundy et al., 2008) studies, including dose proportionality while MCT1 plays a significant role in this improvement (Cundy et al., 2004a; Cundy et al., 2004b).

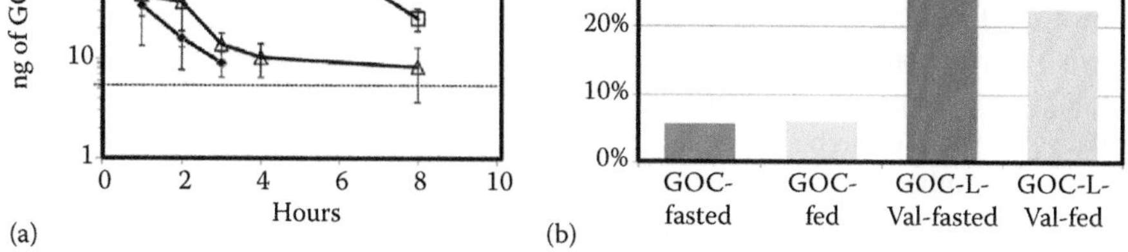

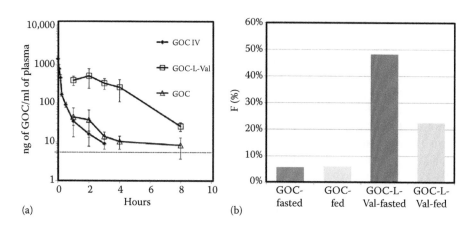

FIGURE 3.2 Plasma levels (a) and systemic oral bioavailability (b) of GOCarb and its L-Valine prodrug following oral administration of 10 mk/kg (n = 5). (Reproduced from Gupta, D., Varghese Gupta, S., Dahan, A., Tsume, Y., Hilfinger, J., Lee, K. D., Amidon, G. L., *Molecular Pharmaceutics*, 10, 512–522, 2013, with permission.)

An additional transporter that was exploited as a potential target for improved absorption of prodrugs is the sodium-dependent bile acid transporter (ASBT) (Balakrishnan and Polli, 2006), and significantly improved absorption of the antiviral agent acyclovir (Tolle-Sander et al., 2004) and the GABA analogue gabapentin (Rais et al., 2011) have been reported. Other transporters have also been targeted as noted above. Overall, this modern approach for oral prodrug design allows a more mechanistic and intelligent strategy to enable increased intestinal absorption of poorly permeable compounds. Since intestinal permeability is, alongside the drug solubility, the most important factor governing drug absorption following oral administration (Amidon et al., 1995; Dahan et al., 2009; Dahan et al., 2010; Lennernas, 1998), the improved permeability achieved by this approach may enhance drug-like properties and "developability" (Lipinski et al., 2001; Sun et al., 2004), thereby allowing new orally administered treatment options.

TARGETING ENZYMES IN PRODRUG DESIGN

After absorption, a subsequent essential step in effective prodrug therapy is the activation (hydrolysis) of the prodrug to the active therapeutic agent. The most important enzymes involved in the bioconversion of ester-based prodrugs include paraoxonase, carboxylesterase, acetylcholinesterase, and cholinesterase (Landowski et al., 2006; Liederer and Borchardt, 2006; Satoh and Hosokawa, 1998). However, in the classical/traditional approach for prodrug design, the activation mechanism was often overlooked, and as long as the parent drug could be regenerated, the activation was considered successful, and the enzymes responsible for this activation did not capture much further attention. As noted above, the activation process is not necessarily specific, yet a good knowledge of the activating enzyme(s) will help to rationally design successful prodrugs. Hence, the identification of enzymes responsible for activating different classes of prodrugs, particularly in humans, can provide important new targets for the design of more effective therapeutic agents.

Valacyclovir is the 5′-valyl ester prodrug of the antiviral drug acyclovir. Valacyclovir increased the oral bioavailability of its parent drug acyclovir by three- to fivefold (Weller et al., 1993). This improved absorption provided by the prodrug has been shown to be attributable to carrier-mediated intestinal transport of the prodrug via hPEPT1 (Balimane et al., 1998; Han et al., 1998). As such, valacyclovir represents a successful example for the modern transporter-targeted prodrug approach. However, the efficiency of valacyclovir as an antiviral drug relies also on the rapid in vivo conversion of valacyclovir to acyclovir. Given the importance of nucleoside analogs in pharmacotherapy, the identification of the activation mechanism(s) of valacyclovir was of high significance. First, it has been shown in several studies that enzymatic (rather than chemical) hydrolysis of valacyclovir is the predominant in vivo activation mechanism in rats, primates, and humans (Burnette and de Miranda, 1994; de Miranda and Burnette, 1994; Soul-Lawton et al., 1995). Moreover, valacyclovir was found to be relatively stable in the GI milieu, accompanied by high susceptibility to intracellular enzymatic hydrolysis (Sinko and Balimane, 1998). Also, Burnette et al. (1995) purified and sequenced several peptide fragments of the major polypeptide from a purified preparation of a putative novel protein from rat liver.

However, in 2003, Kim et al. (2003) succeeded in purifying, identifying, and characterizing the human enzyme that activates valacyclovir to acyclovir, named valacyclovirase, a serine hydrolase containing a catalytic triad S122-H255-D227 (Lai et al., 2008). Further characterization studies have found that valacyclovirase is one of the primary enzymes activating the amino acid ester prodrug with high and specific preference for amino acid esters as substrates that are attributed to the critical residue D123 forming electrostatic interaction with the α-amino group of substrates. Valacyclovirase contains a large leaving group accommodating a groove, which accommodates various leaving groups, including nucleoside analogues as well as simple alcohols, such as methanol, ethanol, and benzyl alcohol (Gupta et al., 2009; Kim et al., 2004a; Kim et al., 2004b; Landowski et al., 2006; Sun et al., 2010b).

As opposed to the traditional low attention the activation step used to receive, it is essentially the unique and one of the most critical processes for a prodrug to exert a therapeutic effect. If the activating enzyme(s) are identified, it will be possible to design prodrugs to target these enzymes, which will significantly increase the chances for the effective production of the active parent drug. Although the amino acid ester prodrug strategy has been applied to many nucleoside analogues and was successful in improving oral absorption by targeting PEPT1, the activation step of these prodrugs was not well studied and was considered to be nonspecific until the identification of valacyclovirase. This was further exploited as is presented hereinafter.

The positively charged (in physiological pH) guanidino functionality is well known for its important biological roles in vivo; many biologically active receptors show affinity for the L-arginine residue attributable to strong electrostatic interaction between the positively charged guanidino group and the negatively charged carboxylate in the active site of the receptor. Hence, when rationally designing an inhibitor, the guanidine functionality is frequently selected to mimic the arginine residue of the endogenous substrate and secure the affinity of the drug to the target (Sun et al., 2011). Guanidino-containing drug molecules include the antidiabetic drug metformin, the H_2-receptor antagonist famotidine, the aminoglycoside antibiotic drug streptomycin, the anticoagulant thrombin inhibitor argatroban, and others. However, guanidino-containing compounds are frequently associated with low oral bioavailability; inherent polarity and positive charge in the gastrointestinal tract make it difficult for them to be orally absorbed by passive diffusion. For instance, while the classical approach for prodrug design was successful in enhancing the oral absorption of oseltamivir carboxylate by making the simple ethyl ester, this strategy failed when applied for its guanidine analogue guanidino oseltamivir carboxylate (Li et al., 1998). Several other attempts to mask the guanidino group by classical prodrugs can be found in the literature with varying degrees of success (Clement et al., 2005; Huttunen et al., 2009; Maryanoff et al., 2006; Saulnier et al., 1994). The modern prodrug approach, targeting PEPT1 for intestinal transport, may be a promising strategy to increase the oral absorption of guanidine-containing molecules.

A unique approach was taken to evaluate the feasibility of this strategy, the double-targeted prodrug approach. In this approach, both transport and activation processes are accounted for at the initial prodrug design stage (Figure 3.3). A series of amino acid esters of a model guanidine-containing compound,

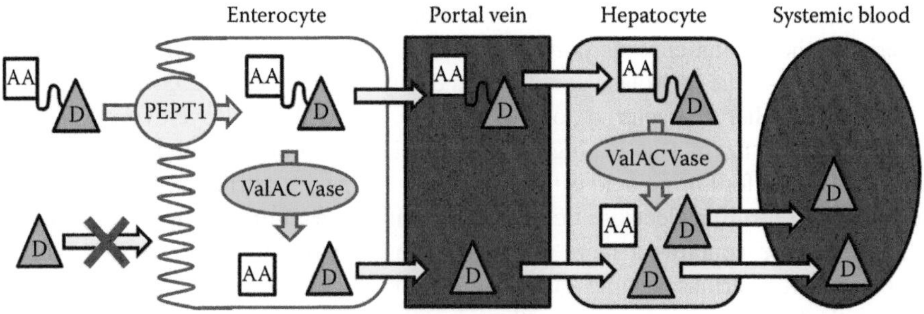

FIGURE 3.3 Illustration of the "double targeted" prodrug approach, accounting for both transport via PEPT1 and activation via valacyclovirase. (Developed by Sun, J., Dahan, A., Amidon, G. L., *Journal of Medicinal Chemistry*, 53, 624–632, 2010a.)

[3-(hydroxymethyl)phenyl]guanidine (3-HPG), was synthesized and evaluated for both transport and activation (Sun et al., 2010a; Sun et al., 2010b). Compared to the parent molecule, the valine and the isoleucine esters exhibited significant increased Caco-2 and rat intestinal permeability that was shown to be mediated by PEPT1 (Figure 3.4). Remarkably, these L-amino acid prodrugs of 3-HPG were shown to be effectively activated by valacyclovirase with K_m values in the range of the positive control valacyclovir, thereby liberating the parent moiety (Sun et al., 2010a). At the same time, the possibility that other enzymes can also contribute to the activation of amino acid ester prodrugs cannot be ruled out. These novel studies, in which both transport and activation processes are taken into consideration at the earliest stages, represent the next step in the modern approach to drug delivery using prodrugs, which may greatly minimize the empirical elements of the development and hence may result in better products with more predictable performance in comparison to the current practice.

In an additional example, we have designed a novel type of prodrugs, substituting the *sn-2* positioned fatty acid of a phospholipid by the nonsteroidal anti-inflammatory drug indomethacin through a linker (Dahan et al., 2007; Dahan et al., 2008; Dahan and Hoffman, 2007; Dvir et al., 2007; Dvir et al., 2006). Physiologically, the *sn-2* positioned fatty acid is cleaved by the enzyme phospholipase A_2 (PLA_2), liberating a free fatty acid and a lysophospholipid as the lipolysis products. The substitution of the *sn-2* positioned fatty acid by a drug moiety was designed to target PLA_2 as the activating enzyme for this class of prodrugs. Although it was reported that PLA_2 strictly requires a fatty acid at the *sn-2* position (Kurz and Scriba, 2000), we have found that, depending on the number of carbons in the linker, PLA_2 was able to recognize and activate the phospholipidic prodrugs of indomethacin; in vitro incubation of the prodrug with the 5-carbon linker with the enzyme showed 60% activation while shorter linkers were significantly less susceptible for activation by PLA_2 (Dahan et al., 2007). Subsequent in vivo investigations in rats revealed that following oral administration there was no absorption of the intact prodrugs; however, the prodrug with the 5-carbon linker was continuously activated by PLA_2 throughout the intestinal tract, resulting in a controlled release profile of the liberated free indomethacin in the systemic circulation (Dahan et al., 2007).

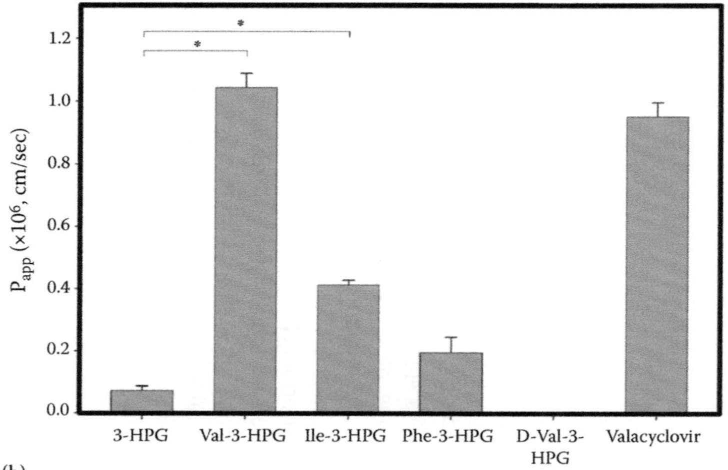

(b)

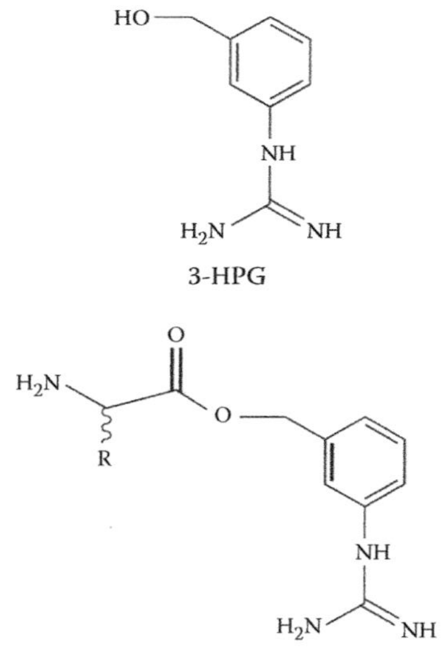

	R
Val-3-HPG	$CH(CH_3)_2$
Ile-3-HPG	$CH(CH_3)CH_2CH_3$

(a)

	K_m (μM)	V_{max} (nmol/min/μg)	k_{cat} (s^{-1})	k_{cat}/K_m ($mM^{-1}\cdot s^{-1}$)
Val-3-HPG (5a)	46 ± 5	321 ± 9	154 ± 4	3370 ± 460
Ile-3-HPG (5b)	9.0 ± 1.2	30 ± 1	14 ± 1	1580 ± 260
Phe-3-HPG (5c)	207 ± 16	718 ± 16	345 ± 8	1660 ± 160
Valacyclovir	68 ± 4	120 ± 2	58 ± 1	850 ± 66

(c)

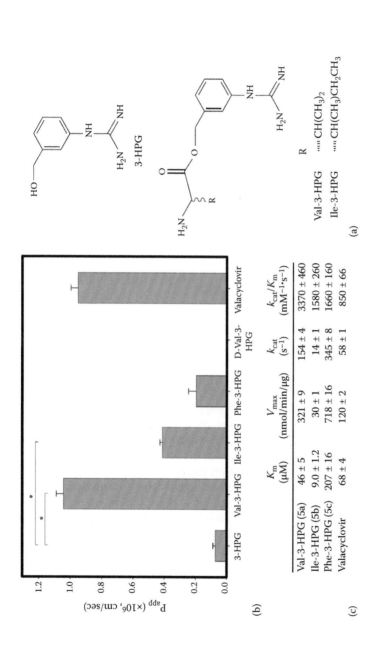

FIGURE 3.4 Molecular structure of zanamivir and its L-valyl prodrug (a), and the permeability of zanamivir and its amino acid prodrug across Caco-2 monolayers (b), and in the single-pass rat jejunal perfusion method (c). (Reproduced from Sun, J., Dahan, A., Amidon, G. L., *Journal of Medicinal Chemistry*, 53, 624–632, with permission.)

This research shows the advantage of rational activating-enzyme targeted design of prodrugs, which minimizes the empirical elements of the activation process and allows better control of the liberation of the free active drug moiety from the intact prodrug.

In an additional interesting study, Sabit et al. were trying to achieve site-specific activation and targeting of human cytomegalovirus (HCMV) protease (Sabit, 2013). The main goal of this study was to develop ganciclovir (GCV) prodrug substrates for a specific HCMV-encoded protease. For that purpose, a series of mono alanine ester prodrugs of ganciclovir with the α-amino group of alanine blocked by different protection groups were synthesized. The esterase activity of the more stable HCMV A143T/A144T protease mutant was evaluated, and it was found that it has esterase activity toward the above specific small ester compounds. An additional group of molecules based on mono amino acid and dipeptide prodrugs of GCV were also synthesized and evaluated for hydrolysis by the A143T/A144T protease mutant and also by caco-2 cell homogenates, human liver microsomes (HLMs), and rat and human plasma. A dipeptide prodrug of ganciclovir, Ac-L-Gln-L-Ala-GCV, was found as a potential selective prodrug candidate. These studies demonstrated that α-amino substituted alanine esters of GCV and dipeptide prodrugs of GCV have potential for HCMV prodrug targeting (Sabit, 2013).

CONCLUSIONS

For many years, the prodrug approach, in general, used to be viewed as a last option strategy—almost an act of desperation after all other possible solutions were exhausted; this is no longer the case. In fact, taking the prodrug approach should be considered very early on in the development process. Indeed, as noted above, the prodrug approach has become more and more popular and successful.

The molecular revolution has significantly changed the pharmaceutical sciences in general and the way we use the prodrug approach in particular. While the classic prodrug approach was focused on altering various physiochemical parameters, for example, lipophilicity and charge state, the modern approach considers molecular/cellular factors, for example, membrane influx/efflux transporters and cellular protein expression and distribution. An a priori mechanistic design that aims to enable absorption by specific transports as well as activation by specific enzymes, may greatly improve the process efficiency and allow for novel oral treatment options. Minimizing the empirical elements by taking the targeted prodrug approach promotes an intelligent and powerful process as the outcomes may be significantly more predictable; knowledge of the prodrug activating enzyme(s) in preclinical animals and their counterpart(s) in humans may improve the translation of preclinical data to clinical trial design, potentially speeding the prodrug development process and lowering its cost. In addition, good knowledge of the transporter(s) and enzyme(s) involved in the absorption and activation may allow the prediction and recognizing potential competition-based drug–drug interactions. A critical aspect that was not covered in this paper is the site-specific targeting potential; a prodrug designed to be activated by a specific enzyme that is overexpressed in the target site may allow the targeting of the free drug to the site of action, resulting in improved efficacy and reduced toxicity.

Overall, in the coming years, more and more information will undoubtedly become available regarding intestinal transporters and potential enzymes that may be exploited for the targeted modern prodrug approach. Hence, the concept of prodrug design can no longer be viewed as merely a chemical modification to solve problems associated with parent compounds. Rather, it opens promising opportunities for precise and efficient drug delivery as well as enhancement of treatment options and therapeutic efficacy. In our opinion, the novel "double targeted" approach presented above, in which both transporters for intestinal permeability and enzymes for activation are accounted for, represents the direction for significant exploitation of the molecular revolution in oral drug delivery via prodrugs. The simultaneous utilization of all three approaches described in this chapter—that is, using the computational approaches for rational design that will allow targeting of a prodrug to a certain transporter for enhanced absorption followed by targeting an enzyme for enhanced/predicted activation—represents a considerably important future direction that will significantly advance the field.

ACKNOWLEDGMENT

This work was supported by the Binational Science Foundation (BSF), Grant No. 2015365.

REFERENCES

Amidon, G. L., Leesman, G. D., Elliott, R. L., 1980. Improving intestinal absorption of water-insoluble compounds: A membrane metabolism strategy. *Journal of Pharmaceutical Sciences* 69, 1363–1368.

Amidon, G. L., Lennernas, H., Shah, V. P., Crison, J. R., 1995. A theoretical basis for a biopharmaceutic drug classification: The correlation of in vitro drug product dissolution and in vivo bioavailability. *Pharmaceutical Research* 12, 413.

Anderson, C. M. H., Grenade, D. S., Boll, M., Foltz, M., Wake, K. A., Kennedy, D. J., Munck, L. K. et al., 2004. H+/amino acid transporter 1 (PAT1) is the imino acid carrier: An intestinal nutrient/drug transporter in human and rat. *Gastroenterology* 127, 1410–1422.

Aoki, F. Y., Doucette, K. E., 2001. Oseltamivir: A clinical and pharmacological perspective. *Expert Opinion on Pharmacotherapy* 2, 1671–1683.

Bai, J. P. F., Amidon, G. L., 1992. Structural specificity of mucosal-cell transport and metabolism of peptide drugs: Implication for oral peptide drug delivery. *Pharmaceutical Research* 9, 969–978.

Balakrishnan, A., Polli, J. E., 2006. Apical sodium dependent bile acid transporter (ASBT, SLC10A2): A potential prodrug target. *Molecular Pharmaceutics* 3, 223–230.

Balimane, P. V., Tamai, I., Guo, A., Nakanishi, T., Kitada, H., Leibach, F. H., Tsuji, A., Sinko, P. J., 1998. Direct evidence for peptide transporter (PepT1)-mediated uptake of a nonpeptide prodrug, valacyclovir. *Biochemical and Biophysical Research Communications* 250, 246–251.

Beaumont, K., Webster, R., Gardner, I., Dack, K., 2003. Design of ester prodrugs to enhance oral absorption of poorly permeable compounds: Challenges to the discovery scientist. *Current Drug Metabolism* 4, 461–485.

Bernard, T., 2009. Prodrugs: Bridging pharmacodynamic/pharmacokinetic gaps. *Current Opinion in Chemical Biology* 13, 338–344.

Brandsch, M., Knütter, I., Bosse-Doenecke, E., 2008. Pharmaceutical and pharmacological importance of peptide transporters. *Journal of Pharmacy and Pharmacology* 60, 543–585.

Burnette, T. C., de Miranda, P., 1994. Metabolic disposition of the acyclovir prodrug valaciclovir in the rat. *Drug Metabolism and Disposition* 22, 60–64.

Burnette, T. C., Harrington, J. A., Reardon, J. E., Merrill, B. M., de Miranda, P., 1995. Purification and characterization of a rat liver enzyme that hydrolyzes valaciclovir, the L-valyl ester prodrug of acyclovir. *Journal of Biological Chemistry* 270, 15827–15831.

Cao, X., Gibbs, S., Fang, L., Miller, H., Landowski, C., Shin, H.-C., Lennernas, H. et al., 2006. Why is it challenging to predict intestinal drug absorption and oral bioavailability in human using rat model. *Pharmaceutical Research* 23, 1675–1686.

Cass, L., Efthymiopoulos, C., Bye, A., 1999. Pharmacokinetics of zanamivir after intravenous, oral, inhaled or intranasal administration to healthy volunteers. *Clinical Pharmacokinetics* 36, 1–11.

Clement, B., Mau, S., Deters, S., Havemeyer, A., 2005. Hepatic, extrahepatic, microsomal, and mitochondrial activation of the N-hydroxylated prodrugs benzamidoxime, guanoxabenz, and Ro 48-3656 ([[1-[(2s)-2-[[4-[(hydroxyamino)iminomethyl]benzoyl]amino]-1-oxopropyl]-4-piperidinyl]oxy]-acetic acid). *Drug Metabolism and Disposition* 33, 1740–1747.

Cundy, K. C., Annamalai, T., Bu, L., De Vera, J., Estrela, J., Luo, W., Shirsat, P. et al., 2004a. XP13512, a novel gabapentin prodrug: II. Improved oral bioavailability, dose proportionality, and colonic absorption compared with gabapentin in rats and monkeys. *Journal of Pharmacology and Experimental Therapeutics* 311, 324–333.

Cundy, K. C., Branch, R., Chernov-Rogan, T., Dias, T., Estrada, T., Hold, K., Koller, K. et al., H., Zerangue, N., Zhou, C. X., Barrett, R. W., Gallop, M. A., 2004b. XP13512, a novel gabapentin prodrug: I. Design, synthesis, enzymatic conversion to gabapentin, and transport by intestinal solute transporters. *Journal of Pharmacology and Experimental Therapeutics* 311, 315–323.

Cundy, K. C., Sastry, S., Luo, W., Zou, J., Moors, T. L., Canafax, D. M., 2008. Clinical pharmacokinetics of XP13512, a novel transported prodrug of gabapentin. *The Journal of Clinical Pharmacology* 48, 1378–1388.

Dahan, A., Duvdevani, R., Dvir, E., Elmann, A., Hoffman, A., 2007. A novel mechanism for oral controlled release of drugs by continuous degradation of a phospholipid prodrug along the intestine: In vivo and in vitro evaluation of an indomethacin–lecithin conjugate. *Journal of Controlled Release* 119, 86–93.

Dahan, A., Duvdevani, R., Shapiro, I., Elmann, A., Finkelstein, E., Hoffman, A., 2008. The oral absorption of phospholipid prodrugs: In vivo and in vitro mechanistic investigation of trafficking of a lecithin-valproic acid conjugate following oral administration. *Journal of Controlled Release* 126, 1–9.

Dahan, A., Hoffman, A., 2007. Mode of administration-dependent brain uptake of indomethacin: Sustained systemic input increases brain influx. *Drug Metabolism and Disposition* 35, 321–324.

Dahan, A., Khamis, M., Agbaria, R., Karaman, R., 2012. Targeted prodrugs in oral drug delivery: The modern molecular biopharmaceutical approach. *Expert Opinion on Drug Delivery* 9, 1001–1013.

Dahan, A., Miller, J. M., Amidon, G. L., 2009. Prediction of solubility and permeability class membership: Provisional BCS classification of the world's top oral drugs. *The AAPS Journal* 11, 740–746.

Dahan, A., Miller, J. M., Hilfinger, J. M., Yamashita, S., Yu, L. X., Lennernas, H., Amidon, G. L., 2010. High-permeability criterion for BCS classification: Segmental/pH dependent permeability considerations. *Molecular Pharmaceutics* 7, 1827–1834.

Dawood, F., Jain, S., Finelli, L., Shaw, M., Lindstrom, S., Garten, R., Gubareva, L., Xu, X., Bridges, C., Uyeki, T., 2009. Emergence of a novel swine-origin influenza A (H1N1) virus in humans. *New England Journal of Medicine* 360, 2605–2615.

de Miranda, P., Burnette, T. C., 1994. Metabolic fate and pharmacokinetics of the acyclovir prodrug valaciclovir in cynomolgus monkeys. *Drug Metabolism and Disposition* 22, 55–59.

Dvir, E., Elman, A., Simmons, D., Shapiro, I., Duvdevani, R., Dahan, A., Hoffman, A., Friedman, J. E., 2007. DP-155, a lecithin derivative of indomethacin, is a novel nonsteroidal antiinflammatory drug for analgesia and Alzheimer's disease therapy. *CNS Drug Reviews* 13, 260–277.

Dvir, E., Friedman, J. E., Lee, J. Y., Koh, J. Y., Younis, F., Raz, S., Shapiro, I. et al., 2006. A novel phospholipid derivative of indomethacin, DP-155, shows superior safety and similar efficacy in reducing brain amyloid β in an Alzheimer's disease model. *Journal of Pharmacology and Experimental Therapeutics* 318, 1248–1256.

Ettmayer, P., Amidon, G. L., Clement, B., Testa, B., 2004. Lessons learned from marketed and investigational prodrugs. *Journal of Medicinal Chemistry* 47, 2393–2404.

Ezra, A., Hoffman, A., Breuer, E., Alferiev, I. S., Mönkkönen, J., El Hanany-Rozen, N., Weiss, G. et al., 2000. A peptide prodrug approach for improving bisphosphonate oral absorption. *Journal of Medicinal Chemistry* 43, 3641–3652.

Fleisher, D., Bong, R., Stewart, B. H., 1996. Improved oral drug delivery: Solubility limitations overcome by the use of prodrugs. *Advanced Drug Delivery Reviews* 19, 115–130.

Ganapathy, M. E., Ganapathy, V., 2005. Amino acid transporter ATB0,+ as a delivery system for drugs and prodrugs. *Current Drug Targets—Immune, Endocrine & Metabolic Disorders* 5, 357–364.

Giacomini, K., Huang, S., Tweedie, D., Benet, L., Brouwer, K., Chu, X., Dahlin, A. et al., 2010. Membrane transporters in drug development. *Nature Reviews Drug Discovery* 9, 215–236.

Gupta, D., Gupta, S. V., Lee, K.-D., Amidon, G. L., 2009. Chemical and enzymatic stability of amino acid prodrugs containing methoxy, ethoxy and propylene glycol linkers. *Molecular Pharmaceutics* 6, 1604–1611.

Gupta, D., Varghese Gupta, S., Dahan, A., Tsume,Y., Hilfinger, J., Lee, K.-D., Amidon, G. L., 2013. Increasing oral absorption of polar neuraminidase inhibitors: A prodrug transporter approach applied to oseltamivir analogue. *Molecular Pharmaceutics* 10, 512–522.

Halestrap, A., Meredith, D., 2004. The SLC16 gene family—From monocarboxylate transporters (MCTs) to aromatic amino acid transporters and beyond. *Pflügers Archiv European Journal of Physiology* 447, 619–628.

Han, H.-K., de Vrueh, R. L. A., Rhie, J. K., Covitz, K.-M. Y., Smith, P. L., Lee, C.-P., Oh, D.-M., Sadee, W., Amidon, G. L., 1998. 5′-Amino acid Esters of antiviral nucleosides, acyclovir, and AZT are absorbed by the Intestinal PEPT1 peptide transporter. *Pharmaceutical Research* 15, 1154–1159.

Han, H. K., Amidon, G. L., 2000. Targeted prodrug design to optimize drug delivery. *AAPS PharmSci* 2, E6.

Hatanaka, T., Haramura, M., Fei, Y.-J., Miyauchi, S., Bridges, C. C., Ganapathy, P. S., Smith, S. B., Ganapathy, V., Ganapathy, M. E., 2004. Transport of amino acid-based prodrugs by the Na+- and Cl-- coupled amino acid transporter ATB0,+ and expression of the transporter in tissues amenable for drug delivery. *Journal of Pharmacology and Experimental Therapeutics* 308, 1138–1147.

Huttunen, K. M., Mannila, A., Laine, K., Kemppainen, E., Leppanen, J., Vepsalainen, J., Jarvinen, T., Rautio, J., 2009. The first bioreversible prodrug of metformin with improved lipophilicity and enhanced intestinal absorption. *Journal of Medicinal Chemistry* 52, 4142–4148.

Huttunen, K. M., Raunio, H., Rautio, J., 2011. Prodrugs—From serendipity to rational design. *Pharmacological Reviews* 63, 750–771.

Jappar, D., Hu, Y., Smith, D. E., 2011. Effect of dose escalation on the in vivo oral absorption and disposition of glycylsarcosine in wild type and pept1 knockout mice. *Drug Metabolism and Disposition* 39, 2250–2257.

Jonker, J. W., Schinkel, A. H., 2004. Pharmacological and physiological functions of the polyspecific organic cation transporters: OCT1, 2, and 3 (SLC22A1-3). *Journal of Pharmacology and Experimental Therapeutics* 308, 2–9.

Kikuchi, A., Tomoyasu, T., Tanaka, M., Kanamitsu, K., Sasabe, H., Maeda, T., Odomi, M., Tamai, I., 2009. Peptide derivation of poorly absorbable drug allows intestinal absorption via peptide transporter. *Journal of Pharmaceutical Sciences* 98, 1775–1787.

Kim, I., Chu, X.-Y., Kim, S., Provoda, C. J., Lee, K.-D., Amidon, G. L., 2003. Identification of a human valacyclovirase. *Journal of Biological Chemistry* 278, 25348–25356.

Kim, I., Crippen, G. M., Amidon, G. L., 2004a. Structure and specificity of a human valacyclovir activating enzyme: A homology model of BPHL. *Molecular Pharmaceutics* 1, 434–446.

Kim, I., Song, X., Vig, B. S., Mittal, S., Shin, H.-C., Lorenzi, P. J., Amidon, G. L., 2004b. A novel nucleoside prodrug-activating enzyme: Substrate specificity of biphenyl hydrolase-like protein. *Molecular Pharmaceutics* 1, 117–127.

Koepsell, H., Lips, K., Volk, C., 2007. Polyspecific organic cation transporters: Structure, function, physiological roles, and biopharmaceutical implications. *Pharmaceutical Research* 24, 1227–1251.

Kurz, M., Scriba, G. K. E., 2000. Drug–phospholipid conjugates as potential prodrugs: Synthesis, characterization, and degradation by pancreatic phospholipase A2. *Chemistry and Physics of Lipids* 107, 143–157.

Lai, L., Xu, Z., Zhou, J., Lee, K.-D., Amidon, G. L., 2008. Molecular basis of prodrug activation by human valacyclovirase, an α-amino acid ester hydrolase. *Journal of Biological Chemistry* 283, 9318–9327.

Landowski, C. P., Lorenzi, P. L., Song, X., Amidon, G. L., 2006. Nucleoside ester prodrug substrate specificity of liver carboxylesterase. *Journal of Pharmacology and Experimental Therapeutics* 316, 572–580.

Landowski, C. P., Vig, B. S., Song, X., Amidon, G. L., 2005. Targeted delivery to PEPT1-overexpressing cells: Acidic, basic, and secondary floxuridine amino acid ester prodrugs. *Molecular Cancer Therapeutics* 4, 659–667.

Le, Q. M., Kiso, M., Someya, K., Sakai, Y. T., Nguyen, T. H., Nguyen, K. H. L., Pham, N. D. et al., Avian flu: Isolation of drug-resistant H5N1 virus. *Nature* 437, 1108.

Lee, V. H. L., Chu, C., Mahlin, E. D., Basu, S. K., Ann, D. K., Bolger, M. B., Haworth, I. S. et al., 1999. Biopharmaceutics of transmucosal peptide and protein drug administration: Role of transport mechanisms with a focus on the involvement of PepT1. *Journal of Controlled Release* 62, 129–140.

Lennernas, H., 1998. Human intestinal permeability. *Journal of Pharmaceutical Sciences* 87, 403–410.

Li, F., Maag, H., Alfredson, T., 2008. Prodrugs of nucleoside analogues for improved oral absorption and tissue targeting. *Journal of Pharmaceutical Sciences* 97, 1109–1134.

Li, W., Escarpe, P. A., Eisenberg, E. J., Cundy, K. C., Sweet, C., Jakeman, K. J., Merson, J. et al., 1998. Identification of GS 4104 as an orally bioavailable prodrug of the influenza virus neuraminidase inhibitor GS 4071. *Antimicrobial Agents and Chemotherapy* 42, 647–653.

Liederer, B. M., Borchardt, R. T., 2006. Enzymes involved in the bioconversion of ester-based prodrugs. *Journal of Pharmaceutical Sciences* 95, 1177–1195.

Lipinski, C. A., Lombardo, F., Dominy, B. W., Feeney, P. J., 2001. Experimental and computational approaches to estimate solubility and permeability in drug discovery and development settings. *Advanced Drug Delivery Reviews* 46, 3–26.

Majumdar, S., Duvvuri, S., Mitra, A. K., 2004. Membrane transporter/receptor-targeted prodrug design: Strategies for human and veterinary drug development. *Advanced Drug Delivery Reviews* 56, 1437–1452.

Martinez, M. N., Amidon, G. L., 2002. A mechanistic approach to understanding the factors affecting drug absorption: A review of fundamentals. *Journal of Clinical Pharmacology* 42, 620–643.

Maryanoff, B. E., McComsey, D. F., Costanzo, M. J., Yabut, S. C., Lu, T., Player, M. R., Giardino, E. C., Damiano, B. P., 2006. Exploration of potential prodrugs of RWJ-445167, an oxyguanidine-based dual inhibitor of thrombin and factor Xa. *Chemical Biology & Drug Design* 68, 29–36.

Miller, J. M., Dahan, A., Gupta, D., Varghese, S., Amidon, G. L., 2010. Enabling the intestinal absorption of highly polar antiviral agents: Ion-pair facilitated membrane permeation of zanamivir heptyl ester and guanidino oseltamivir. *Molecular Pharmaceutics* 7, 1223–1234.

Mittal, S., Song, X., Vig, B. S., Landowski, C. P., Kim, I., Hilfinger, J. M., Amidon, G. L., 2005. Prolidase, a potential enzyme target for melanoma: Design of proline-containing dipeptide-like prodrugs. *Molecular Pharmaceutics* 2, 37–46.

Mizuno, N., Niwa, T., Yotsumoto, Y., Sugiyama, Y., 2003. Impact of drug transporter studies on drug discovery and development. *Pharmacological Reviews* 55, 425–461.

Qiu, A., Jansen, M., Sakaris, A., Min, S. H., Chattopadhyay, S., Tsai, E., Sandoval, C., Zhao, R., Akabas, M. H., Goldman, I. D., 2006. Identification of an intestinal folate transporter and the molecular basis for hereditary folate malabsorption. *Cell* 127, 917–928.

Rais, R., Fletcher, S., Polli, J. E., 2011. Synthesis and in vitro evaluation of gabapentin prodrugs that target the human apical sodium-dependent bile acid transporter (hASBT). *Journal of Pharmaceutical Sciences* 100, 1184–1195.

Rautio, J., Kumpulainen, H., Heimbach, T., Oliyai, R., Oh, D., Jarvinen, T., Savolainen, J., 2008. Prodrugs: Design and clinical applications. *Nature Reviews Drug Discovery* 7, 255–270.

Sabit, H., Dahan, A., Sun, J., Provoda, C.J., Lee, K.-D., Hilfinger, J.H., Amidon, G.L., 2013. Cytomegalovirus protease targeted prodrug development. *Molecular Pharmaceutics* 10, 1417–1424.

Satoh, T., Hosokawa, M., 1998. The mammalian carboxylesterases: From molecules to functions. *Annual Review of Pharmacology and Toxicology* 38, 257–288.

Saulnier, M. G., Frennesson, D. B., Deshpande, M. S., Hansel, S. B., Vyas, D. M., 1994. An efficient method for the synthesis of guanidino prodrugs. *Bioorganic & Medicinal Chemistry Letters* 4, 1985–1990.

Shugarts, S., Benet, L., 2009. The role of transporters in the pharmacokinetics of orally administered drugs. *Pharmaceutical Research* 26, 2039–2054.

Sinko, P. J., Balimane, P. V., 1998. Carrier-mediated intestinal absorption of valacyclovir, the L-valyl ester prodrug of acyclovir. 1. Interactions with peptides, organic anions and organic cations in rats. *Biopharmaceutics & Drug Disposition* 19, 209–217.

Song, X., Lorenzi, P. L., Landowski, C. P., Vig, B. S., Hilfinger, J. M., Amidon, G. L., 2005. Amino acid ester prodrugs of the anticancer agent gemcitabine: Synthesis, bioconversion, metabolic bioevasion, and hPEPT1-mediated transport. *Molecular Pharmaceutics* 2, 157–167.

Soul-Lawton, J., Seaber, E., On, N., Wootton, R., Rolan, P., Posner, J., 1995. Absolute bioavailability and metabolic disposition of valaciclovir, the L-valyl ester of acyclovir, following oral administration to humans. *Antimicrobial Agents and Chemotherapy* 39, 2759–2764.

Stella, V. J., 2010. Prodrugs: Some thoughts and current issues. *Journal of Pharmaceutical Sciences* 99, 4755–4765.

Stella, V. J., Nti-Addae, K. W., 2007. Prodrug strategies to overcome poor water solubility. *Advanced Drug Delivery Reviews* 59, 677–694.

Sun, D., Yu, L., Hussain, M., Wall, D., Smith, R., Amidon, G., 2004. In vitro testing of drug absorption for drug 'developability' assessment: Forming an interface between in vitro preclinical data and clinical outcome. *Current opinion in Drug Discovery and Development* 7, 75–85.

Sun, J., Dahan, A., Amidon, G. L., 2010a. Enhancing the intestinal absorption of molecules containing the polar guanidino functionality: A double-targeted prodrug approach. *Journal of Medicinal Chemistry* 53, 624–632.

Sun, J., Dahan, A., Walls, Z. F., Lai, L., Lee, K.-D., Amidon, G. L., 2010b. Specificity of a prodrug-activating enzyme hVACVase: The leaving group effect. *Molecular Pharmaceutics* 7, 2362–2368.

Sun, J., Miller, J. M., Beig, A., Rozen, L., Amidon, G. L., Dahan, A., 2011. Mechanistic enhancement of the intestinal absorption of drugs containing the polar guanidino functionality. *Expert Opinion on Drug Metabolism & Toxicology* 7, 313–323.

Tamai, I., 2012. Oral drug delivery utilizing intestinal OATP transporters. *Advanced Drug Delivery Reviews*, in press.

Thwaites, D. T., Anderson, C. M. H., 2011. The SLC36 family of proton-coupled amino acid transporters and their potential role in drug transport. *British Journal of Pharmacology* 164, 1802–1816.

Tolle-Sander, S., Lentz, K. A., Maeda, D. Y., Coop, A., Polli, J. E., 2004. Increased acyclovir oral bioavailability via a bile acid conjugate. *Molecular Pharmaceutics* 1, 40–48.

Tsuda, M., Terada, T., Irie, M., Katsura, T., Niida, A., Tomita, K., Fujii, N., Inui, K.-I., 2006. Transport characteristics of a novel peptide transporter 1 substrate, antihypotensive drug midodrine, and its amino acid derivatives. *Journal of Pharmacology and Experimental Therapeutics* 318, 455–460.

Tsuji, A., 1999. Tissue selective drug delivery utilizing carrier-mediated transport systems. *Journal of Controlled Release* 62, 239–244.

Tsume, Y., Hilfinger, J., Amidon, G., 2011. Potential of amino acid/dipeptide monoester prodrugs of floxuridine in facilitating enhanced delivery of active drug to interior sites of tumors: A two-tier monolayer in vitro study. *Pharmaceutical Research* 28, 2575–2588.

Tsume, Y., Hilfinger, J. M., Amidon, G. L., 2008. Enhanced cancer cell growth inhibition by dipeptide prodrugs of floxuridine: Increased transporter affinity and metabolic stability. *Molecular Pharmaceutics* 5, 717–727.

Varghese Gupta, S., Gupta, D., Sun, J., Dahan, A., Tsume, Y., Hilfinger, J., Lee, K.-D., Amidon, G. L., 2011. Enhancing the intestinal membrane permeability of zanamivir: A carrier mediated prodrug approach. *Molecular Pharmaceutics* 8, 2358–2367.

Varma, M., Ambler, C., Ullah, M., Rotter, C., Sun, H., Litchfield, J., Fenner, K., El-Kattan, A., 2010. Targeting intestinal transporters for optimizing oral drug absorption. *Current Drug Metabolism* 11, 730–742.

Weller, S., Blum, M., Doucette, M., Burnette, T., Cederberg, D., de Miranda, P., Smiley, M., 1993. Pharmacokinetics of the acyclovir pro-drug valaciclovir after escalating single- and multiple-dose administration to normal volunteers. *Clinical Pharmacology and Therapeutics* 54, 595–605.

Zhao, R., Diop-Bove, N., Visentin, M., Goldman, I. D., 2011. Mechanisms of membrane transport of folates into cells and across epithelia. *Annual Review of Nutrition* 31, 177–201.

4 Gastroretentive Delivery
Physicochemical, Biopharmaceutical, Technological, and Regulatory Considerations

Yuvraj Singh, Vivek K. Pawar, Mohini Chaurasia, and Manish K. Chourasia

CONTENTS

INTRODUCTION

Oral route has turned out to be the single most effective way of conveying medicaments since inception of drug delivery due to variety of reasons, even if we exclude the supreme convenience it offers to a patient undergoing treatment (after all, nothing seems easier than taking a tablet and gulping it down with a glass of water). Nonetheless, oral drug delivery sometimes becomes unmanageable due to complex physiology of gastrointestinal tract (GIT) [1]. Add to it the occasional multiple dosage regimen essential for dispensing an active ingredient in therapeutic concentrations, and we see that modest concept of oral drug delivery begins losing its simplistic efficiency. Retrospective analysis reveals majority of drugs in use today that are administered through oral route are of a weakly basic nature, probably due to small intestine being the major absorptive site, which is attributable to its massively enhanced surface area. The explanation offered for this historic trend has farfetched consequences as it makes it rudimentary for mainstream drugs (unless other absorptive sites are proposed) intended to be given through the oral route to be available as a molecular dispersion in and around the vicinity of small intestine. This implies that any sporadic events leading to delay or sometimes even failure of drug release from oral dosage form around intestine may cause loss of therapeutic action. Oral sustained drug delivery system (OSDDS) was subsequently developed as a promising alternative drug delivery system due to several advantages offered, including improved bioavailability, higher patient compliance, and reduced adverse effects and toxicity. However, drug absorption form GIT can still be variable and unsatisfactory among different individuals, which ultimately compromises overall efficiency of OSDDS [2].

Variability in performance of OSDDS in maximum circumstances is precipitated by unpredictable gastric retention time (GRT), which does not allow OSDDS to stay at the absorption site until complete release of its drug content; with the process reported as premature gastric emptying of OSDDS. Bioavailability of pharmaceutical dosage forms is considerably affected by unpredictable GRT [3]. Short GRT contributes to incomplete absorption of the released drug from OSDDS, which ultimately leads to decreased efficacy. The fed and fasted states of stomach affect the GRT and hence exert direct influence on bioavailability of OSDDS [4].

To overcome these drawbacks, scientists have come up with an elegant solution in the form of gastroretentive drug delivery systems (GRDDS), which can meliorate the performance pitfalls of OSDDS. GRDDS enables OSDDS to remain in gastric region

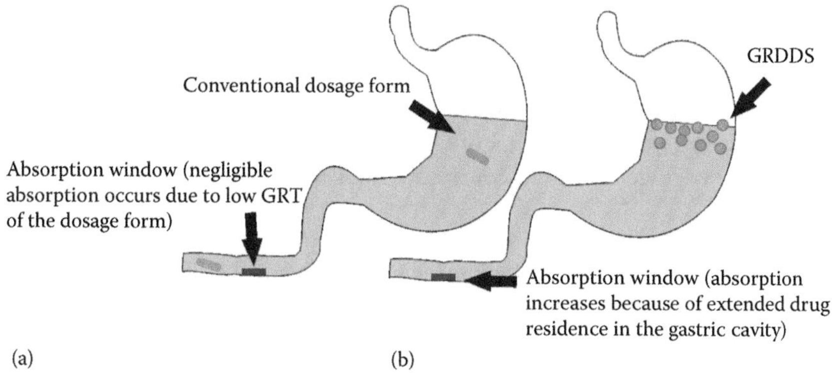

FIGURE 4.1 (a) Absorption criteria from a conventional drug delivery system; often dosage forms prematurely evacuate from the stomach due to unpredictable gastric motility, which can curtail amount of drug released at preferred absorption sites, reducing potential bioavailability of candidate drug (b). GRDDS, owing to several mechanisms, tend to affix/prolong GRT due to which drug is released in the gastric cavity for longer periods, raising probability of absorption through appropriate window.

until complete release of drug takes place. An optimum GRDDS can be defined as "a system which is retained in stomach for a sufficient time interval against all physiological barriers, releasing active moiety in a controlled manner, and finally metabolized in the body" [5]. It is imperative to note that formulating a GRDDS does not restrict drug absorption to stomach only. GRDDS technologically ensures that dosage form stays in stomach for an extended period of time so that a drug released in the stomach is distributed among gastric fluids and moves along with gastric flux, getting absorbed at locations where it is most suitable (including the stomach for certain drugs) ruling out any hasty exit or avoidance of absorptive sites. Several GRDDS have been developed in last two decades to prolong GRT; the main aim being focused on improving performance of OSDDS along with optimizing therapy so as to attain significant patient compliance [6–8]. Figure 4.1 shows absorption pattern of a drug candidate in case of conventional systems and GRDDS after oral administration.

Apart from improving efficacy of OSDDS, there are several other reasons as well, which call for an increase in GRT of a drug delivery systems viz. drugs acting locally in the gastric cavity like amoxicillin for *H. pylori* infection [9], drugs that are poorly soluble and unstable at alkaline pH (ranitidine and captopril) [10,11], and candidates that are primarily absorbed from stomach or have a narrow absorption window [12].

GIT PHYSIOLOGY

The GIT on average is a 9 meter long tube that starts from the mouth and ends at the anus running throughout the body. The GIT is not a uniform entity. Its biologic construction varies immensely. The pH of luminal fluid circulating through GIT spans from a very acidic 1 in the stomach to an alkaline pH of 8 in the distal portion of the ileum and colon. Scatter of membrane transporters, type of epithelial cells, absorption characteristics, and distribution of microbial flora is different in each portion of GIT. This correspondingly leads to specified functions particular to that portion only; important facets of GIT are expanded here to obtain an idea of roles these play in determining course of OSDDS and GRDDS once inside the body.

Anatomically, as in Figure 4.2, GIT consists of esophagus, stomach, small intestine (consisting of the duodenum, jejunum, and ileum), and large intestine (consisting of the cecum, appendix, colon, and rectum). The stomach is located in left upper division of abdominal cavity straightaway beneath the diaphragm. Size of the stomach varies according to its fed or fasted condition, usually 1500 ml following a meal and 25–50 ml after gastric emptying. Structurally, it can be differentiated into three parts, namely the fundus, body, and antrum (or pylorus). Stomach secretes protein-processing enzymes, such as pepsin and hydrochloric acid, which are partly responsible for providing a stern defense against ingested microbes and partly for breaking down and dissolving food. Food is ground down by powerful contractions of the stomach wall, termed peristalsis, which results in conversion of food into chime, a thick slimy gruel. Fundus and body regions

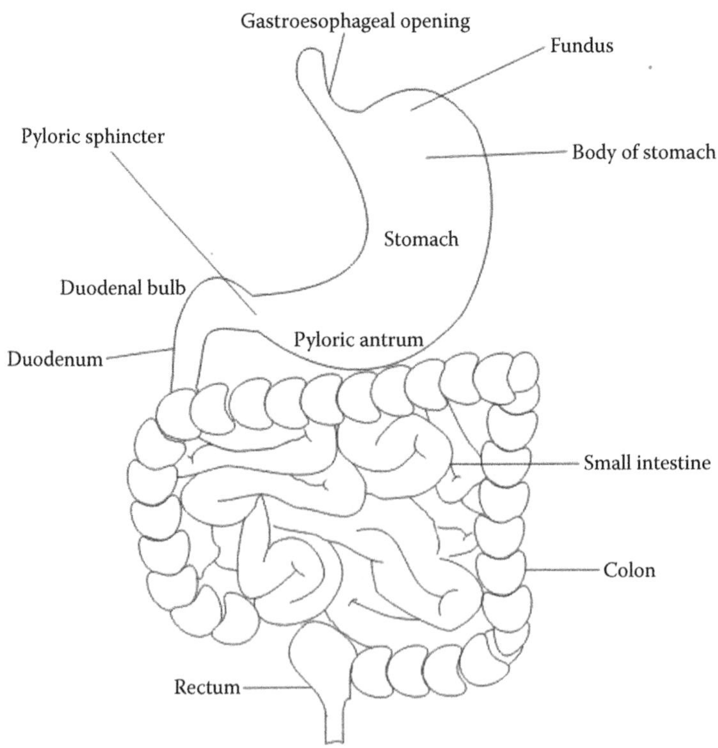

FIGURE 4.2 Anatomy of the human digestive system.

(the proximal stomach) act as a reservoir for ingested materials whereas the antrum or distal region performs the mixing and churning with chime to reduce size of food particles and act as a pump to achieve gastric emptying. Pylorus is bound by a tiny pyloric sphincter, which is a portal into duodenum and further lying small intestine. Size of this sphincter varies in direct correlation to fed or fasted state of the stomach. The pylorus acts as a screen ensuring that contents of stomach do not move into small intestine before they have attained a very minute dimension smaller than the pyloric cutoff of around 10 mm. In fasted state, pylorus is relaxed, having a diameter of approximately 15 mm. The pylorus opens into duodenum, which is first part of the small intestine. Duodenum is responsible for chemical breakdown of food substances. It is also a secretory site for cholecystokinin, pepsin, and mucin. Many drugs, including β adrenergic blockers, such as propranolol and metoprolol [13], are preferentially absorbed from this site. The jejunum and small intestine directly follow the duodenum and serve as principal site of nutrient absorption. Pharmaceutically speaking, the ileum is largest site of drug absorption in GIT. Folds offered by villi on which several microvilli are themselves folded upon amplify the available surface area many hundredfold in comparison to stomach even when it is bloated to its full capacity. Majority of absorptive and efflux protein transporters line up in/or between the enterocytes, which make up more than 99% of the ileal epithelial cell lining. It also localizes the microfold cell, M-cells found in *payer patches*; these subserve special absorptive characteristics not found in other cells. It thus becomes easy to realize potential of small intestine in determining bioavailability of drugs [14].

Ileum terminates into the ileo-cecal valve, which, like the pylorus, is a restrictive junction and prevents regurgitation or movement of food from distal to proximal direction. Colon or large intestine is the terminal portion of GIT and is the site of water reabsorption. Its epithelial lining is different from that of previous sections, and it docks undigested solid content until it is excreted. The innocuous and conducive environment existing in large intestine harbors a variety of microbiota, which ferment food content in a symbiotic manner, yielding minor nutrients. The flora offers opportunities for targeted delivery by carrying out enzymatic reactions exclusive to the colon. Sulfasalazine immediately comes to mind as a prodrug, which yields 5-aminosalicylic acid due to action of azo-reductase generated by microflora. Colon targeting is exploited in treatment of local infections, such as Crohn's disease, colon cancer, and amoebiasis. Table 4.1 elaborates anatomical and physiological features of human GIT along with absorptive pathways for drugs and nutrients.

Importance of diving into relevant anatomy and physiology of GIT can only be realized by laying a cursory introspection in concept of gastric emptying and GRT. The rate of gastric emptying and GRT are two faces of the same coin. They convey a similar idea. GRT, as discussed previously, expresses duration of time for which a dosage form lies in the stomach before being expelled to the ileal portion whereas rate of gastric emptying captures the notion of speed with which the emptying process takes place. The transit time of content present in GIT is more or less fixed in ileum (3–4 hours) and is rather short for a drug to be absorbed substantially if it happens to be present in an aggregated

TABLE 4.1
List of Anatomical Sections of the Human GIT along with Their Physiological Characteristics

Anatomical Section	Average Length of the Section (cm)	Mechanism of Drug Absorption	pH	Food Transit Time (h)
Oral cavity	14–20	Through passive diffusion	5.4–6.8	0.1–0.3
Esophagus	26	–	5–6	Very short
Stomach	22	Through passive diffusion	1.2–3.5	0.3–4.0
Duodenum	26	Through passive diffusion, active transport, pinocytosis, convective transport, facilitated transport	4.6–6.0	1–2
Jejunum	300	Through passive diffusion, pinocytosis, active transport	6.3–7.3	–
Ileum	300	Through passive diffusion, pinocytosis, convective transport, active transport, facilitated transport, ion pair	7.6	1–8
Cecum	8–30	Through passive diffusion, pinocytosis convective transport, active transport	7.5–8.0	Short
Colon	150	Through passive diffusion	7.9–8.0	4–22
Rectum	14–18	Through passive diffusion, pinocytosis convective transport	7.5–8.0	Variable

state or an undispersed form. Translocation in the colon can take up to 24 hours, but its relevance with respect to drug absorption is limited. GRT thus becomes a very prominent factor in absorption of drugs. An extended GRT for a conventional drug (not undergoing any special absorptive processes) ensures that the drug reaches its preeminent absorptive site in a physical form that would undergo absorption without much hindrance. The GRT of a human is highly variable even when same drug is under consideration. Stomach undergoes nonperiodic, frequent peristaltic contractions, which are themselves initiated by a variety of external and internal stimuli, creating a very complex and unpredictable pattern of gastric emptying.

Configuration of gastrointestinal transit and emptying depends considerably on whether the patient is in a fasted or fed state. Fed and fasted states of stomach affect bioavailability of orally administered drugs due to inconsistency of gastrointestinal motility and secretions. Fasted state is characterized by a series of interdigestive electrical events and cycles that propogate through the stomach and intestine. This interdigestive series is frequently termed the *interdigestive myoelectric cycle* or migrating motor complex (MMC) and is composed of four consecutive phases: basal (Phase I), preburst (Phase II), burst (Phase III), and Phase IV intervals [15].

Phase I lasts for 45 to 60 minutes and is a quiescent period with very rare contractions. Phase II continues further for 30 to 45 minutes with generation of sporadic action potential and contractions. Intensity and frequency of contractions increase gradually as Phase II progresses. In terms of magnitude, the biggest contractions are those attained in Phase III. Phase II also marks the time period in which secretion of bile begins. The fluid content of food ingested also begins to be discharged into portions distal to its current location. Mucus and particle discharge (derived from food taken) might also occur during latter periods of Phase II. Phase III (burst phase) lasts for 5 to 15 minutes. In this, four to five intense and regular contractions per minute occur for a short period due to a housekeeper wave, which sweeps out all undigested material from stomach to the small intestine. There seems to be some sort of synchronization in propulsion of Phase III; a new housekeeper wave arises at duodenum as the other one is dying down at terminal junction of ileum. Mucus secretion and particle discharge continues during Phase III. Phase IV follows for 0 to 5 minutes and happens in between Phases III and I and acts as a transition phase between the first and the fourth phases. MMC sometimes moves directly from Phase III to Phase I, bypassing Phase IV. As OSDDS can be administered in any phase of MMC, the kinetics of gastric emptying become highly variable.

Consider an example of a conventional sustained-release tablet expected to dissolve arbitrarily within 4 hours so as to attain a duration of action of 6 hours. If, in any instance, the dosage form is administered in a fasted state (remember, the GIT at this point has an expanded pyloric sphincter), coinciding with the advent of housekeeper wave; one can anticipate it to be rapidly emptied into small intestine within 30 minutes of administration. This is followed by a fixed transit period of 3 hours through ileum, which means there is a huge likelihood that dosage form would be evicted from its primary absorption site even before it has released its entire drug content, leading to loss of therapy and failure of dosage form. Major absorptive portion of intestine for many drugs, for example, ranitidine [16] and metformin [17], is the proximal region [18] of the small intestine; however in most instances of oral delivery an OSDDS usually travels beyond this major absorptive window before undergoing sufficient disaggregation, and the drug carried by it remains unabsorbed despite best intentions of the formulation. This is just one random scenario explained in brief. Multiply the countless different permutations that a person might subject himself or herself to before taking a dosage form and the role played by fluctuating GRT in shortcomings of OSDDS and the thrust of formulation scientists in generating reliable GRDDS becomes very apparent.

In fed state, MMC is substituted by irregular contractions, which have the effect of mixing intestinal contents and propelling intestinal flow toward colon in short intervals. The fed state is composed of 5–10 minutes of motor activity, which occurs after ingestion of a meal and remains until gastric emptying is completed. Time period of fed activity depends upon the amount of food taken, which usually persists for 2–6 hours and sometimes for 3–4 hours with phasic contractions similar to Phase II of MMC.

Unless absorption of a drug candidate is very slow, gastric emptying is expected to be a rate-determining step in absorption of drugs irrespective of their chemical nature, whether they are weak acids, weak bases, or neutral compounds. Gastric emptying justifies much of the observed variation in drug absorption. Interestingly, gastric emptying is influenced by many factors, such as emotional state, pain, posture, autonomic and hormonal activity, food, the volume, pH, composition, viscosity and temperature of the contents, surface active agents, and bile salts [19]. Gastric emptying of nondisintegrating solids is significant enough to consider their incorporation in biopharmaceutical testing of GRDDS. Different factors that affect GRT are summarized in Table 4.2 [20].

Increasing GRT has an overall positive effect on bioavailability of many drugs. This, however, does not always hold true as a reduction in bioavailability is possible if the GRT is extended in case of certain drugs. A clinically relevant illustration

TABLE 4.2
Factors Affecting Gastric Emptying

Factor	Comment/Remark
	Dosage Form–Related Factors
Size of the dosage form	Dosage forms having size larger than the valve of the pyloric sphincter can be retained in the gastric cavity.
Shape of dosage form	Ring- and tetrahedron-shaped dosage forms have longer GRT.
Density of the dosage form	A dosage form can be retained in the gastric cavity if it has lower or higher density than gastric fluid.
	Food-Related Factors
Fed and fasted state	GIT motility is high under the fasted state in comparison to the fed state, so any dosage formm if administered under the fasted state, can rapidly leave the gastric cavity.
Nature of meal	Indigestible polymers and fatty acid salts significantly increase the GRT. Highly viscous meals increase the GRT in comparison to less viscous fluid meals. Diets high in fats, triglycerides, and carbs reduce the rate of gastric emptying partly due to simulation of postprandial response, which includes secretion of bile (causes reduction in gastric motility), and partly due to elevation of osmotic pressure.
Caloric content	Diets high in protein and fat content can increase the GRT.
Frequency of feed	Frequent administration of meals can increase the GRT.
	Factors Related to the Patient
Gender	Males have less mean ambulatory GRT (3.4 ± 0.6 hours) compared to female counterparts (4.6 ± 1.2 hours) regardless of their weight, height, and body surface.
Age	Longer GRT is observed in elderly people.
Posture	Supine and upright ambulatory states of the patient affect the GRT.
Concomitant drug administration	Anticholinergics like atropine and propantheline and opiates like codeine cisapride help in prolongation of GRT. Prokinetic agents like metoclopramide and cisapride accelerate gastric emptying.
Disease state	GRT can increase during gastric ulcer, diabetes, and hypothyroidism whereas it can decrease in case of hyperthyroidism and duodenal ulcers.
GIT fluid volume	GRT will be low if the volume of GIT fluid is above the resting volume (25 to 50 ml).

would be proton pump inhibitors (PPIs) (pantoprazole, omeprazole, rabeprazole) used as a first choice in treatment of gastric and duodenal ulcers. PPIs are acid labile because they are protonated to their active configuration in acidic environment of stomach. This ionized form of drug is incapable of being absorbed and is subsequently wasted away leading to loss of therapeutic action. Marketed preparations are hence formulated with enteric coating to protect their degradation in stomach. Since enteric coating is tested to maintain its integrity for up to 2 hours in simulated gastric media, it is a common practice followed by doctors to prescribe PPIs early in the morning before any food consumption. Food is expected to delay gastric emptying for more than 2 hours, thereby raising the chance of gastric degradation of PPI.

Common inference therefore seems to be that a predictable GRT is more crucial than a prolonged one, keeping individual drug candidate in mind for ensuring efficacy of an OSDDS. GRDDS are designed to prolong gastric retention time of OSDDS. Not every drug is suited for a gastroretentive dosage form, and hence careful evaluation of physicochemical properties should be attempted before selecting a candidate for formulating into a GRDDS. Formulating a drug into GRDDS must circumvent some major loophole inflicting oral delivery of that drug, and it should not be attempted for the sake of it. An overview of these potential determining physicochemical properties is presented in the next section.

ACTIVE PHARMACEUTICAL INGREDIENTS (API) FOR GASTRORETENTION

GRDDS cannot deliver each and every API in an efficient manner due to the fact that these APIs have distinct physicochemical and biopharmaceutical properties. Major physicochemical issues are pKa, particle size, solubility, and stability of API in gastric environment. These properties must be evaluated during preformulation studies to optimize performance of GRDDS and to find out compatibility of API with GRDDS. Exhaustive knowledge of these properties is necessary because they offer rationale for formulation design.

When an oral dosage form, say a conventional tablet (Figure 4.3) is ingested, it disintegrates and deaggregates to yield a fine powder, which is dissolved in gastric media and moves toward the site of absorption—that is, near the membrane interface. As displayed in Figure 4.3, water or gastric media is drawn into the tablet via capillary action, leading to its swelling and spontaneous breakup. The rough aggregates are further ground down to fine powder by stomach physiology discussed previously. The fine powder is made up by individual drug particles that go into a dissolved state forming a molecular dispersion capable of moving toward the absorption site.

This process of dissolution (movement of any entity from solid to solution form) is quantitated by a modified Noyes Whitney equation; it confers relationship of direct proportionality between rate of dissolution (ds/dt) and the particle size A of the drug molecule undergoing dissolution. $(C_s - C_b)$ stands for

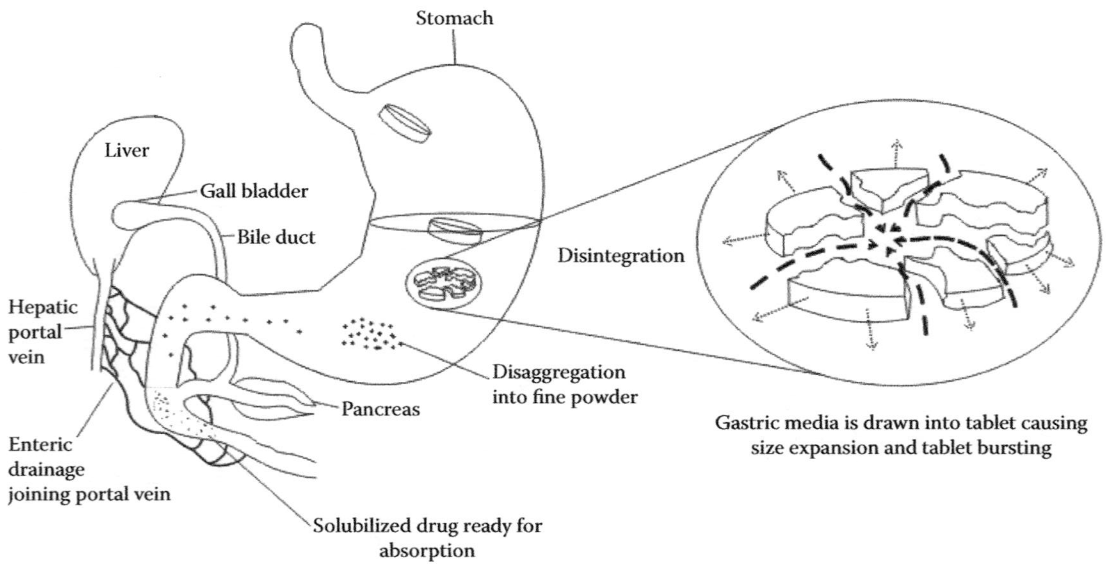

FIGURE 4.3 An artistic impression of tablet breakup in stomach. Disintegration is followed by deaggregation into fine powders, which dissolve rapidly to yield a drug solution ready for absorption.

concentration gradient, V is volume of dissolving fluid, and h is the thickness of saturation layer:

$$\frac{ds}{dt} = \frac{DA(C_s - C_b)}{Vh}$$

Dissolved state of drug is required for diffusion across aqueous unstirred layer (Figure 4.4) present in vicinity of the absorbing surface. Most of the drugs that exist in market today, if we exclude the biotechnologicals and complicated herbal extracts, are ordinarily weak acids, weak bases, or their salts. Thus, predisposition of these drugs to solubilize in aqueous gastric media is dictated by their preferential ionization capability, meaning in order to dissolve the drug dissociate into its constituent ions. Degree of ionization affects speed of drug transport. Ionized species of drug contains a charge and is more water-soluble than nonionized species of drug, which is more lipid-soluble. Extent of ionization of a random drug will depend on both pKa of drug and pH of medium in which drug is to be

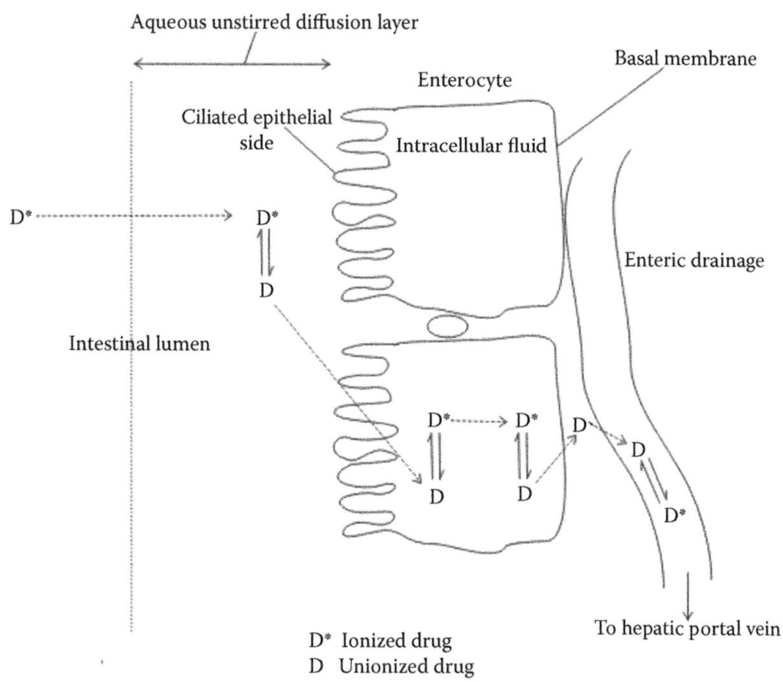

FIGURE 4.4 Pictorial depiction of drug transport across biologic membrane lining the intestine. Dynamic equilibrium between ionized and unionized drug is attained at several sites. Only unionized form partitions across the lipid bilayer whereas ionized form is necessary for drug solubilization and movement in gastric media and blood.

dissolved. Henderson and Hasselbalch used the following expressions pertaining to weak acids and weak bases to describe relationship between pKa, pH, and ratio of ionized to unionized drug, which will exist at that particular pH.

$$\text{For weak acids, } \frac{\text{ionized}}{\text{unionized}} = 10^{(\text{pH}-\text{pKa})}$$

$$\text{For weak bases, } \frac{\text{unionized}}{\text{ionized}} = 10^{(\text{pH}-\text{pKa})}$$

Over-riding theory regarding process of drug transport across a biologic membrane (say a gastric enterocyte in case of GRDDS) requires a drug moiety to be present in a unionized form at the membrane interface, followed subsequently by its partitioning into a lipid bilayer constructing the membrane, repartitioning into intracellular fluid, its translocation across the cell trailed by a repeat of this chain of events on the other side of the cell, leading to expression of drug in the relevant biologic fluid, namely blood on other side of the bimembrane (Figure 4.4). The driving force behind drug transport is Fick's first law of diffusion—that is, the concentration gradient across the barrier until equilibrium is attained. Equilibrium, however, is seldom attained as blood is an excellent sink. Also since only unionized portion of the drug is available for absorption, Fick's first law has to be modified to include the *pH-partition hypothesis*.

According to Henderson–Hasselbalch equation, at any particular pH a fraction of drug is present in unionized form, which diffuses down the gradient. Once inside the absorptive cell, it again attains equilibrium between ionized and unionized states depending upon existing intracellular pH, further reducing amount of drug that can be transferred across basal membrane into bloodstream. The *pH-partition hypothesis* utilizes this concept of successive equilibration to explain selective absorption of drug moieties across GIT. According to *pH-partition hypothesis*, if pH on one side of a cell membrane differs from pH on other side of the membrane, then

a. The drug (weak acid or base) will ionize to different degrees on respective sides of the membrane.
b. The total drug concentrations (ionized plus nonionized drug) on either side of the membrane will be unequal.
c. The compartment in which drug is more highly ionized will contain greater total drug concentration.

For these reasons, a weakly acidic drug (such as aspirin, pKa 3.5) will be rapidly absorbed from stomach (pH 1.2) whereas a weak base (such as quinidine, pKa in vicinity of 9) will be poorly absorbed from stomach [21]. Selection of target drug to be incorporated into GRDDS should probably proceed along these lines only. For example, it would make sense to generate GRDDS of several NSAIDs, like aspirin, ibuprofen, indomethacin, and diclofenac sodium, which show pH-dependent solubility, getting preferentially absorbed from the stomach [22]. Strongly acidic drugs, like penicillin and cromlyn sodium, are ionized in the entire GIT and consequently remain unabsorbed and probably wouldn't be feasible candidates for molding into GRDDS.

BCS Classification

The Biopharmaceutics Classification System (BCS) classification of a drug sometimes serves as a marker for candidate selection in GRDDS. BCS is a method used to differentiate drugs on the basis of their solubility and permeability and acts as a guide for predicting intestinal drug absorption provided by the U.S. Food and Drug Administration. A BCS scheme for correlating in vitro drug dissolution and in vivo bioavailability was recommended centered on recognizing that drug dissolution and gastrointestinal permeability are basic tools supervising rate and extent of drug absorption [23]. The BCS drug classes (Figure 4.5) are defined as following: Case 1: high solubility–high permeability drugs, Case 2: low solubility–high permeability drugs, Case 3: high solubility–low permeability drugs, and Case 4: low solubility–low permeability drugs.

Drugs belonging to BCS Class IV are poor candidates for any sort of oral drug delivery, including GRDDS. By way of their low solubility and permeability, they ensure that they remain undissolved in gastric media incapable of being absorbed. In rare instances, we do come across drugs belonging to Class IV, which have been successfully formulated into GRDDS [24,25]. However, these cases are too few to get any hopes up. Drugs classified in Class I, II, and III are more suited to the GRDDS approach, and literature is loaded with illustrations.

An API having instability at gastric pH would be difficult to deliver through a GRDDS even if it is found to be highly suited to oral delivery after extrapolating its physicochemical properties discussed previously. The PPIs are mostly acid labile, so developing a GRDDS would not be a suitable option, and an enteric coating approach might serve the purpose of oral delivery better.

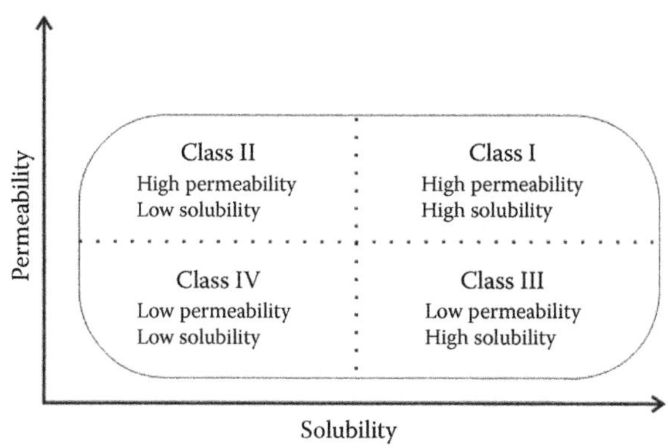

FIGURE 4.5 US-FDA–defined BCS.

Along with physicochemical properties, biopharmaceutical properties of API also contribute a great deal in deciding whether it is to be delivered through GRDDS [26]. Absorption, distribution, metabolism, excretion, half-life (absorption and elimination), therapeutic index, dose size, and first-pass clearance of the API are some fundamental properties. Most of these biopharmaceutical properties are interlinked with physicochemical properties. Absorption of an API in GIT depends upon its relative solubility and stability at various pHs in different regions of the GIT. Stability of molecule might also be affected by enzymatic degradation in GIT. So it is necessary to investigate GIT absorption pattern of API before deciding whether its GRDDS would be of any consequence in improving the bioavailability of a drug.

Half-life and dose size are also important issues and should be monitored before developing GRDDS. Drugs having a short half-life, which necessitate multiple dose therapy, should be converted to GRDDS. Equally, we should refrain from developing a GRDDS for a drug that has an inherently long half-life or a once-a-day dosing regimen unless and until there is a very specific demand for requirement of local action.

First-pass clearance of drugs can be minimized by incorporating into GRDDS because it is well known that P-glycoproteins are available throughout GIT, but

TABLE 4.3
List of APIs Having Potential Candidature for Incorporation into GRDDS

S. No.	API	Therapeutic or Pharmacological Category		Reference
1	Acyclovir	Antiviral	Class III	[28]
2	Atenolol	β1 receptor antagonist	Class III	[29]
3	Furosemide	Loop diuretic	Class IV	[24]
4	Tacrolimus	Immunosuppressant	Class II	[30]
5	Captopril	Angiotensin converting enzyme inhibitor	Class IV	[25]
6	Ranitidine	Histamine H_2-receptor antagonist	Class III	[31]
7	Repaglinide	Oral hypoglycemic agent	Class II	[32]
8	Cisapride	Serotonin 5-HT4 receptor agonist	Class II	[33]
9	Itraconazole	Antifungal	Class II	[34]
10	Metformin	Antidiabetic	Class III	[17]
11	Trimetazidine	Antianginal	Class II	[35]
12	Ciprofloxacin	Fluoroquinolone antibiotic	Class II	[36]
13	Alfuzosin	Alpha-adrenergic receptor blocker	–	[37]
14	Ofloxacin	Fluroquinolone antibiotic	Class I	[7]
15	Levodopa	Antiparkinson agent	Class I	[38]
16	Silymarin	Antioxidant	Class III	[39]
17	Ketoprofen	NSAID	Class I	[40]
18	Verapamil	Calcium channel blocker	Class I	[41]
19	Melatonin	Antioxidant	–	[42]
20	Tetracycline	Antibiotic	Class III	[43]
21	Riboflavin	Vitamin	–	[44]
22	Sotalol	β-adrenergic receptor blocker	Class I	[45]

their availability is higher in distal region (stomach < jejunum < colon) [27]. Thus, bioavailability of drugs that have high first-pass clearance can be increased by limiting their release in gastric cavity. Several drug candidates have been found suitable for incorporation into GRDDS, and a list of such drugs is given in Table 4.3 along with their pharmacological, therapeutic, and BCS classes.

Physicochemical properties of excipients play a major role in performance of drug delivery systems. Therefore, they should be selected on the basis of successful compatibility studies with API. They should not affect physicochemical and therapeutic properties of the incorporated API. Furthermore, the United States Food and Drug Administration (US-FDA)–approved excipients should be incorporated in formulations. US-FDA has developed a database that comprises list of all excipients approved by US-FDA. This database also provides information about the inactive ingredient guide (IIG) and limits of the US-FDA approved excipients.

GASTRORETENTIVE TECHNOLOGIES

We now turn our focus toward differing gastroretentive tools and techniques.

High-Density or Sinking Systems

Density is a major factor to retain dosage forms in the gastric cavity. Its manipulation—that is, increase or decrease in comparison to gastric fluid—can render a system gastroretentive. High-density systems, as the name suggests, are those dosage forms that possess a density higher than gastric fluid (~3 g/cm^3). They generally need to exceed a threshold density of 2.3 to 2.8 g/cm^3 in order to cross the tipping point that allows them to sit in the stomach. High-density systems sink to the bottom of the stomach and get trapped in folds of the antrum and become capable of withstanding peristaltic waves.

Excipients incorporated in high-density systems are barium sulfate, zinc oxide, iron powder, and titanium dioxide. A clinical study suggested that these systems have capability to improve bioavailability of an encapsulated drug in comparison to floating and conventional dosage forms [46]. However, these systems have some drawbacks due to the excipients utilized to formulate them. These excipients can react with other ingredients in the formulation and also with biological fluids. Furthermore, they create issues with respect to quality control in manufacturing and hence have not met with any success in market. Figure 4.6 shows basic principles of different gastroretentive technologies.

Low-Density or Floating Systems

Davis in 1968 first introduced a floating system [47]. Floating systems are the most popular systems among GRDDS. Basically, they have density lower than gastric fluid due to which they stay buoyant over gastric contents. A low-density dosage form remains buoyant for a long time. Along with floating capability, they can release an encapsulated drug in a sustained-release fashion, which helps to reduce dose-dependent adverse effects; decreases dosing frequency; improves patient

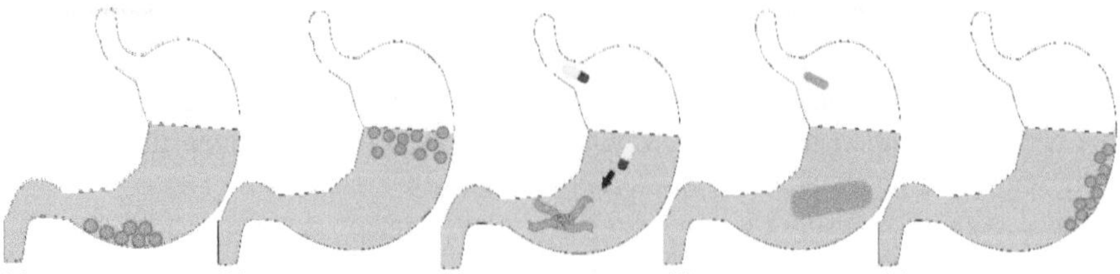

FIGURE 4.6 Basic gastroretentive technologies. (a) High-density systems. (b) Floating systems. (c) Expandable unfolding system: carrier capsule dissolves to release an unfolding system, which is retained in the stomach because of its larger size. (d) Swelling systems. (e) Mucoadhesive system.

compliance; increases bioavailability of such drugs, which are primarily absorbed from stomach; and improves therapeutic effect of short half-life drugs.

Floating systems are characterized by a very important statistic known as floating lag time, which calculates the time differential between the point when dosage form comes in contact with gastric fluid and the point at which it becomes buoyant. Its relevance becomes significant where a larger lag time results in sweeping of the dosage form along with housekeeper wave into the intestine and entire purpose of GRDDS is lost.

These systems have some limitations also, including requirement of high fluid volume in the stomach in order to achieve buoyancy and nonsuitability of drugs that have solubility and stability problems in gastric fluid and for drugs that can cause irritation to gastric mucosa. Floating is sometimes hindered in presence of viscous chime, which causes hindrance in rising and floating of the dosage form. In fact, studies have indicated that floating systems depend heavily on fed state to avoid gastric emptying. The fasted state gastric volume is insufficient for dosage form to attain sufficient buoyancy, and accordingly, they have been purposed to be effective in the fed state only. The target should be to develop a floating system that is independent of food effects. Basically, floating systems can be designed by utilizing two distinct approaches: effervescence and noneffervescence.

Noneffervescent System

These systems are formulated with a high content of gel-forming and highly swellable polymers, including polysaccharides, polystyrene, polycarbophil, polyacrylates, polymethacrylates, and swellable hydrocolloids (hydroxyethyl cellulose, hydroxypropyl cellulose, hydroxypropyl methylcellulose, and sodium carboxymethylcellulose). After reaching the gastric cavity, these systems tend to swell due to hydration followed by gel formation by incorporated polymers. This gelling layer screens the continuous incursion of gastric fluid inside delivery system, which sometimes sustains release of enclosed active moiety. Buoyancy of dosage form is confirmed by trapped air inside the swollen layer, which ultimately reduces density of the dosage form [48].

Floating Tablets

Floating tablets are mainly formulated as single and bilayer systems. Sustained-release matrix in all the systems is developed by employing cellulose derivatives and acrylic polymers, including hydroxypropyl cellulose, hydroxypropyl methylcellulose, crosspovidone, sodium carboxymethyl cellulose, ethyl cellulose, eudragit RS PO, eudragit EPO, sodium alginate, cornstarch, carrageenan, gum guar, and gum arabic. Moreover, bilayer systems additionally comprise an immediate-release layer in order to provide a loading dose to achieve an initial therapeutic concentration. Further, therapeutic concentration is maintained by subsequent release of drug from the sustained-release polymer matrix. The buoyancy is achieved due to swelling of incorporated polymers on contact with gastric fluid, which reduces overall density of the dosage form [49,50].

Hydrodynamically Balanced Systems (HBS)

HBS are single-unit systems, composed of gel-forming hydrophilic polymers, such as hydroxypropyl methylcellulose, hydroxyethyl cellulose, hydroxypropyl cellulose, sodium carboxymethy cellulose, agar, carrageenans, or alginic acid. Generally, these polymers are mixed with an API and administered through a gelatin capsule [51].

Upon administration, the gelatin shell gets dissolved, and a floating mass is formed due to rapid swelling of the incorporated polymers. For an HBS to float, density of dosage form should be less than one. This floating mass is relatively big in size in comparison to valve of the pyloric sphincter due to which its passage through gastric cavity is prohibited. Drug release is controlled by generation of a hydrated boundary at the surface of floating mass, and continued incursion of water within the wet mass maintains buoyancy of the system. HBS gives excellent uniformity of API in polymer matrix and is easy to manufacture. However, hydration of the gelatinous layer may be induced due to entrapped air within the dry mass.

Swelling type systems considerably increase in size and may be problematic if they plug the pyloric sphincter. The delivery system after drug release is expected to be eliminated, but problems do arise if the emptying process is hindered in any case.

Floating Microspheres

Floating microspheres have become increasingly popular in the last two decades, and a lot of research has been done on its formulation and performance evaluation. They are superior to other low-density systems because they float immediately after administration and exclude the concept of floating lag time, which ultimately prevents premature evacuation of system from gastric cavity. Because of their minute size, these regularly get trapped in intestine or folds of antrum, further prolonging their duration of stay in the absorption window. These microspheres are developed by using low-density polymer, which entraps oil or air within the polymeric shell. These microspheres are often called microballoons (hollow microspheres) if air is entrapped in the center of polymeric shell. Floating microspheres are developed by employing polymers, such as albumin, gelatin, starch, cellulosic derivatives, polymethacrylate, polyacrylamine, polyalkylcyanoacrylate, methoxylated pectin, and Eudragit. They have free-flowing properties along with excellent drug loading. The drug is either dispersed or dissolved in polymer matrix. Hollow microspheres are developed by utilizing different solvent evaporation techniques [52]. The drug release depends on plasticizer, polymer ratio, and solvent employed. A simple flow chart depicting sample steps that can be adapted while formulating microballoons is shown in Figure 4.7.

The mechanism behind formation of microspheres is visualized in Figure 4.8. Usually, an organic solvent, like acetone, or a blend of solvents, such as a mixture of DCM and ethanol, is employed to dissolve drug, microballoon forming water-insoluble polymer and sometimes a membrane stabilizing excipient. Mechanical input might be required to form a homogenous organic phase. Upon injecting this organic phase in a surfactant stabilized aqueous solution, the water-soluble ethanol rapidly diffuses outward, creating a tremendous disturbance at the water–oil interface. The insoluble component, like DCM; polymer; and drug are left behind to form spherical droplets. This turbulence raises the entropy of the system to such an extent that it offsets the increased interfacial energy developed due to formation of a new oil–water interface. Any tendency for this nascent interface to coalesce and increase droplet size is prevented due to shielding provided by the surfactants present in solution.

The polymer and drug are dragged to the outer curvature of the droplet with the outward rushing ethanol whereas DCM, which is extremely water-repellant, is left behind and trapped in the interior. Initially, the droplet consists of a thickly

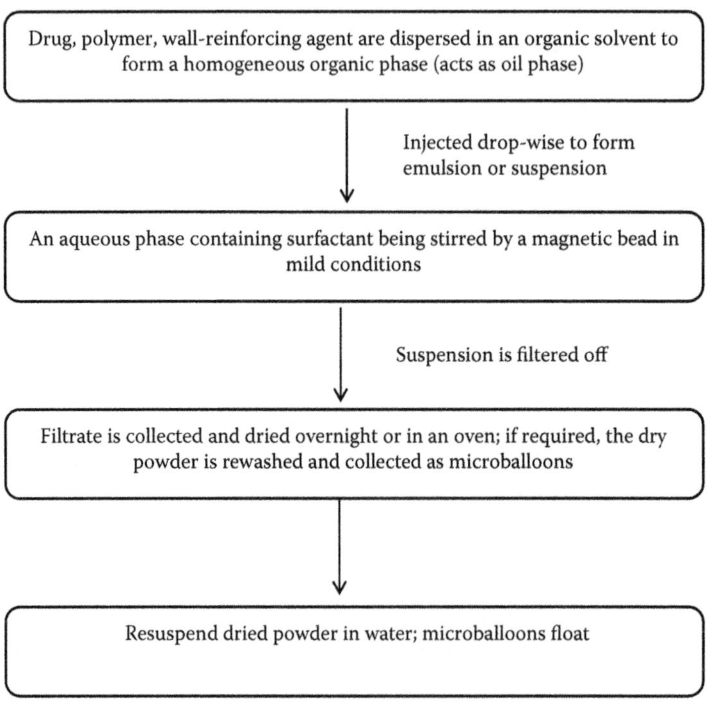

FIGURE 4.7 Schematic diagram of steps employed in forming microballoons.

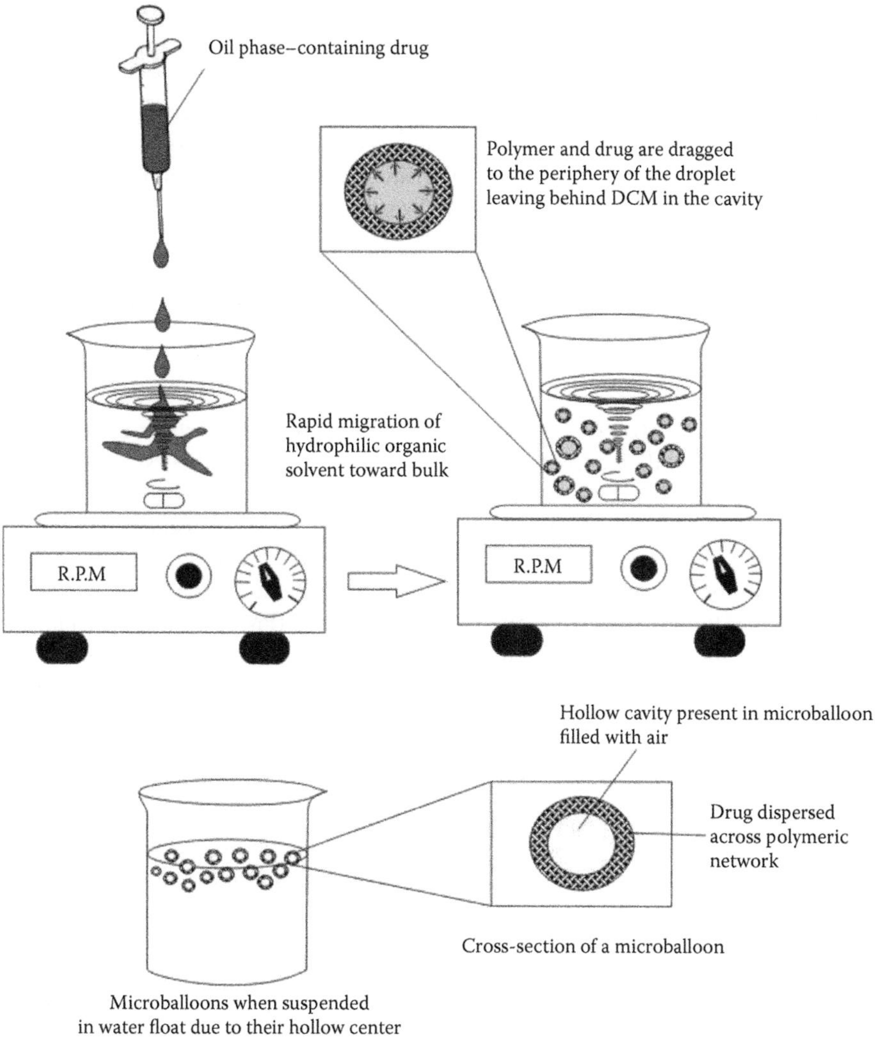

FIGURE 4.8 Mechanistic explanation of microballoon formation and the principle in floating.

concentrated viscous polymeric coating, which hardens with the passage of time whereas highly volatile DCM evaporates, leaving behind a hollow shell filled with air. This structure is similar to that of a normal balloon. A normal balloon floats on water surface based on extension of the *Archimedes principle*: Volume of water displaced by it weighs equal to or more than its entire weight, providing it with an essential up thrust for it to float. Microballoons behave similarly along with added intelligent demeanor of providing controlled drug delivery.

Microballoons, if manufactured from hydrophilic polymers, sometimes clump upon coming in contact with water and start behaving like a single unit dosage form, which can follow all or none of the principles leading to failure of this type of GRDDS. In such cases, a protective filler excipient like Eudragit is mixed in the recipe of microballoons.

Floating microspheres are multiple-unit systems and they have certain advantages over single-unit systems like HBS. Single-unit systems are unreliable and can cause dose dumping because they follow an all-or-none emptying process. Furthermore, single-unit systems sometimes release large amount of drug at a particular site, which can produce local irritation in the gastric cavity whereas multiple-unit systems distribute uniformly through the stomach and reduce chances of intersubject variability in gastric evacuation as only a portion of administered content can be evicted, and any tendency to produce local irritation is mitigated.

Floating Beads

Beads are spherical structures that have been used as an agency for controlling drug delivery. They differ from other carriers with respect to their size and consistency. Beads are usually sized from few hundred microns to several millimeters and could be floating or nonfloating. Floating beads are formulated mainly by employing ionic cross-linking or the ionic gelation process. They are composed of anionic polysaccharides, like pectin and sodium alginate, often requiring supplementation by a swellable polymer, such as HPMC, which expands on contact with water and forms a hydrogel. Low methoxy pectin is gelatinized in presence of divalent cations like Ca^{2+}. Similar to pectin, alginic acid also undergoes a phase transition reaction in presence of divalent cations like Ca^{2+} due to interaction with an available glucuronic acid moiety in structure to form a sequence of interlinked cages with trapped calcium. Sometimes this polyelectrolyte complex requires cross-linking by an aldehyde to further strengthen its integrity and attain a level of control on drug release. Generally, an aqueous solution of anionic polysaccharide is added drop-wise in solution of calcium chloride for development of beads.

Drying of developed beads leads to formation of a porous structure, which ultimately provides high buoyancy. Sometimes a gas-generating agent, like calcium carbonate or sodium tartarate, is added to formulation mixture, which evolves carbon dioxide, leaving behind porous beads, contributing additional buoyancy.

A different technique, termed emulsion extraction, has been developed in past decade [53] to make beads out of amphoteric proteins like casein or gelatin instead of the traditional anionic polysaccharides. Proteins like casein and gelatin have surface activity and are preferentially localized at the air–water interface. They are known to provide a variety of textures by undergoing slight modification. Emulsion extraction utilizes these very surfactant-like properties of proteins to trap drug molecules in porous bead-like structures made out of proteins themselves. Figure 4.9 demonstrates the crude steps that are regularly adapted while preparing beads by this method.

Drug solution is dispersed homogenously with casein and gelatin to form the internal aqueous phase. This aqueous phase is then injected drop-wise into a suitable mineral oil forming the bulk phase. It is herein that the surface-active nature of protein molecules localizes them at oil–water interface and emulsifies the

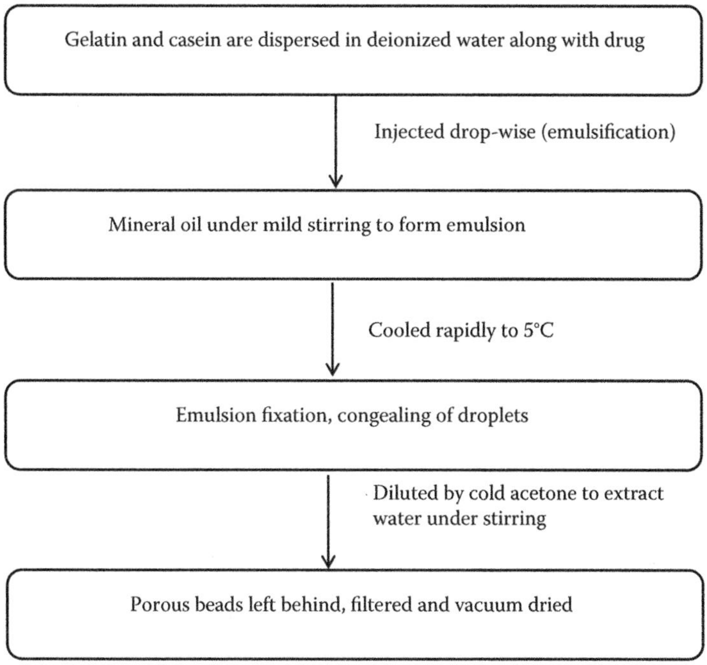
Gelatin and casein are dispersed in deionized water along with drug
Injected drop-wise (emulsification)
Mineral oil under mild stirring to form emulsion
Cooled rapidly to 5°C
Emulsion fixation, congealing of droplets
Diluted by cold acetone to extract water under stirring
Porous beads left behind, filtered and vacuum dried

FIGURE 4.9 Porous beads generated by the emulsion extraction method.

otherwise immiscible oil and water to generate numerous small soft beads, which do not phase separate on standing. Reducing the temperature further congeals the protein droplets. Upon dilution of this fixed water in oil emulsion (W/O) with a water-miscible organic solvent, like acetone, water is drawn out from within the emulsion droplet through the protein boundary into the bulk, leaving behind small hollow pores in bead structure. The beads are subsequently cured, filtered, and dried and float when resuspended.

Floating In Situ Gelling Systems

Floating in situ gelling systems are in a liquid state at room temperature. After administration, these systems swell in gastric cavity and develop a floating layer on top of the gastric fluid. Buoyancy is achieved due to air entrapped within the swelled mass. This system is developed by employing various natural and synthetic polymers, such as alginic acid, pectin, guar gum, gellan gum, xyloglucan, chitosan, and hydroxypropyl methylcellulose. These polymers have unique gelation properties. They can gelatinize in presence of certain cations or upon a change in pH or at particular temperature [54]. The function of floating rafts to not only retain drug, but also act as a barrier for reflux, which is especially important when targeting gastric esophageal reflux disorder.

For a case in point, Rajnikanth et al. [55] developed a floating in situ gelling system using sodium citrate in a gellan gum-amoxicillin dispersion. The calcium carbonate incorporated in the formulation mixture becomes soluble in acidic pH

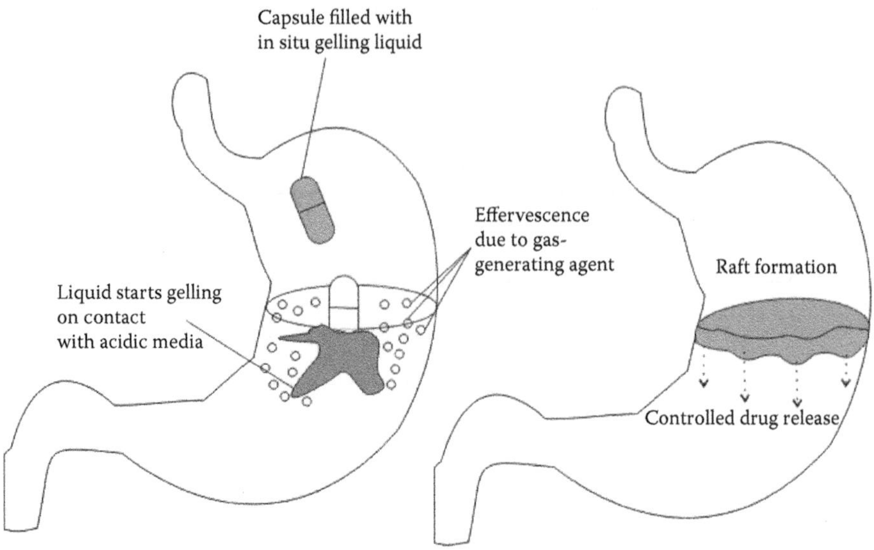

FIGURE 4.10 Floating in situ gelling systems comprising a gelatin capsule as an inert carrier. The formulation mixture, on contact with the acidic pH of the stomach, liberates free calcium ions, which cause gelation. The hydrogel is essentially low density and thereby rises, starts floating on the gastric fluid, and forms a raft capable of being retained. Sometimes a gas-generating agent is added to provide additional buoyancy.

of stomach. The freed-up calcium ions are immediately complexed by sodium citrate. The trapped calcium is slowly rereleased and causes gelation of gellan akin to ionic cross-linking described in the formation of beads. Gelled material floats upward in stomach (Figure 4.10) with a potential to release its drug over a period of time. Calcium carbonate additionally releases carbon dioxide in stomach, thereby making the system buoyant and thus prolonging its residence time.

Floating Granules

Floating granules are generally composed of a lipid carrier like Gelucire 43/01 and glyceryl monosterate in combination with swellable cellulosic polymers like hydroxypropyl methylcellulose, ethylcellulose, hydroxyethyl cellulose, and hydroxypropyl cellulose. They can be prepared by melt granulation and a hot melt extrusion technique. Melt granulation is an emerging technique based on use of binders that have a relatively low melting point (between 50°C and 80°C) and act as a molten binding liquid. Equipment that can be used for melt granulation includes high-shear mixers, fluid bed granulators, and extruders [56]. A sample flowchart drawn in Figure 4.11 lists the steps used to make floating granules via melt homogenization technique.

Buoyancy of the system is achieved due to available lipids on surface of granules, which impart hydrophobicity to the system [16,57]. Buoyancy of system is altered corresponding to density of selected lipid carrier. Since relatively higher

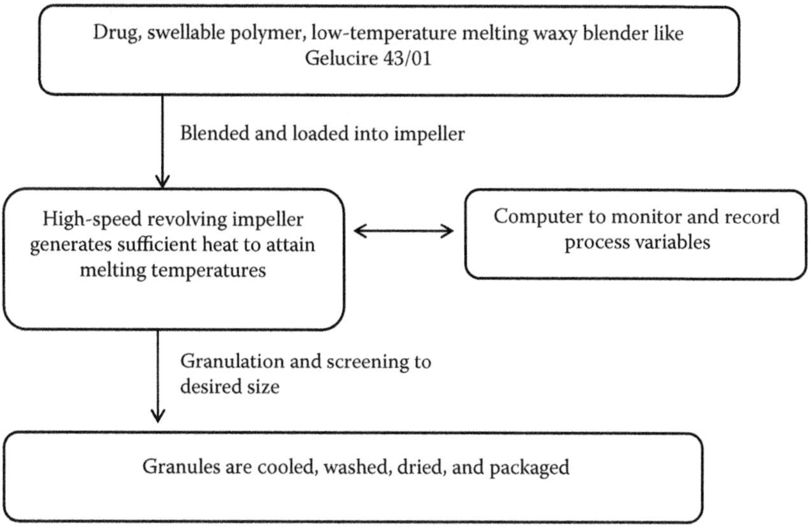

FIGURE 4.11 Floating granules by melt granulation technique.

temperatures are employed during manufacturing process, thermolabile drugs are usually not formulated as floating granules.

Floating Compartmental Systems

Floating compartmental systems are very complex. They are composed of a gas-filled flotation chamber in which the drug is stored in a reservoir. These systems are completely closed and have no contact with gastric fluid except two apertures present on the top and bottom side. The fluid is composed of either air or any other suitable gas or liquid or any solid having suitable specific gravity that helps in floating of the system. Available apertures allow the entrance of gastric fluid inside the floating compartment and subsequent drug release from the system [58].

Effervescent Systems

Effervescent systems are formulated using effervescent components like sodium bicarbonate, citric acid, and tartaric acid. System becomes buoyant due to generation of CO_2 via a reaction between organic acid and a carbonate–bicarbonate alkali. The system can also become buoyant due to incorporation of volatile organic solvents. Along with prolonged buoyancy, they provide sustained release of the encapsulated drug.

Intragastric Floating Tablets

Intragastric floating tablets are prepared by utilizing gas-generating agents like sodium bicarbonate, citric acid, and tartaric acid. These systems also contain some swellable polymer, such as hydroxypropyl methylcellulose and ethylcellulose. These tablets are designed as single-layer, double-layer, and tri-layer tablets. In single-layer tablets, effervescent polymers are mixed with swellable polymers. Double-layer tablets contain a similar layer as single-layer tablets, but they also contain an additional immediate-release layer for the loading dose whereas tri-layer tablets contain an immediate-release layer, an effervescent layer, and a sustained-release layer, which contains drug and swellable polymer(s) to maintain therapeutic dose [59,41].

Intragastric Floating Pills

These floating systems contain a center core of effervescent components like sodium bicarbonate, citric acid, and tartaric acid and an outer layer consisting of a swellable polymer like methocel, ethylcellulose, and polysaccharides like chitosan. Sometimes inner core is divided into two sublayers to avoid contact between two gas-generating agents. The inner sublayer contains sodium bicarbonate whereas the outer sublayer contains tartaric acid and citric acid. System gets buoyant due to generation of CO_2 via gas-generating agents, and outer swellable layer provides sustained release of the entrapped drug.

Volatile Liquid

These systems consist of an inflatable chamber, which contains a volatile liquid like cyclopentane and ether. This volatile liquid evaporates at body temperature and provides flotation to the system. These inflatable systems become deformed upon evaporation of the volatile organic agent but revert to their original shape after a certain time period to cause evacuation of inflatable system from gastric cavity.

Expandable Systems

As the name suggests, expandable systems change their shape and acquire a magnified size once ingested. Expandable systems delay gastric emptying of dosage form by creating an illusion of fed state. The feeling of a filled stomach delays advent of housekeeper wave. Expandable GRDDS achieves three basic shapes (Figure 4.12) during its life span in the gastric cavity.

Initially, it is small enough to enter into the gastric cavity, which is followed by its expandable form preventing its evacuation through the pyloric sphincter, and finally, it is reconverted into a small shape for easy evacuation from the stomach. During this time period, the expandable system completely releases the contained active moiety.

Expandable systems are made with intelligent polymers having unique mechanical shape memory properties, which revert back to their original shape; otherwise, they could be stuck in the stomach forever. These systems are generally administered through a carrier, such as a gelatin capsule shell. At the beginning, they are folded and filled into a gelatin capsule, and afterward, the gelatin capsule gets dissolved, and expandable system regains its mechanical shape. A variety of stimuli can be involved in triggering expansion of dosage form, namely pH or contact with gastric media.

Although this system appears foolproof in guaranteeing gastric retention, careful evaluation should be conducted to ensure proper timing of opening and closure

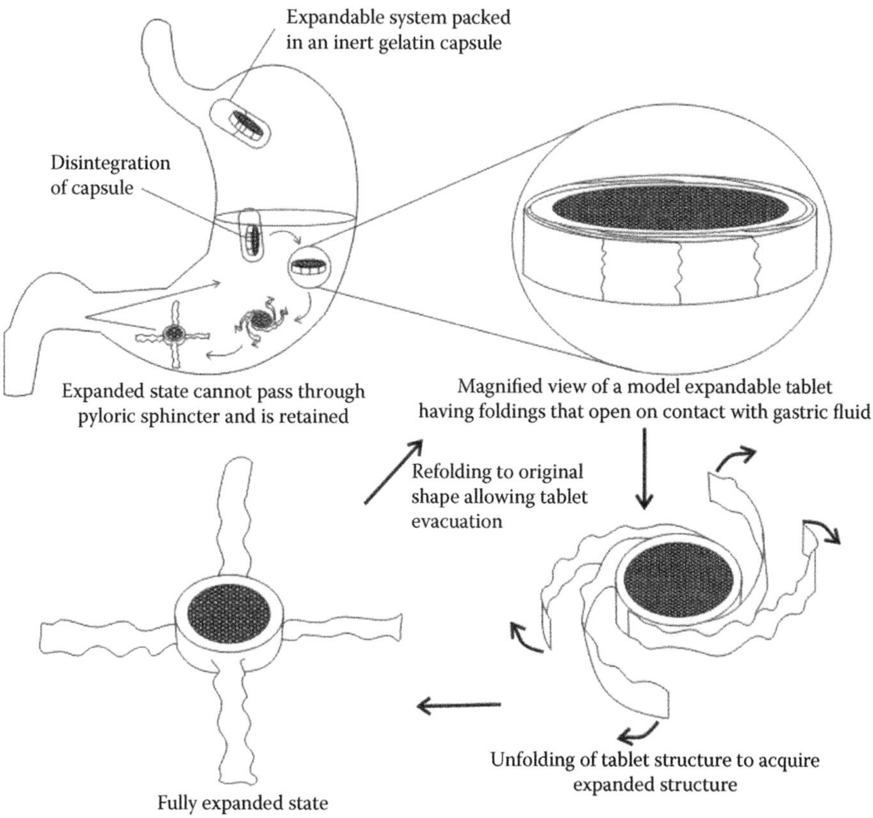

FIGURE 4.12 Shape changes undergone by an expandable system, leading to gastric retention.

of the system. Any discrepancy in opening inside the stomach may lead to failure of expandable system. The system must also not open inadvertently while traversing ileal portion of the GIT, which might cause inflammation and severe pain. Developed system should not intervene in gastric motility and also should not bear sharp edges capable of inducing injury to biological tissues [60]. Occlusion of pylorus or esophagus can sometimes creep into the functioning of expandable systems. Synchronization of dosing intervals also becomes mandatory as it may result in excessive retention, and cumulative accumulation of several dosage units will create a choking hazard.

Swelling Systems

Gastroretention of these floating systems is based upon swelling of incorporated polymers. They swell enough to prevent their expulsion from stomach. The mechanism of retention, however, is not dependent on size alone; the large unit residing in stomach creates an illusion of fed state and delays housekeeping wave. However release of active moiety is dictated by swelling of the selected polymer.

Presence of physical and chemical cross-links in hydrophilic polymer leads to extensive swelling of the polymer. These cross-links preserve three-dimensional structure of polymer by avoiding its dissolution inside the stomach [61].

Superporous Hydrogels

Superporous hydrogels are also swellable systems, but they are very different from conventional hydrogels. These hydrogels have pore sizes ranging from 10 nm to 10 µm, which provides a very rapid water uptake in comparison to conventional systems. Conventional systems may take several hours to achieve an equilibrium state due to which premature evacuation of GRDDS may occur whereas superporous hydrogels achieve equilibrium within a minute because they uptake water via capillary wetting through numerous interconnected open pores (average pore size >100 µm). Furthermore, they swell enough to provide adequate mechanical strength, which assists the system in withstanding high pressure generated due to gastric contraction [62].

Mucoadhesive or Bioadhesive Systems

Mucoadhesive or bioadhesive systems have capability to bind with mucosal surfaces, a property that helps their cohesion to gastric or other GIT mucosal surfaces, assisting them in improving GRT. However, uncontrolled release of mucous might compromise their mucoadhesiveness. Mucoadhesive systems are formulated with natural and synthetic polymers like carbopol, lectins, chitosan, polycarbophil, and more. These polymers have unspecific and specific binding with biological mucus membrane via hydration- or bonding-based adhesive forces and via some receptors, respectively. Mucoadhesive strength of these polymers can be altered in cases of highly hydrated stomach contents. Furthermore, stomach-specific targeting of these systems is quite challenging due to unspecific mucoadhesion of these polymers [63].

Magnetic Systems

Magnetic systems comprise an internal magnet, and its GRT is controlled via an extracorporal magnet. However, these systems have practical problems in terms of application of an external magnet to guide delivery systems to achieve the intended purpose. It is not easy to place an external magnet with perfect precision over stomach, leading to compromised patient compliance [28].

Advanced Systems

Dual Working Systems

Currently, pharmaceutical industries are focused on dual working systems. These systems are formulated in a way that allows them to simultaneously display dual gastroretentive approaches. Basically, these systems are based upon combination of floating and bioadhesion or swelling- and bioadhesion-based gastroretentive approaches [64]. Individually, these contributive technologies have certain demerits of their own; for example, floating tablets mandatorily require a filled stomach to float whereas unpredictable mucus secretion can lead to premature evacuation of mucoadhesive only system. Dual working systems could, in a significant way, overcome these troubles associated with different technologies [65].

For instance, ofloxacin exhibits pH-dependent solubility (more soluble in acidic pH), it has been formulated into GRDDS based on a dual working system [66]. A straightforward method of wet granulation and tablet punching was employed to develop tablets of ofloaxacin. The excipients—more specifically special polymers, namely hydroxyl propyl methyl cellulose, psyllium, and polyvinyl pyrrolidone—were added in tablet mixture in order to accord dual behavior to the finished product. Upon coming in contact with water, the tablet disintegrates into small entities and starts behaving like a multiparticulate system. The polymers either swell up in water or start floating based on any of the principles discussed previously with floating systems. Further including a mucoadhesive polymer in tablet blend confers mucoadhesive properties to the system, and it displays dual behavior.

Floating Osmotic System

These systems depend on osmotic pressure generated inside core of a system to release enclosed drug. Generally, they are formulated in three parts: a central osmotic core containing the drug, an osmotic agent and excipients, a semipermeable membrane that provides shape to the system, and finally, an outer layer composed of gas-generating agents and swelling agents. These systems have an orifice on top and bottom for delivery of drug. Gas-generating and swelling agents present on the outer layer are responsible for floating of system. The drug release from these systems takes place in two steps. First, a saturated solution is formed inside the core of the system due to constant flow of gastric fluid through the semipermeable membrane. Second, an osmotic pressure is generated within the osmotic core to expel out the drug through the orifices. These systems have an advantage over other systems in terms of drug release being independent of physiological principles like pH of the gastric fluid [31].

Floating Pulsatile System

Chronotherapeutic systems have become increasingly important due to synchronization of drug release with biological clock of disease. Generally, these systems have a lag time of 8 to 12 hours in releasing active moiety. One downside with such systems is their propensity for dose dumping if, in any case, the mechanism synchronizing drug release with requirements of body crashes. Floating pulsatile drug delivery systems are proposed to overcome these drawbacks associated with pulsatile systems. They can be retained in gastric cavity for a longer period of time due to floating nature of these systems. These systems have a complex structure consisting of a central core containing drug coated with some hydophillic erodible polymer, which is responsible for the pulsatile release of drug, followed by a floating layer consisting of gas-generating and gel-forming

TABLE 4.4
Gastroretentive Technologies Scaled Up by Pharmaceutical Industries

Product Name and Company	Technology	API
Xifaxan tablets; Lupin, India	Bioadhesive tablets	Rifaximin
Zanocin OD; Ranbaxy, India	Effervescent floating system	Ofloxacin
Conviron; Ranbaxy, India	Colloidal gel-forming floating system	Ferrous sulphate
Inon Ace tablets; Sato Pharma, Japan	Foam-based floating system	Siméthicone
Gabapentin GR; Depomed, United States	Polymer-based swelling technology: AcuForm™	Gabapentin
Prazopress XL; Sun Pharma, India	Effervescent and swelling-based floating system	Prazosin hydrochloride
Cafeclor LP; Galenix, France	Minextab Floating® system	Cefaclor
Cipro XR; Bayer, United States	Erodible matrix–based system	Ciprofloxacin hydrochloride and betaine
Accordion pill; TM Intec Pharma	Expandable film filled in capsule	Single drug or a combination of drugs
Baclofen GRS; Sun Pharma, India	Coated multilayer floating and swelling system	Baclofen
Coreg CR; Glaxosmithkline	Gastroretention with osmotic system	Carvedilol
Madopar; Roche, UK	Floating, CR capsule	Levodopa and benserzide
Liquid Gaviscon; Reckitt Benckiser Healthcare, UK	Effervescent floating liquid alginate preparation	Alginic acid and sodium bicarbonate
Cytotec; Pharmacia Limited, UK	Bilayer floating capsule	Misoprostol
Topalkan; Pierre Fabre Medicament, France	Floating liquid alginate	Aluminum magnesium antacid

agents [67,68]. Table 4.4 comprises gastroretentive approaches taken up by pharmaceutical companies.

CHARACTERIZATION OF GRDDS

In Vitro Evaluation

In vitro evaluation of GRDDS is somewhat different from conventional dosage forms. Analytical specifications for GRDDS should be selected in a proper manner to evaluate their characteristics precisely. The International Conference on Harmonization (ICH) guidelines, "ICH Q6A specifications: test procedures and acceptance criteria for new drug substances and new drug products: chemical substances," should be referenced during selection of general analytical specifications [69]. This guideline provides information about general analytical specifications relevant to specific dosage forms. Furthermore, analytical procedure should be validated according to ICH guideline "Q2 (R1) validation of analytical procedures: text and

TABLE 4.5
List of Some General and Specific In Vitro Analytical Specifications of GRDDS

S. No.	Analytical Specifications	Remarks
	General Tests	
1	Description of dosage form	Detailed description of product should be reported such as physical state, shape, color, etc.
2	Identification test of active moiety and coloring agent if available in composition	–
3	Uniformity of mass or uniformity of content	–
4	pH	–
5	Dissolution	–
6	Assay	–
7	Related substances content	If any
8	Residual solvent content	If any
9	Antimicrobial preservative content	If any
10	Antioxidant preservative content	If any
11	Microbiological limits	–
	Specific Tests	
12	Test for specific gravity	For floating systems
13	Buoyancy/floating ability test	For floating systems
14	Floating lag time	For floating systems
15	Test for swelling index/water uptake	For swelling and expandable systems
16	Test for mucoadhesion	For mucoadhesive systems
17	Texture analysis	For in situ gelling systems

methodology" [70]. In combination with ICH guidelines, pharmacopoeias should also be referred to select analytical specification for a pharmacopoeial product.

Acceptance criteria are specified after selection of analytical specifications. For a new drug delivery system, acceptance criteria can be modified on the basis of experience gained during initial characterization of product. If the product monograph is available in pharmacopoeia, then it is the best reference for selection of acceptance criteria. According to current good manufacturing practices, it is also required to investigate and report critical in-process controls during development of the product that can affect drug product quality and performance. Some general and specific in vitro analytical specifications for GRDDS are summarized in the Table 4.5.

In Vivo Evaluation Criteria

γ-Scintigraphy

An in vivo buoyancy study of various GRDDS can be done with help of γ-scintigraphy. γ-Scintigraphy is a technique in which a radioisotope is administered to humans, and emitted radiation can be detected using an external gamma camera. This external gamma camera can produce two- and three-dimensional images. Usually, a radioisotope like ^{111}In is encapsulated in GRDDS and is administered orally. With the help of radiation generated from the body, gamma detector generates images. We can monitor actual position and GRT of relative GRDDS by interpretation of these images [71]. γ-Scintigraphy, however, requires strict compliance with respect to technical and safety issues, such as related ionization radiations, low resolution, and complex manufacturing of radiopharmaceuticals.

Radiology

X-rays can also be used to determine in vivo buoyancy of GRDDS. Generally, a radio-opaque agent like barium sulfate is formulated with GRDDS, and X-ray images are taken to check position of GRDDS in GIT at various time intervals [38]. In comparison to γ-scintigraphy, radiology is a more safe, simple, and cost-effective process. However, large amount of the radio-opaque agent is required to give better resolution.

Gastroscopy

Gastroscopy is per-oral endoscopy and is considered a minimally invasive technique. It depends on visual inspection of GRDDS in gastric cavity with the aid of some optic fibers and a video camera [72]. It gives detailed information about the administered dosage form. However, expertise is required for interpretation of results. This technique also is susceptible to inducing uncontrolled bleeding and can cause retention of blood and food in stomach and upper GIT.

Magnetic Resonance Imagining (MRI)

MRI is a noninvasive technology and used very frequently for different diagnostic purposes. It works on the basis of a powerful magnetic field to provide detailed images of various parts of the human body. Usually, iron powder is incorporated into GRDDS to take images of administered dosage form in GIT [73]. It is safer than other techniques because harmful radioisotopes are not required for taking images. However, it is not suited to sinking systems due to their iron content.

^{13}C Octanoic Acid Breath Test

In this test, GRDDS is formulated with ^{13}C octanoic acid. After administration, ^{13}C octanoic acid reacts with gastric contents and produces CO_2, which comes out with breath. This CO_2 contains very tiny amounts of constantly liberated carbon ^{13}C until GRDDS is retained in the stomach whereas, in the intestine, ^{13}C octanoic acid does not react as the contents are alkaline and CO_2 is not evolved, leaving us with a very clear demarcating technique.

Ultrasonography

Ultrasonic waves have the capacity to move through biological tissues and other surfaces and can reflect back in response to a change in density. These reflected waves can be used to measure position of any object that reflects them. Electronic sources are used to map a detailed structure of the object. Generally, this technique is used for evaluation of in situ gelling systems, superporous hydrogels, and swelling systems. Mucoadhesive systems can also be evaluated using this technique because these waves can assess the interaction between the gastric wall and the mucoadhesive system.

REGULATORY CONSIDERATIONS

Scale-Up and Postapproval Changes

Scale-up of a developed formulation is required to assess reproducible product quality and adaptability of manufacturing process by prominent machines in production houses. Development of small batches in laboratories is not as difficult as large-scale manufacturing of products at industrial scale. Consequently, much innovative research has been limited to laboratories. For example, industrial scale-up of expandable GRDDS is difficult, and their commercialization is not easy. Therefore, it is necessary to do process validation of the new drug product. The US-FDA provides a guideline for process validation, titled "guidance for industry process validation: general principles and practices" [74]. This guideline provides all relevant information about process validation of a drug product.

Postapproval changes include modification of manufacturing process, analytical procedures, and packaging of drug product after its US-FDA marketing approval. According to US-FDA, it is necessary to produce scale-up data of first three batches during registration of a new drug product. Moreover, after getting marketing authorization, any changes made in drug product, such as excipient(s) or changes in initial material for preparation of active moiety is considered to be a postapproval change, and it is necessary to provide new scale-up data of the modified product to the US-FDA. Scale-up and postapproval change (SUPAC) guidelines are issued by US-FDA, titled "guidance for industry SUPAC-IR/MR: immediate release and modified release solid oral dosage forms manufacturing equipment addendum" to successfully achieve the quality and reproducibility of product [75].

Bioequivalence/Bioavailability Studies

In vivo performance is a major hurdle for market success of GRDDS. There is always a question hovering over successful in vivo performance of GRDDS due to intersubject variability due to alterations of physiology. Currently, several patents have expired between 2008 and 2015, and several more are on verge of expiry. So generic drug manufacturing companies can bypass the overload of bioequivalence studies and minimize regulatory burden. Initially, it is necessary to assess BCS-based class of drug. The US-FDA classifies drugs in four categories based on their solubility and permeability (Figure 4.5). The European Medicines Agency provides guidelines titled "guidelines on investigation of bioequivalence" [76]. According to these guidelines, if a drug product falls into BCS Class I and releases it contents within 15 minutes, there is no need to perform bioequivalence studies. A biowaiver application can be filed for BCS Class I and Class III drugs whereas it is necessary to improve solubility of Class II drugs before filing such a biowaiver application. The US-FDA database "bioequivalence recommendations for specific products" is a good tool for deciding requirements of a bioequivalence study. This database comprises details and protocols of bioequivalence studies registered to the US-FDA. The US-FDA also issues guidelines for bioavailability and bioequivalence studies for orally administered drug products.

CONCLUSION

GRDDS have tremendous potential in delivery of OSDDS. They can improve bioavailability and therapeutic value of various drugs, which have solubility-, stability-, and absorption-related issues in the GIT. However, it is necessary to evaluate physicochemical and biological properties of the API prior to its incorporation in a GRDDS. It is necessary to conceive whether the proposed GRDDS would actually improve therapeutic value of the subjected drug.

Various gastroretentive technologies have been developed, and they can efficiently improve GRT of dosage forms. The associated drawbacks with these technologies can be negated by development of efficient dual working systems. Mucoadhesive-, floating-, and swelling-based systems have gotten priority because they give excellent in vivo performance. An optimized GRDDS should fulfill primary requirements, such as predictable GRT as per the clinical requirement, and the system should be completely biodegradable.

REFERENCES

1. Davis SS. Formulation strategies for absorption windows. *Drug Discovery Today.* 2005;10(4):249–57.
2. Chawla G, Gupta P, Koradia V, Bansal AK. Gastroretention a means to address regional variability in intestinal drug absorption. *Pharmaceutical Technology.* 2003;July:50–68.
3. Bardonnet PL, Faivre V, Pugh WJ, Piffaretti JC, Falson F. Gastroretentive dosage forms: Overview and special case of *Helicobacter pylori. Journal of Controlled Release.* 2006;111(1–2):1–18.
4. Streubel A, Siepmann J, Bodmeier R. Gastroretentive drug delivery systems. *Expert Opinion on Drug Delivery.* 2006;3(2):217–33.
5. Pawar VK, Kansal S, Garg G, Awasthi R, Singodia D, Kulkarni GT. Gastroretentive dosage forms: A review with special emphasis on floating drug delivery systems. *Drug Delivery.* 2011 Feb;18(2):97–110. PubMed PMID: 20958237. Epub 2010/10/21. eng.
6. Mostafavi A, Emami J, Varshosaz J, Davies NM, Rezazadeh M. Development of a prolonged-release gastroretentive tablet formulation of ciprofloxacin hydrochloride: Pharmacokinetic characterization in healthy human volunteers. *International Journal of Pharmaceutics.* 2011;409(1–2):128–36.
7. Chavanpatil M, Jain P, Chaudhari S, Shear R, Vavia P. Development of sustained release gastroretentive drug delivery system for ofloxacin: In vitro and in vivo evaluation. *International Journal of Pharmaceutics.* 2005;304(1–2):178–84.
8. Hu L, Li L, Yang X, Liu W, Yang J, Jia Y et al. Floating matrix dosage form for dextromethorphan hydrobromide based on gas forming technique: In vitro and in vivo evaluation in healthy volunteers. *European Journal of Pharmaceutical Sciences.* 2011;42(1–2):99–105.

9. Awasthi R, Kulkarni GT, Pawar VK, Garg G. Optimization studies on gastroretentive floating system using response surface methodology. *AAPS PharmSciTech.* 2012 Mar;13(1):85–93. PubMed PMID: 22135108. Pubmed Central PMCID: 3299452. Epub 2011/12/03. eng.
10. Kumar P, Singh S, Mishra B. Floating osmotic drug delivery system of ranitidine hydrochloride: Development and evaluation—A technical note. *AAPS PharmSciTech.* 2008;9:480–5.
11. Nur AO, Zhang JS. Recent progress in sustained/controlled oral delivery of captopril: An overview. *International Journal of Pharmaceutics.* 2000;194(2):139–46.
12. Streubel A, Siepmann J, Bodmeier R. Drug delivery to the upper small intestine window using gastroretentive technologies. *Current Opinion in Pharmacology.* 2006;6(5):501–8.
13. Fara JW, Myrback RE, Swanson DR. Evaluation of oxprenolol and metoprolol Oros systems in the dog: Comparison of in vivo and in vitro drug release, and of drug absorption from duodenal and colonic infusion sites. *British Journal of Clinical Pharmacology.* 1985;19 Suppl 2:91S–5S. PubMed PMID: 4005134. Pubmed Central PMCID: PMC1463751. Epub 1985/01/01. eng.
14. Pawar VK, Meher JG, Singh Y, Chaurasia M, Surendar Reddy B, Chourasia MK. Targeting of gastrointestinal tract for amended delivery of protein/peptide therapeutics: Strategies and industrial perspectives. *Journal of Controlled Release.* 2014 12/28/;196:168–83.
15. Pawar VK, Kansal S, Asthana S, Chourasia MK. Industrial perspective of gastroretentive drug delivery systems: Physicochemical, biopharmaceutical, technological and regulatory consideration. *Expert Opinion on Drug Delivery.* 2012 May;9(5):551–65. PubMed PMID: 22512596. Epub 2012/04/20. eng.
16. Patel D, Patel N, Patel V, Bhatt D. Floating granules of ranitidine hydrochloride-gelucire 43/01: Formulation optimization using factorial design. *AAPS PharmSciTech.* 2007 2007/06/01;8(2):E25–E31. English.
17. Nayak A, Jain SK, Pandey RS. Controlling release of metformin HCl through incorporation into stomach specific floating alginate beads. *Molecular Pharmaceutics.* 2011 2011/12/05;8(6):2273–81.
18. Rouge N, Buri P, Doelker E. Drug absorption sites in the gastrointestinal tract and dosage forms for site-specific delivery. *International Journal of Pharmaceutics.* 1996 6/14/;136(1–2):117–39.
19. Prescott LF. Gastric emptying and drug absorption. *British Journal of Clinical Pharmacology.* 1974 Jun;1(3):189–90. PubMed PMID: 22454945. Pubmed Central PMCID: PMC1402550. Epub 1974/06/01. eng.
20. Arora S, Ali J, Ahuja A, Khar RK, Baboota S. Floating drug delivery system: A review. *AAPS PharmSciTech.* 2005;6(3):E372–E90.
21. Shargel LWP, Susanna BC, Yu A. *Applied Biopharmaceutics & Pharmacokinetics* 5th ed: McGraw-Hill Medical; 2005.
22. Singh BN, Kim KH. Floating drug delivery systems: An approach to oral controlled drug delivery via gastric retention. *Journal of Controlled Release.* 2000 2/3/;63(3):235–59.
23. Amidon G, Lennernäs H, Shah V, Crison J. A theoretical basis for a biopharmaceutic drug classification: The correlation of in vitro drug product dissolution and in vivo bioavailability. *Pharmaceutical Research.* 1995 1995/03/01;12(3):413–20. English.
24. Meka L, Kesavan B, Kalamata VN, Eaga CM, Bandari S, Vobalaboina V et al. Design and evaluation of polymeric coated minitablets as multiple unit gastroretentive floating drug delivery systems for furosemide. *Journal of Pharmaceutical Sciences.* 2009;98(6):2122–32.
25. Nur AO, Zhang JS. Captopril floating and/or bioadhesive tablets: Design and release kinetics. *Drug Development and Industrial Pharmacy.* 2000;26(9):965–9.

26. Kagan L, Hoffman A. Systems for region selective drug delivery in the gastrointestinal tract: Biopharmaceutical considerations. *Expert Opinion on Drug Delivery.* 2008;5(6):681–92. PubMed PMID: 18532923.
27. Mouly S, Paine M. P-Glycoprotein increases from proximal to distal regions of human small intestine. *Pharmaceutical Research.* 2003 2003/10/01;20(10):1595–9. English.
28. Groning R, Berntgen M, Georgarakis M. Acyclovir serum concentrations following peroral administration of magnetic depot tablets and the influence of extracorporal magnets to control gastrointestinal transit. *European Journal of Pharmaceutics and Biopharmaceutics.* 1998;46(3):285–91.
29. Rouge N, Allémann E, Gex-Fabry M, Balant L, Cole E, Buri P et al. Comparative pharmacokinetic study of a floating multiple-unit capsule, a high-density multiple-unit capsule and an immediate-release tablet containing 25 mg atenolol. *Pharmaceutica Acta Helvetiae.* 1998;73(2):81–7.
30. Wang YP, Gan Y, Zhang XX. Novel gastroretentive sustained-release tablet of tacrolimus based on self-microemulsifying mixture: In vitro evaluation and in vivo bioavailability test. *Acta Pharmacologica Sinica.* 2011;32:1294–302.
31. Kumar P, Singh S, Mishra B. Floating Osmotic Drug Delivery System of Ranitidine Hydrochloride: Development and Evaluation—A Technical Note. *AAPS PharmSciTech.* 2008 2008/06/01;9(2):480–5. English.
32. Jain SK, Awasthi AM, Jain NK, Agrawal GP. Calcium silicate based microspheres of repaglinide for gastroretentive floating drug delivery: Preparation and in vitro characterization. *Journal of Controlled Release.* 2005;107(2):300–9.
33. Wei Z, Yu Z, Bi D. Design and evaluation of a two-layer floating tablet for gastric retention using cisapride as a model drug. *Drug Development and Industrial Pharmacy.* 2001;27(5):469–74. PubMed PMID: 11448055.
34. Madgulkar A, Kadam S, Pokharkar V. Studies on formulation development of mucoadhesive sustained release itraconazole tablet using response surface methodology. *AAPS PharmSciTech.* 2008 2008/09/01;9(3):998–1005. English.
35. Abdelbary A, El-Gazayerly O, El-Gendy N, Ali A. Floating tablet of trimetazidine dihydrochloride: An approach for extended release with zero-order kinetics. *AAPS PharmSciTech.* 2010 2010/09/01;11(3):1058–67. English.
36. Srinatha A, Pandit JK. Multi-unit floating alginate system: Effect of additives on ciprofloxacin release. *Drug Delivery.* 2008;15(7):471–6. PubMed PMID: 18712625.
37. Liu Q, Fassihi R. Zero-order delivery of a highly soluble, low dose drug alfuzosin hydrochloride via gastro-retentive system. *International Journal of Pharmaceutics.* 2008;348(1–2):27–34.
38. Klausner EA, Eyal S, Lavy E, Friedman M, Hoffman A. Novel levodopa gastroretentive dosage form: In-vivo evaluation in dogs. *Journal of Controlled Release.* 2003;88(1):117–26.
39. Garg R, Gupta GD. Preparation and evaluation of gastroretentive floating tablets of silymarin. *Chemical and Pharmaceutical Bulletin.* 2009;57(6):545–9.
40. El-Kamel AH, Sokar MS, Al Gamal SS, Naggar VF. Preparation and evaluation of ketoprofen floating oral delivery system. *International Journal of Pharmaceutics.* 2001;220(1–2):13–21.
41. Patel A, Modasiya M, Shah D, Patel V. Development and In Vivo Floating Behavior of Verapamil HCl Intragastric Floating Tablets. *AAPS PharmSciTech.* 2009 2009/03/01;10(1):310–5. English.
42. El-Gibaly I. Development and in vitro evaluation of novel floating chitosan microcapsules for oral use: Comparison with non-floating chitosan microspheres. *International Journal of Pharmaceutics.* 2002;249(1–2):7–21.

43. Hejazi R, Amiji M. Stomach-specific anti-*H. pylori* therapy. I: Preparation and characterization of tetracyline-loaded chitosan microspheres. *International Journal of Pharmaceutics*. 2002;235(1–2):87–94.
44. Sato Y, Kawashima Y, Takeuchi H, Yamamoto H, Fujibayashi Y. Pharmacoscintigraphic evaluation of riboflavin-containing microballoons for a floating controlled drug delivery system in healthy humans. *Journal of Controlled Release*. 2004;98(1):75–85.
45. Chueh HR, Zia H, Rhodes CT. Optimization of sotalol floating and bioadhesive extended release tablet formulations. *Drug Development and Industrial Pharmacy*. 1995;21(15):1725–47.
46. Simoni P, Cerrè C, Cipolla A, Polimeni C, Pistillo A, Ceschel G et al. Bioavailability study of a new, sinking, enteric-coated ursodeoxycholic acid formulation. *Pharmacological Research*. 1995;31(2):115–9.
47. Davis DW. Method of swallowing a pill. US Patent, 3, 418, 999, December 31, 1968.
48. Talukder R, Fassihi R. Gastroretentive Delivery Systems: A Mini Review. *Drug Development and Industrial Pharmacy*. 2004;30(10):1019–28. PubMed PMID: 15595568.
49. Streubel A, Siepmann J, Bodmeier R. Floating matrix tablets based on low density foam powder: Effects of formulation and processing parameters on drug release. *European Journal of Pharmaceutical Sciences*. 2003;18(1):37–45.
50. Narendra C, Srinath MS, Babu G. Optimization of bilayer floating tablet containing metoprolol tartrate as a model drug for gastric retention. *AAPS PharmSciTech*. 2006 2006/06/01;7(2):E23–E9. English.
51. Dorożyński P, Jachowicz R, Kulinowski P, Kwieciński S, Szybiński K, Skórka T et al. The Macromolecular polymers for the preparation of hydrodynamically balanced systems—Methods of evaluation. *Drug Development and Industrial Pharmacy*. 2004;30(9):947–57. PubMed PMID: 15554219.
52. Soppimath KS, Kulkarni AR, Rudzinski WE, Aminabhavi TM. Microspheres as floating drug-delivery systems to increase gastric retention of drugs. *Drug Metabolism Reviews*. 2001;33(2):149–60. PubMed PMID: 11495501.
53. Bulgarelli E, Forni F, Bernabei MT. Effect of matrix composition and process conditions on casein-gelatin beads floating properties. *Int J Pharm*. 2000 Apr 5;198(2):157–65. PubMed PMID: 10767565.
54. Rajinikanth PS, Mishra B. Floating in situ gelling system for stomach site-specific delivery of clarithromycin to eradicate *H. pylori*. *Journal of Controlled Release*. 2008;125(1):33–41.
55. Rajinikanth PS, Balasubramaniam J, Mishra B. Development and evaluation of a novel floating in situ gelling system of amoxicillin for eradication of Helicobacter pylori. *International Journal of Pharmaceutics*. 2007 4/20/;335(1–2):114–22.
56. Mašić I, Ilić I, Dreu R, Ibrić S, Parojčić J, Đurić Z. An investigation into the effect of formulation variables and process parameters on characteristics of granules obtained by in situ fluidized hot melt granulation. *International Journal of Pharmaceutics*. 2012 2/28/;423(2):202–12.
57. Shimpi S, Chauhan B, Mahadik KR, Paradkar A. Preparation and evaluation of diltiazem hydrochloride-gelucire 43/01 floating granules prepared by melt granulation. *AAPS PharmSciTech*. 2004 2004/09/01;5(3):51–6. English.
58. Krögel I, Bodmeier R. Development of a multifunctional matrix drug delivery system surrounded by an impermeable cylinder. *Journal of Controlled Release*. 1999;61(1–2):43–50.
59. Raut Desai S, Rohera BD. Formulation, in vitro evaluation and study of variables on tri-layered gastro-retentive delivery system of diltiazem HCl. *Drug Development and Industrial Pharmacy*. 1–10. PubMed PMID: 23369093.

60. Klausner EA, Lavy E, Friedman M, Hoffman A. Expandable gastroretentive dosage forms. *Journal of Controlled Release*. 2003;90(2):143–62.
61. Gröning R, Cloer C, Georgarakis M, Müller RS. Compressed collagen sponges as gastroretentive dosage forms: In vitro and in vivo studies. *European Journal of Pharmaceutical Sciences*. 2007;30(1):1–6.
62. Park H, Park K, Kim D. Preparation and swelling behavior of chitosan-based superporous hydrogels for gastric retention application. *Journal of Biomedical Materials Research Part A*. 2006;76A(1):144–50.
63. Chun M-K, Sah H, Choi H-K. Preparation of mucoadhesive microspheres containing antimicrobial agents for eradication of H. pylori. *International Journal of Pharmaceutics*. 2005;297(1–2):172–9.
64. Umamaheshwari RB, Jain S, Jain NK. A New Approach in Gastroretentive Drug Delivery System Using Cholestyramine. *Drug delivery*. 2003;10(3):151–60. PubMed PMID: 12944135.
65. Singh Y, Singh M, Meher JG, Pawar VK, Chourasia MK. Trichotomous gastric retention of amorphous capecitabine: An attempt to overcome pharmacokinetic gap. *International Journal of Pharmaceutics*. 2015;478(2):811–21.
66. Chavanpatil MD, Jain P, Chaudhari S, Shear R, Vavia PR. Novel sustained release, swellable and bioadhesive gastroretentive drug delivery system for ofloxacin. *International Journal of Pharmaceutics*. 2006;316(1–2):86–92.
67. Zou H, Jiang X, Kong L, Gao S. Design and evaluation of a dry coated drug delivery system with floating–pulsatile release. *Journal of Pharmaceutical Sciences*. 2008;97(1):263–73.
68. Badve SS, Sher P, Korde A, Pawar AP. Development of hollow/porous calcium pectinate beads for floating-pulsatile drug delivery. *European Journal of Pharmaceutics and Biopharmaceutics*. 2007;65(1):85–93.
69. Pileni MP. *Structure and reactivity in reverse micelles*. 1989.
70. Rinaudc M, Pavlov G, Desbrieres J. Solubilization of chitosan in strong acid medium. *International Journal of Polymer Analysis and Characterization*. 1999;5(3):267–76.
71. Goole J, Van Gansbeke B, Pilcer G, Deleuze P, Blocklet D, Goldman S et al. Pharmacoscintigraphic and pharmacokinetic evaluation on healthy human volunteers of sustained-release floating minitablets containing levodopa and carbidopa. *International Journal of Pharmaceutics*. 2008;364(1):54–63.
72. Klausner E, Lavy E, Barta M, Cserepes E, Friedman M, Hoffman A. Novel Gastroretentive Dosage Forms: Evaluation of Gastroretentivity and Its Effect on Levodopa Absorption in Humans. *Pharmaceutical research*. 2003 2003/09/01;20(9):1466–73. English.
73. Dorożyński P, Kulinowski P, Jachowicz R, Jasiński A. Development of a system for simultaneous dissolution studies and magnetic resonance imaging of water transport in hydrodynamically balanced systems: A technical note. *AAPS PharmSciTech*. 2007 2007/03/01;8(1):E109–E12. English.
74. Guidance for Industry Process Validation: General Principles and Practices. Center for Drug Evaluation and Research (CDER), U.S. Department of Health and Human Services, Food and Drug Administration, (2011). Available at: http://www.fda.gov/downloads/Drugs/GuidanceComplianceRegulatoryInformation/Guidances/UCM070336.pdf.
75. Guidance for Industry SUPAC-IR/MR: Immediate Release and Modified Release Solid Oral Dosage Forms Manufacturing Equipment Addendum Center for Drug Evaluation and Research (CDER), U.S. Department of Health and Human Services, Food and Drug Administration, (1999). Available at: http://wwwfdagov/downloads/Drugs/GuidanceComplianceRegulatoryInformation/Guidances/UCM070637.
76. Guideline on the investigation of bioequivalence. Committee for medicinal products for human use (chmp), european medicines agency, (2008). Available at: http://www.Ema.Europa.Eu/pdfs/human/qwp/140198enrev1.Pdf.

5 Invasive versus Noninvasive Delivery of Insulin

Sandra Soares, Ana Costa, Pedro Fonte, and Bruno Sarmento

CONTENTS

INTRODUCTION

Insulin is a therapeutic protein widely used for diabetes mellitus management, being used as insulin replacement in Type 1 diabetes mellitus (T1DM) patients or adjuvant of oral antidiabetic agents in Type 2 diabetes mellitus (T2DM). It is preferably administered by subcutaneous (SC) injection because of limited pharmacokinetics (PK), especially due to low absorption caused by high molecular weight and hydrophilicity. Nevertheless, due to some advances, new needle-free systems that enable insulin delivery through oral, nasal, pulmonary, and transdermal routes have been developed, offering patients more comfort during administration.

However, the big challenge of achieving a worthy bioavailability (BA) through noninvasive formulations remains. It is crucial that a new insulin delivery system presents a BA high enough to overcome the bias related to an unconventional therapeutic compared to a well-established route of administration, such as SC insulin injection. In parallel, its efficacy in the metabolic control and the undesired hypoglycemic events are some concerns to take into account. The frequency of administration, convenience of application, easy handling, cost-effectiveness ratio, and concerns about long-term effects are key points to convince diabetic patients adhering to any insulin therapy, so a great effort has been made to find different insulin delivery system options.

In this chapter, the available invasive and noninvasive routes of administration to deliver insulin in the body are focused on. In addition, the delivery systems used on both routes are also discussed.

INSULIN DELIVERY THROUGH INVASIVE ROUTE

Insulin is usually administered through SC injections in different body areas, such as upper arms, thighs, or abdomen (Gómez-Pérez and Rull 2005; Guerci and Sauvanet 2005). It can be administered through syringes or by insulin pen injection. However, pen devices present several advantages over syringes because they present more comfort during administration, are easier to use, and allow accurate insulin dose administration. They are more reliable since they have an automated stopping system, which ensures the proper insulin dose delivery. In these devices, insulin can be supplied in prefilled pens or in disposable cartridges (Stewart, Wilson, and Rider 2004; Lteif and Schwenk 1999; Flood 2006). Nonetheless, both systems may cause lipodystrophy and require needles for insulin delivery, enabling its reuse during administration and, consequently, the increased possibility of blood viral infections, namely human immunodeficiency virus.

Insulin can be also administered through infusion pumps, allowing continuous insulin administration during the day despite the discomfort felt by patients (Flood 2006).

Therefore, there are different insulin analogs (IA) able to be delivered through the SC route, which present several PK and pharmacodynamics (PD) profiles according to patients' needs.

Insulin Analogs

Insulin was discovered in 1922, and it was obtained from animal sources, namely pig and cow (Burge, Rassam, and Schade 1998; Pillai and Panchagnula 2001). Despite that remarkable step in diabetes therapy, it presented some limitations because insulin from animal sources presents structural differences from human insulin, creating higher risks of immunogenicity problems. Furthermore, insulin requires a purification process during its manufacturing, being usually contaminated with foreign proteins, inducing antibodies formation (Burge, Rassam, and Schade 1998). With the development of biotechnology, insulin started to be produced through recombinant DNA (rDNA) technology. Regular human insulin (RHI) was the first IA marketed, but another analogs were developed with the purpose of satisfying different diabetic patients' needs in order to have better glycemic control in different daily situations (prandial or postprandial) with fewer side effects and with high patient compliance. Each IA presents some structural changes when compared with RHI, affecting its PK and PD properties, so IA are usually classified in terms of duration of activity, insulin peak concentration, and onset of action (Rys et al. 2011). In Table 5.1, the different IAs, their PK profile, and structural modification regarding human insulin along with some important features are described.

Rapid-Acting Insulin Analogs

Rapid-acting IAs are characterized by their fast onset of action as they are able to be administered 5 minutes before a meal and to have a short duration of action, reaching the insulin peak higher than other analogs (Gómez-Pérez and Rull 2005), mimicking the endogenous postprandial insulin better than RHI (Rolla 2008). These analogs differ from human insulin by the modification of one or two amino acids (see Table 5.1), which occur in the end of the B-chain, allowing the decrease of the hexameric form (Home 2012) and, consequently, the reduction of propensity of insulin self-aggregation. After SC administration, insulin forms monomers (Rolla 2008) that are able to be rapidly absorbed into the bloodstream.

The first rapid-acting IA to reach the market was insulin lispro (ILis) (Burge, Rassam, and Schade 1998). It demonstrates comparable glucose control as well the same incidence of severe hypoglycemia events as RHI (Eli Lilly and Company 2013). Due to its short duration of action, it causes better postprandial glucose (PPG) and glycated hemoglobin (HbA_{1c}) control, especially when administered two times a day, combined with neutral protamine hagerdorn (NPH), regarding the usual diabetic regimen (combination of RHI and NPH) (Sargin et al. 2003; Hoffman et al. 2002).

Insulin aspart (IAsp) is produced by recombinant technology using *Sacharomyces cerevisae*, and it was showed to be a good tool for mealtime coverage as it is able to reduce the PPG, improving overall glycemic control and HbA_{1c} in both types of diabetes (Lindholm, McEwen, and Riis 1999; Mannucci, Monami, and Marchionni 2009; Home, Barriocanal, and Lindholm 1999; Home, Lindholm, and Riis 2000). It has also associated with fewer nocturnal hypoglycemic events, improving patients' quality of life (Home et al. 2006).

In parallel, insulin glulisine (IGlu) is another novel rapid-acting IA able to mimic physiologic insulin better than RHI with a shorter duration of action but with a faster onset of action in both types of diabetes (Dailey et al. 2004; EMA 2013). A study proved the efficiency and safety of IGlu by showing that analogs combined with NPH provide better glucose control in T2DM compared to RHI (Dailey et al. 2004). It was also associated with a better PPG and less risk of hypoglycemic events, one of the main concerns among T2DM patients (Rayman, Profozic, and Middle 2007). Despite this, analogs have not shown significant improvements in HbA_{1c} levels; compared to RHI in T2DM (Rayman, Profozic, and Middle 2007) it was shown to be equivalent or better at efficiently reducing HbA_{1c} levels in T1DM when administrated at premeal times (Garg, Rosenstock, and Ways 2005).

Among rapid-acting IAs, it was verified that they have similar PK and PD, but IGlu has a faster onset of action (Home 2012; Luzio et al. 2008; Heise et al. 2007),

TABLE 5.1
Different Types of IA, PK Parameters, Structural Modifications from Human Insulin and Remarks

	Pharmacokinetics Parameters	Structural Modifications	Remarks	Ref.
Insulin lispro Humalog® Eli Lilly (Indianapolis, IN)	Onset: 15 minutes Peak: 30–70 minutes Duration of action: 2–5 hours	Inversion of two amino acid residues: proline and lysine at positions B28 and B29, respectively	When intramuscularly injected has identical effect. Low variability on absorption rate when compared with RHI after injection in different body areas. Gives to patient a better quality life when compared with regular insulin. After administration patient must start to eat immediately. Can be mixed only with NPH insulin. Can be delivered 15 minutes before the meal or immediately after starting the meal. Onset do not significantly depends on the local of injection.	(Gómez-Pérez and Rull 2005; EMA 2013; Eli Lilly and Company 2013; Burge, Rassam, and Schade 1998)
Insulin aspart Novolog® and NovoRapid® Novo Nordisk (Bagsvaerd, Denmark)	Onset: 10–20 minutes Peak: 1–3 hours Duration of action: 3–5 hours	Substitution of proline at position 28 of B-chain by aspartic acid	Lower incidence of hypoglycemia. Allows a postprandial administration, nonetheless preprandial administration is preferable. Gives to patient a better quality of life comparatively to RHI. Significantly less intra-individual variability than RHI for reaching the maximum concentration. Can only be mixed with NPH.	(EMA 2013; Novo Nordisk 2013; Rolla 2008)

(Continued)

TABLE 5.1 (CONTINUED)
Different Types of IA, PK Parameters, Structural Modifications from Human Insulin and Remarks

	Pharmacokinetics Parameters	Structural Modifications	Remarks	Ref.
Insulin glulisine Apidra® Sanofi-Aventis (Paris, France)	Onset (min): 5–15 minutes Peak (h): 0.5–2 hours Duration of action: 3–5 hours	Double substitution at B-chain: lysine for asparagine at position 3 and glutamate for lysine at position 29	Treatment flexibility: can be delivered 15 minutes before or 20 minutes after starting the meal. Shorter duration of activity and faster onset than RHI and slight faster onset than other short-acting IA. Low plasma protein binding. Reduced hypoglycemic events.	(Hahr and Molitch 2010; EMA 2013; Home 2012; Sanofi-Aventis 2009)
Regular insulin Humulin® R Eli Lilly (Indianapolis, IN)	Onset: 15–30 minutes[a] Peak: 2–3 hours[a] Duration of action: 6–8 hours[a]	Similar to human insulin	Should be administrated 30 minutes before meal. Can be used in adults and children with T1DM and T2DM. U-500 allows the insulin-resistance patients management.	(de La Peña et al. 2011; Eli Lilly and Company 2013; Howey et al. 1994; Burge, Rassam, and Schade 1998)
NPH insulin Humulin N Eli Lilly (Indianapolis, IN)	Onset:1.0 ± 0.2 hours[b] Duration of action: 19.8 ± 5.8 hours[b]	Addition of protamine to regular insulin	Can be mixed with short- and rapid-acting IA. Variable peak increasing the risk of hypoglycemic events. Significant within-patient variability. Possibility of more than one daily administration.	(Abrahamson 2010; Hahr and Molitch 2010; Lepore et al. 2000; Eli Lilly and Company 2013; Wang, Carabino, and Vergara 2003)

(Continued)

TABLE 5.1 (CONTINUED)
Different Types of IA, PK Parameters, Structural Modifications from Human Insulin and Remarks

	Pharmacokinetics Parameters	Structural Modifications	Remarks	Ref.
Insulin Glargine Lantus® Sanofi-Aventis (Paris, France)	Onset: 1.5 ± 0.3 hours[c] Peak: No peak Duration of action: 20.5 ± 3.7 hours[c]	Replacement of asparagine at A21 position by a glicine and addition of 2 arginine residues at C-terminal position of B-chain	Peakless activity of IGlar, reducing the hypoglycemic effect. Allow to maintain the blood glucose control with less hypoglycemic events and weight gain. Less intersubject variability than NPH in T1DM but upper than IDet. Due to its acid pH, it cannot be mixed with other insulin types with a neutral pH and cause pain during injection.	(Hahr and Molitch 2010; Gómez-Pérez and Rull 2005; Rosenstock et al. 2000; Garg et al. 2004; Lepore et al. 2000; Heinemann 2008; DailyMed 2013)
Insulin Detemir Levemir® Novo Nordisk (Bagsvaerd, Denmark)	Onset: 1.6 ± 1.1 hours[d] Peak: 6–8 hours Duration of action: 19.9 ± 3.2 hours[d]	Remotion of threonine a B30 position and acylation of lysine with a carbon fatty acid chain (myristic acid) at position B29	Soluble at neutral pH. Reversible binding between insulin and albumin. The binding of IDet to albumin is not modified by substances capable of release free fatty acids such heparin or beta agonists. Allows to reduce the night hypoglycemic effect and has less variability with FBG. Depending on patient needs, it should be administered once or twice a day. Provides a good glucose control, with less hypoglycemic events.	(Hahr and Molitch 2010; Gómez-Pérez and Rull 2005; Heise et al. 2004; Plank et al. 2005; Novo Nordisk 2013; Nasrallah and Reynolds 2012)

(Continued)

TABLE 5.1 (CONTINUED)
Different Types of IA, PK Parameters, Structural Modifications from Human Insulin and Remarks

	Pharmacokinetics Parameters	Structural Modifications	Remarks	Ref.
Insulin degludec Tresiba® Novo Nordisk (Bagsvaerd, Denmark)	Onset: 30–90 minutes Peak: No peak Duration of action: Over 42 hours	Removal of last amino acid threonine at B30 position and the addition of hexadecandoioc fatty acid to lysine B29, using glutamic acid as a spacer	Long-time acting profile. Longer half-life than other long-acting IA. PK suitable to gives a daily flexible insulin-dosing regimens, improving the acceptance of insulin therapy, especially in patients with unpredictable lifestyles. Allows to maintain the glycemic control with a fixed dose. Decrease the hypoglycemic events, especially the nocturnal hypoglycemic, improving patients compliance. Can be coformulated in a soluble form with IAsp.	(Niskanen et al. 2012; Wakil and Atkin 2012; Novo Nordisk 2013; Nasrallah and Reynolds 2012; Heller et al. 2012; EMA 2013)

[a] Obtained for subcutaneous injection of 10U RHI in healthy nondiabetic men (Howey et al. 1994).
[b] Obtained for subcutaneous injection of 0.3 U/kg NPH in T1DM (Lepore et al. 2000).
[c] Obtained for subcutaneous injection of 0.3 U/kg IGlar in T1DM (Lepore et al. 2000).
[d] Obtained for subcutaneous injection of 0.4 U/kg IDet in T1DM (Plank et al. 2005).

which can be explained by the type of formulation: IAsp and ILis contain zinc in their formulations to improve their stability, which promotes the hexamer formation, delaying their dissociation and insulin absorption (Howey et al. 1994) whereas IGlu contains polysorbate 20, a surfactant agent able to reduce the unfolding protein, facilitating its dissociation when subcutaneously delivered (Home 2012; Luzio et al. 2008). However, this faster onset of IGlu is not clinically relevant (Heise et al. 2007; Home 2012).

Short-Acting Insulin Analogs

RHI is the only short-acting IA available on the market, and it is obtained through rDNA technology using *Escherichia coli* bacteria, being the end product structurally similar to human insulin.

RHI is available in two different doses (100 units/mL [U-100] and 500 units/mL [U-500]), or it can be mixed with isophane insulin, being used to improve blood glucose control in adults and children with both types of diabetes (Eli Lilly and Company 2013). Nonetheless, only U-500 enables the treatment of patients with insulin resistance (Eli Lilly and Company 2013) because a single dose is able to deliver a large amount of insulin with a short volume. Despite being used for many years at mealtimes, it presents a relatively slow onset and needs to be administrated 30 minutes before meals (Dailey et al. 2004), so this analog has been replaced by rapid-acting IA.

Intermediate-Acting Insulin

Isophane insulin or NPH is the only intermediate-acting IA available on the market, which results from the addition of protamine to RHI (Hahr and Molitch 2010), yielding a microcrystalline suspension for SC administration (Norrman, Hubálek, and Schluckebier 2007).

Due to the presence of protamine, which is responsible for stabilizing insulin in a hexameric form and, consequently, for prolonging its effect, it presents a duration of effect longer than RHI but even slower than long-acting-IA. (IGlar has zinc in its formulation, but the long-acting profile is also due to structural modifications of insulin.) Therefore, NPH presents a variable peak (see Table 5.1), likely increasing the hypoglycemic risk, mainly at night, so patients must receive it twice daily to have desirable glucose control (Rolla 2008). Also, when badly resuspended, NPH insulin can lead to a different rate of absorption, which results in irregular glucose levels (Jehle et al. 1999).

Long-Acting Insulin Analogs

Long-acting IAs provide daily blood glucose control, being considered as basal insulin. There are some strategies that prolong the time action of insulin, such as the addition of stabilizing agents, such as protamine or zinc, which stabilize insulin in a hexameric form, delay its absorption, and increase its time action (Rosenstock et al. 2000).

Another approach is the addition of positively charged amino acids at the C-terminal portion of the B-chain, which originate a shift in the isoelectric point from pH 5.4 toward pH 6.7. This modification allows the maintenance of IA in a soluble form at acid pH (Rolla 2008; Wang, Carabino, and Vergara 2003), so after administration through SC tissue, it precipitates at physiologic pH, delaying its absorption and prolonging the effect (Wang, Carabino, and Vergara 2003). Insulin glargine (IGlar) is a long-acting IA formulated by the change of some amino acid sequences of regular insulin as described in Table 5.1 (Hahr and Molitch 2010). IGlar formulation also contains zinc, which is responsible for stabilizing insulin in hexameric form (Gómez-Pérez and Rull 2005).

Several studies have demonstrated the good glycemic control achieved by IGlar alongside the decrease in weight gain in both T1DM and T2DM patients (Rosenstock et al. 2000; Garg et al. 2004). IGlar was also shown to be peakless over 24 hours, providing a basal insulin for both types of diabetes (McKeage and Goa 2001), and once-daily basal IGlar had more of an effect on reducing the fasting blood glucose (FBG) with lower insulin doses than NPH insulin (Rosenstock et al. 2000).

To also prolong the long-time action of insulin, a nonesterified fatty acid molecule can be reversibly coupled to the insulin molecule. It is the case of insulin detemir (IDet) (Rolla 2008), which is useful as a basal insulin for treatment of both diabetes types (Keating 2012). IDet was shown to be able to maintain glycemic control in T1DM patients with less variable duration of action and time effect profile than NPH. It was also demonstrated that FBG levels decreased significantly without increasing nocturnal hypoglycemia (Plank et al. 2005). In the case of T2DM, IDet combined with IAsp showed better glycemic control with lower weigh gain and less variation in prandial glucose and risk of nocturnal hypoglycemic events, constituting an option for combined traditional regimens, such as NPH and RHI (Rašlová et al. 2004; EMA 2013).

When IDet was compared with IGlar and NPH insulin, it was verified as a more predictable effect on glycemic control because IDet is formulated in solution, remaining in that state after administration in the SC tissue until interacting with the insulin receptor whereas the IGlar form microprecipitates after SC administration, which must be redissolved to be absorbed. As precipitation and redissolution steps present different individual rates, IGar presents an inherent variability on PK and PD (Heise et al. 2004; Guerci and Sauvanet 2005).

Recently, a novel, once-daily, ultralong-acting basal insulin was discovered and developed by Novo Nordisk (Bagsvaerd, Denmark), and it is known as insulin degludec (IDeg). Due to its structural modification, it allows the self-association of IDeg, leading to the formation of multihexamers able to form a SC depot, which is slowly absorbed into the bloodstream (Wakil and Atkin 2012).

It has already been approved in Europe and Japan for T1DM and T2DM as it offers good advantages compared to other long-acting IA: more than 42 hours of duration of action (Novo Nordisk 2013; EMA 2013), better glycemic control, and better flat time action profile (Wakil and Atkin 2012). There are also studies that reported lower hypoglycemic events in T2DM (Garber et al. 2012) and nocturnal hypoglycemic episodes and good glucose control in T1DM (Heller et al. 2012) as well when compared with IGlar.

Biphasic Insulin

The different IAs provide efficient glucose control in different situations: long-acting IA enables a basal insulin delivery during the day while short-acting IA allows insulin level coverage after meal ingestion. In order to avoid several and distinct administrations during the day, premixed insulins, also called as biphasic insulins, were developed, containing, in the same formulation, a mixture of short-acting IA with basal insulin (Rizvi and Ligthelm 2007). Table 5.2 shows the different biphasic insulin formulations available on the market.

Biphasic human insulin (BHI) is constituted by a mixture of NPH insulin with soluble RHI (see Table 5.2). It is characterized by a delayed onset of action, so its administration must be 30 minutes before a meal (EMA 2013) in order to avoid hyperglycemia after meal intake and posterior hypoglycemia events (Home, Barriocanal, and Lindholm 1999; Raja-Khan, Warehime, and Gabbay 2007). Nevertheless, there are other biphasic IAs with some advantages regarding BHI, mainly because they present rapid onset of action and short duration of action, so they may be administered as late as 15 minutes before meal or even immediately after (EMA 2013; Novo Nordisk 2013), allowing a better meal schedule. Neutral protamine lispro (NPL) is constituted by ILisp mixed with ILisp crystallized with protamine, which forms crystals responsible for its delayed absorption and long-acting effect (Gómez-Pérez and Rull 2005). Similarly, the aspart and crystallized aspart-protamine mixture is constituted by fast-acting IA and IAsp in a free state with a crystallized IAsp-protamine complex, which presents a PK profile similar to NPH insulin (Gómez-Pérez and Rull 2005; EMA 2013).

The mixture of different insulin types simplifies diabetes management in terms of number of administrations and reducing the errors related to two separate

TABLE 5.2
Marketed Biphasic Insulin Formulations

Brand Name	Company	Available Marketed Formulation	Delivery Device	Ref.
Humalog® Mix	Eli Lilly (Indianapolis, IN)	75% of NPL and 25% of ILisp 50% of NPL and 50% of ILisp	Vials, cartridges, or prefilled	(Eli Lilly and Company 2013; EMA 2013)
Mixtard®	Novo Nordisk (Bagsvaerd, Denmark)	10% RHI and 90% NPH 20% RHI and 80% NPH 30% RHI and 70% NPH 40% RHI and 60% NPH 50% RHI and 50% NPH	Vials, cartridges, or prefilled pens	(EMA 2013)
NovoMix® NovoLog® Mix	Novo Nordisk	70% IAsp protamine suspension and 30% IAsp 50% IAsp protamine suspension and 50% IAsp 30% IAsp protamine suspension and 70% IAsp	Cartridges or prefilled pen in the case of NovoMix; Vials and prefilled pens for NovoLog Mix	(EMA 2013; Novo Nordisk 2013)
Ryzodeg®	Novo Nordisk	70% IDeg and 30% IAsp	Prefilled pen	(EMA 2013)

administrations (Gómez-Pérez and Rull 2005). Providing a basal and mealtime insulin delivery, these mixtures are usually administered twice a day during breakfast and dinner. Several studies in T2DM described that biphasic insulin combined with oral therapy had the ability to reduce PPG (Malone et al. 2005; Raskin et al. 2007; Halimi et al. 2005) and nocturnal hypoglycemia (Malone et al. 2005; Davidson et al. 2009) and to improve HbA_{1c} levels (Malone et al. 2005; Raskin et al. 2007; Raskin et al. 2005), compared to other insulin therapy regimens.

Biphasic insulin aspart 30 (BIAsp 30) is the most studied biphasic insulin. Compared to BHI and biphasic insulin Lispro 25, BIAsp 30 was shown to be more effective in terms of PPG control in T2DM subjects (McSorley et al. 2002; Kapitza, Rave et al. 2004; Hermansen et al. 2002); however, studies reported minor hypoglycemic episodes (Raskin et al. 2007; Raskin et al. 2005) and an increased weight gain (Raskin et al. 2007).

There is a shortage of studies relative to the use of biphasic insulin in T1DM, maybe due to the fact that these patients require different doses of prandial insulin, which must be independent of basal insulin (Rizvi and Ligthelm 2007). A 12-week study performed by Chen et al. showed that BIAsp 30 administered three times a day was able to improve the long-term glycemic control with significant HbA_{1c} improvement compared to human insulin (Chen et al. 2006). Moreover, Boehm et al. also showed that BIAsp 30 reduced the PPG when injected two times a day (Boehm et al. 2002). Furthermore, the risk of hypoglycemic episodes and premeal blood glucose control and the overall glycemic control of Humalog® Mix50 was equivalent to human insulin when administrated as a basal bolus regimen, suggesting the ability of that formulation to maintain insulin levels between meals (Herz et al. 2002).

Recently, Novo Nordisk developed a new product for T1DM and T2DM adults, which was approved by EMA in 2013 (EMA 2013). It contains a soluble mixture of IDeg coformulated with IAsp, providing, at the same time, prandial and postprandial glycemic control (Novo Nordisk 2013). Relatively to BIAsp 30, it showed a 58% lower rate of hypoglycemic events, which was considered beneficial to patients (Niskanen et al. 2012).

Biphasic insulin is a good option for T2DM patients, providing, at the same time, basal and mealtime insulin coverage with a better mimic of physiologic insulin (Rizvi and Ligthelm 2007). These mixtures are intended to be administered at breakfast and dinner, constituting a good option when optimal glycemic control is not achieved or in the case of patients with complex diabetic therapeutic regimens. They don't require insulin mixtures; however, due to the fixed proportion of each component of the mixture, it is impossible to make adjustments, reducing the flexibility of dose regimens (Rizvi and Ligthelm 2007).

Sometimes, patients can require supplementation with short-acting IA in cases of extreme hyperglycemia, such as stress or sickness. When the period between meals is too long, early morning and postlunch hyperglycemia are possible to occur, which are solved with distinct doses of short-acting and basal insulin at different times (Rizvi and Ligthelm 2007).

Biphasic insulins can be supplied in disposable and multidose prefilled pens, in cartridges or vials with disposable needles for being delivered through reusable pens or syringes for SC injection (see Table 5.2).

NONINVASIVE INSULIN DELIVERY SYSTEMS

Oral Insulin Delivery Systems

The most desirable administration route for insulin delivery is the oral route because it is totally noninvasive, economic, painless, and easy to handle without using complicated delivery devices or needles, so it is the most propitious approach to catch patient compliance (Soares, Costa, and Sarmento 2012).

As insulin is transported immediately to the liver through a portal vein after its absorption at the gastrointestinal tract (GIT), the oral route allows a better mimic of physiologic insulin and consequently allows better glucose control, decreasing peripheral hyperinsulinemia with fewer hypoglycemic events, also preventing weight gain (Arbit and Kidron 2009). Despite these advantages, when administered by the oral route, insulin faces enzymatic or physical barriers, which lead to poor BA.

Insulin, as well as dietary proteins, is cleaved in the GIT by enzymes into amino acids, which may be absorbed by the intestinal epithelium. Therefore, orally delivered proteins result in a very low BA, usually less than 1%–2% (Pauletti et al. 1996). In fact, enzymes present in the GIT are the most important barrier to insulin oral delivery. The major proteases include pepsin in the stomach and trypsin, chymotrypsin, and carboxypeptidases in the small intestine, responsible for about 20% of protein enzymatic digestion (Pauletti et al. 1996). The remainder of the degradation occurs at the brush border membrane or even within the enterocytes. Furthermore, there is also an insulin-specific enzyme, called insulin-degrading enzyme, located in the cytosol, constituting the majority of insulin-degrading activity (Bai and Chang 1995). During past years, many attempts have been made in order to overcome insulin enzymatic digestion, but it remains a difficult challenge because only one or two of these enzymes are needed to compromise insulin structure, leading to denaturation and biological inactivity.

Another important barrier to insulin uptake is the intestinal epithelium itself because it constitutes a physical barrier that is made of a single layer of columnar cells supported by the *lamina propria* and *muscularis mucosa*. The tight junctions (*zona occludens*) between those cells also prevent insulin transport by the paracellular pathway. The *microvilli* present on the apical surface of epithelial cells is able to increase the absorptive intestinal area by about twofold (Wang 1996), but it also contains proteases that break down the protein structure. On the epithelium surface, there is a layer of mucus, containing glycoproteins, enzymes, electrolytes, and water, and glycocalyx (Carino and Mathiowitz 1999), which represent additional physical barriers to insulin uptake. Furthermore, the absence of selective mechanisms for insulin uptake and its unpredictable transit time in the GIT also constitute important barriers.

Due to all the barriers that insulin faces in the GIT, its intestinal uptake is negligible. Therefore, a proper delivery system able to overcome all these barriers and improve insulin oral BA is needed. Several strategies, such as using absorption enhancers, protease inhibitors, enteric coatings, modified insulin molecules, and also micro and nanoparticle encapsulation of insulin, may be used. The latter is the most commonly and effectively used strategy to protect insulin from the harsh environment of the GIT and promote its intestinal uptake, translocation, and transport to the target site (Florence 2004). The intestinal uptake of insulin encapsulated into nanoparticles may occur by paracellular transport or by transcellular transport, which may be included the transport via M cells of Peyer's patches (Aprahamian et al. 1987; Michel et al. 1991). Figure 5.1 shows the different pathways that insulin-loaded nanoparticles may follow to cross the intestinal epithelium. Generally, nanoparticles lower than 100 nm follow the transcellular pathway, and others higher than 500 nm are taken up by M cells of Peyer's patches in the ileum distal portion of the small intestinal mucosa (Florence 1997, 2005; Jani et al. 1990). The interaction of insulin nanoparticles with the intestinal epithelium are regulated by the carrier and the intestinal mucosa characteristics. Furthermore, the mucus layer and the transit time of nanoparticles may change their interaction with the intestinal epithelium. Mucus may be important to improve the passage across different mucus layers of hydrophilic nanoparticles (Kamba et al. 2000; Florence and Hussain 2001). The interactions of

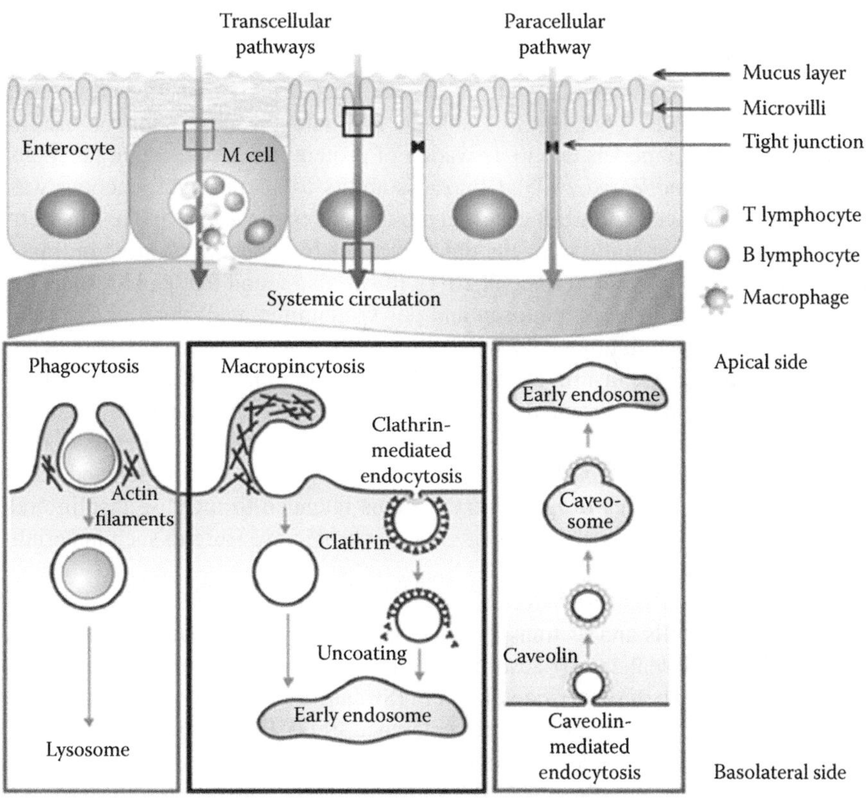

FIGURE 5.1 Routes for insulin nanoparticle translocation through the intestinal epithelium. Schematic focus on phagocytosis, macropinocytosis, and caveolin-mediated endocytosis. (Reprinted with permission from M.-C. Chen, K. Sonaje, K.-J. Chen, and H.-W. Sung, *Biomaterials*, 32, 36, 9826–9838, 2011.)

insulin nanoparticles with the intestinal epithelium may be electrostatic or by specific ligands, depending on the nanoparticle composition or structure, which define the absorption mechanism (Florence and Hussain 2001). Insulin nanoparticles, after absorption, pass through the lymphatic to systemic circulation or are translocated to plasma cells for targeting specific receptors in peripheral tissues, including muscle, fat tissue, liver, and spleen (Jani et al. 1989, 1990; Ebel 1990).

The intestinal uptake of insulin may occur by paracellular transport, which is one of the available pathways via which drugs permeate the intestine. Indeed, this pathway is interesting because the proteases activity between enterocytes is reduced (Shakweh, Ponchel, and Fattal 2004). The paracellular transport may occur due to structural reorganization of tight junction proteins or by decrease in the extracellular concentration of calcium ions, which affects myosin phosphorylation, facilitating insulin absorption (Schipper et al. 1997). Furthermore, formulations containing absorption enhancers, such as chitosan, polyacrylates, and thiomers, are able to improve paracellular transport (Dodane, Amin Khan, and Merwin 1999; Pauletti et al. 1996; Hochman and Artursson 1994). However, insulin uptake through this pathway is limited since tight junctions represent only <1% of the intestinal mucosal surface. In functionalized nanoparticles of chitosan and methyl methacrylate, N-dimethylaminoethyl methacrylate hydrochloride and N-trimethylaminoethyl methacrylate chloride, chitosan was able to facilitate the absorption of insulin through cell culture models due to activation of protein kinase C in tight junctions (Smith, Dornish, and Wood 2005). Chitosan's ability to disrupt tight junctions was studied in a Caco-2 cell culture at gene and protein expression levels, and results were found suggesting that chitosan opens tight junctions by inducing changes in transmembrane CLDN4 protein (Yeh et al. 2011). It was also found that a pH-responsive nanoparticle system made of chitosan and poly(γ-glutamic acid) may infiltrate the mucus layer and open tight junctions and, after infiltration, due to its pH-sensitivity, disintegrate and release insulin directly into systemic circulation (Sung et al. 2012). The N-diethyl methyl chitosan, also has the ability to open tight junctions, facilitating the intestinal uptake of insulin in normal and diabetic rats (Avadi et al. 2005). Overall, it is necessary to explore the different characteristics of chitosan and other materials used to produce drug delivery systems intended to increase insulin oral BA. However, possible toxicity problems due to chronic exposure to such materials may be addressed.

Transcellular transport is characterized by the internalization of insulin into vesicles in epithelial cells and its transport into systemic circulation (Jung et al. 2000). Insulin may be internalized by absorptive cells through clathrin-mediated endocytosis, in vesicles with diameter size of 60 nm (Swaan 1998), or even through phagocytosis, which is a less common process (Florence 1997). Furthermore, potocytosis, based on clathrin-independent endocytosis, may occur for vesicles of 500 nm. Besides the available intestinal area to insulin uptake by transcellular transport, its permeation remains negligible mainly due to its hydrophilicity and high molecular weight. However, insulin may transcellularly permeate the intestinal epithelium by active transport using proper carriers (Fasano 1998). Once more, nanoparticles come to the front line on promoting insulin intestinal uptake. Thus, hydrophobic nanoparticles may permeate through epithelial cells by passive diffusion; however, insulin, as other hydrophilic proteins, is not expected to permeate by passive diffusion (Camenisch et al. 1998). The internalization of insulin-loaded alginate nanoparticles in intestinal cells of Wistar rats was evaluated (Woitiski et al. 2010). Nanoparticles were internalized in enterocytes of different cross-sections of rat small intestinal mucosa, and transcellular transport was the predominant mechanism by which nanoparticles facilitated insulin absorption. In another study, a complex of hydrogels of insulin and transferrin molecules, in a Caco-2 cell monolayer, showed that this conjugate could increase the permeability of insulin through the epithelial barrier by receptor-mediated transcytosis (Kavimandan, Losi, and Peppas 2006). Furthermore, the conjugated transferrin was shown to protect insulin from proteolytic enzymes, thus increasing the BA of orally administered insulin. Multilayered nanoparticles of insulin encapsulated into a core of alginate and dextran sulfate nucleating around calcium and bound to poloxamer, stabilized by chitosan, and coated with albumin, were used in permeability studies in a Caco-2 cell monolayer, in a Caco-2/HT-29 coculture, and in an excised intestinal mucosa of Wistar rats (Woitiski et al. 2011). Nanoparticles containing insulin showed a twofold enhancement of permeability across a Caco-2 cell monolayer compared to an insulin solution and fourfold through mucus secreting Caco-2/HT-29 coculture and fourfold through excised intestinal mucosa. Thus, mucus seems to play an important role in the effectiveness of insulin delivery systems. In the same study, it was also found that labeled insulin and nanoparticles inside the enterocytes, suggest the transcellular pathway is indeed the main pathway of insulin uptake.

Peyer's patches also play an important role in insulin nanoparticle uptake due to the presence of M cells of lymphoid follicle-associated epithelium. These cells increase the ability of nanoparticles to permeate the intestinal epithelium through a transcytotic route (Ermak and Giannasca 1998). In fact, Peyer's patches are able to uptake particles up to 15 μm (O'Hagan 1996), and small particles are taken up to a higher extent than larger particles. The permeation process may occur through the contact of nanoparticles with projections of M cells via both specific and nonspecific receptor-mediated mechanisms along the apical membrane. In addition, these cells have the ability to transport nanoparticles by clathrin-mediated endocytosis (Neutra et al. 1987; Frey et al. 1996), macropinocytosis (Owen 1977), or even by phagocytosis (Jepson et al. 1993). The nonspecific mechanisms of nanoparticle uptake through M cells, strongly depends on its characteristics, such as hydrophobicity or surface charge to selectively interact with these cells (Clark, Jepson, and Hirst 2001). The uptake of nanoparticles by M cells is facilitated by the reduced levels of membrane enzymatic activity and lack of mucus (Florence 2004). In fact, the translocation by Peyer's patches is indeed the fastest process for particle absorption, being a promising pathway for insulin uptake (Jani et al. 1990). It was studied the location and mechanism of fluorescein isothiocyanate (FITC)-insulin absorption, and it was found fluorescence through the ileum tissue in M cells (Sarmento et al. 2007). It was also reported that FITC-insulin encapsulated in nanoparticles consisting of a blend of poly(-ε-caprolactone) and a polycationic nonbiodegradable polyester (Eudragit RS), was able to reduce glycemia in diabetic rats in a dose-dependent manner (maximal at 100 IU/kg) for a prolonged period of time (Damge, Maincent, and Ubrich 2007). FITC-insulin–loaded nanoparticles adhered strongly to intestinal mucosa and the released or still encapsulated FITC-insulin were mainly taken up by the Peyer's patches. Insulin-loaded nanoparticles with an alginate-dextran sulfate core, complexed with a chitosan-polyethylene glycol-albumin shell, also reduced glycemia in diabetic rats and was taken up by Peyer's patches (Reis et al. 2008). Other studies reported that the translocation of insulin nanoparticles through M cells can be related to a longer hypoglycemic response in diabetes (Ma, Lim, and Lim 2005; Sarmento et al. 2007).

Absorption enhancers are able to improve the intestinal uptake of drugs by increasing their paracellular and transcellular transport. They may have different mechanisms of action, such as decrease in mucus viscosity, changes in membrane fluidity, leakage of proteins through membranes, and opening of tight junctions (Mahato et al. 2003). Some nonspecific absorption enhancers may be bile salts, surfactants, fatty acids, chelators, salicylates, and *zonula occludens* toxin. These substances are used in delivery systems in which they are used, for instance, as a physical mixture in capsules or tablets or even by encapsulation into nanoparticles. The latter seems to be a safer strategy since nanoparticles allow a more localized action of absorption enhancers than physical mixtures that spread absorption enhancers all over the intestine, thus avoiding more severe toxicity.

Bile salts in mixed micellar systems were able to improve insulin absorption by paracellular transport (Lane, O'Driscoll, and Corrigan 2005). The enhancer N-lauryl-β-D-maltopyranoside is also able to open the tight junctions (Uchiyama et al. 1999). A dose-related pharmacological effect of insulin in w/o/w multiple emulsions incorporating 2% eicosapentaenoic acid or docosahexaenoic acid (Morishita et al. 2000) was reported. In another study, oral administered insulin-loaded enteric-coated capsules containing sodium salicylate significantly decreased the plasma glucose levels and improved hypoglycemia relative to a SC injection (Hosny, Al-Shora, and Elmazar 2002). Similar levels of serum glucose concentrations in diabetic rats were verified after a parenteral injection of insulin and after oral coadministration of insulin and *zonula occludens* toxin (Fasano and Uzzau 1997). Chitosan may affect both paracellular and transcellular transport of drugs. Results obtained in a HT-29 cell model suggested that the reversible and rapid absorption-enhancing effect of chitosan was due to modifications in intracellular pH caused by activation of a chloride-bicarbonate exchanger, resulting in the tight junctions opening (Rosenthal et al. 2012). Octylglucoside also has the ability to enhance insulin permeability, possibly through the paracellular pathway in T-84 and Caco-2 monolayers (Tirumalasetty and Eley 2006). More recently, cell-penetrating peptides, such as HIV-1, penetratin, and oligoarginine, have been regarded as useful substances to improve the intestinal absorption of biodrugs (Khafagy and Morishita 2012).

It is well known that the absorption and stability of insulin is improved when absorption enhancers and protease inhibitors are coadministered (Carino and Mathiowitz 1999; Maroni et al. 2011). A pulsatile oral delivery system composed of insulin with sodium glycocholate as an absorption enhancer and camostat mesilate as a protease inhibitor are proven to be a potential candidate for insulin delivery in the colon (Del Curto et al. 2009). Nanoparticles containing chitosan and diethylene triamine pentaacetic acid to take advantage of its ability to disrupt tight junctions and inhibit intestinal proteases by chelating divalent metal ions, proven to enhance insulin uptake (Su et al. 2012). In another study, the administration in situ of an insulin solution containing or not sodium glycocholate, sodium caprate, or Na_2EDTA as absorption enhancers and with or without protease inhibitors, such as aprotinin, to colonic and rectal loops of fasted rats, showed that the absorption enhancers better increased insulin efficacy in the colon than in the small intestine (Morishita et al. 1993). Chronic toxicity is another factor that requires attention as the prolonged use of absorption enhancers could increase the ability of pathogen agents, toxins, or other compounds to permeate the intestinal wall and cause toxic effects. Protease inhibitors, which are used to improve the insulin oral absorption, can inhibit some digestive enzymes responsible for cleavage of proteins present in food.

The use of substances generally recognized as safe (GRAS) or registered pharmacopoeial excipients combined with drugs have been used to improve insulin absorption. Such mixtures are able to be formulated in a gastro-resistant capsule with a pH-dependent dissolution profile, allowing protection of the drug in acid pH and release at intestinal pH. It is the case of Capsulin™ developed by Diabetology Ltd. (St. Helier, United Kingdom). By the employment of Axcess™ Oral Delivery System technology, the drug is mixed with absorption enhancers and solubilizers and formulated into an enteric-coated capsule, allowing drug absorption into the intestinal wall (Diabetology Ltd. 2013).

There are two types of Capsulin formulations under Phase 2 clinical trials: Capsulin OAD (oral antidiabetic), which is suitable for T2DM (Diabetology Ltd. 2013), and Capsulin IR (insulin replacement) indicated for T1DM or late-stage T2DM. Capsulin in T2DM showed a glucose control effect during a period of time over 6 hours with a small plasma insulin concentration with decreasing of HbA_{1c} levels, triglycerides, and weight (Luzio et al. 2010). Furthermore, T1DM patients showed that insulin peak is reached 80–90 minutes after ingestion (Whitelaw et al. 2005). Beyond Capsulin safety and tolerability in T1DM subjects, it was also demonstrated to produce glycemic control in a dose-dependent manner with constant increasing plasmatic insulin levels during 30–120 minutes, providing blood glucose control during an extended period of time after administration (Diabetology Ltd. 2013).

ORMD-0801 is a product developed by Oramed Pharmaceuticals Inc. (Jerusalem, Israel) where insulin is coformulated with adjuvants in an enteric-coated capsule (Oramed Pharmaceuticals Inc.). These adjuvants are able to protect insulin from enzymatic degradation and improve the intestinal absorption of insulin (Sabetsky and Ekblom 2010; Eldor, Kidron, and Arbit 2010). This system is suitable for T2DM, mainly in the early stage of diseases, providing additional insulin doses that allow pancreas respite (Oramed Pharmaceuticals Inc.). This delivery system has been shown to be well tolerated without several and accumulative adverse effects (Kidron et al. 2010; Eldor, Kidron, and Arbit 2010), maintaining insulin biological activity after delivery (Eldor, Kidron, and Arbit 2010). A 6-week Phase 2b study carried out in T2DM subjects demonstrated that ORMD-0801, when administered at bedtime, was able to reduce FBG, HbA_{1c} and peptide C (Kidron et al. 2010). It was proposed by Oramed Pharmaceuticals that the introduction of ORMD-0801 as a complement agent of SC insulin injections in T1DM would be able to reduce the daily injections and help to reduce the fluctuations of glucose levels (Oramed Pharmaceuticals Inc.).

A study in T1DM patients showed that ORMD-0801 is safe and effective with an oral preprandial administration, being able to prevent the increasing glucose levels in fasting T1DM patients (Eldor et al. 2010).

The use of delivery agents or carriers without pharmacological properties to avoid insulin degradation and enable its transport across the intestinal wall through passive transcellular transport is the strategy used by Eligen® Technology. It is a platform created by Emisphere Technology Inc. (Cedar Knolls, NJ) for protein and peptide delivery, where delivery agents can interact in a weak and noncovalent manner with the drug, increasing its lipophilicity and stability (Arbit and Kidron 2009; Emisphere Technologies Inc. 2013; Singh and Majuru 2003). It was described that intestinal absorption doesn't cause any histological changes to the intestinal epithelium, and after the drug–carrier complex reaches the intracellular space, they dissociate, so the free drug acquires its native conformation and passes directly into the bloodstream (Emisphere Technologies Inc. 2013; Singh and Majuru 2003).

One of the Eligen Technology agents for insulin delivery is sodium N-[8-(2-hydroxybenzoyl) amino] caprylate (SNAC), which was demonstrated to allow an insulin permeability 10 times higher in a Caco-2 cell monolayer (Malkov et al. 2005). When orally administered in nondiabetic subjects, insulin was absorbed in the GIT in a biological form, decreasing the blood glucose levels in a dose-dependent manner (Kidron et al. 2004).

This system showed a rapid onset with a fast insulin peak in Phase 1 clinical studies (Hoffman and Qadri 2008); however, the formulation appears to cause nausea and requires high amounts of delivery agents regarding insulin doses, which is inconvenient for patients (Park, Kwon, and Park 2011). A Phase 2 clinical trial performed in T2DM subjects with a regimen of metformin alone showed better glycemic control over Eligen Technology combined with metformin (Hoffman and Qadri 2008), and afterward no more information about its clinical development stage was found.

Bows Pharmaceuticals AG (Zug, Switzerland) uses natural polysaccharides as a drug delivery system, due to their biodegradable, biocompatible, nontoxic, and nonimmunogenic properties (BOWS Pharmaceuticals AG). Orin Pharmaceuticals AG (Zug, Switzerland), through a license agreement with Bows Pharmaceuticals AG, uses a dextran matrix capsule to formulate RHI. When dextran is degraded by the intestinal mucosa enzymes, it allows an appropriate target for local absorption (Sabetsky and Ekblom 2010; BOWS Pharmaceuticals AG 2013). They revealed two studies: one for estimating the oral insulin absorption post dose-relative BA and a second one to achieve the lowest dose that enables a significantly lowering of postprandial blood glucose, but no more information is available (ClinicalTrials.gov).

Another company, Merrion Pharmaceuticals, Ltd. (Dublin, Ireland) developed the Gipet® Technology, which uses drug absorption enhancers with the ability to form micelles, which facilitate drug transport across the duodenal cell membrane (Merrion Pharmaceuticals Ltd.). That matrix is constituted by GRAS excipients, namely medium-chain fatty acids (Arbit and Kidron 2009) and physically mixed with insulin and formulated in an enteric-coated tablet (Merrion Pharmaceuticals Ltd.). Once at the duodenum, the tablet dissolves itself and coreleases insulin and excipients, resulting in insulin absorption (Merrion Pharmaceuticals Ltd.). A partnership was established between Merrion Pharmaceuticals and Novo Nordisk where

Gipet Technology was used to deliver a new, long-acting oral IA patented Novo Nordisk analog (NN1956), and in 2013, a single Phase I clinical trial was completed (ClinicTrials.gov 2013; Clinic trials at Novo Nordisk 2013).

Diasome Pharmaceuticals, Inc. (Conshohocken, PA) developed an oral hepatic-directed vesicle insulin (HDV-I) delivery system, where insulin is entrapped into liposomes, forming a hepatic-directed vesicle (HDV). In its phospholipid bilayer, it contains a hepatocyte-targeting molecule (HTM) to deliver insulin directly to hepatocytes, having the ability to cross biological membranes due to their small size, avoiding insulin degradation (Diasome Pharmaceuticals Inc. 2013; Geho et al. 2009; Arbit and Kidron 2009). Studies showed that single doses of oral HDV-I combined with oral antidiabetic drug (OAD) therapy was able to reduce the PPG in T2DM (Schwartz et al. 2008). A 14-day study in T1DM subjects showed that oral HDV-I was able to reduce the mean daily seven-point blood glucose in a significant manner, compared to SC RHI (Schwartz et al. 2009).

Biocon (Bangalore, India) developed a new oral IA, In-105 (Arbit and Kidron 2009), which is in Phase 3 of clinical development in T2DM subjects (Biocon Biopharmaceuticals 2013). It is manufactured by the combination of RHI with a short chain of methoxypolyethylene glycol derivative by a covalent binding (Dave et al. 2008). In T2DM patients poorly controlled with metformide, IN-105 was demonstrated to have a decreasing of PPG levels in a dose-dependent manner. The insulin maximum concentration was reached at 20 minutes, and the insulin levels disappeared from the bloodstream around 80 minutes after administration (Iyer et al. 2009).

Access Pharmaceuticals Inc. (Dallas, TX) developed a new oral approach based on the "Trojan horse strategy," which uses the natural uptake mechanism of vitamin B12 to promote insulin absorption (Access Pharmaceuticals 2013). The Cobalamin™ (vitamin B12 or its analogs) forms conjugates directly with the drug or can be combined with polymers containing the drug. Eventually, it can be on the surface of drug-loaded nanoparticles. Through the intrinsic factor mediation, the Cobalamin is linked to the intrinsic factor receptor, allowing the coabsorption of Cobalamin and drugs across the intestinal wall by a mediated endocytotic process (Access Pharmaceuticals 2013). Nevertheless, the use of vitamin B12 conjugates has some limitations, particularly the low transport capacity of the system, presenting a low BA for proteins and the possibility of conjugate degradation at the GIT. Furthermore, the probability of loss of intrinsic factor activity and loss of drug activity caused by covalent binding are also some drawbacks of such a system (Chalasani, Russell-Jones, Jain et al. 2007). Thus, the use of hydrophilic nanocarriers, such those based on dextran has been used as they have the capacity to protect insulin against enzymes with a proper release profile (Chalasani, Russell-Jones, Jain et al. 2007; Chalasani, Russell-Jones, Yandrapu et al. 2007).

In vivo studies showed that oral insulin containing vitamin B12–dextran nanoparticle conjugates were able to reduce glucose levels in a dose-dependent manner with a slow onset and prolonged duration of action (Chalasani, Russell-Jones, Jain et al. 2007; Chalasani, Russell-Jones, Yandrapu et al. 2007).

In general, most of the mentioned delivery systems are in Phase 1 or 2 of clinical development so that information such as changes of PK parameters caused by drugs and/or food interactions, interindividual variability of glucodynamic parameters, and reproducibility of insulin absorption needs to be further evaluated.

Buccal Insulin Delivery Systems

A good noninvasive route of administration that presents some advantages for insulin delivery is the buccal route, as buccal mucosa has a thin vascularized layer, providing a high absorption area and direct access to the bloodstream, which allows an increase of BA of macromolecules. Unlike the oral route, where insulin absorption occurs at the intestinal epithelium, this route avoids the enzymatic degradation along the stomach and intestinal tract (Khafagy et al. 2007; Heinemann and Jacques 2009; Generex Biotechnology Corp.). However, buccal mucosa present different histology among different areas (sublingual, palate, and cheek mucosa), and consequently, a different permeability rate may occur. Another drawback is the continuous release of saliva, constituting a barrier to drug absorption (Heinemann and Jacques 2009).

RapidMist™ is a safe and easy-to-use drug delivery system created by Generex Biotechnology Corp. (Toronto, Canada), which can be used for drug delivery through buccal mucosa without deposition of the drug in the lungs (Generex Biotechnology Corp.; Bernstein 2008). That metered dose spray allows the delivery of the drug in a precise manner without the pain of daily SC injections (Bernstein 2008). Oral-lyn® uses the technology RapidMist for RHI delivery (Heinemann and Jacques 2009), where insulin is formulated in a liquid with a mixture of GRAS excipients and small amounts of absorption enhancers, particularly surfactants, which are important to solubilize and stabilize insulin in formulation and promote its absorption through buccal mucosa (Generex Biotechnology Corp.). Each administration allows only 10% of absorption (1 IU of insulin) whereas SC injections allow 20%–40% of insulin absorption; therefore that system is suitable for both types of diabetic patients in prandial situations (Heinemann and Jacques 2009; Bernstein 2008). Therefore, the use of Oral-lyn for meal coverage can require several consecutive administrations, so it may be considered a time-consuming system. This system is being marketed and is also in Phase III clinical trials in several countries (Heinemann and Jacques 2009).

PharmFilm® Drug Delivery Technology is a new buccal system under clinical development developed by Monosol Rx (Warren, NJ) in partnership with Midatech Group (Abingdon, United Kingdom) (Monosol Rx). That technology employs the Midatech Group's system, which is based on three-layered gold nanoparticles: the most internal layer is constituted by a gold core, an intermediate portion formed by linkers, and a hydrosoluble outer layer composed of ligands that enable specific targeting to cells or tissues. These nanoparticles are stable, allowing the formation of covalent bonds with several bioactive molecules, enabling its administration. Due to their small size, they present high mobility through the membranes and are eliminated by renal and biliary excretion without accumulative effects (Midatech Ltd.).

Thus, PharmFilm drug delivery technology was designed to allow drug administration at therapeutic levels with low doses and fast onset of action, enabling the administration of either low or high dose regimens. That technology is suitable for buccal insulin delivery through a small and thin film, which easily dissolves in the mouth enabling insulin delivery with reproducible doses. As it doesn't present any taste, it is suitable for patients for whom administration presents some complications, namely pediatric, geriatric, and psychiatric subjects. Phase 1 clinical trials of this system showed positive results in terms of safety, BA, and PK parameters (Monosol Rx).

Pulmonary Insulin Delivery Systems

We can find several inhaled insulin products in all development stages. Exubera® (Nektar Therapeutics (San Francisco, CA), the first inhaled insulin product on the market, was available in August 2006. Despite the high levels of acceptability and satisfaction demonstrated by those involved in clinical trials (Freemantle et al. 2005; Bellary and Barnett 2006; Gerber et al. 2001; Rosenstock et al. 2004), Exubera received some complaints and was withdrawn in October 2007. Outwardly, its device was considered large and complicated, associated with the need for training and time-consuming handling. It also presented unconventional units, which could lead to confusion and erroneous administration. It was actually more costly because it needed a higher amount of insulin to produce the same effect as a SC injection and because it was not covered by all insurance plans. Furthermore, the recommendation for regular assessment of pulmonary functions (e.g., spirometry) within the first 6 months and annually thereafter was another drawback able to affect a patient's life on multiple levels, such as economical, emotional, and comfort.

The formulation of Exubera consists of a dry powder composed of rRHI, sodium citrate, mannitol, glycine, and sodium hydroxide, available in blisters of 1 mg and 3 mg. Exubera showed a rapid onset of action that was comparable with injected rapid-acting IAsp (Forst et al. 2009) and significantly faster than both RHI and ILis (32 vs. 48 and 41 minutes, respectively). It revealed a duration of action between that of ILis and RHI ($313 < 387 < 415$ minutes) with a relative bioefficacy of 10% (vs. RHI) and 11% (vs. ILis) (Rave et al. 2005). Maximal metabolic activity achieved with 6 mg of insulin via Exubera was lower than that of ILis (18 U) but comparable to that of RHI (18 U), which justifies the equivalence that 1 mg of inhaled insulin corresponds to 3 IU SC RHI.

It was demonstrated that inhaled insulin using Exubera was rapidly and reproducibly absorbed (Gelfand, Schwartz, and Horton 2000), well tolerated, and comparable in glycemic control to a conventional SC insulin regimen in both T1DM and T2DM patients (Quattrin et al. 2004; Hollander et al. 2004). Overall, hypoglycemia events occurred with the same incidence for Exubera or SC RHI treatment. However, in T2DM patients poorly controlled with OAD therapy, the addition of Exubera was associated with a higher rate of hypoglycemia than a second OAD agent (Pfizer).

Long-term safety studies reported some respiratory effects (Skyler et al. 2008; Rosenstock et al. 2008), specifically the decrease of forced expiratory volume in 1 second (FEV_1) and the diffusing capacity of the lung for carbon monoxide (DLCO) in Exubera-treated patients. These changes were small and considered reversible upon treatment, nonprogressive, nonpathological, and not associated with the increased antibody levels that occur within the first months of treatment. Furthermore, clinical data do not suggest any correlation between the increased antibody levels with increased HbA_{1c} levels, insulin doses, or hypoglycemia rates (Heinemann and Heise 2004).

Afrezza® (MannKind Corporation, Valencia, CA) can be the next inhaled insulin on the market. It represents the combination between the Technosphere® insulin formulation and the Dreamboat™ inhaler device, both technologies developed by MannKind Corp.

Mannkind's inhalable formulation consists of Technosphere's technologies that stabilize insulin in its monomeric form unlike other formulations in which insulin is formulated as a hexamer. Furthermore, Technosphere particles are formed by fumaryl diketopiperazine (FDKP) molecules (a novel excipient of MannKind Corp.) that self-assemble into plates, yielding a structure with a large surface area and that is highly porous (internal porosity of 70% approx.) with a median aerodynamic diameter of 2 to 2.5 μm (10% of the particles are <1 μm, 90% <5 μm) (Richardson and Boss 2007). Technosphere insulin is characterized by a low-density dry powder predominantly composed of insulin and FDKP (1:9 ratio by dry weight) and polysorbate 80, able to be uniformly distributed and deposited throughout the lungs (Cassidy et al. 2011). FDKP is highly soluble at physiologic pH and allows a rapid dissolution of microparticles in the lung, consequently providing rapid insulin absorption (Potocka et al. 2010). It was demonstrated that the rapid insulin permeation across the alveolar surface into the bloodstream occurred naturally due to rapid dissolution of microparticles that instantaneously form a high local concentration gradient (Angelo et al. 2009). MannKind's inhaler, a device for premetered, single-dose cartridges, also brings an attractive design (small, light, and discreet) with a very patient-friendly usage (Leone-Bay et al. 2010). These unique characteristics differentiate it from all other insulin forms, inhaled or injected. Afrezza is characterized by a rapid absorption profile with a maximum concentration occurring at 15 minutes approximately, a duration of insulin action of about 2 hours, and a faster time action profile compared with all other insulin forms (Markey 2011; Steiner et al. 2002). Therefore, it can provide glycemic control with lower risk of hypoglycemia, less weight gain, and improved PPG control when compared with conventional SC insulin as verified in clinical trials with both T1DM and T2DM patients (Kapsner et al. 2009; Rosenstock et al. 2010).

Afrezza achieved an insulin BA of 20%–25% (Rave et al. 2009) and an interindividual variability of 19.6% compared with 50.1% of SC insulin (Potocka, Baughman, and Derendorf 2011). The safety and tolerability profile has been comparable with conventional treatments, but it is affected by the higher incidence of cough, reported as mild and transient in nature, and by nonprogressive and reversible pulmonary function changes (Raskin et al. 2012; Petrucci et al. 2009). Nonetheless, it was already demonstrated that inhaled insulin by Afrezza was well tolerated without serious safety concerns during 4 years of treatment (Rossiter et al. 2009).

The AERx® insulin diabetes management system (AERx iDMS, Aradigm Corp.) consists of a system for delivering inhaled insulin into the deep peripheral parts of the lung via the inhaler AERx Essence®. Such a device is a microprocessor-controlled inhaler that enables fine particle aerosol generation with a mass median aerodynamic diameter of 2–3 um from prepackaged single-use dosage forms with four different insulin doses (0.3–1.8 U/kg) available (Brunner et al. 2001). The date, time, breathing parameters during delivery, and amount of delivered insulin are recorded electronically, allowing an assessment of dosage, breathing maneuvers, and patient compliance (Farr et al. 2000; Thipphawong et al. 2002).

Trial studies demonstrated a more rapid onset of action (Patton, Bukar, and Nagarajan 1999), similar efficacy and safety of intensified insulin treatment between inhaled insulin via AERx iDMS and SC insulin injections (Hermansen et al. 2004) in a linear dose-response relationship (Brunner et al. 2001). A reduced BA was found, about 8%, indicating insulin loss most likely due to loss from the device itself, particle deposition in the mouth and throat or particles that are exhaled, and possibly from intrapulmonary degradation.

The relative biopotency over 6 hours was 13%. Overall, insulin inhaled via the AERx iDMS system was well tolerated and showed similar PK/PD measures and lower (however, not statistically significant) intraindividual variability compared to SC insulin administration (Kapitza, Hompesch et al. 2004).

Another developed approach using aerosolization of liquid insulin formulations was developed by Aerogen (Dangan, Ireland). The Aerodose insulin inhaler consists of the OnQ™ technology, a system that allows a low-velocity aerosol generation optimized for deep lung deposition as a result of the formation of consistently sized droplets (approx. 4 μm of mean size) by a vibrational element acting as a micropump (Aerogen Inc. 2013). The inhaler device developed by Aerogen exhibited significantly shorter time-to-peak insulin levels and metabolic effects compared with SC RHI (Kapitza, Heise et al. 2004). Interestingly, altering the aerosolization times (2 vs. 4 seconds) had an impact on the metabolic effect opposite to particle sizes changing (fine or very fine, 4.4 or 3.5 μm, respectively), which is an indicator of the optimization of delivery parameters for further clinical testing. Studies revealed a comparable dose–response profile on the overall glucose lowering effect between inhaled insulin via Aerodose and SC RHI (Kim et al. 2003), which facilitates the direct dosing conversion ratio among doses. The BA values found, 18%–22% in T1DM patients and 16% in T2DM (Perera et al. 2002), represent greater achievements compared with other inhaled insulin systems, but it requires further studies with a larger number of subjects, including long-term studies, to assess the efficacy and safety of this delivery system.

The Advanced Inhalation Research (AIR®) insulin system (Alkermes, Dublin, Ireland) is a technology based on the deep lung delivery of dry powder aerosols with particularly large low-density particles. These porous particles with low density (<0.1 g/cm^2) and large geometric (10–20 μm) but small aerodynamic diameter (1–3 μm) are easily dispersible, and therefore, AIR insulin can be aerosolized using a simple breath-actuated inhaler (Edwards et al. 1997; Wolzt et al. 2008), which is easy to teach and use (Ellis, Gemperline, and Garg 2007). Clinical data showed better PK/PD properties comparable to ILis (Muchmore et al. 2007; Gross, Nakano, Colon-Vega, Ortiz-Carasquillo et al. 2009). AIR insulin also showed dose interchangeability and reproducibility across a range of doses (de La Peña et al. 2009). Outcomes from a multicenter study (n = 137, T1DM patients) revealed that 80% preferred AIR inhaled insulin to injected insulin, attending its reduced impact on their lifestyles, easier blood sugar control, and comfort (Hayes, Muchmore, and Schmitke 2007). Long-term studies (Gross, Nakano, Colon-Vega, Ortiz-Carasquillo, Ferguson et al. 2009; Ang et al. 2009) confirmed the tolerability of AIR insulin, revealing similar incidence of hypoglycemia and more frequent cough (not always clinically relevant), compared to SC insulin treatment groups. Despite comparable glycemic control and a greater decrease in pulmonary functions (FEV_1 and DLCO) verified in these studies, in a 6-month trial (Comulada et al. 2009), AIR insulin treatment exhibited body weight decrease in T1DM patients.

The company KOS (Cranbury, NJ) developed a regular insulin preparation intended to be conveyed by a simple, robust, and inexpensive metered-dose inhaler (MDI). Studies with healthy subjects, inhalation of different insulin doses had a linear dose–response relationship and induced rapid onset of action, achieving a biopotency ranging between 10% and 15% compared to SC regular insulin (Kapitza et al. 2003).

Other innovative technology was developed by Epic Therapeutics (Norwood, MA), using protein matrix microspheres known as ProMaxx®. These systems are produced by a temperature-controlled precipitation from an aqueous insulin solution in the presence of polyethylene glycol without additional excipients. Such technology is differentiated by its robust formulation process that allows protein preservation and produces a consistent narrow size distribution of 1–3 μm sized microspheres. Furthermore, this process results in a dry formulation based on more than 95% of insulin (White et al. 2007). First trials with ProMaxx inhaled insulin using a breath-actuated dry powder inhaler (DPI) confirmed its faster onset of action, similar duration of action and metabolic effect, with 12% of BA comparing with SC RHI (Heise et al. 2009).

Nasal Insulin Delivery Systems

A few years ago, two intranasal ultra-rapid-acting insulin products reached Phase 2 of clinical trials, demonstrating that insulin can be noninvasively administrated through the nose, enabling a friendly strategy to improve patient compliance. Nevertheless, nasal insulin delivery had a more ashamed development mainly due to poor permeability through the mucosa, susceptibility to the enzymatic barrier, low retention time, and fast mucociliary clearance, requiring formulations with high protein concentrations to satisfy acceptable dose volume limits (100 and 200 mL per nostril), and unavoidable adverse effects inherently related to this route (e.g., sneezing, runny nose, watering eyes, unpleasant taste or smell, headache, and nasal congestion) (Mitchell et al. 2008).

One of them was an insulin nasal named Nasulin™ and developed by CPEX Pharmaceuticals (Wilmington, DE). Nasulin is a nasal formulation of rRHI, containing polysorbate 20, sorbitan monolaurate, cottonseed oil, and CPE-215™ (cyclopentadecalactone), a new compound that enhances absorption of molecules across mucous membranes (Stote et al. 2011). Nasulin promotes a rapid absorption of insulin that results in an onset of action at 10–20 minutes and peaks at around 30–50 minutes (Leary et al. 2005, 2006; Stote et al. 2009) during 100–120 minutes (Leary et al. 2008), providing insulin coverage while food is being absorbed and will not be present before subsequent meals. Therefore, it revealed a promising profile able to mimic the initial spike of insulin produced by the pancreas in response to a meal even faster than fast-acting injectable insulin. Previous studies in healthy volunteers and T1DM patients have estimated a relative BA of 10%–20% compared to SC insulin (Leary et al. 2005, 2006). Nasulin administration also showed proportional and linear dose responses at 0.7% and 1.0% concentrations, achieved with repeated administrations, in which time to maximal serum insulin concentration remained unaltered (Stote et al. 2010). This makes possible the availability of multiple strengths and enhanced titration flexibility. In the initial Phase 1 and 2 studies, Nasulin appeared to be well-tolerated in healthy volunteers and diabetes patients at doses up to 100 U. Administration site reactions were the most adverse effects reported despite that they lasted only a few minutes and disappeared with continued dosing. They were transient (5–20 minutes) with mild severity and included site irritation, sneezing, increased lacrimation, throat irritation, dysgeusia, headache, cough, nasal congestion, ocular hyperemia, nasal discharge, and mucosal paresthesia. Furthermore, several patients have experienced hypoglycemic events (Stote et al. 2010) that increased in a dose-dependent manner. For example, for a dual nostril administration of 50, 75, and 100 U, the occurrence of hypoglycemia was 12.5%, 31.3%, and 43.8%, respectively (Stote et al. 2011). Additionally, intrasubject variability observed with Nasulin administrations varied between 33% and 47% (Leary et al. 2008). After 15 completed clinical trials with approximately 390 subjects, including one Phase 2 trial, the Nasulin program were suspended in 2010. This decision was taken after a Phase 2 study, designed to assess the glycemic control in T2DM patients (n = 94, 6 weeks) treated with basal IGlar and Nasulin (50 or 100 U) or placebo three times daily prior to meals. Several uncertainties arose regarding further development because subjects in the placebo group spent less time (p = 0.2) reaching euglycemia compared to subjects in the Nasulin group (CPEX Pharmaceuticals Inc. 2010).

Nastech Pharmaceutical Company Inc. also developed a rapid-acting intranasal insulin formulation, currently licensed by Marina Biotech Inc. (Bothell, WA). Results from the last Phase 2 clinical trial (n = 29 T2DM) demonstrated that their intranasal insulin was superior to usual therapy (OAD medicines and/or basal insulin) and noninferior to IAsp (NovoLog®). Data showed that the time to maximum concentration for intranasal insulin was even faster (30 minutes) than for insulin aspart (90 minutes). More notably, Nastech's intranasal insulin also showed a statistically significant reduction in the incidence of hypoglycemia (3% vs. 21%, p = 0.025) (Nastech Pharmaceutical Inc. 2008). Currently Marina Biotech believes in further development of the intranasal insulin clinical program, once several trials showed evidence of its tolerability, rapid PK profile, stability at room temperature and potential use on Alzheimer's and other CNS diseases (Marina Biotech 2011).

Recently, the therapeutic potential of an intranasally administered insulin formulation gained a new direction toward treatment of cognitive impairments (Shemesh et al. 2012; Schiöth et al. 2012). As demonstrated by a recent pilot clinical trial (n = 104, 4 months), intranasal insulin treatment (20 and 40 IU) improved delayed memory and also preserved general cognition ($p < 0.05$ for both) in adults with amnestic mild cognitive impairment or Alzheimer's disease (Craft et al. 2012). These results support longer clinical trials of intranasal insulin treatment, which are already ongoing and focused on diseases affected by neurocognitive functions.

Transdermal Insulin Delivery Systems

Skin is a good route for drug delivery due to its large surface, which allows the absorption of many drugs without the first-pass effect of liver and GIT degradation. In the case of diabetes therapy, it is considered to be a noninvasive and painless approach as it avoids the use of needles and consequently the fear of injections of patients (Khafagy et al. 2007; Silpi, Manish, and Kumar 2011). However, *stratum corneum*, the skin's outer layer, has corneocytes, constituting a barrier for drug absorption, especially for hydrophilic macromolecules (Khafagy et al. 2007; Lassmann-Vague and Raccah 2006). Thus, as insulin presents low skin permeability, an effort has been made to create new approaches for overcoming this issue.

One approach is the use of microneedles, which are systems based on needles fabricated on a microscale with sizes less than 1 mm, which enables the administration of drugs (McAllister et al. 2003). Due to its small size, it pierces the *stratum corneum* with 10–15 μm of thickness, forming micropores where drugs, such as insulin, can cross the skin layers until they reach the bloodstream. Since microneedles don't reach the nervous ending at the dermis, they are painless and are considered to be minimally invasive, constituting a good approach to replacing the SC injections (McAllister et al. 2003; Shivanand, Binal, and Viral 2009; Khafagy et al. 2007).

Beyond the size, which has a high influence on drug delivery, other important factors are the geometry and sharpness of the microneedle tips since they may influence the force that is required for the microneedles to perforate the skin (van der Maaden, Jiskoot, and Bouwstra 2012).

There are four types of microneedles which are classified according to their approach for drug delivery (see Figure 5.2), being solid, hollow, and dissolving, and the most microneedle types described for in vitro and in vivo studies of transdermal insulin delivery (Martanto et al. 2004; Gupta, Felner, and Prausnitz 2009; Davis et al. 2005; Migalska et al. 2011).

To achieve better transdermal insulin delivery, the combination of microneedles with traditional patches has been regarded (Roxhed et al. 2008). That hybrid system allows the combination of each system's advantages, namely the ability of needles to insert drugs into the skin with the capacity of easy-to-use, painless, and controlled drug release properties provided by the traditional transdermal patch (McAllister et al. 2003; Silpi, Manish, and Kumar 2011).

V-Go™ is a marketed system approved by the Food and Drug Administration (FDA) and the European Medicines Agency (EMA), developed by Valeritas Inc. (Bridgewater, NJ), which combines the use of microneedles and h-Patch™ technology, a transdermal patch that enables drug release into SC tissue (Touch Digital Media Ltd. 2007; Valeritas Inc. 2013). That device is characterized by its small size, disposability, low weight, and easy application on the body by removing the adhesive strip (Touch Digital Media Ltd. 2007; Valeritas Inc. 2013). That system doesn't require any electronic source, pumps, or needles for insulin delivery, but a second system called EZ Fill is needed to fill the insulin reservoir (Valeritas Inc. 2013; Touch Digital Media Ltd. 2007). It allows basal and continuous SC infusion of rapid-acting IA or on-demand bolus insulin, being suitable for T2DM, which requires several daily insulin doses (see Table 5.3) (Touch Digital Media Ltd. 2007; Valeritas Inc. 2013). After removal of

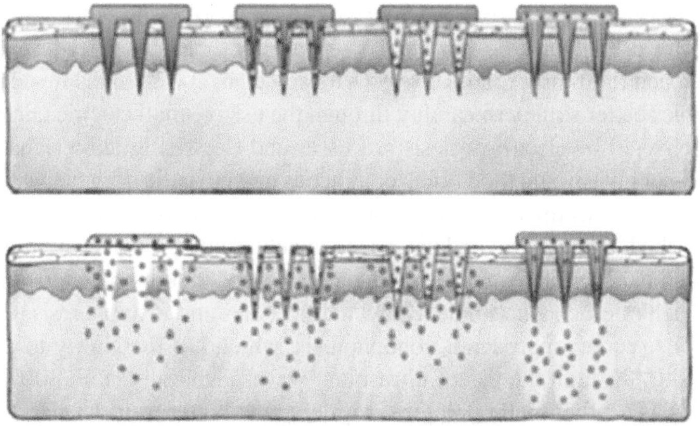

FIGURE 5.2 Different types of microneedles (MN). (a) Application of microneedles at stratum corneum and (b) drug release into dermis layer. Solid microneedles are first inserted to create micropores where the drug is delivered from formulation. The drug can be coated at the microneedle surface where the drug coating dissolves the microneedle into the skin. The dissolving microneedles are constituted by biodegradable compounds where drugs are entrapped and released after microneedle dissolution. Liquid formulations can be delivered through the skin by a hollow microneedle. (Reprinted with permission from Y.-C. Kim, J.-H. Park, and M. R. Prausnitz, *Advanced Drug Delivery Reviews*, 64, 14, 1547–1568, 2012.)

TABLE 5.3
Features of V-Go Disposable Insulin Delivery System

Preset basal insulin dosage	20 units/24 hours (0.83 units/hour) 30 units/24 hours (1.25 units/hour) 40 units/24 hours (1.67 units/hour)
On-demand insulin dosage	All V-Go options allow an increment of 2-Unit bolus on-demand to cover insulin needs during mealtime, until maximum of 36 Units
Insulin type	A U-100 fast-acting should be used with V-Go: Humalog (Eli Lilly) and Novolog (Novo Nordisk)
Special features	Does not require external sources or needles for insulin delivery; Easy-to-use, disposable, and discreet device; Only used during 24 hours; Is not suitable for people who requires less than 2 units on-demand or regular adjustments on insulin basal rate; Requires a second device for V-Go insulin fill; A separate medical prescription is required for fast-acting IA; The system is applied by pressing the bottom, and when microneedle is correctly inserted the device makes an audible click; A second bottom is required for 2-unit on-demand.

the h-patch from the skin, the microneedles retract, and the system cannot be reused (Valeritas Inc. 2013; Touch Digital Media Ltd. 2007; Amin et al. 2008).

The use of electric currents or ultrasounds has been studied as an alternative approach for transdermal delivery (Khafagy et al. 2007). In the first case, iontophoresis enables better skin permeability through the use of small electric currents and the drug is delivered by electro-osmosis processes and electromigration (Khafagy et al. 2007). This noninvasive method offers continuous and pulsatile drug delivery, being able to be combined with microneedles in order to have a synergic effect for insulin delivery as described in an in vitro and in vivo study published by Chen et al. In this study, insulin-loaded nanovesicles were driven into deep layers of skin with a good permeability rate through microchannels induced by microneedles and iontophoresis (Chen et al. 2009).

The second approach is sonophoresis, which has the ability to deliver drugs into the skin through the use of ultrasound waves (Khafagy et al. 2007). It can be combined with other methodologies in order to get better transdermal drug permeability, such as iontophoresis or chemical enhancers (Polat, Blankschtein, and Langer 2010; Mitragotri 2000); however, frequency, intensity, ultrasound energy dose, distance of the transducer from the skin as well as pulse length are important parameters that need attention for sonophoresis efficiency (Saroha, Sharma, and Yadav 2011).

Sonophoresis can be divided into high-frequency sonophoresis (HFS) or low-frequency sonophoresis (LFS), according to the frequency above 0.7 MHz or between 20 and 100 kHz, respectively (Polat, Blankschtein, and Langer 2010; Polat et al. 2011). HFS was shown to be able to improve the permeability of drugs with low molecular weight (Polat et al. 2011). Nevertheless, LFS was shown to be more effective for administration of hydrophilic macromolecules than HFS (Mitragotri, Blankschtein, and Langer 1995).

It is believed that the sonophoresis mechanism is due to a cavitation effect, which is characterized by the growing and oscillation of the air pocket present at *stratum corneum*, being responsible for lipid bilayer disorganization, which leads to enhancement of skin permeability (Polat et al. 2011; Mitragotri, Blankschtein, and Langer 1995), and this effect decreases with the increase of ultrasound frequency, so FFS are able to allow skin permeation of large molecules (Mitragotri, Blankschtein, and Langer 1995).

U-Strip™ is a needle-free system developed by Transdermal Specialties Inc. for insulin delivery, which uses alternating ultrasound waves, namely Ultrasound Sawtooth Waveforms, to enlarge the pore of skin from 50 μm to 100 μm, enabling macromolecule permeability through the skin (Transdermal Specialties Inc.). Currently in Phase III clinical trial, it is constituted by a patch (Insulin Patch™), where insulin is stored, a battery, and a transducer coupler snapped on the patch connected with a sonic applicator control unit, which allows programming the frequency and drug dosage adjustments for basal or mealtime insulin, according to the patient's needs (see Table 5.4) (Transdermal Specialties Inc.).

Transferosome is another approach for transdermal delivery of a range of small molecules, peptides, proteins, and vaccines (Benson 2006). They are vesicles with elasticity, flexibility, and deformability properties, which are able to squeeze themselves and pass over skin pores even with a smaller size than transferosome itself (Kulkarni et al. 2011; Wadhwa et al. 2012). Furthermore, they protect the drug against degradation and can act as a depot (Kulkarni et al. 2011).

TABLE 5.4
Features of U-Strip Insulin Delivery System

Insulin dosage	25 units (Insulin Patch U-25) 50 units (Insulin Patch U-50) 100 units (Insulin Patch U-100) 150 units (Insulin Patch U-150)
Insulin type	ILis
Application	Insulin Patch U-25 and U-50 for T2DM in combination with oral meds Insulin Patch U-100 and U-150 for T1DM
Insulin delivery regiment	Basal for Insulin Patch U-25, U-50, and U-100 Basal and bolus for meals in the case of insulin patch U-150
Programmable insulin delivery	Basal range: 0 to 1.1 U/min Bolus range: 1 to 4.0 U/min
Special feature	Totally noninvasive without using needles Can be worn on the arm and waist Contains an easy-to-use touch screen control Glucose data registration during 60 days Avoid peaks of glucose during day and night Provides sound alarm Provides daily information about dosages and glucose data to patient Allows monitoring by physicians

The skin permeability occurs through a transcellular route. Since transepidermal hydration is a drive force to conduct transferosomes into deep layers, it must be hydrated, so they can follow the natural gradient of water (Kulkarni et al. 2011; Wadhwa et al. 2012). Developed by IDEA AG (Munich, Germany), they are constituted by a phospholipid component to assemble the lipid bilayer, and surfactants. The flexibility and stability of transferosomes can be controlled through the mixture of surfactants used at an appropriate rate (Kulkarni et al. 2011; Wadhwa et al. 2012).

Insulin can also be also delivered through the skin by its encapsulation into transferosomes, namely Transfersulin® (Kulkarni et al. 2011), constituting a good alternative approach for the invasive route. It was shown that an optimized transferosomal gel containing insulin was able to decrease the blood glucose level after 24 hours of transdermal administration in alloxan-induced diabetic rats (Malakar et al. 2012). When the system is properly optimized, it allows insulin skin absorption with an efficacy rate above 50% (Gangwar et al. 2012; Cevc et al. 1998). Despite these results, further information about its status of development is not known, maybe because it was abandoned due to the possibility of phospholipids to suffer oxidation, which is a drawback of transferosome use on insulin delivery.

CONCLUSION AND FUTURE PROSPECTS

Diabetes mellitus is a metabolic disease, and its treatment requires patient adherence and management. Patients must embrace a lifestyle with proper physical exercise, control of food intake, especially carbohydrates, and pharmacological treatment.

Furthermore, physicians have an important role in encouraging patients to adhere to healthy lifestyles, train them to measure and control daily glucose levels by themselves, and give the best pharmacological treatment taking into account the specificities of each diabetic patient. OAD are usually used for diabetes management, especially at T2DM; however, in the case of insulin resistance and T1DM, insulin therapy is the best option.

Insulin is usually administered by the SC route; however, different noninvasive routes have been explored to find an alternative to the invasive route of insulin administration. The oral route seems to be the preferable route mainly because of its easy handling, convenience, and comfort avoiding the use of needles and improving patient compliance. Different delivery systems have been developed to administer insulin by a noninvasive route, such as the use of particulate carriers, which protect insulin and deliver it in a controlled manner, which seems to be promising and useful for diabetes treatment. None of those attempts can be considered to be a good alternative to the invasive route mainly due to poor insulin BA. Further developments need to be made to develop a noninvasive delivery system that can reach the market in the near future. In addition, the toxicity profile of some excipients and formulations needs to be also assessed.

ACKNOWLEDGMENTS

The authors acknowledge the financial support received from *Fundação para a Ciência e Tecnologia* (FCT, Portugal) through NanoFreeze project (PTDC/SAL FCT/104492/2008) and SFRH/BD/78127/2011 PhD grant.

LIST OF ABBREVIATIONS

AERx-iDMS	AERx® Insulin Diabetes Management System
AIR	Advances inhalation research
BA	Bioavailability
BHI	Biphasic human insulin
BIAsp 30	Biphasic insulin aspart 30
DLCO	Diffusion capacity of the lung for carbon monoxide
DPI	Dry powder inhaler
EMA	European Medicines Agency
FBG	Fasting blood glucose
FDA	Food and Drug Administration
FDKP	Fumaryl diketopiperazina
FITC	Fluorescein isothiocyanate
GIT	Gastrointestinal tract
GRAS	Generally recognized as safe
HbA_{1c}	Glycated hemoglobin
HDV	Hepatic-directed vesicle
HDV-I	Hepatic-directed vesicle insulin
HFS	High-frequency sonophoresis
HTM	Hepatocyte-targeting molecule

IA	Insulin analog
IAsp	Insulin aspart
IDeg	Insulin degludec
IDet	Insulin detemir
IGlar	Insulin glargine
IGlu	Insulin glulisine
ILis	Insulin lispro
LFS	Low-frequency sonophoresis
MDI	Metered-dose inhaler
NPH	Neutral protamine hagerdorn
NPL	Neutral protamine lispro
OAD	Oral antidiabetic drugs
PD	Pharmacodynamics
PEG	Poly(ethylene glycol)
PK	Pharmacokinetics
PLA	Poly(lactic acid)
PLGA	Poly(lactic-co-glycolic acid)
PPG	Postprandial glucose
rDNA	Recombinant DNA
RHI	Regular human insulin
SC	Subcutaneous
SLN	Solid lipid nanoparticle
SNAC	N-[8-(2-hydroxybenzoyl) amino] caprylate
T1DM	Type 1 diabetes mellitus
T2DM	Type 2 diabetes mellitus

REFERENCES

Abrahamson, M. J. 2010. Basal insulins: Pharmacological properties and patient perspectives. *Primary Care Diabetes* 4, Supplement 1 (0):S19–S23.

Access Pharmaceuticals, I. 2013. [cited March 18, 2013]. Available from http://www.accesspharma.com.

Aerogen Inc. 2013. *OnQ™ technology* 2013 [cited June 10, 2013]. Available from http://www.aerogen.com/on-q.html.

Amin, A., T. Shah, J. Patel, and A. Gajjar. 2008. Non invasive insulin—Annual update on non-invasive insulin delivery technologies. *Drug Delivery Technology* 8:43–48.

Ang, E., M. K. Lawrence, C. R. Heilmann, J. A. Ferguson, J. A. Tobian, D. M. Webb, and P. Y. Berclaz. 2009. Safety and efficacy of AIR inhaled insulin compared with subcutaneous insulin in patients having diabetes and asthma: A 12-month, randomized, noninferiority trial. *Diabetes Technology & Therapeutics* 11 (Suppl 2):S35–44.

Angelo, R., K. Rousseau, M. Grant, A. Leone-Bay, and P. Richardson. 2009. Technosphere insulin: Defining the role of Technosphere particles at the cellular level. *Journal of Diabetes Science and Technology* 3 (3):545–554.

Aprahamian, M., C. Michel, W. Humbert, J. P. Devissaguet, and C. Damge. 1987. Transmucosal passage of polyalkylcyanoacrylate nanocapsules as a new drug carrier in the small intestine. *Biology of the Cell* 61 (1–2):69–76.

Arbit, E., and M. Kidron. 2009. Oral insulin: The rationale for this approach and current developments. *Journal of Diabetes Science and Technology* 3 (3):562–567.

Avadi, M. R., A. Jalali, A. M. Sadeghi, K. Shamimi, K. H. Bayati, E. Nahid, A. R. Dehpour, and M. Rafiee-Tehrani. 2005. Diethyl methyl chitosan as an intestinal paracellular enhancer: Ex vivo and in vivo studies. *International Journal of Pharmaceutics* 293 (1–2):83–89.

Bai, J. P., and L. L. Chang. 1995. Transepithelial transport of insulin: I. Insulin degradation by insulin-degrading enzyme in small intestinal epithelium. *Pharmaceutical Research* 12 (8):1171–1175.

Bellary, S., and A. H. Barnett. 2006. Inhaled insulin (Exubera®): Combining efficacy and convenience. *Diabetes and Vascular Disease Research* 3 (3):179–185.

Benson, H. A. E. 2006. Transfersomes for transdermal drug delivery. *Expert Opinion on Drug Delivery* 3 (9):727–737.

Bernstein, G. 2008. Delivery of insulin to the buccal mucosa utilizing the RapidMist™ system. *Expert Opinion on Drug Delivery* 5 (9):1047–1055.

Biocon Biopharmaceuticals. 2013. [cited March 18, 2013]. Available from http://www.biocon.com.

Boehm, B. O., P. D. Home, C. Behrend, N. M. Kamp, and A. Lindholm. 2002. Premixed insulin aspart 30 vs. premixed human insulin 30/70 twice daily: A randomized trial in Type 1 and Type 2 diabetic patients. *Diabetic Medicine* 19 (5):393–399.

BOWS Pharmaceuticals AG. 2013. [cited March 13, 2013]. Available from http://www.bowspharma.com/default_files/Page346.htm.

Brunner, G. A., B. Balent, M. Ellmerer, L. Schaupp, A. Siebenhofer, J. H. Jendle, J. Okikawa, and T. R. Pieber. 2001. Dose-response relation of liquid aerosol inhaled insulin in Type I diabetic patients. *Diabetologia* 44 (3):305–308.

Burge, M. R., A. G. Rassam, and D. S. Schade. 1998. Lispro insulin: Benefits and limitations. *Trends in Endocrinology & Metabolism* 9 (8):337–341.

Camenisch, G., J. Alsenz, H. van de Waterbeemd, and G. Folkers. 1998. Estimation of permeability by passive diffusion through Caco-2 cell monolayers using the drugs' lipophilicity and molecular weight. *European Journal of Pharmaceutical Sciences* 6 (4):317–324.

Carino, G. P., and E. Mathiowitz. 1999. Oral insulin delivery. *Advanced Drug Delivery Reviews* 35 (2–3):249–257.

Cassidy, J., N. Amin, M. Marino, M. Gotfried, T. Meyer, K. Sommerer, and R. Baughman. 2011. Insulin lung deposition and clearance following Technosphere® insulin inhalation powder administration. *Pharmaceutical Research* 28 (9):2157–2164.

Cevc, G., D. Gebauer, J. Stieber, A. Schätzlein, and G. Blume. 1998. Ultraflexible vesicles, Transfersomes, have an extremely low pore penetration resistance and transport therapeutic amounts of insulin across the intact mammalian skin. *Biochimica et Biophysica Acta (BBA)—Biomembranes* 1368 (2):201–215.

Chalasani, K. B., G. J. Russell-Jones, A. K. Jain, P. V. Diwan, and S. K. Jain. 2007. Effective oral delivery of insulin in animal models using vitamin B12-coated dextran nanoparticles. *Journal of Controlled Release* 122 (2):141–150.

Chalasani, K. B., G. J. Russell-Jones, S. K. Yandrapu, P. V. Diwan, and S. K. Jain. 2007. A novel vitamin B12-nanosphere conjugate carrier system for peroral delivery of insulin. *Journal of Controlled Release* 117 (3):421–429.

Chen, H., H. Zhu, J. Zheng, D. Mou, J. Wan, J. Zhang, T. Shi, Y. Zhao, H. Xu, and X. Yang. 2009. Iontophoresis-driven penetration of nanovesicles through microneedle-induced skin microchannels for enhancing transdermal delivery of insulin. *Journal of Controlled Release* 139:63–72.

Chen, J. W., T. Lauritzen, A. Bojesen, and J. S. Christiansen. 2006. Multiple mealtime administration of biphasic insulin aspart 30 versus traditional basal-bolus human insulin treatment in patients with type 1 diabetes. *Diabetes, Obesity and Metabolism* 8 (6):682–689.

Chen, M.-C., K. Sonaje, K.-J. Chen, and H.-W. Sung. 2011. A review of the prospects for polymeric nanoparticle platforms in oral insulin delivery. *Biomaterials* 32 (36):9826–9838.

Clark, M. A., M. A. Jepson, and B. H. Hirst. 2001. Exploiting M cells for drug and vaccine delivery. *Advanced Drug Delivery Reviews* 50 (1–2):81–106.
Clinic trials at Novo Nordisk 2013. http://www.novonordisk-trials.com/ (accessed March 14, 2013).
ClinicalTrials.gov. 2013. [cited August 22, 2013]. Available from http://clinicaltrials.gov.
Comulada, A. L., E. Renard, M. Nakano, N. Rais, X. Mao, D. M. Webb, and Z. Milicevic. 2009. Efficacy and safety of AIR inhaled insulin compared to insulin lispro in patients with type 1 diabetes mellitus in a 6-month, randomized, noninferiority trial. *Diabetes Technology & Therapeutics* 11 Suppl 2:S17–25.
CPEX Pharmaceuticals Inc. 2010. *Form 10-K annual report: United States securities and exchange comission* 2010 [cited June 10, 2013]. Available from http://www.faqs.org /sec-filings/110331/CPEX-Pharmaceuticals-Inc_10-K.
Craft, S., L. D. Baker, T. J. Montine, S. Minoshima, G. S. Watson, A. Claxton, M. Arbuckle et al. 2012. Intranasal insulin therapy for Alzheimer disease and amnestic mild cognitive impairment: A pilot clinical trial. *Archives of Neurology* 69 (1):29–38.
Dailey, G., J. Rosenstock, R. G. Moses, and K. Ways. 2004. Insulin glulisine provides improved glycemic control in patients with type 2 diabetes. *Diabetes Care* 27 (10):2363–2368.
DailyMed. 2013. [cited February 17, 2013]. Available from http://dailymed.nlm.nih.gov/dailymed /about.cfm.
Damge, C., P. Maincent, and N. Ubrich. 2007. Oral delivery of insulin associated to polymeric nanoparticles in diabetic rats. *Journal of Controlled Release* 117 (2):163–170.
Dave, N., P. Hazra, A. Khedkar, H. S. Manjunath, H. Iyer, and S. Suryanarayanan. 2008. Process and purification for manufacture of a modified insulin intended for oral delivery. *Journal of Chromatography A* 1177 (2):282–286.
Davidson, J. A., A. Liebl, J. S. Christiansen, G. Fulcher, R. J. Ligthelm, P. Brown, T. Gylvin, and R. Kawamori. 2009. Risk for nocturnal hypoglycemia with biphasic insulin aspart 30 compared with biphasic human insulin 30 in adults with type 2 diabetes mellitus: A meta-analysis. *Clinical Therapeutics* 31 (8):1641–1651.
Davis, S. P., W. Martanto, M. G. Allen, and M. R. Prausnitz. 2005. Hollow metal microneedles for insulin delivery to diabetic rats. *IEEE Transactions on Biomedical Engineering* 52 (5):909–915.
de La Peña, A., M. Riddle, L. A. Morrow, H. H. Jiang, H. Linnebjerg, A. Scott, K. M. Win et al. 2011. Pharmacokinetics and pharmacodynamics of high-dose human regular U-500 insulin versus human regular U-100 insulin in healthy obese subjects. *Diabetes Care* 34 (12):2496–2501.
de La Peña, A., M. Seger, K. Rave, L. Heinemann, B. Silverman, and D. B. Muchmore. 2009. AIR insulin capsules of different dose strengths may be combined to yield equivalent pharmacokinetics and glucodynamics. *Diabetes Technology & Therapeutics* (Suppl 2):S75–80.
Del Curto, M. D., A. Maroni, A. Foppoli, L. Zema, A. Gazzaniga, and M. E. Sangalli. 2009. Preparation and evaluation of an oral delivery system for time-dependent colon release of insulin and selected protease inhibitor and absorption enhancer compounds. *Journal of Pharmaceutical Sciences* 98 (12):4661–4669.
Diabetology Ltd. 2013. [cited March 13, 2013]. Available from http://www.diabetology.co.uk.
Diasome Pharmaceuticals Inc. 2013. [cited March 18, 2013]. Available from http://www .diasome.com/main3.swf.
Dodane, V., M. Amin Khan, and J. R. Merwin. 1999. Effect of chitosan on epithelial permeability and structure. *International Journal of Pharmaceutics* 182 (1):21–32.
Ebel, J. P. 1990. A method for quantifying particle absorption from the small intestine of the mouse. *Pharmaceutical Research* 7 (8):848–851.

Edwards, D. A., J. Hanes, G. Caponetti, J. Hrkach, A. Ben-Jebria, M. L. Eskew, J. Mintzes, D. Deaver, N. Lotan, and R. Langer. 1997. Large porous particles for pulmonary drug delivery. *Science* 276 (5320):1868–1872.

Eldor, R., E. Arbit, Y. Miteva, R. Freier, and M. Kidron. 2010. *Oral insulin: Type I diabetes (T1DM) patient response upon preprandial administration* 2010 [cited March 13, 2013]. Available from http://oramed.com/ufiles/ADA%20poster%202010.pdf.

Eldor, R., M. Kidron, and E. Arbit. 2010. Open-label study to assess the safety and pharmacodynamics of five oral insulin formulations in healthy subjects. *Diabetes, Obesity and Metabolism* 12 (3):219–223.

Eli Lilly and Company. 2013. *Information for the patient 3ml prefilled insulin delivery device, Humulin® N Pen NPH human insulin (rDNA ORIGIN) isophane suspension 100 Units per ml (U-100)* 2009 [cited February 17, 2013]. Available from http://pi.lilly.com/us/humulinn-pen.pdf.

———. 2013. *Patient information, Humulin® (HU-mu-lin) R Regular U-500 (concentrated) insulin human injection, USP (rDNA origin)* 2011 [cited February 19, 2013]. Available from http://pi.lilly.com/us/humulin-r-u500-ppi.pdf.

———. 2013. *Patient information, Humulin® R Regular insulin human injection, USP (rDNA origin) 100 Units per ml (U-100)* 2011 [cited February 17, 2013]. Available from http://pi.lilly.com/us/humulin-r-ppi.pdf.

———. 2013. *Highlights of prescribing information* 2012 [cited February 17, 2013]. Available from http://pi.lilly.com/us/humalog-pen-pi.pdf.

———. 2013. *Instructions for use HUMALOG® Mix50/50™ KwikPen™ 50% insulin lispro protamine suspension and 50% insulin lispro injection (rDNA origin)* 2012 [cited March 24, 2013]. Available from http://pi.lilly.com/us/humalog5050-kwikpen-um.pdf.

———. 2013. *Instructions for use HUMALOG® Mix75/25™ KwikPen™ 75% insulin lispro protamine suspension and 25% insulin lispro injection (rDNA origin)* 2012 [cited March 24, 2013]. Available from http://pi.lilly.com/us/humalog7525-kwikpen-um.pdf.

Ellis, S. L., K. A. Gemperline, and S. K. Garg. 2007. Review of phase 2 studies utilizing the AIR particle technology in the delivery of human insulin inhalation powder versus subcutaneous regular or lispro insulin in subjects with type 1 or type 2 diabetes. *Diabetes Technology & Therapeutics* (Suppl 1):S48–56.

EMA. 2013. *Apidra: EPAR—Product information* 2011 [cited February 17, 2013]. Available from http://www.ema.europa.eu/docs/en_GB/document_library/EPAR_-_Product_Information/human/000557/WC500025250.pdf.

———. 2013. *Humalog: EPAR—Product information* 2011 [cited February 17, 2013]. Available from http://www.ema.europa.eu/docs/en_GB/document_library/EPAR_-_Product_Information/human/000088/WC500050332.pdf.

———. 2013. *Levemir: EPAR—Product information* 2012 [cited February 19, 2013]. Available from http://www.ema.europa.eu/ema/index.jsp?curl=pages/medicines/human/medicines/000528/human_med_000884.jsp&mid=WC0b01ac058001d124.

———. 2013. *Mixtard: EPAR—Product information* 2012 [cited March 26, 2013]. Available from http://www.ema.europa.eu/docs/en_GB/document_library/EPAR_-_Product_Information/human/000428/WC500029822.pdf.

———. 2013. *NovoMix: EPAR—Product information* 2012 [cited March 22, 2013]. Available from http://www.ema.europa.eu/docs/en_GB/document_library/EPAR_-_Product_Information/human/000308/WC500029441.pdf.

———. 2013. *NovoRapid: EPAR—Product information* 2012 [cited February 17, 2013]. Available from http://www.ema.europa.eu/docs/en_GB/document_library/EPAR_-_Product_Information/human/000258/WC500030372.pdf.

———. 2013. 2013 [cited April 5, 2013]. Available from http://www.ema.europa.eu/ema.

———. 2013. *Ryzodeg: EPAR—Product information* 2013 [cited April 4, 2013]. Available from http://www.ema.europa.eu/docs/en_GB/document_library/EPAR_-_Product_Information/human/002499/WC500139011.pdf.

———. 2013. *Tresiba: EPAR—Product information* 2013 [cited April 5, 2013]. Available from http://www.ema.europa.eu/docs/en_GB/document_library/EPAR_-_Product_Information/human/002498/WC500138940.pdf.

Emisphere Technologies Inc. 2013. 2013 [cited March 13, 2013]. Available from http://www.emisphere.com/index.html.

Ermak, T. H., and P. J. Giannasca. 1998. Microparticle targeting to M cells. *Advanced Drug Delivery Reviews* 34 (2–3):261–283.

Farr, S. J., A. McElduff, L. E. Mather, J. Okikawa, M. E. Ward, I. Gonda, V. Licko, and R. M. Rubsamen. 2000. Pulmonary insulin administration using the AERx system: Physiological and physicochemical factors influencing insulin effectiveness in healthy fasting subjects. *Diabetes Technology & Therapeutics* 2 (2):185–197.

Fasano, A. 1998. Innovative strategies for the oral delivery of drugs and peptides. *Trends in Biotechnology* 16 (4):152–157.

Fasano, A., and S. Uzzau. 1997. Modulation of intestinal tight junctions by Zonula occludens toxin permits enteral administration of insulin and other macromolecules in an animal model. *The Journal of Clinical Investigation* 99 (6):1158–1164.

Flood, T. 2006. Advances in insulin delivery systems and devices: Beyond the vial and syringe. *Insulin* 1 (3):99–108.

Florence, A. T. 1997. The oral absorption of micro- and nanoparticulates: Neither exceptional nor unusual. *Pharmaceutical Research* 14 (3):259–266.

———. 2004. Issues in oral nanoparticle drug carrier uptake and targeting. *Journal of Drug Targeting* 12 (2):65–70.

———. 2005. Nanoparticle uptake by the oral route: Fulfilling its potential? *Drug Discovery Today: Technologies* 2 (1):75–81.

Florence, A. T., and N. Hussain. 2001. Transcytosis of nanoparticle and dendrimer delivery systems: Evolving vistas. *Advanced Drug Delivery Reviews* 50 Suppl 1:S69–89.

Forst, T., C. Hohberg, T. Schöndorf, M. Borchert, S. Forst, W. Roth, B. Dehos, and A. Pfützner. 2009. Time-action profile and patient assessment of inhaled insulin via the Exubera device in comparison with subcutaneously injected insulin aspart via the FlexPen device. *Diabetes Technology & Therapeutics* 11 (2):87–92.

Freemantle, N., L. Blonde, D. Duhot, M. Hompesch, R. Eggertsen, F. D. R. Hobbs, L. Martinez, S. Ross, B. Bolinder, and E. Stridde. 2005. Availability of inhaled insulin promotes greater perceived acceptance of insulin therapy in patients with type 2 diabetes. *Diabetes Care* 28 (2):427–428.

Frey, A., K. T. Giannasca, R. Weltzin, P. J. Giannasca, H. Reggio, W. I. Lencer, and M. R. Neutra. 1996. Role of the glycocalyx in regulating access of microparticles to apical plasma membranes of intestinal epithelial cells: Implications for microbial attachment and oral vaccine targeting. *The Journal of Experimental Medicine* 184 (3):1045–1059.

Gangwar, M., R. Singh, R. K. Goel, and G. Nath. 2012. Recent advances in various emerging vescicular systems: An overview. *Asian Pacific Journal of Tropical Biomedicine* 2 (2, Supplement):S1176–S1188.

Garber, A. J., A. B. King, S. D. Prato, S. Sreenan, M. K. Balci, M. Muñoz-Torres, J. Rosenstock, L. A. Endahl, A. M. O. Francisco, and P. Hollander. 2012. Insulin degludec, an ultra-longacting basal insulin, versus insulin glargine in basal-bolus treatment with mealtime insulin aspart in type 2 diabetes (BEGIN Basal-Bolus Type 2): A phase 3, randomised, open-label, treat-to-target non-inferiority trial. *The Lancet* 379 (9825):1498–1507.

Garg, S., J. Rosenstock, and K. Ways. 2005. Optimized Basal-bolus insulin regimens in type 1 diabetes: Insulin glulisine versus regular human insulin in combination with Basal insulin glargine. *Endocrine Practice* 11 (1):11–17.

Garg, S. K., P. A. Gottlieb, M. E. Hisatomi, A. D'Souza, A. J. Walker, K. E. Izuora, and H. P. Chase. 2004. Improved glycemic control without an increase in severe hypoglycemic episodes in intensively treated patients with type 1 diabetes receiving morning, evening, or split dose insulin glargine. *Diabetes Research and Clinical Practice* 66 (1):49–56.

Geho, W. B., H. C. Geho, J. R. Lau, and T. Gana. 2009. Hepatic-directed vesicle insulin: A review of formulation development and preclinical evaluation. *Journal of Diabetes Science and Technology* 3 (6):1451–1459.

Gelfand, R. A., S. L. Schwartz, and M. Horton. 2000. Pharmacological reproducibility of inhaled human insulin dosed pre-meal in patients with type 2 DM. *Diabetologia* 43 (Suppl 1):A202.

Generex Biotechnology Corp. 2013. [cited March 22, 2013]. Available from http://www.generex.com/index.php.

Gerber, R. A., J. C. Cappelleri, I. A. Kourides, and R. A. Gelfand. 2001. Treatment satisfaction with inhaled insulin in patients with type 1 diabetes: A randomized controlled trial. *Diabetes Care* 24 (9):1556–1559.

Gómez-Pérez, F. J., and J. A. Rull. 2005. Insulin therapy: Current alternatives. *Archives of Medical Research* 36 (3):258–272.

Gross, J. L., M. Nakano, G. Colon-Vega, R. Ortiz-Carasquillo, F. J. A., S. Althouse, J. A. Tobian, P. Y. Berclaz, and Z. Milicevic. 2009. Initiation of prandial insulin therapy with AIR inhaled insulin or insulin lispro in patients with type 2 diabetes: A randomized noninferiority trial. *Diabetes Technology & Therapeutics* (Suppl 2):S27–S34.

Gross, J. L., M. Nakano, G. Colon-Vega, R. Ortiz-Carasquillo, J. A. Ferguson, S. Althouse, J. A. Tobian, P. Y. Berclaz, and Z. Milicevic. 2009. Two-year efficacy and safety of AIR inhaled insulin in patients with type 1 diabetes: An open-label randomized controlled trial. *Diabetes Technology & Therapeutics* (Suppl 2):S5–S16.

Guerci, B., and J. P. Sauvanet. 2005. Subcutaneous insulin: Pharmacokinetic variability and glycemic variability. *Diabetes & Metabolism* 31 (4, Part 2):4S7–4S24.

Gupta, J., E. Felner, and M. Prausnitz. 2009. Minimally invasive insulin delivery in subjects with type 1 diabetes using hollow microneedles. *Diabetes Technology & Therapeutics* 11 (6):329–337.

Hahr, A., and M. Molitch. 2010. Optimizing insulin therapy in patients with type 1 and type 2 diabetes mellitus: Optimal dosing and timing in the outpatient setting. *Disease-a-month: DM* 56 (3):148–162.

Halimi, S., P. Raskin, A. Liebl, R. Kawamori, G. Fulcher, and G. Yan. 2005. Efficacy of biphasic insulin aspart in patients with type 2 diabetes. *Clinical Therapeutics* 27, Supplement 2 (0):S57–S74.

Hayes, R. P., D. Muchmore, and J. Schmitke. 2007. Effect of inhaled insulin on patient-reported outcomes and treatment preference in patients with type 1 diabetes. *Current Medical Research and Opinion* 23 (2):435–442.

Heinemann, L. 2008. Variability of insulin action: Does it matter? *Insulin* 3 (1):37–45.

Heinemann, L., and T. Heise. 2004. Review: Current status of the development of inhaled insulin. *The British Journal of Diabetes & Vascular Disease* 4 (5):295–301.

Heinemann, L., and Y. Jacques. 2009. Oral and buccal insulin: A critical reappraisal. *Journal of Diabetes Science and Technology* 3 (3):568–584.

Heise, T., A. Brugger, C. Cook, U. Eckers, A. Hutchcraft, L. Nosek, K. Rave et al. 2009. PROMAXX® inhaled insulin: Safe and efficacious administration with a commercially available dry powder inhaler. *Diabetes, Obesity and Metabolism* 11 (5):455–459.

Heise, T., L. Nosek, B. B. Rønn, L. Endahl, L. Heinemann, C. Kapitza, and E. Draeger. 2004. Lower within-subject variability of insulin Detemir in comparison to NPH insulin and insulin Glargine in people with type 1 diabetes. *Diabetes* 53 (6):1614–1620.

Heise, T., L. Nosek, H. Spitzer, L. Heinemann, E. Niemöller, A. D. Frick, and R. H. A. Becker. 2007. Insulin glulisine: A faster onset of action compared with insulin lispro. *Diabetes, Obesity and Metabolism* 9 (5):746–753.

Heller, S., J. Buse, M. Fisher, S. Garg, M. Marre, L. Merker, E. Renard et al. 2012. Insulin degludec, an ultra-longacting basal insulin, versus insulin glargine in basal-bolus treatment with mealtime insulin aspart in type 1 diabetes (BEGIN Basal-Bolus Type 1): A phase 3, randomised, open-label, treat-to-target non-inferiority trial. *The Lancet* 379 (9825):1489–1497.

Hermansen, K., M. Colombo, H. Storgaard, A. Østergaard, K. Kølendorf, and S. Madsbad. 2002. Improved postprandial glycemic control with biphasic insulin Aspart relative to biphasic insulin Lispro and biphasic human insulin in patients with type 2 diabetes. *Diabetes Care* 25 (5):883–888.

Hermansen, K., T. Rönnemaa, A. H. Petersen, S. Bellaire, and U. Adamson. 2004. Intensive therapy with inhaled insulin via the AERx insulin diabetes management system: A 12-week proof-of-concept trial in patients with type 2 diabetes. *Diabetes Care* 27 (1):162–167.

Herz, M., V. Arora, B. Sun, S. C. Ferguson, G. B. Bolli, and B. M. Frier. 2002. Basal-bolus insulin therapy in Type 1 diabetes: Comparative study of pre-meal administration of a fixed mixture of insulin lispro (50%) and neutral protamine lispro (50%) with human soluble insulin. *Diabetic Medicine* 19 (11):917–923.

Hochman, J., and P. Artursson. 1994. Mechanisms of absorption enhancement and tight junction regulation. *Journal of Controlled Release* 29 (3):253–267.

Hoffman, A., and B. Qadri. 2008. Eligen insulin—A system for the oral delivery of insulin for diabetes. *IDrugs: The Investigational Drugs Journal* 11 (6):433–441.

Hoffman, R. M., J. H. Shah, C. S. Wendel, W. C. Duckworth, K. D. Adam, S. U. Bokhari, C. Dalton, and G. H. Murata. 2002. Evaluating once- and twice-daily self-monitored blood glucose testing strategies for stable insulin-treated patients with type 2 diabetes: The diabetes outcomes in veterans Study. *Diabetes Care* 25 (10):1744–1748.

Hollander, P. A., L. Blonde, R. Rowe, A. E. Mehta, J. L. Milburn, K. S. Hershon, J. L. Chiasson, and S. R. Levin. 2004. Efficacy and safety of inhaled insulin (Exubera) compared with subcutaneous insulin therapy in patients with type 2 diabetes: Results of a 6-month, randomized, comparative trial. *Diabetes Care* 27 (10):2356–2362.

Home, P. D. 2012. The pharmacokinetics and pharmacodynamics of rapid-acting insulin analogues and their clinical consequences. *Diabetes, Obesity and Metabolism* 14 (9):780–788.

Home, P. D., L. Barriocanal, and A. Lindholm. 1999. Comparative pharmacokinetics and pharmacodynamics of the novel rapid-acting insulin analogue, insulin aspart, in healthy volunteers. *European Journal of Clinical Pharmacology* 55 (3):199–203.

Home, P. D., P. Hallgren, K. H. Usadel, T. Sane, J. Faber, V. Grill, and H. H. Friberg. 2006. Pre-meal insulin aspart compared with pre-meal soluble human insulin in type 1 diabetes. *Diabetes Research and Clinical Practice* 71 (2):131–139.

Home, P. D., A. Lindholm, and A. Riis. 2000. Insulin aspart vs. human insulin in the management of long-term blood glucose control in Type 1 diabetes mellitus: A randomized controlled trial. *Diabetic Medicine* 17 (11):762–770.

Hosny, E. A., H. I. Al-Shora, and M. M. Elmazar. 2002. Oral delivery of insulin from enteric-coated capsules containing sodium salicylate: Effect on relative hypoglycemia of diabetic beagle dogs. *International Journal of Pharmaceutics* 237 (1–2):71–76.

Howey, D. C., R. R. Bowsher, R. L. Brunelle, and J. R. Woodworth. 1994. [Lys(B28), Pro(B29)]-human insulin: A rapidly absorbed analogue of human insulin. *Diabetes* 43 (3):396–402.

Iyer, H., A. Khedkar, M. Verma, S. Krishnamurthy, and A. Anand. 2013. *A dose escalation study of IN-105 (insulin analogue) tablets in type 2 diabetes mellitus subjects* 2009 [cited March 18, 2013]. Available from http://professional.diabetes.org/Abstracts_Display.aspx?TYP=1&CID=73505.

Jani, P., G. W. Halbert, J. Langridge, and A. T. Florence. 1989. The uptake and translocation of latex nanospheres and microspheres after oral administration to rats. *The Journal of Pharmacy and Pharmacology* 41 (12):809–812.

———. 1990. Nanoparticle uptake by the rat gastrointestinal mucosa: Quantitation and particle size dependency. *The Journal of Pharmacy and Pharmacology* 42 (12):821–826.

Jehle, P. M., C. Micheler, D. R. Jehle, D. Breitig, and B. O. Boehm. 1999. Inadequate suspension of neutral protamine Hagendorn (NPH) insulin in pens. *The Lancet* 354 (9190):1604–1607.

Jepson, M. A., N. L. Simmons, T. C. Savidge, P. S. James, and B. H. Hirst. 1993. Selective binding and transcytosis of latex microspheres by rabbit intestinal M cells. *Cell and Tissue Research* 271 (3):399–405.

Jung, T., W. Kamm, A. Breitenbach, E. Kaiserling, J. X. Xiao, and T. Kissel. 2000. Biodegradable nanoparticles for oral delivery of peptides: Is there a role for polymers to affect mucosal uptake? *European Journal of Pharmaceutics and Biopharmaceutics* 50: 147–160.

Kamba, M., Y. Seta, A. Kusai, M. Ikeda, and K. Nishimura. 2000. A unique dosage form to evaluate the mechanical destructive force in the gastrointestinal tract. *International Journal of Pharmaceutics* 208 (1–2):61–70.

Kapitza, C., T. Heise, R. S. Fishman, D. A. Shapiro, V. Gopalakrishnan, K. Rave, S. Bott, A. D. Perera, and L. Heinemann. 2004. Impact of particle size and aerosolization time on the metabolic effect of an inhaled insulin aerosol. *Diabetes Technology & Therapeutics* 6 (2):119–127.

Kapitza, C., T. Heise, M. McGovern, E. Cefali, A. Buchwald, and L. Heinemann. 2003. Time-action profile of a new pulmonary insulin applied with a metered-dose inhaler. *Diabetes* 52 (Suppl 1):A91.

Kapitza, C., M. Hompesch, B. Scharling, and T. Heise. 2004. Intrasubject variability of inhaled insulin in type 1 diabetes: A comparison with subcutaneous insulin. *Diabetes Technology & Therapeutics* 6 (4):466–472.

Kapitza, C., K. Rave, K. Ostrowski, T. Heise, and L. Heinemann. 2004. Reduced postprandial glycaemic excursion with biphasic insulin Aspart 30 injected immediately before a meal. *Diabetic Medicine* 21 (5):500–501.

Kapsner, P., R. Bergenstal, M. Rendell, C. P. Howard, A. H. Boss, and P. Chang. 2009. Comparative efficacy and safety of Technosphere® insulin and a rapid-acting analog both given with glargine in subjects with T1DM in a 52-week study. *Diabetologia* 52 (S1):Abstract #982.

Kavimandan, N. J., E. Losi, and N. A. Peppas. 2006. Novel delivery system based on complexation hydrogels as delivery vehicles for insulin-transferrin conjugates. *Biomaterials* 27 (20):3846–3854.

Keating, G. M. 2012. Insulin Detemir: A review of its use in the management of diabetes mellitus. *Drugs* 72 (17):2255–2287.

Khafagy, E.-S., and M. Morishita. 2012. Oral biodrug delivery using cell-penetrating peptide. *Advanced Drug Delivery Reviews* 64 (6):531–539.

Khafagy, E.-S., M. Morishita, Y. Onuki, and K. Takayama. 2007. Current challenges in noninvasive insulin delivery systems: A comparative review. *Advanced Drug Delivery Reviews* 59:1521–1546.

Kidron, M., S. Dinh, Y. Menachem, R. Abbas, B. Variano, M. Goldberg, E. Arbit, and H. Bar-On. 2004. A novel per-oral insulin formulation: Proof of concept study in non-diabetic subjects. *Diabetic Medicine* 21 (4):354–357.

Kidron, M., R. Eldor, M. Yanitsa, R. Freier, and E. Arbit. 2013. *Extended exposure to an oral insulin formulation yields decreased insulin secretion in Type II diabetes subjects* 2010 [cited March 13, 2013]. Available from http://oramed.com/ufiles/DT_Nov2010handout_Nov172010.pdf.

Kim, D., S. Mudaliar, S. Chinnapongse, N. Chu, S. M. Boies, T. Davis, A. D. Perera, R. S. Fishman, D. A. Shapiro, and R. Henry. 2003. Dose-response relationships of inhaled insulin delivered via the aerodose insulin inhaler and subcutaneously injected insulin in patients with type 2 diabetes. *Diabetes Care* 26 (10):2842–2847.

Kim, Y.-C., J.-H. Park, and M. R. Prausnitz. 2012. Microneedles for drug and vaccine delivery. *Advanced Drug Delivery Reviews* 64 (14):1547–1568.

Kulkarni, P. R., J. D. Yadav, K. A. Vaidya, and P. P. Gandhi. 2011. Transferosomes: An emerging tool for transdermal drug delivery. *International Journal of Pharmaceutical Science and Research* 2 (4):735–741.

Lane, M. E., M. O'Driscoll, and O. I. Corrigan. 2005. Quantitative estimation of the effects of bile salt surfactant systems on insulin stability and permeability in the rat intestine using a mass balance model. *Journal of Pharmacy and Pharmacology* 57 (2):169–175.

Lassmann-Vague, V., and D. Raccah. 2006. Alternatives routes of insulin delivery. *Diabetes & Metabolism* 32 (5):513–522.

Leary, A. C., M. Dowling, K. Cussen, J. O'Brien, and R. M. Stote. 2008. Pharmacokinetics and pharmacodynamics of intranasal insulin spray (Nasulin™) administered to healthy male volunteers: Influence of the nasal cycle. *Journal of Diabetes Science and Technology* 2 (6):1054–1060.

Leary, A. C., R. M. Stote, H. J. Breedt, J. O'Brien, and B. Buckley. 2005. Pharmacokinetics and pharmacodynamics of intranasal insulin administered to healthy subjects in escalating doses. *Diabetes Technology & Therapeutics* 7 (1):124–130.

Leary, A. C., R. M. Stote, K. Cussen, J. O'Brien, W. P. Leary, and B. Buckley. 2006. Pharmacokinetics and pharmacodynamics of intranasal insulin administered to patients with type 1 diabetes: A preliminary study. *Diabetes Technology & Therapeutics* 8 (1):81–88.

Leone-Bay, A., R. Baughman, C. Smutney, and J. Kocinsky. 2010. Innovation in drug delivery by inhalation. In *Orally Inhaled & Nasal Drug Products: Innovations from Major Delivery System Developers*, edited by F. F. Publishing: ONdrugDelivery.

Lepore, M., S. Pampanelli, C. Fanelli, F. Porcellati, L. Bartocci, A. Di Vincenzo, C. Cordoni, E. Costa, P. Brunetti, and G. B. Bolli. 2000. Pharmacokinetics and pharmacodynamics of subcutaneous injection of long-acting human insulin analog glargine, NPH insulin, and ultralente human insulin and continuous subcutaneous infusion of insulin lispro. *Diabetes* 49:2142–2148.

Lindholm, A., J. McEwen, and A. P. Riis. 1999. Improved postprandial glycemic control with insulin aspart. A randomized double-blind cross-over trial in type 1 diabetes. *Diabetes Care* 22 (5):801–805.

Lteif, A. N., and W. F. Schwenk. 1999. Accuracy of pen injectors versus insulin syringes in children with type 1 diabetes. *Diabetes Care* 22 (1):137–140.

Luzio, S., R. Peter, G. J. Dunseath, L. Mustafa, and D. R. Owens. 2008. A comparison of preprandial insulin glulisine versus insulin lispro in people with Type 2 diabetes over a 12-h period. *Diabetes Research and Clinical Practice* 79 (2):269–275.

Luzio, S. D., G. Dunseath, A. Lockett, T. P. Broke-Smith, R. R. New, and D. R. Owens. 2010. The glucose lowering effect of an oral insulin (Capsulin) during an isoglycaemic clamp study in persons with type 2 diabetes. *Diabetes, Obesity and Metabolism* 12 (1):82–87.

Ma, Z., T. M. Lim, and L. Y. Lim. 2005. Pharmacological activity of peroral chitosan-insulin nanoparticles in diabetic rats. *International Journal of Pharmaceutics* 293 (1–2):271–280.

Mahato, R. I., A. S. Narang, L. Thoma, and D. D. Miller. 2003. Emerging trends in oral delivery of peptide and protein drugs. *Critical Reviews in Therapeutic Drug Carrier Systems* 20 (2–3):153–214.

Malakar, J., S. O. Sen, A. K. Nayak, and K. K. Sen. 2012. Formulation, optimization and evaluation of transferosomal gel for transdermal insulin delivery. *Saudi Pharmaceutical Journal* 20 (4):355–363.

Malkov, D., R. Angelo, H. Wang, E. Flanders, H. Tang, and I. Gomez-Orellana. 2005. Oral delivery of insulin with the eligen technology: Mechanistic studies. *Current Drug Delivery* 2 (2):191–197.

Malone, J. K., S. Bai, B. N. Campaigne, J. Reviriego, and B. Augendre-Ferrante. 2005. Twice-daily pre-mixed insulin rather than basal insulin therapy alone results in better overall glycaemic control in patients with Type 2 diabetes. *Diabetic Medicine* 22 (4):374–381.

Mannucci, E., M. Monami, and N. Marchionni. 2009. Short-acting insulin analogues vs. regular human insulin in type 2 diabetes: A meta-analysis. *Diabetes, Obesity and Metabolism* 11 (1):53–59.

Marina Biotech. 2011. [cited June 9, 2013]. Available from http://www.marketwire.com/press-release/marina-biotech-granted-patent-rights-china-intranasal-insulin-delivery-formulations-nasdaq-mrna-1588245.htm.

Markey, K. A. 2011. MannKind Corporation update report. New York: Griffin Securities Equities Research.

Maroni, A., L. Zema, M. D. Del Curto, A. Foppoli, and A. Gazzaniga. 2011. Oral colon delivery of insulin with the aid of functional adjuvants. *Advanced Drug Delivery Reviews.*

Martanto, W., S. Davis, N. Holiday, J. Wang, H. Gill, and M. Prausnitz. 2004. Transdermal delivery of insulin using microneedles in vivo. *Pharmaceutical Research* 21 (6):947–952.

McAllister, D., P. Wang, S. Davis, J.-H. Park, P. Canatella, M. Allen, and M. Prausnitz. 2003. Microfabricated needles for transdermal delivery of macromolecules and nanoparticles: Fabrication methods and transport studies. *Proceedings of the National Academy of Sciences* 100 (24):13755–13760.

McKeage, K., and K. L. Goa. 2001. Insulin Glargine: A review of its therapeutic use as a long-acting agent for the management of type 1 and 2 diabetes mellitus. *Drugs* 61 (11):1599–1624.

McSorley, P. T., P. M. Bell, L. V. Jacobsen, A. Kristensen, and A. Lindholm. 2002. Twice-daily biphasic insulin aspart 30 versus biphasic human insulin 30: A double-blind crossover study in adults with type 2 diabetes mellitus. *Clinical Therapeutics* 24 (4):530–539.

Merrion Pharmaceuticals Ltd. 2013. [cited March 14, 2013]. Available from http://www.merrionpharma.com.

Michel, C., M. Aprahamian, L. Defontaine, P. Couvreur, and C. Damge. 1991. The effect of site of administration in the gastrointestinal tract on the absorption of insulin from nanocapsules in diabetic rats. *Journal of Pharmacy and Pharmacology* 43 (1):1–5.

Midatech Ltd. 2013. [cited March 22, 2013]. Available from http://www.midatechgroup.com.

Migalska, K., D. Morrow, M. Garland, R. Thakur, A. Woolfson, and R. Donnelly. 2011. Laser-engineered dissolving microneedle arrays for transdermal macromolecular drug delivery. *Pharmaceutical Research* 28 (8):1919–1930.

Mitchell, R. L., H. R. Costantino, A. Sileno, T. Duffy, G. Brandt, and S. C. Quay. 2008. Intranasal insulin: PK profile designed specifically for prandial treatment of Type 2 Diabetes. *Drug Development Research* 69 (3):143–152.

Mitragotri, S. 2000. Synergistic effect of enhancers for transdermal drug delivery. *Pharmaceutical Research* 17 (11):1354–1359.

Mitragotri, S., D. Blankschtein, and R. Langer. 1995. Ultrasound-mediated transdermal protein delivery. *Science* 269 (5225):850–853.

Monosol Rx. 2013. [cited March 22, 2013]. Available from http://www.monosolrx.com/index.htms.

Morishita, M., M. Kajita, A. Suzuki, K. Takayama, Y. Chiba, S. Tokiwa, and T. Nagai. 2000. The dose-related hypoglycemic effects of insulin emulsions incorporating highly purified EPA and DHA. *International Journal of Pharmaceutics* 201 (2):175–185.

Morishita, M., I. Morishita, K. Takayama, Y. Machida, and T. Nagai. 1993. Site-dependent effect of aprotinin, sodium caprate, Na2EDTA and sodium glycocholate on intestinal absorption of insulin. *Biological & Pharmaceutical Bulletin* 16 (1):68–72.

Muchmore, D. B., B. Silverman, A. De La Peña, and J. Tobian. 2007. The AIR inhaled insulin system: System components and pharmacokinetic/glucodynamic data. *Diabetes Technology & Therapeutics* (Suppl 1):S41–S47.

Nasrallah, S. N., and L. R. Reynolds. 2012. Insulin Degludec, the new generation basal insulin or just another basal insulin? *Clinical Medicine Insights: Endocrinology and Diabetes* 2012 (5):31–37.

Nastech Pharmaceutical Inc. 2013. *Nastech announces positive intranasal insulin data at American Diabetes Association Meeting* 2008 [cited June 9, 2013]. Available from http://investor.nastech.com/phoenix.zhtml?c=83674&p=irol-newsArticle&ID=1163556&highlight=.

Neutra, M. R., T. L. Phillips, E. L. Mayer, and D. J. Fishkind. 1987. Transport of membrane-bound macromolecules by M cells in follicle-associated epithelium of rabbit Peyer's patch. *Cell and Tissue Research* 247 (3):537–546.

Niskanen, L., L. A. Leiter, E. Franek, J. Weng, T. Damci, M. Muñoz-Torres, J.-P. Donnet, L. Endahl, T. V. Skjøth, and A. Vaag. 2012. Comparison of a soluble co-formulation of insulin degludec/insulin aspart vs biphasic insulin aspart 30 in type 2 diabetes: A randomised trial. *European Journal of Endocrinology* 167 (2):287–294.

Norrman, M., F. Hubálek, and G. Schluckebier. 2007. Structural characterization of insulin NPH formulations. *European Journal of Pharmaceutical Sciences* 30 (5):414–423.

Novo Nordisk. 2013. [cited February 17, 2013]. Available from http://www.novonordisk.com.

———. 2013. *Highlights of prescribing information* 2010 [cited March 31, 2013]. Available from http://www.novo-pi.com/novologmix7030.pdf.

———. 2013. *Endocrinologic and metabolic drug advisory committee. Insulin degludec and insulin degludec/insulin aspart treatment to improve glycemic control in patients with diabetes mellitus* 2012 [cited February 19, 2013]. Available from http://www.fda.gov/downloads/AdvisoryCommittees/CommitteesMeetingMaterials/Drugs/EndocrinologicandMetabolicDrugsAdvisoryCommittee/UCM327017.pdf.

———. 2013. *Novolog® insulin aspart (rDNA origin) injectin* 2013 [cited February 17, 2013]. Available from http://www.novo-pi.com/novolog.pdf.

O'Hagan, D. T. 1996. The intestinal uptake of particles and the implications for drug and antigen delivery. *Journal of Anatomy* 189 (Pt 3):477–482.

Oramed Pharmaceuticals Inc. 2013. [cited March 13, 2013]. Available from http://www.oramed.com.

Owen, R. L. 1977. Sequential uptake of horseradish peroxidase by lymphoid follicle epithelium of Peyer's patches in the normal unobstructed mouse intestine: An ultrastructural study. *Gastroenterology* 72 (3):440–451.

Park, K., I. C. Kwon, and K. Park. 2011. Oral protein delivery: Current status and future prospect. *Reactive and Functional Polymers* 71 (3):280–287.

Patton, J. S., J. Bukar, and S. Nagarajan. 1999. Inhaled insulin. *Advanced Drug Delivery Reviews* 35 (2–3):235–247.

Pauletti, G. M., S. Gangwar, G. T. Knipp, M. M. Nerurkar, F. W. Okumu, K. Tamura, T. J. Siahaan, and R. T. Borchardt. 1996. Structural requirements for intestinal absorption of peptide drugs. *Journal of Controlled Release* 41 (1–2):3–17.

Perera, A. D., C. Kapitza, L. Nosek, R. S. Fishman, D. A. Shapiro, T. Heise, and L. Heinemann. 2002. Absorption and metabolic effect of inhaled insulin: Intrapatient variability after inhalation via the aerodose insulin inhaler in patients with type 2 diabetes. *Diabetes Care* 25 (12):2276–2281.

Petrucci, R., N. Amin, P. Lovertin, A. Boss, and R. P. 2009. Pulmonary function tests remain similar in patients who received Technosphere insulin and in patients currently receiving standard antidiabetic therapy. *Diabetologia* 52 (S1):S361 Abstract #919.

Pfizer. 2013. [cited June 10, 2013]. Available from http://dailymed.nlm.nih.gov/dailymed/fda/fdaDrugXsl.cfm?id=7043.

Pillai, O., and R. Panchagnula. 2001. Insulin therapies—Past, present and future. *Drug Discovery Today* 6 (20):1056–1061.

Plank, J., M. Bodenlenz, F. Sinner, C. Magnes, E. Görzer, W. Regittnig, L. A. Endahl, E. Draeger, M. Zdravkovic, and T. R. Pieber. 2005. A double-blind, randomized, dose-response study investigating the pharmacodynamic and pharmacokinetic properties of the long-acting insulin analog detemir. *Diabetes Care* 28 (5):1107–1112.

Polat, B. E., D. Blankschtein, and R. Langer. 2010. Low-frequency sonophoresis: Application to the transdermal delivery of macromolecules and hydrophilic drugs. *Expert Opinion on Drug Delivery* 7 (12):1415–1432.

Polat, B. E., D. Hart, R. Langer, and D. Blankschtein. 2011. Ultrasound-mediated transdermal drug delivery: Mechanisms, scope, and emerging trends. *Journal of Controlled Release* 152 (3):330–348.

Potocka, E., R. A. Baughman, and H. Derendorf. 2011. Population pharmacokinetic model of human insulin following different routes of administration. *The Journal of Clinical Pharmacology* 51 (7):1015–1024.

Potocka, E., J. P. Cassidy, P. Haworth, D. Heuman, S. van Marle, and R. A. Baughman. 2010. Pharmacokinetic characterization of the novel pulmonary delivery excipient fumaryl diketopiperazine. *Journal of Diabetes Science and Technology* 4 (5):1164–1173.

Quattrin, T., A. Bélanger, N. J. Bohannon, S. L. Schwartz, and E. P. I. S. Group. 2004. Efficacy and safety of inhaled insulin (Exubera) compared with subcutaneous insulin therapy in patients with type 1 diabetes: Results of a 6-month, randomized, comparative trial. *Diabetes Care* 27 (11):2622–2627.

Raja-Khan, N., S. S. Warehime, and R. A. Gabbay. 2007. Review of biphasic insulin aspart in the treatment of type 1 and 2 diabetes. *Vascular Health and Risk Management* 3 (6):919–935.

Raskin, P., E. Allen, P. Hollander, A. Lewin, R. A. Gabbay, P. Hu, B. Bode, and A. Garber. 2005. Initiating insulin therapy in type 2 diabetes: A comparison of biphasic and basal insulin analogs. *Diabetes Care* 28 (2):260–265.

Raskin, P., S. Heller, M. Honka, P. C. Chang, A. H. Boss, P. C. Richardson, and N. Amin. 2012. Pulmonary function over 2 years in diabetic patients treated with prandial inhaled Technosphere Insulin or usual antidiabetes treatment: A randomized trial. *Diabetes, Obesity and Metabolism* 14 (2):163–173.

Raskin, P. R., P. A. Hollander, A. Lewin, R. A. Gabbay, B. Bode, and A. J. Garber. 2007. Basal insulin or premix analogue therapy in type 2 diabetes patients. *European Journal of Internal Medicine* 18 (1):56–62.

Rašlová, K., M. Bogoev, I. Raz, G. Leth, M. A. Gall, and N. Hâncu. 2004. Insulin detemir and insulin aspart: A promising basal-bolus regimen for type 2 diabetes. *Diabetes Research and Clinical Practice* 66 (2):193–201.

Rave, K., S. Bott, L. Heinemann, S. Sha, R. H. A. Becker, S. A. Willavize, and T. Heise. 2005. Time-action profile of inhaled insulin in comparison with subcutaneously injected insulin lispro and regular human insulin. *Diabetes Care* 28 (5):1077–1082.

Rave, K., E. Potocka, A. H. Boss, M. Marino, D. Costello, and R. Chen. 2009. Pharmacokinetics and linear exposure of AFRESA™ compared with the subcutaneous injection of regular human insulin. *Diabetes, Obesity and Metabolism* 11 (7):715–720.

Rayman, G., V. Profozic, and M. Middle. 2007. Insulin glulisine imparts effective glycaemic control in patients with Type 2 diabetes. *Diabetes Research and Clinical Practice* 76 (2):304–312.

Reis, C. P., F. J. Veiga, A. J. Ribeiro, R. J. Neufeld, and C. Damge. 2008. Nanoparticulate biopolymers deliver insulin orally eliciting pharmacological response. *Journal of Pharmaceutical Sciences* 97 (12):5290–5305.

Richardson, P. C., and A. H. Boss. 2007. Technosphere® insulin technology. *Diabetes Technology & Therapeutics* 9 (Suppl 1):S65–S72.

Rizvi, A. A., and R. J. Ligthelm. 2007. The use of premixed insulin analogues in the treatment of patients with type 2 diabetes mellitus: Advantages and limitations. *Insulin* 2 (2):68–79.

Rolla, A. 2008. Pharmacokinetic and pharmacodynamic advantages of insulin analogues and premixed insulin analogues over human insulins: Impact on efficacy and safety. *The American Journal of Medicine* 121 (6, Supplement):S9–S19.

Rosenstock, J., J. Cappelleri, B. Bolinder, and R. Gerber. 2004. Patient satisfaction and glycemic control after 1 year with inhaled insulin (Exubera) in patients with type 1 or type 2 diabetes. *Diabetes Care* 27 (6):1318–1323.

Rosenstock, J., W. T. Cefalu, P. A. Hollander, A. Belanger, F. G. Eliaschewitz, J. L. Gross, S. S. Klioze, L. B. S. Aubin, H. Foyt, M. Ogawa, and W. T. Duggan. 2008. Two-year pulmonary safety and efficacy of inhaled human insulin (Exubera) in adult patients with type 2 diabetes. *Diabetes Care* 31 (9):1723–1728.

Rosenstock, J., D. L. Lorber, L. Gnudi, C. P. Howard, D. W. Bilheimer, P. C. Chang, R. E. Petrucci, A. H. Boss, and P. C. Richardson. 2010. Prandial inhaled insulin plus basal insulin glargine versus twice daily biaspart insulin for type 2 diabetes: A multicentre randomised trial. *The Lancet* 375 (9733):2244–2253.

Rosenstock, J., G. Park, J. Zimmerman, and U. S. I. G. T. D. I. Group. 2000. Basal insulin glargine (HOE 901) versus NPH insulin in patients with type 1 diabetes on multiple daily insulin regimens. U.S. Insulin Glargine (HOE 901) Type 1 Diabetes Investigator Group. *Diabetes Care* 23 (8):1137–1142.

Rosenthal, R., D. Gunzel, C. Finger, S. M. Krug, J. F. Richter, J. D. Schulzke, M. Fromm, and S. Amasheh. 2012. The effect of chitosan on transcellular and paracellular mechanisms in the intestinal epithelial barrier. *Biomaterials* 33 (9):2791–2800.

Rossiter, A., N. Amin, R. Harris, A. H. Boss, and P. C. Richardson. 2009. Pulmonary safety of inhaled Technosphere® Insulin therapy in adults with diabetes using high-resolution computerized tomography of the chest. *Diabetologia* 52 (S1):Abstract #921.

Roxhed, N., B. Samel, L. Nordquist, P. Griss, and G. Stemme. 2008. Painless drug delivery through microneedle-based transdermal patches featuring active infusion. *IEEE Transactions on Biomedical Engineering* 55 (3):1063–1071.

Rys, P., O. Pankiewicz, K. Łach, A. Kwaskowski, I. Skrzekowska-Baran, and M. T. Malecki. 2011. Efficacy and safety comparison of rapid-acting insulin aspart and regular human insulin in the treatment of type 1 and type 2 diabetes mellitus: A systematic review. *Diabetes & Metabolism* 37 (3):190–200.

Sabetsky, V., and J. Ekblom. 2010. Insulin: A new era for an old hormone. *Pharmacological Research* 61 (1):1–4.

Sanofi-Aventis. 2009. *Highlights of prescribing information.* [cited February 18, 2013]. Available from http://products.sanofi.us/apidra/apidra.pdf.

Sargin, H., M. Sargin, Y. Altuntaş, A. M. Şengül, E. Orbay, S. Seber, S. Uçak, and A. Yayla. 2003. Comparison of lunch and bedtime NPH insulin plus mealtime insulin Lispro therapy with premeal regular insulin plus bedtime NPH insulin therapy in type 2 diabetes. *Diabetes Research and Clinical Practice* 62 (2):79–86.

Sarmento, B., A. Ribeiro, F. Veiga, P. Sampaio, R. Neufeld, and D. Ferreira. 2007. Alginate/chitosan nanoparticles are effective for oral insulin delivery. *Pharmaceutical Research* 24 (12):2198–2206.

Saroha, K., B. Sharma, and B. Yadav. 2011. Sonophoresis: An advanced tool in transdermal drug delivery system. *International Journal of Current Pharmaceutical Research* 3 (3):89–97.

Schiöth, H., S. Craft, S. Brooks, W. Frey, II, and C. Benedict. 2012. Brain insulin signaling and Alzheimer's disease: Current evidence and future directions. *Molecular Neurobiology* 46 (1):4–10.

Schipper, N. G. M., S. Olsson, J. A. Hoogstraate, A. G. deBoer, K. M. Varum, and P. Artursson. 1997. Chitosans as absorption enhancers for poorly absorbable drugs 2: Mechanism of absorption enhancement. *Pharmaceutical Research* 14 (7):923–929.

Schwartz, S., B. Geho, L. Rosenberg, and J. Lau. 2013. *Single-blind, placebo-controlled, dose-ranging trial of oral HDV-insulin in patients with type 2 diabetes mellitus* 2008 [cited March 18, 2013]. Available from http://professional.diabetes.org/Content/Posters/2008/p426-P.pdf.

———. 2013. *A two-week randomized active comparator study of two HDV-insulin routes (SC and Oral) and SC human insulin in patients with Type 1 diabetes mellitus* 2009 [cited March 18, 2013]. Available from http://professional.diabetes.org/Content/Posters/2008/p417-P.pdf.

Shakweh, M., G. Ponchel, and E. Fattal. 2004. Particle uptake by Peyer's patches: A pathway for drug and vaccine delivery. *Expert Opinion on Drug Delivery* 1 (1):141–163.

Shemesh, E., A. Rudich, I. Harman-Boehm, and T. Cukierman-Yaffe. 2012. Effect of intranasal insulin on cognitive function: A systematic review. *Journal of Clinical Endocrinology & Metabolism* 97 (2):366–376.

Shivanand, P., P. Binal, and D. Viral. 2009. Microneedles: Progress in developing new technology for painless drug delivery. *International Journal of PharmTech Research* 1 (4):1279–1282.

Silpi, C., B. Manish, and T. Kumar. 2011. Microneedles in transdermal drug delivery: An unique painless option. *International Research Journal of Pharmacy* 2 (4):72–78.

Singh, B., and S. Majuru. 2003. Oral delivery of therapeutic macromolecules: A perspective using the Eligen™ technology. *Drug Delivery Technology* 3 (4):58–62.

Skyler, J. S., P. A. Hollander, L. Jovanovic, S. Klioze, A. Krasner, R. J. Riese, J. Reis, P. Schwartz, and W. Duggan. 2008. Safety and efficacy of inhaled human insulin (Exubera®) during discontinuation and readministration of therapy in adults with type 1 diabetes: A 3-year randomized controlled trial. *Diabetes Research and Clinical Practice* 82 (2):238–246.

Smith, J. M., M. Dornish, and E. J. Wood. 2005. Involvement of protein kinase C in chitosan glutamate-mediated tight junction disruption. *Biomaterials* 26 (16):3269–3276.

Soares, S., A. Costa, and B. Sarmento. 2012. Novel non-invasive methods of insulin delivery. *Expert Opinion on Drug Delivery* 9 (12):1539–1558.

Steiner, S., A. Pfützner, B. R. Wilson, O. Harzer, L. Heinemann, and K. Rave. 2002. Technosphere/Insulin—Proof of concept study with a new insulin formulation for pulmonary delivery. *Experimental and Clinical Endocrinology & Diabetes* 110 (1):17–21.

Stewart, K. M., M. F. Wilson, and J. M. Rider. 2004. Insulin delivery devices. *Journal of Pharmacy Practice* 17 (1):20–28.

Stote, R., T. Marbury, L. Shi, M. Miller, and P. Strange. 2010. Comparison pharmacokinetics of two concentrations (0.7% and 1.0%) of Nasulin, an ultra-rapid-acting intranasal insulin formulation. *Journal of Diabetes Science and Technology* 4 (3):603–609.

Stote, R., M. Miller, T. Marbury, L. Shi, and P. Strange. 2011. Enhanced absorption of Nasulin™, an ultrarapid-acting intranasal insulin formulation, using single nostril administration in normal subjects. *Journal of Diabetes Science and Technology* 5 (1):113–119.

Stote, R., S. Schwartz, C. Dehn, and P. Strange. 2009. Two randomized crossover glucose clamp studies of Nasulin™ and lispro. San Francisco, November 5–7.

Su, F.-Y., K.-J. Lin, K. Sonaje, S.-P. Wey, T.-C. Yen, Y.-C. Ho, N. Panda, E.-Y. Chuang, B. Maiti, and H.-W. Sung. 2012. Protease inhibition and absorption enhancement by functional nanoparticles for effective oral insulin delivery. *Biomaterials* 33 (9):2801–2811.

Sung, H. W., K. Sonaje, Z. X. Liao, L. W. Hsu, and E. Y. Chuang. 2012. pH-responsive nanoparticles shelled with chitosan for oral delivery of insulin: From mechanism to therapeutic applications. *Accounts of Chemical Research*.

Swaan, P. W. 1998. Recent advances in intestinal macromolecular drug delivery via receptor-mediated transport pathways. *Pharmaceutical Research* 15 (6):826–834.

Thipphawong, J., B. Otulana, P. Clauson, J. Okikawa, and S. J. Farr. 2002. Pulmonary insulin administration using the AERx® insulin diabetes system. *Diabetes Technology & Therapeutics* 4 (4):499–504.

Tirumalasetty, P. P., and J. G. Eley. 2006. Permeability enhancing effects of the alkylglycoside, octylglucoside, on insulin permeation across epithelial membrane in vitro. *Journal of Pharmacy & Pharmaceutical Sciences* 9 (1):32–39.

Touch Digital Media Ltd. 2013. *US Endocrino Disease 2007. V-Go™—A novel device for delivering basal–bolus insulin therapy to patients with type 2 diabetes mellitus* 2007 [cited February 25, 2013]. Available from http://www.touchendocrinology.com/articles/v-go-novel-device-delivering-basal-bolus-insulin-therapy-patients-type-2-diabetes-mellitus?page=0,1.

Transdermal Specialties Inc. 2013. [cited March 6, 2013]. Available from http://www.transdermalspecialties.com.

Uchiyama, T., T. Sugiyama, Y. S. Quan, A. Kotani, N. Okada, T. Fujita, S. Muranishi, and A. Yamamoto. 1999. Enhanced permeability of insulin across the rat intestinal membrane by various absorption enhancers: Their intestinal mucosal toxicity and absorption-enhancing mechanism of n-lauryl-beta-D-maltopyranoside. *Journal of Pharmacy and Pharmacology* 51 (11):1241–1250.

Valeritas Inc. 2013. [cited February 25, 2013]. Available from https://www.valeritas.com.

———. 2013. *V-Go disposable insulin delivery device* [cited February 25, 2013]. Available from https://www.go-vgo.com.

———. 2013. *Instruction for patient use* 2011 [cited February 22, 2013]. Available from https://www.go-vgo.com/docs/pdf/Instructions-for-Patient-Use-h.pdf.

van der Maaden, K., W. Jiskoot, and J. Bouwstra. 2012. Microneedle technologies for (trans) dermal drug and vaccine delivery. *Journal of Controlled Release* 161 (2):645–655.

Wadhwa, S., S. Rawat, S. Singhal, N. Saini, and M. Khichi. 2012. Transferosome: A versatile tool for transdermal drug delivery. *Journal of Pharmacy Research* 5 (1):610–615.

Wakil, A., and S. L. Atkin. 2012. Efficacy and safety of ultra-long-acting insulin degludec. *Therapeutic Advances in Endocrinology and Metabolism* 3 (2):55–59.

Wang, F., J. M. Carabino, and C. M. Vergara. 2003. Insulin glargine: A systematic review of a long-acting insulin analogue. *Clinical Therapeutics* 25 (6):1541–1577.

Wang, W. 1996. Oral protein drug delivery. *Journal of Drug Targeting* 4 (4):195–232.

White, S., L. R. Brown, J. McGeehan, K. Hogeland, A. Brugger, and J. Troeger. 2007. The science and technology of the PROMAXX biotechnology platform. *Respiratory Drug Delivery Europe* 1:51–58.

Whitelaw, D., C. Kelly, W. Ironmonger, C. Cunliffe, R. New, and J. Phillips. 2013. *Absorption of orally ingested insulin in human type I diabetic subjects: Proof of concept study* 2005 [cited March 13, 2013]. Available from http://www.diabetology.co.uk/ADA%20poster%20June%2005.pdf.

Woitiski, C. B., R. J. Neufeld, F. Veiga, R. A. Carvalho, and I. V. Figueiredo. 2010. Pharmacological effect of orally delivered insulin facilitated by multilayered stable nanoparticles. *European Journal of Pharmaceutical Sciences* 41 (3–4):556–563.

Woitiski, C. B., B. Sarmento, R. A. Carvalho, R. J. Neufeld, and F. Veiga. 2011. Facilitated nanoscale delivery of insulin across intestinal membrane models. *International Journal Pharmaceutics* 412 (1–2):123–131.

Wolzt, M., A. de la Peña, P.-Y. Berclaz, F. S. Tibaldi, J. R. Gates, and D. B. Muchmore. 2008. AIR inhaled insulin versus subcutaneous insulin: Pharmacokinetics, glucodynamics, and pulmonary function in asthma. *Diabetes Care* 31 (4):735–740.

Yeh, T. H., L. W. Hsu, M. T. Tseng, P. L. Lee, K. Sonjae, Y. C. Ho, and H. W. Sung. 2011. Mechanism and consequence of chitosan-mediated reversible epithelial tight junction opening. *Biomaterials* 32 (26):6164–6173.

6 The Artificial Pancreas

Joseph Shivers, Jennifer Lane, Eyal Dassau, and Howard Zisser

CONTENTS

TYPE 1 DIABETES

Type 1 diabetes is an autoimmune disease in which the insulin-producing beta cells in the pancreas are destroyed by the body's immune system. Insulin is a growth hormone that enables cells to take up glucose, which can be used immediately for energy or stored for future use. When insulin production is low or absent, as in patients with type 1 diabetes, glucose accumulates in the blood and is partially filtered out by the kidneys, leading to excessive urination and thirst. Instead of metabolizing glucose, the body metabolizes fats and creates byproducts called ketones. The buildup of these ketones can lead to a toxic condition called diabetic ketoacidosis, marked by nausea, weakness, confusion, and high levels of glucose and ketones in the blood and urine. Diabetic ketoacidosis can quickly lead to coma and death if it is not treated with exogenous insulin. Thus, until insulin was discovered in the early 20th century, the diagnosis of type 1 diabetes was usually a sentence of death within months. The most frequent complications of type 1 diabetes are those involving long-term exposure to high glucose levels (hyperglycemia)—for example, kidney failure, blindness, neuropathy, impotence, heart disease, stroke—or acute exposure to low glucose levels brought on by insulin overdose (hypoglycemia)—for example, seizure, coma.

DISCOVERY OF INSULIN

The name "insulin" was introduced by both Jean de Meyer in 1909 and by Sir Edward Albert Sharpey-Schafer in 1913 (1). Shafer used the word to describe the hypothetical substance produced by the islets of Langerhans—collections of cells distributed throughout the pancreas. (The specific source of insulin was later found to be the beta cells, one of several endocrine cell types in the islets.) In the years that followed, the focus of the research turned to the hormone produced by the islets, insulin. In 1921, Frederick Banting and Charles Best in Toronto, Canada, successfully extracted insulin, which they called "isletin," and administered it to a dog that had been given diabetes by the removal of its pancreas (Figure 6.1). Following the

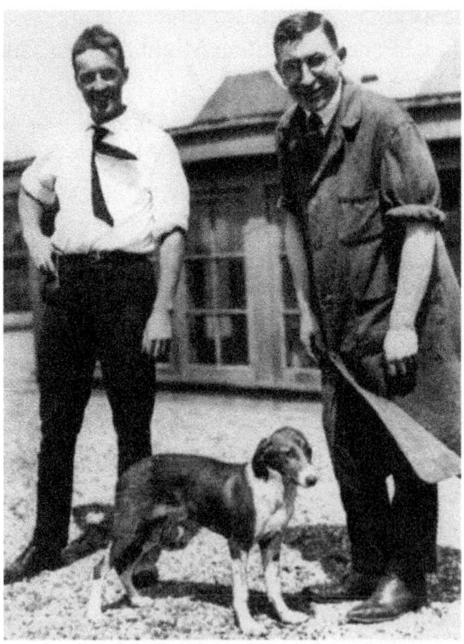

FIGURE 6.1 Banting (right) and medical student Best (left) standing with one of the diabetic dogs used in experiments with insulin. (Image courtesy of University of Toronto Archives.)

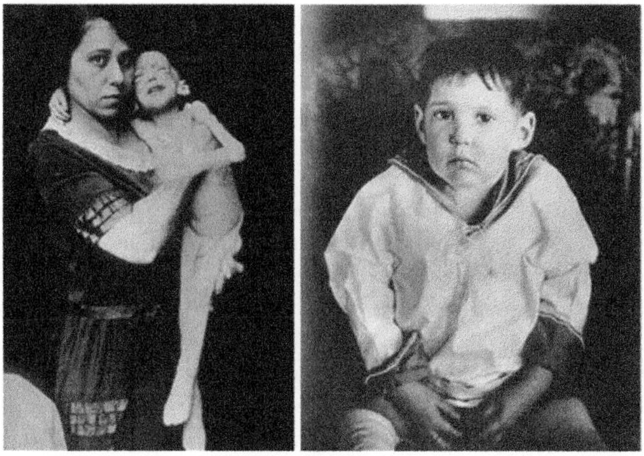

FIGURE 6.2 Leonard Thompson, the first human to receive insulin as treatment for diabetes, depicted before and after treatment. (Copyright Eli Lilly and Company. All Rights Reserved. Photo courtesy of Eli Lilly and Company Archives.)

insulin injection, the dog's blood glucose dropped from 200 mg/dl to 120 mg/dl (2). This dog, much like the dogs in several subsequent experiments, died soon after the surgery and insulin injection. However, Banting and Best continued to work toward a more pure extract. Finally, on January 11, 1922, Leonard Thompson, a 14-year-old boy, became the first person to ever receive an injection of insulin to treat diabetes. Although the serum was seen to moderately lower his blood glucose levels, 440 mg/dl to 320 mg/dl, the effect was not grand enough to justify further administration. After further purification of the serum by James Collip, treatment for the 14-year-old boy resumed and led to immediate improvement in the boy's health (Figure 6.2). The next day, Thompson's blood glucose dropped from 520 mg/dl to 120 mg/dl, his renal glucose excretion decreased from 71.1 g to 8.7 g, and acetone bodies disappeared from his urine. It was the first successful clinical test of using insulin to treat diabetes (3). In May 1922, the Toronto group began collaboration with Eli Lilly and Co. to start mass production of what they now called insulin (1).

TIGHT GLYCEMIC CONTROL

Modern insulin therapy is designed to mimic the physiological secretion of insulin. A healthy pancreas secretes insulin at a low basal rate throughout the day and night and in higher amounts at meals and other periods of energy storage. A portion of secreted insulin is taken up by the portal vein, where it promotes glucose storage in the liver. The other half circulates throughout the bloodstream and acts on various organs and tissues involved in energy balance (e.g., fat, muscles). This pathway of endogenous insulin is not perfectly matched by insulin that is injected subcutaneously. Subcutaneous insulin forms a depot that takes a relatively long time to enter the bloodstream and to fully clear the body. Subcutaneously delivered insulin also has a much lower proportional effect on the liver. Despite these limitations, subcutaneous insulin can still be delivered in a quasiphysiological pattern of basal dosage (for round-the-clock insulin needs) and bolus dosage (for meals or to correct excessively high glucose levels).

Insulin Delivery

The most common way for people with diabetes to deliver insulin is with multiple daily injections of long- and short-acting insulin formulations. Long-acting insulin formulations range from having a peak effect in 2–3 hours and a total duration of action of 8–10 hours to having a nearly stable action profile for over 20 hours. Short-acting insulin formulations have a peak of activity in 30–90 minutes and a duration of action of 4–6 hours (4). To estimate mealtime insulin needs, people with diabetes must somehow assess the size and type of every meal. The standard way to calculate mealtime insulin is by "carbohydrate counting"—estimating a meal's carbohydrate content and then applying a predetermined insulin-to-carbohydrate ratio. This process is imperfect at best because carbohydrate content can be difficult to estimate and is not the only relevant variable. Fats, proteins, fiber, and other factors, such as time of day, amount eaten, and rate of ingestion, also affect glycemic response.

In order to determine their insulin dosages and to detect unexpected glycemic changes, people with diabetes are encouraged to perform self-monitoring of blood glucose several times a day. Self-monitoring of blood glucose (SMBG) involves pricking the finger to draw capillary blood, testing the blood with an electrochemical strip and a hand-held meter, and interpreting the result, which appears on the meter within several seconds after testing. Blood glucose meters became popular in the 1980s. Prior to this, people with diabetes mainly assessed their glucose control with urine tests, which were generally less precise and less timely than SMBG. The combination of basal-bolus insulin therapy and frequent SMBG facilitates intensive control of blood glucose levels.

Advantages and Disadvantages of Tight Glycemic Control

Intensive glycemic control has been proven to decrease the risk of long-term complications of diabetes. The Diabetes Control and Complications Trial (DCCT) that took place from 1983 to 1993 was the first of its kind, a massive randomized controlled trial comparing the effects of standard control of blood glucose versus intensive control of the complications of diabetes (5). The goal in the intensive therapy group was to keep levels of hemoglobin A1c (a marker of glucose exposure in the past 3 months) as close as possible to 6.0% or lower, which corresponds to a mean blood glucose of 100–152 mg/dl (6). The goal in the control therapy group included only two daily insulin injections, urine glucose monitoring or SMBG no more than twice daily, and no goal A1c. Relative to standard therapy, intensive therapy reduced the development and progression of eye disease by 76%, kidney disease by 50%, and nerve disease by 60%. When the DCCT ended in 1993, the conventional treatment group was taught intensive therapy, and all future care for both groups was transferred to the patients' own health care providers. After this transition period, an observational follow-up study titled Epidemiology of Diabetes Interventions and Complications (EDIC) took place to evaluate intensive blood glucose control's long-term effects on cardiovascular disease in those same patients. The EDIC study found a reduction in cardiovascular disease by 42% and a 57% reduction in nonfatal heart attack and stroke or death from cardiovascular causes (5,7).

The main side effect of tight glycemic control is low blood glucose (hypoglycemia), typically defined as blood glucose below 60–80 mg/dl. Hypoglycemic episodes can result in confusion, seizures, or even death due to neuroglycopenia. The brain uses glucose as its primary source of energy. This makes the glucose that is brought by the bloodstream to the brain exceedingly important. If the brain has no glucose delivery via the bloodstream to use as energy, patients can suffer cognitive, physiological, and symptomatic changes. The results can include major vascular events such as stroke, myocardial infarction, acute cardiac failure, ventricular arrhythmias, coma, or even death (8,9). In children, hypoglycemia exposure may be associated with long-term cognitive impairment (10,11).

Some researchers have suggested that A1c may not be the best indicator of good glycemic control because it is only an average and does not account for high and low glycemic swings, which may contribute to the vascular complications of diabetes (12). Thus, some clinicians emphasize that the avoidance of hypo- and hyperglycemia, not simply a reduction in average glucose, should be the focus of treatment (13).

DEVELOPMENT OF GLYCEMIC CONTROL THERAPIES

Since publication of the DCCT in 1993, people living with diabetes have sought out more precise and convenient tools to achieve near-normal glycemia and delay progression of diabetes complications.

Insulin Pumps

Insulin pumps are one such tool that has been shown to facilitate tighter blood glucose control, relative to multiple daily injections (14); many patients also find pumps more convenient since they eliminate the need for daily injections and can simplify dose calculations. Insulin pump therapy, also called continuous subcutaneous insulin infusion therapy (CSII), involves subcutaneous infusion of short-acting insulin. A preprogrammed basal rate of insulin is infused at all times (usually in microdoses every few minutes), and bolus insulin doses can be delivered by the patient at any time. The pump system consists of the pump itself, which has a user interface on the front for adjustment of insulin dosages; a disposable reservoir that holds the insulin and is inserted into the pump; and a disposable infusion set that consists of tubing and a cannula that is inserted under the skin. The first commercial insulin pump was introduced in 1978 and named the autosyringe or "Big Blue Brick" (15) (Figure 6.3); today's pumps are much smaller and smarter (Figure 6.4). Most pumps still use infusion sets, but some "patch pumps" attach directly to patients' bodies. Patch pumps deliver insulin directly from the pump reservoir through a small cannula without tubing.

New insulin pumps are customizable and user-friendly. Pumps can be preprogrammed to hold one or more basal insulin rates so that the user may constantly

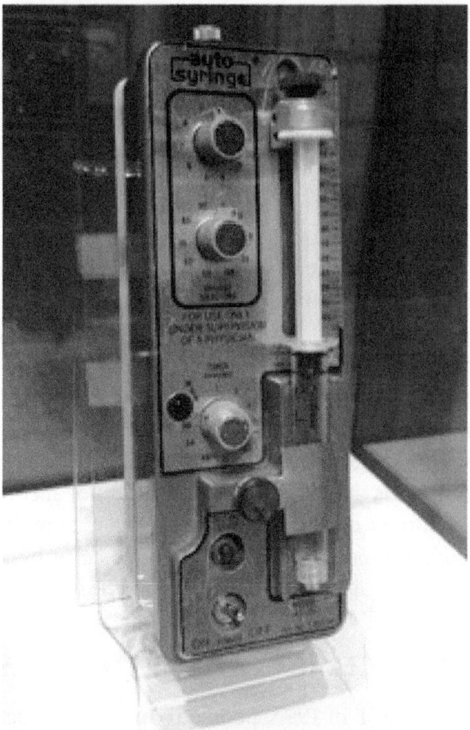

FIGURE 6.3 The Autosyringe ("Big Blue Brick"), the first commercially available insulin pump. (Copyright Eli Lilly and Company. All Rights Reserved. Photo courtesy of Eli Lilly and Company Archives.)

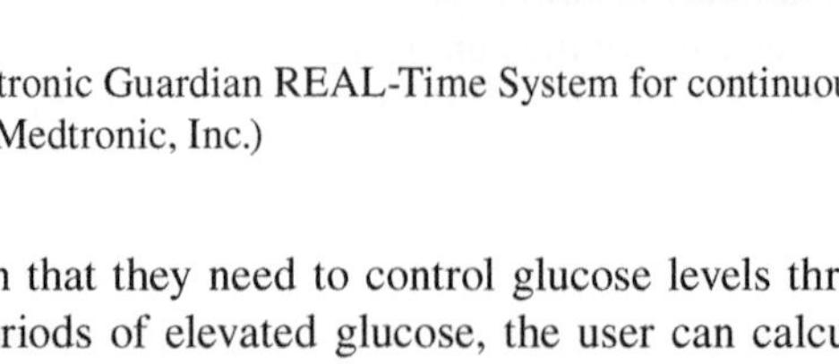

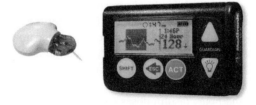

FIGURE 6.4 Medtronic Guardian REAL-Time System for continuous glucose monitoring. (Image courtesy of Medtronic, Inc.)

receive the insulin that they need to control glucose levels throughout the day. At meals or other periods of elevated glucose, the user can calculate his or her own dosage or take advantage of the "bolus calculator" feature that is now available on most pumps. Bolus calculators use individualized ratios to determine insulin dosage based on the user's blood glucose level and the carbohydrate content of a recent or upcoming meal. Many pumps also have the ability to change the shape or duration of the bolus. For example, a square-wave bolus is used to deliver the bolus over an extended period of time, and a dual-wave bolus is broken down into two smaller boluses: a standard bolus given immediately and a square-wave bolus given for the next few hours (16). Currently, more than half a dozen manufacturers supply insulin pumps worldwide with Medtronic MiniMed leading in the United States and Roche (formerly Disetronic) leading the market outside the United States.

CONTINUOUS GLUCOSE MONITORS

Continuous glucose monitors have been commercially available since 1999 with the launch of the MiniMed (Northridge, CA) continuous glucose monitoring system. A continuous glucose monitor (CGM) is a therapeutic device that measures the concentration of glucose in a patient's subcutaneous (interstitial) fluid and displays an estimate of blood glucose to the user. The CGM consists of a sensor (an electrochemical electrode), a transmitter (which analyzes and wirelessly broadcasts data from the sensor), and a receiver (which displays the real-time glucose value as well as recent trends). The sensor is inserted in the subcutaneous layer and can be worn there for days at a time (Figure 6.5).

Available continuous glucose monitors do not estimate blood glucose as accurately as blood glucose meters can measure it, so CGMs are approved only as adjuncts to self-monitoring of blood glucose, not as a replacement. (Periodic blood glucose meter tests are also required to calibrate the CGM.) Compared to SMBG alone, adjunctive use of continuous glucose monitors has been shown to help patients lower A1c while still reducing time spent in hypoglycemia (14). CGM use has been recommended for children and adults looking to gain tighter control of blood glucose levels and in patients looking to detect nocturnal hypoglycemia, transient early-morning hyperglycemia ("the dawn phenomenon"), postprandial hyperglycemia, and loss of the symptoms of mild-to-moderate hypoglycemia, such as sweatiness and shakiness (hypoglycemia unawareness) (17).

Sensor-Augmented Pumping

Some patients use both insulin pump therapy and CGM—a pairing that is sometimes called sensor-augmented pumping. As of this writing, two commercially available pumps can also act as CGM receivers so that the user needs only one hand-held

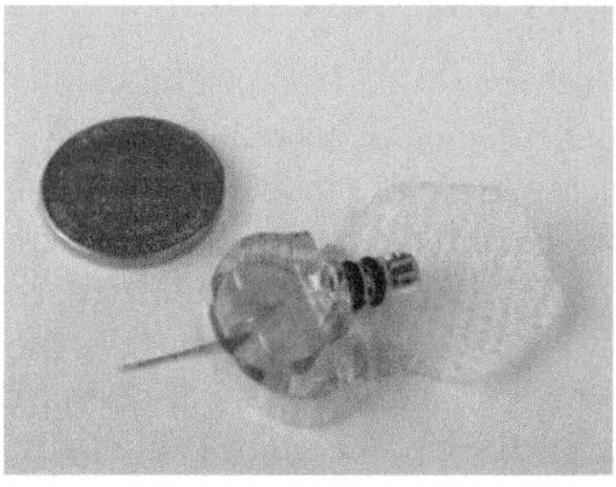

FIGURE 6.5 Medtronic subcutaneous glucose sensor. (Image courtesy of Medtronic, Inc.)

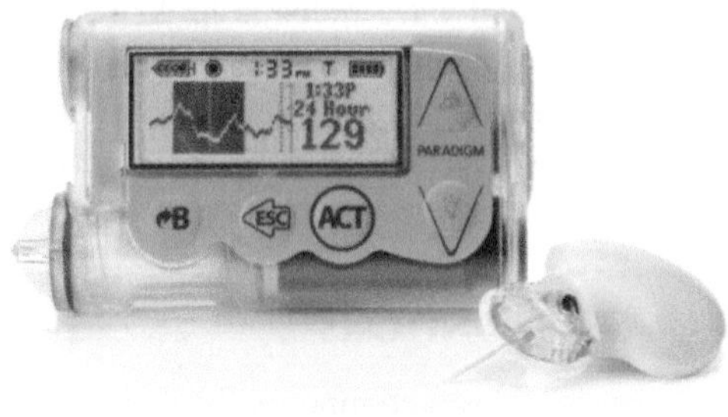

FIGURE 6.6 Medtronic Paradigm Revel insulin pump. (Image courtesy of Medtronic, Inc.)

device to view his or her glucose data and program insulin doses: the Animas Vibe and the Medtronic Paradigm Veo (or its U.S. variant, the Paradigm Revel). The Veo (but not the Revel) has a "low glucose suspend" feature, described at length below, which temporarily shuts off insulin delivery when the sensor detects hypoglycemia. However, currently, commercially available pumps cannot autonomously increase insulin dose, attenuate insulin dose without full suspension, or suspend insulin delivery predictively while readings are trending down (15) (Figure 6.6).

While insulin pumps and continuous glucose monitors improve glycemic control, patients still play an involved role in managing their diabetes. Patients must set their basal rates, calculate nutritional content and administer boluses for meals, frequently monitor their blood glucose levels, and adjust their insulin therapy to avoid hyper- and hypoglycemia. The ideal solution to this would be to implement a "closed-loop" system that would work as an artificial pancreas. This system would allow communication between an insulin pump and a glucose sensor and react to these variations in measured glucose by responding quickly to cover insulin needs. For example, when blood glucose levels exceed normal levels after a meal, the system would automatically correct by administering insulin, mimicking the action of the pancreatic beta cells (15). The artificial pancreas would free the patient from carbohydrate counting, performing tedious calculations, and constantly checking his or her blood glucose throughout the day. It could increase the safety, healthfulness, and ease of living with diabetes.

HISTORY OF THE ARTIFICIAL PANCREAS

Arnold Kadish designed the first closed-loop insulin pump device. This pump both detected blood glucose and provided continuous insulin to the body. It was the size of a large backpack and was worn on the back with tubing running to the arm (Figure 6.7). Unfortunately, Kadish did not gain much interest in his product due to its impracticality for daily use (15). Greater attention was given to the second closed-loop system, the Biostator, which was developed in 1974 (Figure 6.8). The Biostator was a dual-chambered pump with the capability of delivering either insulin or dextrose. The computer-controlled pump worked by continually withdrawing blood and putting it through a glucose analyzer to establish the blood glucose concentration.

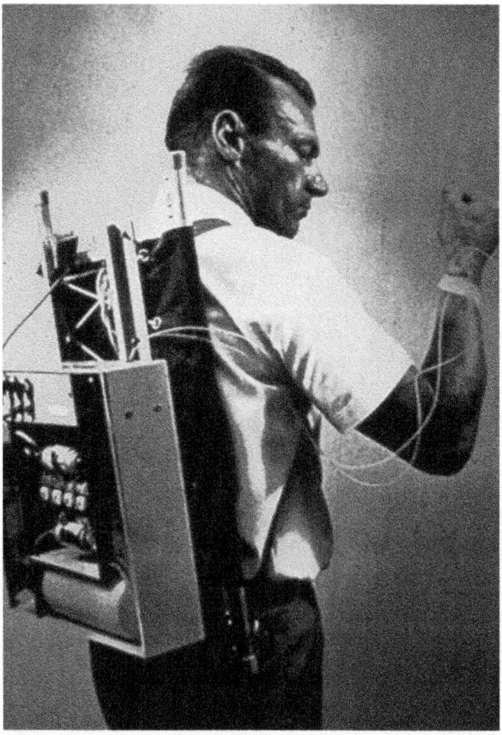

FIGURE 6.7 Closed-loop system introduced by Arnold Kadish, MD, in the early 1960s. (From Bode BW, Sabbah HT, Gross TM, Fredrickson LP, and Davidson PC, *Diabetes Metab Res Rev.*, 18, S14–20, 2002.)

The Biostator's computer used a set algorithm to determine how much insulin or dextrose was needed, and the determined amount of drug was given to the patient through an infusion pump. The system also had a printer that printed out continuous blood glucose recordings (15). The original Biostator had a 5- to 6-minute delay between withdrawing the blood and recording of glucose analysis by the computer, required 70 ml of blood for a 24-hour period, and was the size of a small refrigerator. Due to these drawbacks, the Biostator was overhauled: The size was taken down to that of a portable television, the lag time was decreased to 90 seconds, and the blood consumption was lowered to 50 ml in a 24-hour period (18). Despite these improvements, the Biostator was not practical for long-term use.

Both Kadish's model and the Biostator used the intravenous route of glucose sensing and insulin infusion. However, due to the risks of thrombosis, phlebitis, and infection, more practical means of insulin delivery began to be pursued. Then, in 1979, subcutaneous insulin infusion was proven effective in adults (19) and in adolescents (20). These discoveries led to the widespread use of subcutaneous insulin pumps, which have become the standard method of insulin delivery in artificial pancreas research.

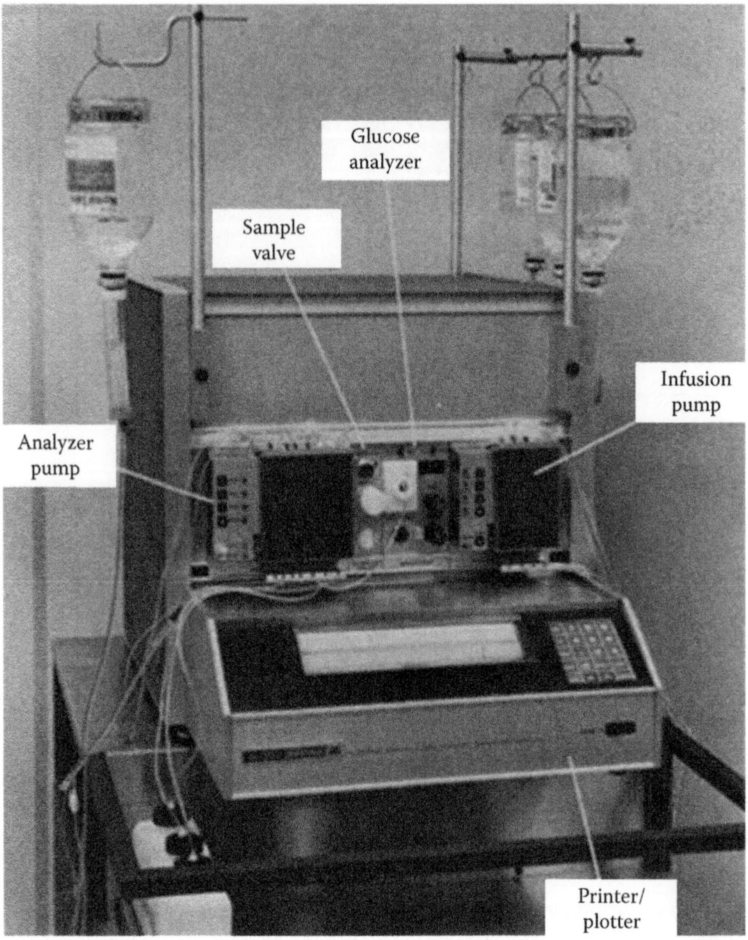

FIGURE 6.8 The Biostator closed-loop system, developed in 1974. (From Fogt EJ, Dodd LM, Jenning EM, Clemens AH, *Clin Chem.*, 24, 8, 1366–72, 1978.)

MODERN AP

Artificial pancreas research continued at a relatively slow pace for the next several decades but reached a turning point in 2006 when the Juvenile Diabetes Research Foundation (now called simply JDRF) launched its Artificial Pancreas Project (21). In the years since, JDRF has supported closed-loop research with tens of millions of dollars as well as high-level advocacy efforts, including four public workshops on artificial pancreas research conducted with the U.S. Food and Drug Administration and National Institutes of Health (in 2005, 2008, 2010, and 2013). The National Institutes of Health (NIH) is itself a major funder of closed-loop research (roughly $18 million in fiscal year 2010 alone) (22), and the Food and Drug Administration (FDA) has designated the development of an artificial pancreas as one of its critical

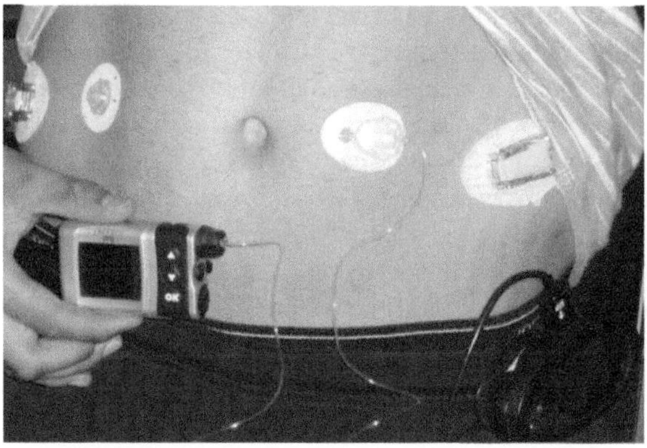

FIGURE 6.9 Devices used in clinical trial for the Artificial Pancreas (AP) Project. Continuous glucose monitor and insulin pump are paired with the AP algorithm to instruct insulin delivery. (Image courtesy of Sansum Diabetes Research Institute.)

path initiatives (23). The FDA's most significant recent action came in late 2012, when the agency published a guidance document on the clinical trials required for approval of an artificial pancreas device system (24) (Figure 6.9). This document is generally viewed as more conducive to research and commercialization than the previous draft version. The revisions were likely a response to Congressional and public enthusiasm for speedy development of an artificial pancreas given the many unmet clinical needs in type 1 diabetes care (25).

CLINICAL UNMET NEEDS

Benefits of intensive treatment for type 1 diabetes were proven in DCCT and EDIC. Since then, tight control has been facilitated with the use of CGMs and insulin pump technology. However, even with the use of new technology, hypo- and hyperglycemic episodes and long-term complications are still dangers associated with diabetes. Diabetes management also still demands a great deal of time and effort from patients and their families. Some patients find that pumps and CGMs make their lives more flexible and free, but other people believe that modern technologies introduce more challenges than they solve.

Hypoglycemia

Studies have shown that the use of continuous glucose monitors and/or insulin pumps has provided a benefit when it comes to hypoglycemia avoidance (26,27). Continuous glucose monitors can provide the patient with awareness of his or her hypoglycemia, and insulin pumps allow for several basal rates to be set to allow for better control throughout the day. Although these tools may give patients greater flexibility with their diabetes, they are by no means a complete solution. Hypoglycemia continues to be a major cause of death in patients living with diabetes. According to recent estimates, hypoglycemia accounts for 6% to 10% of mortality in type 1 diabetes (28,29). One of the most terrifying risks is hypoglycemia's association with the spontaneous overnight death in type 1 diabetes (dead-in-bed syndrome) (9)—a phenomenon that has been estimated to account for 6% of deaths among type 1 diabetes patients younger than 40 (30). In 2012, a case study of a 23-year-old man with a history of type 1 diabetes discussed the cause of his death. This 23-year-old man was found in his bed unresponsive and undisturbed. It was initially hypothesized that his death was due to nocturnal hypoglycemia, and upon further investigation, the man's retrospective CGM confirmed hypoglycemia as cause of death (9). Hypoglycemic seizures and comas, while not fatal, are traumatic and alarmingly common. In a study of a nationwide registry of clinical centers (Helmsley Charitable Trust's T1D Exchange), 7% of patients reported a severe hypoglycemic episode within the past year (31).

Hyperglycemia

Along with hypoglycemia, the second most common emergency associated with type 1 diabetes is diabetic ketoacidosis (DKA) resulting from a shortage of insulin, causing hyperglycemia and eventually the burning of fatty acids that produce acidic ketone bodies. Although hypoglycemia is more common, DKA is associated with a higher risk of mortality. DKA is most commonly a result of discontinuation of insulin treatment either intentionally or unintentionally or from high insulin demands at times such as illness or pregnancy. Patients using subcutaneous insulin infusion (CSII) are claimed to have increased risk of developing DKA due to pump line occlusions, disconnection, or device malfunction. However, studies have provided conflicting evidence (32).

Long-Term Complications

Another persistent concern in type 1 diabetes care is long-term complications. One hope for closed-loop systems is that they could help people lower their A1c, which was shown to reduce the incidence of complications in DCCT and EDIC (5). However, as noted above, many believe that large, frequent, and/or rapid changes in glucose levels (hypo-/hyperglycemic spikes) are significant contributors to the vascular complications of diabetes, independent of average hyperglycemic exposure as indicated by A1c (12,33,34). Thus, reducing "glycemic variability" is a major goal of many modern treatment regimens. Unfortunately, temporary hyperglycemic spikes are sometimes unavoidable; hyperglycemic spikes are particularly likely after meals (Figure 6.10). A closed-loop glucose control system could potentially stabilize glucose swings and increase the time spent in near-normoglycemia, often called "time in range" or "time in zone." In this way, the artificial pancreas could potentially further decrease the incidence of long-term complications even beyond the benefits achieved with current best practices.

Diabetes self-management involves constant vigilance and discipline even with the use of new technologies. Pumps and CGMs address some challenges of diabetes, but they also introduce hassles, such as the need for frequent replacement, the risk of technical problems, and the potential for alarm fatigue (the tendency to not respond

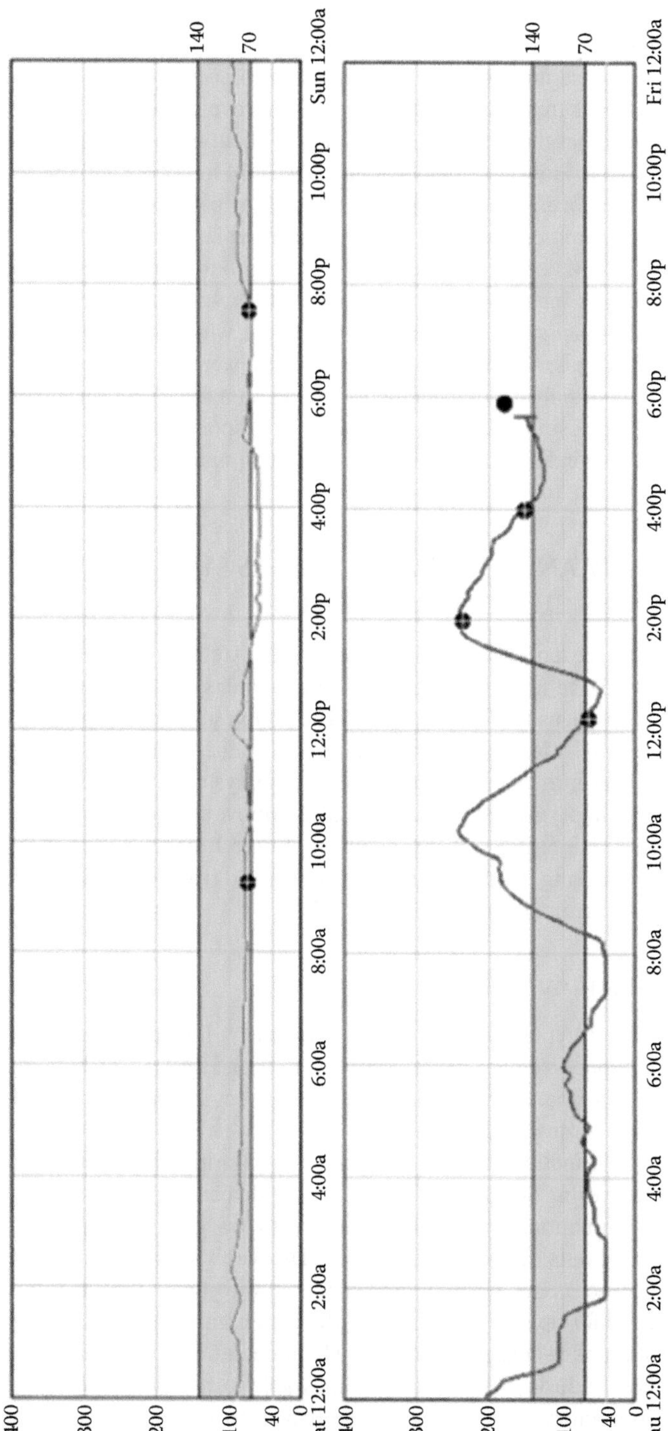

FIGURE 6.10 Documented postprandial hyperglycemia. (Image courtesy of Sansum Diabetes Research Institute.)

appropriately to alarms due to their frequency or inaccuracy) (35). These hassles can, in turn, decrease quality of life (QoL). Technical advances, such as insulin pumps and continuous glucose monitors, are used in order to decrease hassle, to lower the amount of time spent treating diabetes, and to improve the quality of life. Some studies have shown that the use of CGM, with or without insulin pump therapy, can improve QoL (36–39). However, many patients try CGM for a time and then decrease or stop their use even in clinical trial settings (40). Many past users say that they want CGM to become more accurate, affordable, comfortable, and easy to use (41). As new and updated CGMs come out, these demands begin to be met, but perhaps even more people would be interested in using CGMs if they were integrated with insulin pumps into closed-loop systems, and perhaps people who already use pumps and CGMs would have higher quality of life if they had fewer daily responsibilities and uncertainties in their diabetes management. Indeed, in a European survey of people with type 1 diabetes using CSII (n = 132), 75% of respondents expressed intent to use an AP. Most respondents said that they anticipate improvements in both glucose control and ease of use (42).

HOW AND WHY AN ARTIFICIAL PANCREAS SYSTEM MIGHT ADDRESS CLINICAL UNMET NEEDS

Artificial pancreas systems can be classified by the extent to which they automate diabetes control (43). In a similar way, artificial pancreas systems can be classified by the clinical challenges that they address. The simplest closed-loop products will reduce hypoglycemia. More complex systems will reduce both hypoglycemia and hyperglycemia. The most sophisticated closed-loop systems will not only reduce hypoglycemia and hyperglycemia, they will also remove the need for most or all of the tasks involved in intensive self-management of type 1 diabetes, for example, frequent glucose monitoring, mealtime insulin dosage, and troubleshooting or frequent replacement of the medical equipment involved.

Hypoglycemia-Mitigating Systems

The chief purpose of hypoglycemia-reducing systems will be to decrease the likelihood of severe hypoglycemic events. During or in anticipation of hypoglycemia, these systems will suspend or attenuate insulin delivery so that any period of low glucose is cut short (or avoided altogether).

The most basic functionality for a hypoglycemia-mitigating system is for the pump to stop delivering insulin when the sensor detects hypoglycemia—a "low glucose suspend" functionality. The first pump with low glucose suspend, the Veo, is already available outside the United States. The Veo's suspend feature activates when sensor glucose passes below a user-specified threshold, and insulin delivery remains suspended for up to 2 hours or until the patient turns it back on. The 2-hour limit is to prevent under-dosage of insulin, which could lead to hyperglycemia and even diabetic ketoacidosis. The pump becomes able to resuspend insulin delivery after a 4-hour refractory period. Several published prospective and observational studies indicate that the Veo reduces exposure to hypoglycemia without increasing the risk of severe hyperglycemia (44–47). However, regulators have identified several risks, including the possibility that erroneous pump suspension could lead to diabetic ketoacidosis. The U.S. Food and Drug Administration therefore required the Veo's manufacturer to perform an additional randomized, controlled trial of the low glucose suspend function's safety and efficacy (48,49). As of this writing, the FDA is reviewing the manufacturer's regulatory submission for a device similar to the Veo (Minimed 530G), which would become the first low-glucose-suspend device to be sold in the United States. Notably, the agency has indicated that it might approve devices that significantly reduce hypoglycemia even if the result is a higher A1c (24).

The next level of automation is to suspend or attenuate insulin delivery before low glucose even occurs. Such a system could minimize exposure to hypoglycemia, further reducing the risk of a severe adverse event. It might even decrease the chances that a patient's blood glucose would drift low in the first place, since each hypoglycemic event increases the risk of subsequent hypoglycemia (50). Predictive action would also reduce the number of hypoglycemia alarms, thus easing alarm fatigue and potentially allowing patients and their loved ones to sleep with fewer interruptions. Dr. Bruce Buckingham and colleagues have studied a system with "predictive low glucose suspend." In two short-term inpatient studies, different implementations of the system have used a prediction horizon of 30–45 minutes and succeeded in preventing 60%–80% of hypoglycemic events that otherwise would likely have occurred (51,52). More recently, the same group has tested three different predictive algorithms in a 21-night randomized trial in the home setting (n = 19). For the final algorithm tested, incidence of nocturnal hypoglycemia below 70 mg/dl occurred in 30% of 37 nights without intervention but only 16% of 77 intervention nights (53). Medtronic, the manufacturer of the system, has announced plans to submit a predictive low-glucose-suspend product for approval internationally in the near future in advance of filing with the U.S. FDA (54).

The most sophisticated hypoglycemia-preventing systems will be able to decrease insulin delivery partially so that full suspension is not required as often. Relative to pumps with low glucose suspend and predictive low glucose suspend, these hypoglycemia minimizers would limit the risks of subsequent hyperglycemia and ketoacidosis (43).

Hypoglycemia–Hyperglycemia Minimizing Systems

Beyond hypoglycemia minimizers will come systems that minimize both hypoglycemia and hyperglycemia. Such devices would introduce the ability to increase insulin delivery during (and in anticipation of) high glucose excursions. Patients would still need to practice tight glycemic control on their own as they do with current sensor-augmented pump therapy; hypoglycemia–hyperglycemia minimizers would simply help to mitigate glycemic extremes in either direction. In JDRF's control-to-range trial, such a system performed with moderate success at seven research centers around the world (n = 53) (55,56). Preliminary clinical research has also been conducted on a hypo-/hyperglycemia-minimizing system developed by Animas to see how well it can react to glycemic changes (57).

"Normoglycemia" Systems

The step after hypoglycemia–hyperglycemia minimization will be to target a tighter range of "normoglycemia," enabling fully closed-loop control overnight and for much of the day. Under fasting and sedentary conditions, these hybrid closed-loop systems will improve the safety and effectiveness of tight glycemic control, and they will also reduce the hour-by-hour burdens of glucose monitoring and insulin adjustment. However, open-loop treatment modifications would likely still be necessary for meals, exercise, and other glycemic disturbances.

In many ways, nighttime is the ideal scenario for automated insulin delivery. Sleeping patients and their families might not respond to crises, such as the severe hypoglycemia that precedes seizures and dead-in-bed syndrome (9), even if such events generate CGM alarms (58). Knowing this, many people wake up nightly to check their own or their loved one's glucose levels. An automatic system to prevent overnight hypoglycemic events could therefore save lives and/or significantly ease burdens of care.

An overnight closed-loop system could also be a boon for reducing hyperglycemia. In several clinical trials comparing open-loop to closed-loop control, closed-loop control has been shown to reduce patients' exposure to overnight hyperglycemia (59–61). One advantage of closed-loop systems is that they can finely adjust insulin delivery in ways that would be impossible to program prospectively and impractical to perform manually. In other words, closed-loop systems can use variability in insulin dosage to reduce variability in glucose levels. Decreasing overnight hyperglycemia might also promote better glycemic control during the daytime. A widespread clinical observation is that when nighttime glycemic control is good, glucose levels on the following day tend to be closer to target and more predictable.

The chief downside of overnight closed-loop control is the risk of insulin overdose and hypoglycemia. The risk is arguably greater than it would be during the day since sleeping patients would be less likely to detect system errors and respond to them. However, if closed-loop systems are designed safely, this risk of overnight hypoglycemia could be equivalent to (or less than) the risk associated with current sensor-augmented pump therapy.

Fully Closed-Loop Systems

The ideal artificial pancreas would, in addition to promoting safe and effective glycemic control overnight, also take over nearly all of the daily burdens of diabetes management. A "fully closed-loop" subcutaneous insulin delivery system would automatically maintain glucose in a safe range for 24 hours a day, and it would require human intervention only to replace the disposable components every few days and to address rare emergencies (e.g., system malfunction or damage, abnormal glycemic fluctuations). However, inpatient experiments to date have not demonstrated that a system of this type could be safe and effective outside strictly controlled settings. Especially significant challenges have been presented by large meals (62) and bouts of exercise (when glucose levels might fall so quickly that patients require hypoglycemia-rescue therapy in the form of glucose or glucagon) (63,64). What's more, in free-living conditions, meals might be much larger and exercise might be more intense than in clinical studies to date. Additional challenges would be presented by stress, sickness, and technical problems. These challenges can of course be mitigated—for example, with manual premeal boluses or open-loop therapy adjustments around periods of exercise—but at the expense of the wearer's time and effort, decreasing the appeal and benefits of the closed-loop system.

Some believe that fully closed-loop insulin delivery will become possible with the ongoing enhancements in CGM and subcutaneous insulin dosage that are described below. In other views, systems delivering solely subcutaneous insulin can never be made safe and effective enough for full automation due to inherent delays and uncertainties in insulin uptake. Thus, many groups are investigating the concomitant use of noninsulin hormones and/or alternative routes of insulin delivery (e.g., intravenous or intraperitoneal delivery from an implantable pump). A fully implantable artificial pancreas would remove the hassles and risks associated with disposable components used for subcutaneous insulin delivery and glucose sensing. Thus, in some ways, a fully implantable system would solve most clinical problems associated with modern type 1 diabetes management. However, the process of periodic implantation and explantation would introduce its own risks—a trade-off that many people might find unacceptable. Some believe that the ideal scenario is for many different closed-loop products to be available so that patients and health care providers can choose the functionalities that they think best (65).

Most clinical trials of the artificial pancreas have enrolled nonpregnant adults with type 1 diabetes, but closed-loop glucose control could benefit many other groups as well. Children and adolescents have used artificial pancreas devices in a variety of studies. In general, young patients' experience with closed-loop control has been similar to the experiences of adults in closed-loop studies (66). In current clinical practice, the American Diabetes Association has recommended that children and adolescents with type 1 diabetes seek less-strict A1c targets than adults. These higher targets are largely a result of concerns about hypoglycemia in the developing brain and the behavioral challenges of diabetes management for parents and/or patients (67). However, an artificial pancreas could potentially enable tighter glucose control and decrease the stress that is characteristic of pediatric type 1 diabetes (68,69), so such a device is highly desired among families with type 1 diabetes.

In pregnant women with type 1 diabetes, tight glucose control is especially challenging but especially important. Due to continuous hormonal changes, pregnant women may need significantly different regimens of insulin delivery from one week to the next (70). Many clinicians also recommend lower blood glucose targets than in typical type 1 diabetes management because even small amounts of hyperglycemia are thought to increase the risk of pregnancy complications, such as large birth weight (macrosomia) (71). On the other hand, severe hypoglycemia is an even greater risk than usual since the health of the fetus is at stake. Pregnant women with type 1 diabetes are thus often encouraged to follow a strict low-carbohydrate diet in order to minimize glycemic swings. However, in published studies of closed-loop control in pregnancy, patients did not follow such a strict diet, and the target glucose range was relatively wide: 63–140 mg/dl (72,73). The systems in these trials achieved a mean time in target range of more than 80%, but the authors acknowledge that ensuring the health of the fetus may require meeting more ambitious targets: 60–99 mg/dl while fasting and <130 mg/dl after meals (72,73). For pregnant women seeking such tight control, the utility of artificial pancreas devices still remains to be tested.

People with type 1 diabetes are not the only ones who can benefit from tight glycemic control. Patients in the intensive care unit (ICU) often experience stress hyperglycemia as a result of illness or injury. At extreme levels, this hyperglycemia can prolong healing time and promote infection whereas intensive insulin therapy has been shown beneficial in several different ICU patient populations with and without diabetes (74–76). Thus, despite ongoing debate about the optimal glycemic targets, some degree of inpatient glucose control is recommended by the leading clinical societies and performed throughout the world (77–79). For nurses to monitor blood glucose and adjust insulin delivery throughout the day is, unfortunately, labor-intensive and subject to human error. However, these drawbacks can be eased with an artificial pancreas. Takahashi and colleagues have achieved good glycemic control in Japanese sepsis patients using a closed-loop device that intravenously monitors blood glucose and intravenously delivers insulin and glucose (75). In the United States and Europe, fully closed-loop control devices are not yet available, but several products can calculate insulin dosage based on glucose measurements and patient characteristics (80–82). At least one company has developed a system that integrates a dosage algorithm with an insulin infusion pump so that hospital staffers need only to measure glucose levels and confirm the algorithm's recommended dosage (83). Various inpatient CGM systems are also available or in development (84–86). If and when inpatient CGMs become widely used, the next logical step would be integration with control algorithms and insulin delivery devices to create closed-loop systems for the hospital.

RECENT DATA AND TRENDS

Closed-loop glucose control has been achieved many times in inpatient settings, but the critical tests will occur in the free-living conditions of daily life. In the FDA's guidance document on clinical trials of artificial pancreas device systems, the agency calls for pivotal trials in real-world settings (24). Thus several artificial pancreas research groups have begun transitioning toward simulated outpatient settings and, in some cases, even the home environment.

Outpatient Closed-Loop Studies

In one of the most prominent examples of outpatient closed-loop research, a multinational consortium led by Drs. Moshe Philip, Tadej Battelino, and Thomas Danne has performed overnight control among adolescents ($n = 56$) at diabetes camps (59). Dr. Roman Hovorka and his team at Cambridge University have initiated three crossover-design studies of their artificial pancreas system in patients' homes for 3 weeks at a time: overnight control in adolescents ($n = 16$), overnight control in adults ($n = 24$), and day-and-night control in adults ($n = 18$). Meanwhile, a study group including researchers from France (University of Montpellier), Italy (Universities of Pavia and Padova), and the United States (Universities of Virginia and Santa

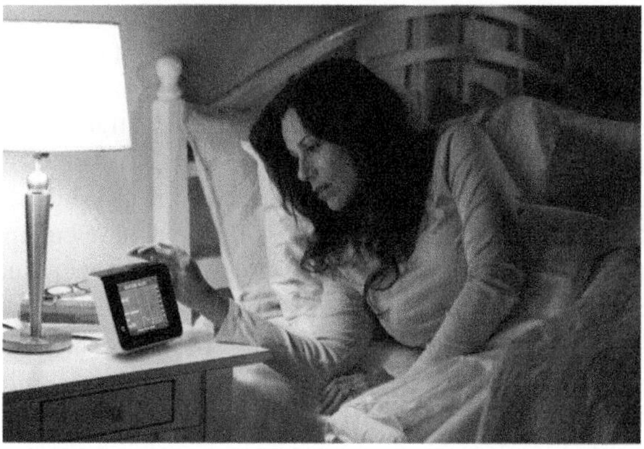

FIGURE 6.11 mySentry Remote Glucose Monitor. (Image courtesy of Medtronic, Inc.)

Barbara, and Sansum Diabetes Research Institute) is performing outpatient research with a range-control system that automatically adjusts insulin delivery between meals (87). Some of the most ambitious and promising research in free-living conditions is being performed in Boston by Dr. Edward Damiano and colleagues, whose bihormonal system for round-the-clock closed-loop control is described here in the section on glucagon (64).

Outpatient closed-loop studies do not necessarily require remote monitoring, but several researchers have developed or proposed remote-monitoring systems to ensure patient safety (59,88–90). Remote monitoring might become a common feature of diabetes management even before closed-loop systems do. For example, Medtronic already markets a bedside outpost that allows nocturnal CGM values to be monitored from up to 50 feet away (Figure 6.11) (91). During diabetes emergencies, remote-monitoring products could quickly alert family members, caregivers, and health care providers; during normal circumstances, these systems could simply promote peace of mind. The legal liabilities and sociopolitical implications of remote diabetes monitoring have not yet been fully explored. However, whatever else their benefits and drawbacks, remote monitoring will likely remain a key aspect of artificial pancreas research.

Improving the Artificial Pancreas Components

At the same time as outpatient studies are performed, many companies and academic groups are at work to improve the underlying performance of the artificial pancreas' components: for example, continuous glucose monitors, closed-loop control algorithms, and insulin delivery systems.

The accuracy and reliability of continuous glucose monitors have generally improved since these devices became commercially available in 1999 (92,93) albeit with some exceptions when newer sensors appear comparably accurate to old ones (94). Upcoming products look to be even more accurate and reliable, and many manufacturers are designing next-generation CGM devices with a focus on closed-loop applications. (A particular concern for closed-loop control is to minimize the frequency and duration of "large inaccuracy"—sensor errors of 40% or more (95).) For example, Medtronic has partnered with JDRF and the Helmsley Charitable Trust to build a sensing system with two separate types of sensors: a traditional electrochemical sensor and a novel optical sensor (96). The explicit goal of this "orthogonally redundant" setup is to improve accuracy and reliability of CGM used in closed-loop products (97). Researchers from the University of Padova have enhanced a Dexcom CGM with accuracy-improving algorithms to create a prototype "smart sensor" for closed-loop control and other applications (98). Results from early-stage clinical studies can be difficult to interpret since different groups design studies and analyze data in different ways. However, in general, the industry seems to be meeting the demand to improve on today's CGM performance.

The development of implantable CGM has been a goal in diabetes technology for over a decade (99) and remains the objective of many companies and researchers (100–104). Implanted CGMs would use sensors that remained in the body for several months or more at a time. Thus, they would eliminate the need for frequent sensor replacement—a process that requires significant time and effort from patients and one that involves several technical risks (e.g., premature sensor failure, poor sensor performance due to issues at the insertion site). However, implantable CGMs present their own slew of technical challenges, and researchers are still determining how best to improve biocompatibility, power implanted sensors and transmitters, and make the implantation/explantation process minimally invasive.

Another trend in CGM research is to design glucose sensors that are integrated with insulin-delivery catheters (105). Preliminary studies suggest that glucose sensors can function well despite close proximity to insulin infusion (106,107), but further research will be necessary to confirm this. The goal of this research is not to improve CGM performance, per se. However, a "single-port" sensor–catheter device could decrease the hassle of using CGM and pumps, which could encourage wider adoption of modern diabetes technologies (including artificial pancreas products).

Improving the Algorithms Used in Closed-Loop Devices

The most widely used algorithms for closed-loop glucose control fall into a few broad categories. Proportional integrative derivative (PID) controllers calculate insulin dosage using only the current sensor glucose value, the integral of recent glucose values, and the rate of glycemic change (derivative). The simplicity of PID control makes it easy to understand and implement, but PID does not account for the specific behavior of insulin and glucose in humans. Model predictive control (MPC) is more sophisticated; MPC controllers deliver insulin according to predictions of glucose levels in the near future. These predictions are based on a model of insulin–glucose dynamics and are continuously recalculated using input from the sensor. Fuzzy logic controllers use artificial intelligence to recognize glycemic patterns and adjust insulin delivery accordingly. Each strategy has its proponents, and distinctly different algorithms (e.g., PID vs. fuzzy logic) have not yet been compared in head-to-head studies.

It is straightforward to design an algorithm that can control glucose levels when patients are fasting, sedentary, healthy, and calm. In real-life conditions, however, the challenge is far greater. Thus, many groups are trying to both refine their primary control algorithms and develop complementary algorithms that can be used alongside the main algorithm as part of a larger, modular design (108). Research is active on algorithms designed to predict hypoglycemia (109,110), detect meals (111–113), detect exercise (perhaps by integrating the input of a physical activity monitor) (114), reduce insulin delivery when a lot of insulin is already in the body (insulin-on-board constraints) (115–117), adjust the aggressiveness of control at prespecified times (e.g., less aggressive control overnight than during the day) (118), adjust the aggressiveness of control based on short-term changes in patient characteristics (e.g., steroid treatment that increases insulin resistance) (119,120), and/or adjust the aggressiveness of control based on long-term changes in patient characteristics (e.g., weight loss and concomitant increase in insulin sensitivity) (121). For preclinical testing of algorithms and other system features, FDA has accepted the use of a simulator developed by researchers at the University of Virginia and the University of Padova (122). The simulator and its 300 in silico "patients" can be periodically updated to bring the simulations closer to reality (123).

Improving Insulin Delivery Speed

An ongoing effort in diabetes care is to improve the speed and predictability of insulin delivery. In the past two decades, three "rapid-acting" insulin analogs have been developed to improve upon the action profile of regular human insulin (124,125). However, these analogs still take roughly 1 hour to reach peak glycemic effect—a time lag that makes fully closed-loop control quite difficult as noted above. Several companies are working either to reformulate existing insulin products (126) or to develop entirely new analogs for subcutaneous injection (127,128). If these new forms of insulin pass through the gauntlet of drug development and regulatory review, they will likely have applications in closed-loop glucose control.

Developing new forms of insulin is not the only way to increase the speed and consistency of subcutaneous delivery. InsuLine has developed a device to heat the site of insulin infusion, thereby significantly accelerating insulin's pharmacokinetics (129) and pharmacodynamics (130). A downside of this heating patch is that it requires an insulin pump to be attached to an adaptor that includes a rechargeable battery and electronics (131); many people might decide that the marginal benefit is not worth this additional inconvenience. Halozyme is investigating the use of recombinant human hyaluronidase (PH20), which promotes diffusion in the interstitial tissue as an adjunct to insulin therapy. Researchers have found that by injecting PH20 when a patient inserts a new infusion set, they can reduce the intraday variability that is typical with insulin pump therapy. In general, insulin absorption is faster and more predictable on the third day of infusion-set use than the first (132,133). Coadministration of PH20 has been shown to improve the day-one results so that they become equivalent to the day-three results (134). Another way to reduce variability in infusion site performance is to build better infusion sets—a project that Becton Dickinson and Company has undertaken with funding from JDRF (135).

The pharmacokinetics and pharmacodynamics of insulin can also be improved by using a different route of delivery than subcutaneous infusion. For example, intradermal insulin delivery can be achieved with an array of microneedles roughly 1 mm in length. Relative to subcutaneous delivery, intradermal insulin delivery allows peak insulin concentration to be reached in roughly half the time (136). Becton Dickinson is investigating this approach in its aforementioned collaboration with JDRF (135,137).

Intraperitoneal delivery, which has been achieved with both implantable pumps and transcutaneous ports, yields a faster absorption and faster clearance of infused insulin. As part of closed-loop control systems, intraperitoneal insulin delivery has allowed patients to spend significantly more time in the target glucose range (138). Another probable advantage of intraperitoneal delivery is reduced intrapatient variability because—in contrast to subcutaneous and intradermal delivery—the entire infusion system would not need to be replaced every few days. However, thus far, intraperitoneal delivery has not been shown to be fast enough to control large meals and other glycemic challenges in an entirely reactive system (138).

A reasonable prediction is that any insulin-only closed-loop product would require frequent user intervention to be safe and effective in the general population of people with type 1 diabetes. For example, patients might need to perform meal announcement or "open-loop" mealtime insulin boluses. The most straightforward way to deliver these premeal boluses would be with the closed-loop system itself. However, glycemic control might be better with inhalable Technosphere insulin, which reaches its peak glucose-lowering effect roughly 2 hours earlier than subcutaneous regular human insulin and which clears the bloodstream significantly faster (139). Research is underway to determine how meal-time Technosphere affects closed-loop control that is otherwise fully automated (140).

Perhaps the most promising way to enhance insulin action is to supplement the closed-loop system with another glucodynamic hormone. One strategy for bihormonal control is to introduce a hormone that raises blood sugar so that insulin therapy can be made more aggressive without causing rebound hypoglycemia. Glucagon is the prime example of such an anti-insulin hormone. An alternative form of bihormonal control would use a hormone that stabilizes glycemic swings so that insulin therapy doesn't need to be as aggressive. Hormones that stabilize glucose levels in this way include pramlintide (a synthetic version of amylin) as well as liraglutide and exenatide (agonists of the glucagon-like peptide 1 receptor). In bihormonal closed-loop studies to date, the second hormone has been delivered with a separate pump (141,142) or manual injections (136). However, JDRF has funded an insulin manufacturer to develop a dual-chambered pump, laying a foundation for commercialized bihormonal closed-loop products (143).

Glucagon, secreted by the pancreatic alpha cells, is a hormone that raises blood sugar. In response to glucagon, the liver converts stores of glycogen into glucose. Systems that deliver both insulin and glucagon have been used to achieve some of the tightest, safest control seen in single-arm studies (64,144), and insulin-glucagon systems have outperformed both insulin-only closed-loop control (141) and open-loop pump therapy (142). As with insulin-only devices, insulin-glucagon systems are more effective when augmented with premeal boluses that cover a fraction of mealtime carbohydrate content (64).

One caveat with the use of glucagon is that liquid-stable formulations are not currently available (although researchers and companies are working to fill this niche) (145,146). Also, if insulin-delivery algorithms are optimized under conditions when glucagon is available to counteract hypoglycemia, insulin delivery could become dangerously aggressive any time that glucagon delivery malfunctions or the liver's glycogen stores are depleted. Another issue is that glucagon is already secreted by the pancreases of people with type 1 diabetes at abnormally high quantities; some researchers have even proposed that glucagon excess is actually the key problem of type 1 diabetes (147). It is not yet known how the long-term therapeutic use of low-dose glucagon would affect the body's own hormonal secretions, if at all.

Pramlintide is a synthetic version of the hormone amylin. In people without diabetes, amylin and insulin are co-secreted by the beta cells in equimolar quantities. The therapeutic reintroduction of amylin in type 1 diabetes therefore makes intuitive sense, and clinical results have been encouraging: pramlintide therapy has been shown to reduce glycemic variability for patients using insulin therapy, in part by suppressing postprandial glucagon and delaying gastric emptying (148). The clinical use of pramlintide is currently rare, in part because the drug is complicated to dose and is associated with gastric side effects. However, some researchers have begun studying pramlintide in bihormonal artificial pancreas systems in the hope that the benefits of closed-loop control could outweigh pramlintide's drawbacks. In a 24-hour, crossover-design closed-loop study, participants with type 1 diabetes ($n = 8$) experienced smaller glycemic excursions and a longer time to peak postprandial glucose when they received mealtime pramlintide injections than when they did not. The authors noted that pramlintide is currently available only in injections but that, if subsequent closed-loop studies show promise, researchers may develop ways for pramlintide to be delivered with a dual-chambered pump or as a coformulation with insulin (136).

Besides pramlintide, the glucose-stabilizing hormone that has received most attention for bihormonal control is liraglutide. Liraglutide is an analog of glucagon-like peptide 1 (GLP-1), an "incretin" hormone released during digestion. One effect of native GLP-1 is to stimulate glucose-dependent insulin secretion in order to counteract increases in blood glucose after meals. For this reason, liraglutide was originally developed as a treatment to improve glycemic control in people with type 2 diabetes. However, liraglutide may also be beneficial in type 1 diabetes. In a pilot clinical trial among people with type 1 diabetes, liraglutide was shown to reduce glycemic variability and enable people to reach a lower A1c without a significant increase in the duration of hypoglycemia (149). Liraglutide's mechanism of action in type 1 diabetes is not fully understood, but it is thought to involve the inhibition of glucagon secretion (149). The drug is not currently labeled for people with type 1 diabetes. However, liraglutide's manufacturer, Novo Nordisk, is funding clinical research to gain FDA approval for this population (150). Meanwhile, in anticipation of approval, at least one research group has begun testing the use of liraglutide in a bihormonal artificial pancreas (151).

A "Bridge to a Cure"

Technologies for closed-loop glucose control, also called artificial pancreas device systems, have the potential to make insulin delivery safer, more effective, and more convenient. These devices do not represent a true cure for type 1 diabetes. However, as a "bridge to a cure," they could improve the lives of millions. Thousands of patients worldwide are already using insulin pumps with low glucose suspend, a safety feature that represents the first step toward "closing the loop." More sophisticated closed-loop products are being developed and will likely become available within the next few years. However, in order to fully automate insulin delivery, scientists must still overcome several challenges. The biggest challenge is the speed of insulin onset and offset. (Unfortunately, of all the forms of modern insulin delivery that have been studied in clinical trials to date, none appear fast enough to enable safe and widespread use of a fully reactive, single-hormone system.) Scientists are also working to improve the accuracy and reliability of continuous glucose sensors, the predictive power of glucose-control algorithms, and the feasibility of delivering other glucose-affecting hormones besides insulin.

Research on closed-loop control has progressed significantly within the past decade, and work continues at a quick pace with support from the public, the federal government, major diabetes foundations, and the industry. The direct impact of artificial pancreas products will depend on their commercial viability, which will reflect the technologies' quality, their cost, and their public reception. However, the quest to close the loop has already led to many other benefits, such as better glucose sensors, faster insulin delivery, and more robust models of diabetes physiology. These authors hope that the improvements continue and that closed-loop research will be a "rising tide" that benefits the health of all people with type 1 diabetes.

REFERENCES

1. Rosenfeld L. Insulin: Discovery and controversy. *Clin Chem.* 2002 Dec;48(12):2270–88.
2. Banting FG, Best CH. The internal secretion of the pancreas. *J Lab Clin Med.* 1922;7:251–66.
3. Banting FG, Best CH, Collip JB, Campbell WR, Fletcher AA. Pancreatic extracts in the treatment of diabetes mellitus. *Can Med Assoc J.* 1922 Mar;12(3):141–6.
4. Michael J, Fowler M. Diabetes treatment, part 3: Insulin and incretins. *Clin Diabetes.* 2008;26(1):35–9.
5. The effect of intensive treatment of diabetes on the development and progression of long-term complications in insulin-dependent diabetes mellitus. The Diabetes Control and Complications Trial Research Group. *N Engl J Med.* 1993 Sep 30;329(14):977–86.
6. Nathan DM, Kuenen J, Borg R, Zheng H, Schoenfeld D, Heine RJ. Translating the A1C assay into estimated average glucose values. *Diabetes Care.* 2008 Aug;31(8):1473–8.
7. Nathan DM, Cleary PA, Backlund JY, Genuth SM, Lachin JM, Orchard TJ, Raskin P, Zinman B. Intensive diabetes treatment and cardiovascular disease in patients with type 1 diabetes. *N Engl J Med.* 2005 Dec 22;353(25):2643–53.
8. Zammitt NN, Frier BM. Hypoglycemia in type 2 diabetes: Pathophysiology, frequency, and effects of different treatment modalities. *Diabetes Care.* 2005 Dec;28(12):2948–61.
9. Tanenberg RJ, Newton CA, Drake AJ. Confirmation of hypoglycemia in the "dead-in-bed" syndrome, as captured by a retrospective continuous glucose monitoring system. *Endocr Pract.* 2010 Mar–Apr;16(2):244–8.

10. Hershey T, Lillie R, Sadler M, White NH. Severe hypoglycemia and long-term spatial memory in children with type 1 diabetes mellitus: A retrospective study. *J Int Neuropsychol Soc.* 2003 Jul;9(5):740–50.
11. Hershey T, Perantie DC, Wu J, Weaver PM, Black KJ, White NH. Hippocampal volumes in youth with type 1 diabetes. *Diabetes.* 2010 Jan;59(1):236–41.
12. Zaccardi F, Pitocco D, Ghirlanda G. Glycemic risk factors of diabetic vascular complications: The role of glycemic variability. *Diabetes Metab Res Rev.* 2009 Mar; 25(3):199–207.
13. Mazze R, Akkerman B, Mettner J. An overview of continuous glucose monitoring and the ambulatory glucose profile. *Minn Med.* 2011 Aug;94(8):40–4.
14. Pickup JC, Freeman SC, Sutton AJ. Glycaemic control in type 1 diabetes during real time continuous glucose monitoring compared with self monitoring of blood glucose: Meta-analysis of randomised controlled trials using individual patient data. *BMJ.* 2011 Jul;343:d3805.
15. Alsaleh FM, Smith FJ, Keady S, Taylor KM. Insulin pumps: From inception to the present and toward the future. *J Clin Pharm Ther.* 2010 Apr;35(2):127–38.
16. Skyler JS, Kruger DF, Matheson D, Parkin CG. Is there a place for insulin pump therapy in your practice? *Clinical Diabetes.* 2007;25:50–6.
17. Klonoff DC, Buckingham B, Christiansen JS, Montori VM, Tamborlane WV, Vigersky RA, Wolpert H. Continuous glucose monitoring: An Endocrine Society Clinical Practice Guideline. *J Clin Endocrinol Metab.* 2011 Oct;96(10):2968–79.
18. Fogt EJ, Dodd LM, Jenning EM, Clemens AH. Development and evaluation of a glucose analyzer for a glucose controlled insulin infusion system (Biostator). *Clin Chem.* 1978 Aug;24(8):1366–72.
19. Pickup JC, Keen H, Parsons JA, Alberti KG. Continuous subcutaneous insulin infusion: An approach to achieving normoglycaemia. *Br Med J.* 1978 Jan 28;1(6107):204–7.
20. Tamborlane WV, Sherwin RS, Genel M, Felig P. Reduction to normal of plasma glucose in juvenile diabetes by subcutaneous administration of insulin with a portable infusion pump. *N Engl J Med.* 1979 Mar 15;300(11):573–8.
21. Juvenile Diabetes Research Foundation. JDRF Clinical Panel Recommends Next Steps for Artificial Pancreas Clinical Testing Experts Present at FDA-NIH Workshop [press release]. 2010 [updated 2010; cited]; Available from: http://jdrf.org/press-releases/jdrf-clinical-panel-recommends-next-steps-for-artificial-pancreas-clinical-testing/.
22. Hanlon M. Email to: Joseph Shivers Bethesda, MD; 2011.
23. Pinkos A, Heetderks WJ, Irony I, Joffe HV, Schneider B, Zimliki CL. FDA's proactive role in the development of an artificial pancreas for the treatment of diabetes mellitus. *Drug Discovery Today: Technologies.* Elsevier. 2007;4(1):25–8.
24. Guidance for Industry and Food and Drug Administration Staff: The Content of Investigational Device Exemption (IDE) and Premarket Approval (PMA) Applications for Artificial Pancreas Device Systems. In: Services USDoHaH, editor. Silver Spring, Maryland: U.S. Department of Health and Human Services FDA Center for Devices and Radiological Health; 2012.
25. Juvenile Diabetes Research Foundation. In Just 23 Days, Over 100,000 Individuals Sign Petition for the FDA to Advance, Not Delay, the Development of an Artificial Pancreas [press release]. Journal [serial on the Internet]. 2011 Date: Available from: http://jdrf.org/press-releases/u-s-senators-clinicians-people-with-type-1-urge-fda-to-issue-clear-amp-reasonable-guidance-on-artificial-pancreas/.
26. Shalitin S, Phillip M. Hypoglycemia in type 1 diabetes: A still unresolved problem in the era of insulin analogs and pump therapy. *Diabetes Care.* 2008 Feb;31 Suppl 2:S121–4.
27. Battelino T, Phillip M, Bratina N, Nimri R, Oskarsson P, Bolinder J. Effect of continuous glucose monitoring on hypoglycemia in type 1 diabetes. *Diabetes Care.* 2011 Apr;34(4):795–800.

28. Musen G, Jacobson AM, Ryan CM, Cleary PA, Waberski BH, Weinger K, Dahms W et al. Impact of diabetes and its treatment on cognitive function among adolescents who participated in the Diabetes Control and Complications Trial. *Diabetes Care.* 2008 Oct;31(10):1933–8.
29. Feltbower RG, Bodansky HJ, Patterson CC, Parslow RC, Stephenson CR, Reynolds C, McKinney PA. Acute complications and drug misuse are important causes of death for children and young adults with type 1 diabetes: Results from the Yorkshire Register of diabetes in children and young adults. *Diabetes Care.* 2008 May;31(5):922–6.
30. Sovik O, Thordarson H. Dead-in-bed syndrome in young diabetic patients. *Diabetes Care.* 1999 Mar;22 Suppl 2:B40–2.
31. Beck RW, Tamborlane WV, Bergenstal RM, Miller KM, DuBose SN, Hall CA. The T1D Exchange clinic registry. *J Clin Endocrinol Metab.* 2012 Dec;97(12):4383–9.
32. Realsen J, Goettle H, Chase HP. Morbidity and mortality of diabetic ketoacidosis with and without insulin pump care. *Diabetes Technol Ther.* 2012 Dec;14(12):1149–54.
33. Ceriello A. Postprandial hyperglycemia and diabetes complications: Is it time to treat? *Diabetes.* 2005 Jan;54(1):1–7.
34. Hirsch IB. Glycemic variability: It's not just about A1C anymore! *Diabetes Technol Ther.* 2005 Oct;7(5):780–3.
35. Shivers JP, Mackowiak L, Anhalt H, Zisser H. "Turn it off!": Diabetes device alarm fatigue considerations for the present and the future. *J Diabetes Sci Technol.* 2013 May;7(3):789–94.
36. Ruedy KJ, Tamborlane WV. The landmark JDRF continuous glucose monitoring randomized trials: A look back at the accumulated evidence. *J Cardiovasc Transl Res.* 2012 Aug;5(4):380–7.
37. Rubin RR, Peyrot M. Treatment satisfaction and quality of life for an integrated continuous glucose monitoring/insulin pump system compared to self-monitoring plus an insulin pump. *J Diabetes Sci Technol.* 2009 Nov;3(6):1402–10.
38. Polonsky WH, Hessler D. What are the quality of life-related benefits and losses associated with real-time continuous glucose monitoring? A survey of current users. *Diabetes Technol Ther.* 2013 Apr;15(4):295–301.
39. Ritholz MD, Atakov-Castillo A, Beste M, Beverly EA, Leighton A, Weinger K, Wolpert H. Psychosocial factors associated with use of continuous glucose monitoring. *Diabet Med.* 2010 Sep;27(9):1060–5.
40. Ruedy KJ, Tamborlane WV. The landmark JDRF continuous glucose monitoring randomized trials: A look back at the accumulated evidence. *J Cardiovasc Transl Res.* 2012 Aug;5(4):380–7.
41. Shivers J, Close K, Dougan M, Kozak B, Taylor L, Trehan S, Wood R, Wu V, Woolverton G. Cross-sectional survey of patient perspectives on continuous glucose monitoring [abstract]. *Diabetes.* 2011;60(suppl 1):A234.
42. van Bon AC, Brouwer TB, von Basum G, Hoekstra JB, DeVries JH. Future acceptance of an artificial pancreas in adults with type 1 diabetes. *Diabetes Technol Ther.* 2011 Jul;13(7):731–6.
43. Kowalski AJ. Can we really close the loop and how soon? Accelerating the availability of an artificial pancreas: A roadmap to better diabetes outcomes. *Diabetes Technology & Therapeutics.* [Article]. 2009 Apr;11:S113–S9.
44. Choudhary P, Shin J, Wang Y, Evans ML, Hammond PJ, Kerr D, Shaw JA, Pickup JC, Amiel SA. Insulin pump therapy with automated insulin suspension in response to hypoglycemia: Reduction in nocturnal hypoglycemia in those at greatest risk. *Diabetes Care.* 2011 Sep;34(9):2023–5.
45. Agrawal P, Welsh JB, Kannard B, Askari S, Yang Q, Kaufman FR. Usage and effectiveness of the low glucose suspend feature of the Medtronic Paradigm Veo insulin pump. *J Diabetes Sci Technol.* 2011 Sep;5(5):1137–41.

46. Danne T, Kordonouri O, Holder M, Haberland H, Golembowski S, Remus K, Blasig S, Wadien T, Zierow S, Hartmann R, Thomas A. Prevention of hypoglycemia by using low glucose suspend function in sensor-augmented pump therapy. *Diabetes Technol Ther.* 2011 Nov;13(11):1129–34.
47. Ly TT, Nicholas JA, Retterath A, Davis EA, Jones TW. Analysis of glucose responses to automated insulin suspension with sensor-augmented pump therapy. *Diabetes Care.* 2012 Jul;35(7):1462–5.
48. Brazg RL, Bailey TS, Garg S, Buckingham BA, Slover RH, Klonoff DC, Nguyen X, Shin J, Welsh JB, Lee SW. The ASPIRE study: Design and methods of an in-clinic crossover trial on the efficacy of automatic insulin pump suspension in exercise-induced hypoglycemia. *J Diabetes Sci Technol.* 2011 Nov;5(6):1466–71.
49. Garg S, Brazg RL, Bailey TS, Buckingham BA, Slover RH, Klonoff DC, Shin J, Welsh JB, Kaufman FR. Reduction in duration of hypoglycemia by automatic suspension of insulin delivery: The in-clinic ASPIRE study. *Diabetes Technol Ther.* 2012 Mar;14(3):205–9.
50. Dagogo-Jack SE, Craft S, Cryer PE. Hypoglycemia-associated autonomic failure in insulin-dependent diabetes mellitus. Recent antecedent hypoglycemia reduces autonomic responses to, symptoms of, and defense against subsequent hypoglycemia. *J Clin Invest.* 1993 Mar;91(3):819–28.
51. Buckingham B, Cobry E, Clinton P, Gage V, Caswell K, Kunselman E, Cameron F, Chase HP. Preventing hypoglycemia using predictive alarm algorithms and insulin pump suspension. *Diabetes Technol Ther.* 2009;11(2):93–7.
52. Buckingham B, Chase HP, Dassau E, Cobry E, Clinton P, Gage V, Caswell K et al. Prevention of nocturnal hypoglycemia using predictive alarm algorithms and insulin pump suspension. *Diabetes Care.* 2010 May;33(5):1013–7.
53. Buckingham BA, Cameron F, Calhoun P, Maahs DM, Wilson DM, Chase HP, Bequette BW et al. Outpatient safety assessment of an in-home predictive low-glucose suspend system with type 1 diabetes subjects at elevated risk of nocturnal hypoglycemia. *Diabetes Technol Ther.* 2013 Jul 24.
54. Medtronic. 2012 Investor Conference. Thomson Reuters; 2012.
55. Breton M, Farret A, Bruttomesso D, Anderson S, Magni L, Patek S, Dalla Man C et al. Fully integrated artificial pancreas in type 1 diabetes: Modular closed-loop glucose control maintains near normoglycemia. *Diabetes.* 2012 Jun 11.
56. Kovatchev B, Patek S, Dassau E, Doyle FJ, III, Magni L, De Nicolao G, Cobelli C. Control to range for diabetes: Functionality and modular architecture. *J Diabetes Sci Technol.* 2009 Sep;3(5):1058–65.
57. Finan DA, Mackowiak L, McCann TW, Dassau E, Patek SD, Kovatchev BP, Doyle III FJ, Zisser H, Anhalt H, Venugopalan R. Closed-loop performance of the Hypoglycemia-Hyperglycemia Minimizer (HHM) System in a feasibility study. *Diabetes Care* (Accepted). 2013.
58. Buckingham B, Block J, Burdick J, Kalajian A, Kollman C, Choy M, Wilson DM, Chase P. Response to nocturnal alarms using a real-time glucose sensor. *Diabetes Technol Ther.* 2005 Jun;7(3):440–7.
59. Phillip M, Battelino T, Atlas E, Kordonouri O, Bratina N, Miller S, Biester T et al. Nocturnal glucose control with an artificial pancreas at a diabetes camp. *N Engl J Med.* 2013 Feb 28;368(9):824–33.
60. Nimri R, Danne T, Kordonouri O, Atlas E, Bratina N, Biester T, Avbelj M et al. Overnight automated type 1 diabetes control under MD-logic closed-loop system: A randomized crossover trial. *Pediatr Diabetes.* 2013 Feb 28.
61. Hovorka R, Kumareswaran K, Harris J, Allen JM, Elleri D, Xing D, Kollman C et al. Overnight closed loop insulin delivery (artificial pancreas) in adults with type 1 diabetes: Crossover randomised controlled studies. *BMJ.* 2011;342:d1855.

62. van Bon AC, Hermanides J, Koops R, Hoekstra JB, DeVries JH. Postprandial glycemic excursions with the use of a closed-loop platform in subjects with type 1 diabetes: A pilot study. *J Diabetes Sci Technol.* 2010 Jul;4(4):923–8.
63. Van Bon AC, Jonker LD, Koebrugge R, Koops R, Hoekstra JB, DeVries JH. Feasibility of a bihormonal closed-loop system to control postexercise and postprandial glucose excursions. *J Diabetes Sci Technol.* 2012;6(5):1114–22.
64. Russell SJ, El-Khatib FH, Nathan DM, Magyar KL, Jiang J, Damiano ER. Blood glucose control in type 1 diabetes with a bihormonal bionic endocrine pancreas. *Diabetes Care.* 2012 Nov;35(11):2148–55.
65. Weinzimer SA. Closed-loop systems: Diversity and natural selection. *Diabetes Care.* 2012 Nov;35(11):2111–2.
66. Dauber A, Corcia L, Safer J, Agus MS, Einis S, Steil GM. Closed-loop insulin therapy improves glycemic control in children aged <7 years: A randomized controlled trial. *Diabetes Care.* 2012 Oct 1.
67. Silverstein J, Klingensmith G, Copeland K, Plotnick L, Kaufman F, Laffel L, Deeb L et al. Care of children and adolescents with type 1 diabetes: A statement of the American Diabetes Association. *Diabetes Care.* 2005 Jan;28(1):186–212.
68. Whittemore R, Jaser S, Chao A, Jang M, Grey M. Psychological experience of parents of children with type 1 diabetes: A systematic mixed-studies review. *The Diabetes educator.* 2012 Jul-Aug;38(4):562–79.
69. Delamater AM, Patiño-Fernández AM, Smith KE, Bubb J. Measurement of diabetes stress in older children and adolescents with type 1 diabetes mellitus. *Pediatric Diabetes.* 2013 Feb;14(1):50–6.
70. Garcia-Patterson A, Gich I, Amini SB, Catalano PM, de Leiva A, Corcoy R. Insulin requirements throughout pregnancy in women with type 1 diabetes mellitus: Three changes of direction. *Diabetologia.* 2010 Mar;53(3):446–51.
71. Kyne-Grzebalski D, Wood L, Marshall SM, Taylor R. Episodic hyperglycaemia in pregnant women with well-controlled Type 1 diabetes mellitus: A major potential factor underlying macrosomia. *Diabet Med.* 1999 Aug;16(8):702–6.
72. Murphy HR, Elleri D, Allen JM, Harris J, Simmons D, Rayman G, Temple R et al. Closed-loop insulin delivery during pregnancy complicated by type 1 diabetes. *Diabetes Care.* 2011 Feb;34(2):406–11.
73. Murphy HR, Kumareswaran K, Elleri D, Allen JM, Caldwell K, Biagioni M, Simmons D et al. Safety and efficacy of 24-h closed-loop insulin delivery in well-controlled pregnant women with type 1 diabetes: A randomized crossover case series. *Diabetes Care.* 2011 Dec;34(12):2527–9.
74. Furnary AP, Wu Y, Bookin SO. Effect of hyperglycemia and continuous intravenous insulin infusions on outcomes of cardiac surgical procedures: The Portland Diabetic Project. *Endocr Pract.* 2004 Mar-Apr;10 Suppl 2:21–33.
75. Takahashi G, Sato N, Matsumoto N, Shozushima T, Hoshikawa K, Akitomi S, Kikkawa T et al. Preliminary study on glucose control with an artificial pancreas in postoperative sepsis patients. *Eur Surg Res.* 2011 May 17;47(1):32–8.
76. Van den Berghe G, Wouters P, Weekers F, Verwaest C, Bruyninckx F, Schetz M, Vlasselaers D, Ferdinande P, Lauwers P, Bouillon R. Intensive insulin therapy in critically Ill patients. *New England Journal of Medicine.* 2001;345(19): 1359–67.
77. Jacobi J, Bircher N, Krinsley J, Agus M, Braithwaite SS, Deutschman C, Freire AX et al. Guidelines for the use of an insulin infusion for the management of hyperglycemia in critically ill patients. *Crit Care Med.* 2012 Dec;40(12):3251–76.
78. Qaseem A, Chou R, Humphrey LL, Shekelle P. Inpatient glycemic control: Best practice advice from the clinical guidelines committee of the american college of physicians. *Am J Med Qual.* 2013 Jun 7.

79. Moghissi ES, Korytkowski MT, DiNardo M, Einhorn D, Hellman R, Hirsch IB, Inzucchi SE, Ismail-Beigi F, Kirkman MS, Umpierrez GE, American Association of Clinical E, American Diabetes A. American Association of Clinical Endocrinologists and American Diabetes Association consensus statement on inpatient glycemic control. *Endocr Pract.* 2009 May-Jun;15(4):353–69.
80. Juneja R, Roudebush CP, Nasraway SA, Golas AA, Jacobi J, Carroll J, Nelson D, Abad VJ, Flanders SJ. Computerized intensive insulin dosing can mitigate hypoglycemia and achieve tight glycemic control when glucose measurement is performed frequently and on time. *Crit Care.* 2009;13(5):R163.
81. Yamashita S, Ng E, Brommecker F, Silverberg J, Adhikari NK. Implementation of the glucommander method of adjusting insulin infusions in critically ill patients. *Can J Hosp Pharm.* 2011 Sep;64(5):333–9.
82. Dumont C, Bourguignon C. Effect of a computerized insulin dose calculator on the process of glycemic control. *Am J Crit Care.* 2012 Mar;21(2):106–15.
83. Amrein K, Ellmerer M, Hovorka R, Kachel N, Fries H, von Lewinski D, Smolle K, Pieber TR, Plank J. Efficacy and safety of glucose control with Space Glucose Control in the medical intensive care unit—An open clinical investigation. *Diabetes Technol Ther.* 2012 Aug;14(8):690–5.
84. Jax T, Heise T, Nosek L, Gable J, Lim G, Calentine C. Automated near-continuous glucose monitoring measured in plasma using mid-infrared spectroscopy. *J Diabetes Sci Technol.* 2011 Mar;5(2):345–52.
85. Joseph JI, Hipszer B, Mraovic B, Chervoneva I, Joseph M, Grunwald Z. Clinical need for continuous glucose monitoring in the hospital. *J Diabetes Sci Technol.* 2009 Nov;3(6):1309–18.
86. Harvey RA, Dassau E, Zisser H, Seborg DE, Jovanovic L, Doyle FJ. Design of the health monitoring system for the artificial pancreas: Low glucose prediction module. *J Diabetes Sci Technol.* 2012;6(6):1345–54.
87. Kovatchev BP, Renard E, Cobelli C, Zisser HC, Keith-Hynes P, Anderson SM, Brown SA et al. Feasibility of outpatient fully integrated closed-loop control: First studies of wearable artificial pancreas. *Diabetes Care.* 2013 Jul;36(7):1851–8.
88. Dassau E, Jovanovič L, Doyle III FJ, Zisser H. Enhanced 911/GPS Wizard: A telemedicine application for the prevention of severe hypoglycemia—Monitor, alert and locate. *J Diabetes Sci Technol.* 2009;3(6):1501–6.
89. Klonoff DC, Zimliki CL, Stevens LA, Beaston P, Pinkos A, Choe SY, Arreaza-Rubin G, Heetderks W. Innovations in technology for the treatment of diabetes: Clinical development of the artificial pancreas (an autonomous system). *J Diabetes Sci Technol.* 2011 May;5(3):804–26.
90. Cobelli C, Renard E, Kovatchev BP, Keith-Hynes P, Ben Brahim N, Place J, Del Favero S et al. Pilot studies of wearable outpatient artificial pancreas in type 1 diabetes. *Diabetes Care.* 2012 Sep;35(9):e65–7.
91. Kaiserman K, Buckingham BA, Prakasam G, Gunville F, Slover RH, Wang Y, Nguyen X, Welsh JB. Acceptability and utility of the mySentry remote glucose monitoring system. *J Diabetes Sci Technol.* 2013 Mar;7(2):356–61.
92. Udelsman R, Chen H, Loman K, Pitt HA, Saudek CD. Implanted programmable insulin pumps: One hundred fifty-three patient years of surgical experience. *Surgery.* 1997 Dec;122(6):1005–11.
93. Luijf YM, Mader JK, Doll W, Pieber T, Farret A, Place J, Renard E et al. Accuracy and Reliability of Continuous Glucose Monitoring Systems: A Head-to-Head Comparison. *Diabetes Technol Ther.* 2013 May 7.
94. Calhoun P, Lum J, Beck RW, Kollman C. Performance comparison of the Medtronic Sof-Sensor and Enlite glucose sensors in inpatient studies of individuals with type 1 diabetes. *Diabetes Technol Ther.* 2013 Sep.

95. Leelarathna L, Nodale M, Allen JM, Elleri D, Kumareswaran K, Haidar A, Caldwell K et al. Evaluating the accuracy and large inaccuracy of two continuous glucose monitoring systems. *Diabetes Technol Ther.* 2013 Feb;15(2):143–9.
96. Nielsen JK, Christiansen JS, Kristensen JS, Toft HO, Hansen LL, Aasmul S, Gregorius K. Clinical evaluation of a transcutaneous interrogated fluorescence lifetime-based microsensor for continuous glucose reading. *J Diabetes Sci Technol.* 2009 Jan;3(1):98–109.
97. Sorensen W, Anderson M, Sheldon A, Warren J. JDRF through the Joint JDRF-Helmsley Charitable Trust Initiative Partners with Medtronic to Advance Continuous Glucose Monitoring Towards Artificial Pancreas Systems. [News Release] Northridge, CA: Medtronic; 2012 [updated 2012; cited]; Available from: http://newsroom.medtronic.com/phoenix.zhtml?c=251324&p=irol-newsArticle&ID=1769517&highlight=.
98. Facchinetti A, Sparacino G, Guerra S, Luijf YM, DeVries JH, Mader JK, Ellmerer M, Benesch C, Heinemann L, Bruttomesso D, Avogaro A, Cobelli C. Real-time improvement of continuous glucose monitoring accuracy: The smart sensor concept. *Diabetes Care.* 2013 Apr;36(4):793–800.
99. Garg SK, Schwartz S, Edelman SV. Improved glucose excursions using an implantable real-time continuous glucose sensor in adults with type 1 diabetes. *Diabetes Care.* 2004 Mar;27(3):734–8.
100. Colvin AE, Jiang H. Increased in vivo stability and functional lifetime of an implantable glucose sensor through platinum catalysis. *J Biomed Mater Res A.* 2013 May;101(5):1274–82.
101. Muller AJ, Knuth M, Nikolaus KS, Herbrechtsmeier P. First clinical evaluation of a new long-term subconjunctival glucose sensor. *J Diabetes Sci Technol.* 2012 Jul 1;6(4):875–83.
102. Croce RA, Jr., Vaddiraju S, Kondo J, Wang Y, Zuo L, Zhu K, Islam SK, Burgess DJ, Papadimitrakopoulos F, Jain FC. A miniaturized transcutaneous system for continuous glucose monitoring. *Biomed Microdevices.* 2013 Feb;15(1):151–60.
103. Hanashi T, Yamazaki T, Tsugawa W, Ikebukuro K, Sode K. BioRadioTransmitter: A self-powered wireless glucose-sensing system. *J Diabetes Sci Technol.* 2011 Sep;5(5):1030–5.
104. Gough DA, Kumosa LS, Routh TL, Lin JT, Lucisano JY. Function of an implanted tissue glucose sensor for more than 1 year in animals. *Sci Transl Med.* 2010 Jul 28;2(42):42ra53.
105. Heinemann L, Benesch C, DeVries JH. AP@home: A novel European approach to bring the artificial pancreas home. *J Diabetes Sci Technol.* 2011 Nov;5(6):1363–72.
106. Lindpointner S, Korsatko S, Kohler G, Kohler H, Schaller R, Kaidar R, Yodfat O et al. Use of the site of subcutaneous insulin administration for the measurement of glucose in patients with type 1 diabetes. *Diabetes Care.* 2010 Mar;33(3):595–601.
107. Regittnig W, Lindpointner S, Korsatko S, Tutkur D, Bodenlenz M, Pieber TR. Periodic extraction of interstitial fluid from the site of subcutaneous insulin infusion for the measurement of glucose: A novel single-port technique for the treatment of type 1 diabetes patients. *Diabetes Technol Ther.* 2013 Jan;15(1):50–9.
108. Patek S, Magni L, Dassau E, Karvetski C, Toffanin C, De Nicolao G, Del Favero S et al. Modular closed-loop control of diabetes. *IEEE Trans Biomed Eng.* 2012 Apr 3.
109. Harvey RA, Dassau E, Zisser CH, Seborg DE, Jovanovic L, Doyle III FJ. Design of the health monitoring system for the artificial pancreas: Low glucose prediction module. *J Diabetes Sci Technol.* 2012;6(6):1345–54.
110. Daskalaki E, Norgaard K, Zuger T, Prountzou A, Diem P, Mougiakakou S. An early warning system for hypoglycemic/hyperglycemic events based on fusion of adaptive prediction models. *J Diabetes Sci Technol.* 2013;7(3):689–98.
111. Lee H, Buckingham BA, Wilson DM, Bequette BW. A closed-loop artificial pancreas using model predictive control and a sliding meal size estimator. *J Diabetes Sci Technol.* 2009;3(5):1082–90.

112. Dassau E, Bequette BW, Buckingham BA, Doyle III FJ. Detection of a meal using continuous glucose monitoring (CGM): Implications for an Artificial β-cell. *Diabetes Care.* 2008;31(2):295–300.
113. Cameron F, Niemeyer G, Buckingham BA. Probabilistic evolving meal detection and estimation of meal total glucose appearance. *J Diabetes Sci Technol.* 2009;3(5):1022–30.
114. Maahs DM, Mayer-Davis E, Bishop FK, Wang L, Mangan M, McMurray RG. Outpatient assessment of determinants of glucose excursions in adolescents with type 1 diabetes: Proof of concept. *Diabetes Technol Ther.* 2012 Aug;14(8):658–64.
115. Ruiz JL, Sherr JL, Cengiz E, Carria L, Roy A, Voskanyan G, Tamborlane WV, Weinzimer SA. Effect of insulin feedback on closed-loop glucose control: A crossover study. *J Diabetes Sci Technol.* 2012;6(5):1123–30.
116. Dassau E, Zisser H, Harvey RA, Percival MW, Grosman B, Bevier W, Seborg DE, Jovanovič L, Doyle III FJ. Clinical evaluation of a fully automated personalized artificial pancreas with an unannounced meal using mpMPC and insulin-on-board. *Diabetes Care.* (in submission). 2011.
117. Dassau E, Zisser H, Harvey RA, Percival MW, Grosman B, Bevier W, Atlas E et al. Clinical evaluation of a personalized artificial pancreas. *Diabetes Care.* 2013 Apr;36(4):801–9.
118. Grosman B, Dassau E, Zisser HC, Jovanovic L, Doyle III FJ. Zone model predictive control: A strategy to minimize hyper- and hypoglycemic events. *J Diabetes Sci Technol.* 2010 Jul;4(4):961–75.
119. El Youssef J, Castle JR, Branigan DL, Massoud RG, Breen ME, Jacobs PG, Bequette BW, Ward WK. A controlled study of the effectiveness of an adaptive closed-loop algorithm to minimize corticosteroid-induced stress hyperglycemia in type 1 diabetes. *J Diabetes Sci Technol.* 2011 Nov;5(6):1312–26.
120. Finan DA, Zisser H, Jovanovic L, Bevier WC, Seborg DE. Automatic detection of stress states in Type 1 diabetes subjects in ambulatory conditions. *Ind Eng Chem Res.* 2010 Sep 1;49(17):7843–8.
121. Doyle III FJ. Moving the Closed-Loop Artificial Pancreas from the Clinic to the Home: Algorithmic Developments. 12th Annual Diabetes Technology Meeting; 2012 November 8–10, 2012; Bethesda, Maryland. 2012.
122. Kovatchev BP, Breton M, Man CD, Cobelli C. In silico preclinical trials: A proof of concept in closed-loop control of type 1 diabetes. *J Diabetes Sci Technol.* 2009 Jan;3(1):44–55.
123. Patek SD, Bequette BW, Breton M, Buckingham BA, Dassau E, Doyle FJ, III, Lum J, Magni L, Zisser H. In silico preclinical trials: Methodology and engineering guide to closed-loop control in type 1 diabetes mellitus. *J Diabetes Sci Technol.* 2009 Mar;3(2):269–82.
124. Helms KL, Kelley KW. Insulin Glulisine: An Evaluation of Its Pharmacodynamic Properties and Clinical Application. *The Annals of Pharmacotherapy.* 2009 April 1, 2009;43(4):658–68.
125. Homko C, Deluzio A, Jimenez C, Kolaczynski JW, Boden G. Comparison of insulin aspart and lispro: Pharmacokinetic and metabolic effects. *Diabetes Care.* 2003 Jul;26(7):2027–31.
126. Krasner A, Pohl R, Simms P, Pichotta P, Hauser R, De Souza E. A review of a family of ultra-rapid-acting insulins: Formulation development. *J Diabetes Sci Technol.* 2012 Jul;6(4):786–96.
127. Rulls M, Morley A, Poulsen KR, Mersebach FD, Jacobsen LB, Lindegaard J. Company Announcement: The final phase 3a trial for IDegLira completed, and FIAsp approved for phase 3 development. [press release]. Bagsvaerd, Denmark: Novo Nordisk; 2012 [updated 2012 December 19; cited 2013 June 16]; Available from: http://www.novonordisk.com/include/asp/exe_news_attachment.asp?sAttachmentGUID=eb27510c-b564-43b8-a3b0-f9fc2d833f16.

128. Thermalin Diabetes Pipeline. Cleveland, Ohio: Thermalin Diabetes, LLC; [cited 2013 June 16]; Available from: http://www.thermalin.com/pipeline.html.
129. Raz I, Weiss R, Yegorchikov Y, Bitton G, Nagar R, Pesach B. Effect of a local heating device on insulin and glucose pharmacokinetic profiles in an open-label, randomized, two-period, one-way crossover study in patients with type 1 diabetes using continuous subcutaneous insulin infusion. *Clin Ther.* 2009 May;31(5):980–7.
130. Cengiz E, Weinzimer SA, Sherr JL, Tichy E, Martin M, Carria L, Steffen A, Tamborlane WV. Acceleration of insulin pharmacodynamic profile by a novel insulin infusion site warming device. *Pediatr Diabetes.* 2013 May;14(3):168–73.
131. Products. InsuLine Medical; [cited 2013 June 16]; Available from: http://www.insuline-medical.com/products.
132. Swan KL, Dziura JD, Steil GM, Voskanyan GR, Sikes KA, Steffen AT, Martin ML, Tamborlane WV, Weinzimer SA. Effect of age of infusion site and type of rapid-acting analog on pharmacodynamic parameters of insulin boluses in youth with type 1 diabetes receiving insulin pump therapy. *Diabetes Care.* 2009 Feb;32(2):240–4.
133. Luijf YM, Arnolds S, Avogaro A, Benesch C, Bruttomesso D, Farret A, Heinemann L et al. On behalf of the Ap@Home Consortium. Patch pump versus conventional pump: Postprandial glycemic excursions and the influence of wear time. *Diabetes Technol Ther.* 2013 May 7.
134. Muchmore DB, Vaughn DE. Accelerating and improving the consistency of rapid-acting analog insulin absorption and action for both subcutaneous injection and continuous subcutaneous infusion using recombinant human hyaluronidase. *J Diabetes Sci Technol.* 2012 Jul;6(4):764–72.
135. Finn E. JDRF and BD Collaborate to Improve Insulin Pump Delivery [press Release]. Becton Dickinson and Company; 2010 [updated 2010; cited 2013 June 16]; Available from: http://www.bd.com/contentmanager/b_article.asp?Item_ID=24403&ContentType_ID=1&BusinessCode=20008&d=Industry&s=industry&dTitle=&dc=us&dcTitle=United+States.
136. Weinzimer SA, Sherr JL, Cengiz E, Kim G, Ruiz JL, Carria L, Voskanyan G, Roy A, Tamborlane WV. Effect of pramlintide on prandial glycemic excursions during closed-loop control in adolescents and young adults with type 1 diabetes. *Diabetes Care.* 2012 Oct;35(10):1994–9.
137. McVey E, Hirsch L, Sutter DE, Kapitza C, Dellweg S, Clair J, Rebrin K, Judge K, Pettis RJ. Pharmacokinetics and postprandial glycemic excursions following insulin lispro delivered by intradermal microneedle or subcutaneous infusion. *J Diabetes Sci Technol.* 2012 Jul 1;6(4):743–54.
138. Renard E, Place J, Cantwell M, Chevassus H, Palerm CC. Closed-loop insulin delivery using a subcutaneous glucose sensor and intraperitoneal insulin delivery. *Diabetes Care.* 2010 January 2010;33(1):121–7.
139. Rave K, Potocka E, Boss AH, Marino M, Costello D, Chen R. Pharmacokinetics and linear exposure of AFRESA compared with the subcutaneous injection of regular human insulin. *Diabetes Obes Metab.* 2009 Jul;11(7):715–20.
140. Lee JJ, Dassau E, Zisser H, Harvey RA, Jovanovic L, Doyle FJ, III. In silico evaluation of an artificial pancreas combining exogenous ultrafast-acting technosphere insulin with zone model predictive control. *J Diabetes Sci Technol.* 2013;7(1):215–26.
141. Castle JR, Engle JM, Youssef JE, Massoud RG, Yuen KC, Kagan R, Ward WK. Novel use of glucagon in a closed-loop system for prevention of hypoglycemia in type 1 diabetes. *Diabetes Care.* 2010 Jun;33(6):1282–7.
142. Haidar A, Legault L, Dallaire M, Alkhateeb A, Coriati A, Messier V, Cheng P, Millette M, Boulet B, Rabasa-Lhoret R. Glucose-responsive insulin and glucagon delivery (dual-hormone artificial pancreas) in adults with type 1 diabetes: A randomized crossover controlled trial. *CMAJ.* 2013 Mar 5;185(4):297–305.

143. Tandem Diabetes Care Announces Partnership with JDRF to Develop a Novel Dual-Chamber Infusion Pump. San Diego, California: Tandem Diabetes Care; 2013 [updated 2013; cited 2013 June 16]; Available from: http://www.tandemdiabetes.com/News/2013/Tandem-Diabetes-Care-Announces-Partnership-with-JDRF-to-Develop-a-Novel-Dual-Chamber-Infusion-Pump/.
144. El-Khatib FH, Russell SJ, Nathan DM, Sutherlin RG, Damiano ER. A bihormonal closed-loop artificial pancreas for type 1 diabetes. *Sci Transl Med.* 2010;2(27):1–12.
145. Steiner SS, Li M, Hauser R, Pohl R. Stabilized glucagon formulation for bihormonal pump use. *J Diabetes Sci Technol.* 2010 Nov;4(6):1332–7.
146. Ramdial S. Xeris Pharmaceuticals Awarded Phase II Funding of NIH Fast-Track SBIR Grant to Advance Glucagon for the Artificial Pancreas [press release]. Xeris Pharmaceuticals; 2013 [updated 2013; cited 2013 June 16]; Available from: http://xerispharma.com/Artificial_Pancreas_SBIR_Phase_II_OHSU-Xeris.pdf.
147. Unger RH, Cherrington AD. Glucagonocentric restructuring of diabetes: A pathophysiologic and therapeutic makeover. *J Clin Invest.* 2012 Jan 3;122(1):4–12.
148. Hoogwerf BJ, Doshi KB, Diab D. Pramlintide, the synthetic analogue of amylin: Physiology, pathophysiology, and effects on glycemic control, body weight, and selected biomarkers of vascular risk. *Vasc Health Risk Manag.* 2008;4(2):355–62.
149. Varanasi A, Bellini N, Rawal D, Vora M, Makdissi A, Dhindsa S, Chaudhuri A, Dandona P. Liraglutide as additional treatment for type 1 diabetes. *Eur J Endocrinol.* 2011 Jul;165(1):77–84.
150. Nordisk N. The Efficacy and Safety of Liraglutide as Adjunct Therapy to Insulin in the Treatment of Type 1 Diabetes (ADJUNCT ONE). [Study Record]: ClinicalTrials.gov; 2013 [updated 2013; cited 2013 June 16]; Available from: http://clinicaltrials.gov/ct2/show/NCT01836523?term=liraglutide+type+1+diabetes&rank=8.
151. Heptulla R. Liraglutide Versus Insulin Mono-therapy in the Closed Loop Setting. [Study Record] Bronx, New York: ClinicalTrials.gov; 2012 [updated 2012, January 25, 2013; cited 2013 June 16]; Available from: http://clinicaltrials.gov/ct2/show/NCT01755416.

7 Micro/Nano Devices for Drug Delivery

Roya Sheybani and Ellis Meng

CONTENTS

CLINICAL NEED FOR DRUG DELIVERY DEVICES

Effective drug therapy is an essential tool in improving health outcomes in the treatment and management of chronic conditions, such as hypertension, respiratory disease, and diabetes, and therefore, improved methods and technologies for drug delivery are a critical health care need [1]. Chronic conditions affect an estimated 133 million Americans (46% of the population in 2006). This number is estimated to reach 171 million (nearly half the population) by 2030. Statistics gathered in 2006 showed that the management of chronic conditions contributes to an estimated 83% of total health care costs [2], and the average annual health care coverage cost for individuals suffering from a chronic condition is $6,032, five times higher than for healthy individuals [1].

The efficacy of drug therapy in treating these chronic conditions is in part linked to its administration route. Commonly used oral, topical, or intravenous injection administration routes require high systemic doses in order to achieve the intended therapeutic effect at remote sites within the body. Many systemically administered drugs, such as anticancer drugs, antifertility agents, and anti-inflammatory steroids, are associated with severe side effects [3] and therefore dramatically impact the patient's quality of life. Parenteral drug injection uses conventional needles and catheters and requires repeated time- and labor-intensive procedures for chronic treatment. These are associated with frequent clinical visits, lost productivity at the workplace or in the field, low patient compliance, and elevated risk of infection. These methods are also unsuitable for long-term treatment, have a narrow drug therapeutic window, and utilize a complex dosing schedule with combination therapy or labile active ingredients [4]. On the other hand, many emerging pharmaceutical agents, including biologics, biosimilars, and other small molecules, are not suitable for administration through the aforementioned conventional routes [5]. For instance, the past quarter century of outstanding progress in fundamental cancer biology has not translated into comparable advances in the clinic. This discrepancy is in part due to the fact that only between 1 and 10 parts per 100,000 of intravenously administered monoclonal antibodies reach their parenchymal targets in vivo [6]. Commercially available pumps for site-specific delivery are large and bulky, making them unsuitable for pediatrics and smaller patients [5,7,8]. The decades-old mechanisms employed cannot be miniaturized and are inefficient in their use of space. Their incompatibility with new pharmaceuticals has led to recent recalls due to stalling and drug dumping malfunctions [9].

Shortcomings of current methods have motivated efforts to develop implantable site-specific drug delivery systems that minimize side effects, improve safety, and have the potential to be more effective by allowing the use of new and more potent drugs [10]. While certain chronic conditions, such as drug addiction and menopause, have associated static therapeutic windows and may be treated with constant drug administration [11], most chronic conditions have chronobiological pattern in their pathogenesis [12–15]. More importantly, drug dosing affects the therapeutic window. Following successful drug administration, the clinical need for additional pharmacological intervention for certain conditions diminishes transiently while the ratio of risk to benefit dramatically increases [5].

Implantable drug delivery devices seek to mitigate some of challenges facing conventional drug delivery methods by bypassing physiological barriers to enable delivery of new compounds, such as biologics, biosimilars, and other small molecules, directly to the target tissue [16] and to maximize therapeutic efficacy of the drug and limit toxic side effects by delivering the correct amount of drug in the vicinity of the target cells while reducing the drug exposure to the nontarget cells. Site-specific and controlled drug administration avoids the peak and trough time course of drug concentrations in the plasma between successive doses and the corresponding peak and trough pattern of drug action, leading to therapies that mimic the chronobiological pattern of the condition [3,4,16].

Nanotechnologies and microelectromechanical system (MEMS) devices are scaled to allow implantation near the region of interest for localized drug therapy [4]. Moreover, sensors can be incorporated into MEMS devices to monitor the drug release profile and provide useful information for bioengineers and clinicians to optimize the drug therapy for the patients [4].

In this chapter, the requirements for an implantable drug delivery device are considered followed by a discussion on enabling nano/micro technologies. Then nanotechnology and microtechnology devices are reviewed, including examples of research and commercial devices. Microtechnology devices are further categorized based on their actuation method. Suitable materials for device construction and some examples of commercially available MEMS drug delivery systems are discussed. Last, shortcomings of available technology and future trends are addressed.

DRUG DELIVERY DEVICE REQUIREMENTS

In order for a micro/nano device to be suitable for drug delivery, certain requirements must be met. While high volumetric flow rates are not likely to be required of implanted micropumps, precise fluid metering and pressure generation requirements are of great importance since in the body backpressure of up to 25 kPa could be encountered, depending on the delivery site [17]. The device should be capable of delivering precise quantities of a drug at the right time and as close to the treatment site as possible. Other critical requirements include long-term reliability, accuracy, low power consumption, cost, compatibility with an assortment of drug formulations (both existing and new), biocompatibility, and minimal patient intervention following surgical placement [4,17,18]. The overall size of the device is also a major consideration. The device should be as small as possible to allow for ease of implantation and removal (if necessary) requiring only minor surgery and local anesthesia, and not cause any adverse effects after implantation [4]. Some systems may possess many components, including external patches or interfaces.

In many indications, chronic, repeated delivery is required (2–5 years); therefore, the accuracy, precision, and reliability of the device should be maintained over the treatment duration [19]. Drug concentration below or above the therapeutic limits might result in side effects or even cause intoxication [20]. As a consequence, the dose, frequency, duration, oscillatory behavior, toxicity, drug interaction, and allergies must all be considered when designing the device and possibly be customized for patients based on their illness and history [18]. Ideally, a drug can be delivered exclusively to the target tissues, cells, or cellular components, which suggests the need for developing delivery mechanisms that would equal or surpass the selectivity of naturally occurring effectors [3].

Over the last three decades, MEMS and nanotechnology have enabled drug delivery device miniaturization for a number of different applications [4]. Based on the specific clinical indication, design requirements such as flow rate, backpressure, power, efficiency, reliability, size, and cost must be considered and appropriately prioritized to determine the most suitable method of and technology for delivery [17,21].

NANOTECHNOLOGY DEVICES

Nanotechnology devices are typically defined as having at least one dimension in the 1–100 nm range and that the device or its essential components are manmade [6]. The two major classes are nanovectors and nanoporous silicon membranes. Silicon and silica, as well as several polymer-based materials, have been investigated as interesting candidate materials for intravascularly injectable nanovectors and seem promising for clinical translation. A range of drug release time profiles can be achieved by selecting the nanovector material. Biodegradable porosified silicon has rapid kinetics (minutes to hours) versus biodegradable polymers with longer kinetics (weeks to months). Metal-based nanovectors include nanoshells, which comprise a gold layer over a silica core. The nanoshell can be selectively activated through tissue irradiation with near-infrared light by precisely tuning the thickness of this gold layer [6]. Active recognition elements can be added to the surface of a nanovector to attain molecular targeting. This increases specificity at the expense of added complexity in the nanoparticle preparation, increased particle size, and the risk of biological adverse reactions to the targeting agent [6].

Ferrari et al. developed silicon membranes with nanofabricated channels having dimensions in the 5–100 nm range that inhibit passage of immunologic cells, antibodies, and large proteins while being permeable to small molecules, such as oxygen, glucose, and insulin. The group showed that their membranes could outperform controls in terms of insulin-secretion capability over periods of several weeks [22–24]. In 2005, Abraxane®, a 130-nm paclitaxel nanoparticle developed by Patrick Soon-Shiong at American Bioscience Inc. was approved by the Food and Drug Administration (FDA) for the treatment of metastatic breast cancer and non-small cell lung cancer [6,25].

Nanoporous silicon membranes were also developed by Ferrari and coworkers for application as immune-isolating biocapsules and for molecular filtration [26]. iMEDD Inc. has developed nanoporous microparticles to treat systemically accessible solid tumors, specifically the multiple lesion sites associated with metastatic disease (Figure 7.1) [3,27]. Controlled dual-sided, symmetric particulates of porous

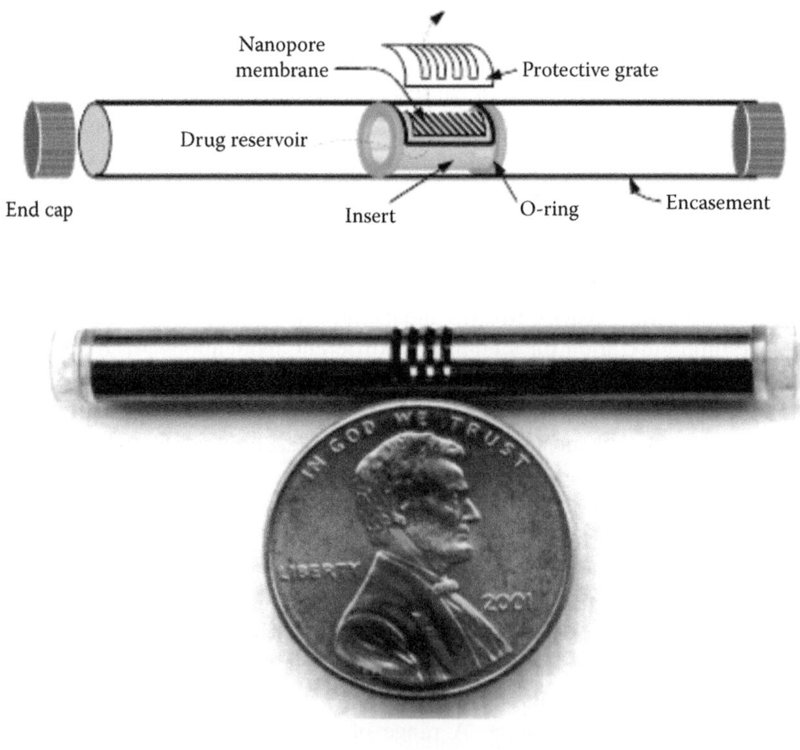

FIGURE 7.1 Implant fitted with nanoporous silicon membrane. (Reprinted from F. Martin et al., *Journal of Controlled Release*, 102, 123–133, 2005, with permission Elsevier.)

silicon from polysilicon have also been fabricated by Smith et al. to enable unidirectional flow of transported drugs, proteins–peptides, and nucleic acids [3,28].

MICROELECTROMECHANICAL SYSTEMS DEVICES

In the early 1980s, Jan Smits developed one of the first micropumps intended for use in controlled insulin delivery systems for maintaining diabetics' blood sugar levels without frequent needle injections [17,29]. This peristaltic pump consisted of three active valves actuated by piezoelectric discs. This publication was first to demonstrate the feasibility of silicon-based micropumps and subsequently inspired extensive research on micropumps [18].

A MEMS drug delivery system typically consists of micropumps, sensors, and control circuitry [20]. These devices can be divided into two categories based on the method by which the drug release is controlled. In passive devices, the device is preprogrammed to release a certain drug dosage profile. This can be achieved whether through passive mechanisms, such as osmosis or in response to an environmental stimulus. Although these systems are generally less complex in terms of design and fabrication, they have limited control of drug delivery. Active mechanisms require an external stimulus, such as an electrical signal, radio frequency wave, or magnetic wave, to alter the behavior of the drug delivery device and cause it to dispense the drug. Active control requires power, and these systems are generally harder to design and fabricate; however, they offer precise metering of the dispensed drug [4].

PASSIVE MEMS MICROPUMPS

Passive mechanisms to control drug delivery are highly dependent on the properties of the fluid to be transported and, therefore, face unique challenges for clinical translation. However, they are generally easier to fabricate [4].

An osmotic flow is generated when two solutions having different solute concentrations are separated by a semipermeable membrane that is impermeable to the solute but allows solvent molecules to pass freely. The osmotic flow across the membrane, from low to high solute concentration, results in development of a hydrostatic pressure difference, which is harnessed to pump the drug [30]. In osmotic micropumps, an osmotic driving agent is placed inside the semipermeable membrane bounded chamber to establish the concentration difference that drives generation of the osmotic pressure (Figure 7.2) [20]. Both liquid and solid drugs can be stored within osmotic micropumps. With solid drugs, a concentrated drug can be stored in minimal space and is dissolved on contact with bodily fluids. Hence, these systems can be considered to be one of the most space-efficient drug delivery technologies [30]. However, although this type of micropump needs no external power (mechanical or electrical), it suffers from low flow rate and low response with long time delay [20]. The rate of delivery cannot be altered or stopped once started. Ryu et al. developed a biodegradable osmotic micropump for controlled release of growth factors (Figure 7.3). The planar device fabricated from poly(lactic-co-glycolic acid) (PLGA) and polyethylene glycol (PEG) is capable of delivering 40 ng/day for 4 weeks [31]. Other examples of osmotic drug delivery devices can be found [30,32,33].

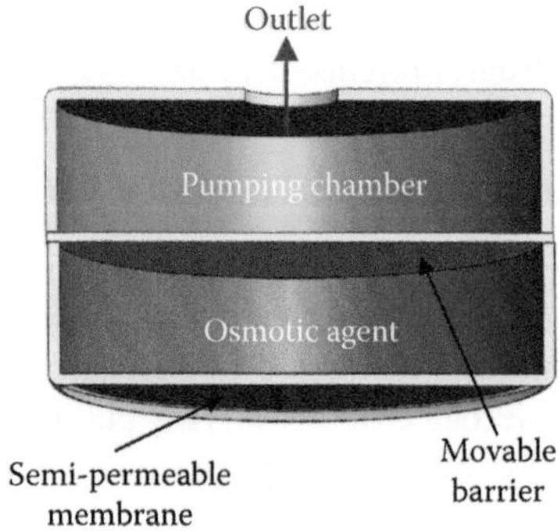

FIGURE 7.2 Schematic of osmotic micropump operation.

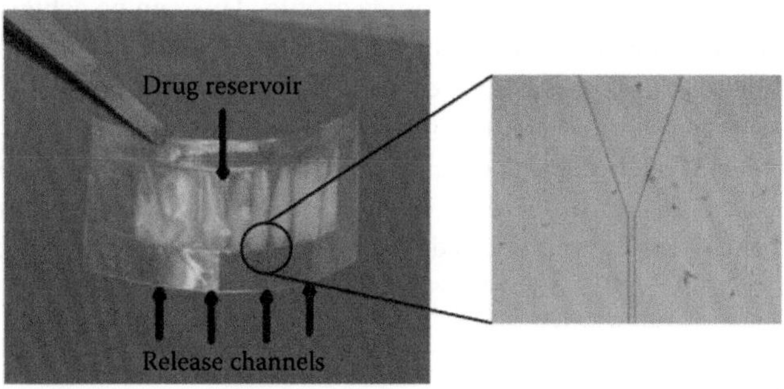

FIGURE 7.3 Photograph of osmotic device and the zoomed-in view of a micro-channel. (Reprinted from W. H. Ryu et al., *Journal of Controlled Release*, 124, 98–105, 2007, with permission Elsevier.)

Another class of passive MEMS drug delivery devices respond to an environmental stimulus. Responsive hydrogels are biocompatible and can be specifically engineered to respond to a variety of factors and marker molecules within the blood, such as temperature, pH, saccharide concentration, and antigen concentration. These factors fluctuate over the course of treatment and, as a result, alter the response of the hydrogel and the delivery rate of drug [4]. Desai et al. created biocapsules bounded by silicon diffusion membranes having uniform pore sizes through which drug release is controlled by diffusion of biological stimulants into the biocapsule [24].

Active MEMS Micropumps

Most active micropumps can be roughly divided into two groups based on their architecture: reciprocating or continuous. Reciprocating micropumps use the oscillatory or rotational movement of mechanical parts to displace fluid. These piston-like micropumps can be further classified intro micro diaphragm and peristaltic types. Micro diaphragm micropumps employ a pump chamber, which is closed with a flexible diaphragm on (at least) one side. Oscillatory movement of the diaphragm generates a two-phase pump cycle with periodic volume changes and, hence, under- and overpressure transients in the pump chamber to force fluid through the inlet into the pump chamber and subsequently transfer it to the outlet. Fluid rectifying check-valves are required at the inlet and outlet to block unwanted reverse flow in the respective pump phases and create unidirectional flow [34]. Alternatively, actuation chambers can be placed in series to create a peristaltic pump and eliminate the need for check-valves. Continuous flow micropumps operate based on a direct transformation of nonmechanical or mechanical energy into a continuous fluid movement. Depending on the specific actuation method, continuous flow micropumps may also require check-valves to prevent fluid backflow. Reviews of MEMS check-valves can be found [35,36].

Active micropumps can be further grouped based on the actuator type as either displacement or dynamic. Displacement microactuators exert pressure forces on the working fluid using one or more moving boundaries [17] and include piezoelectric, thermopeumatic, thermal/shape memory alloy (SMA), electrostatic, electromagnetic, ionic conductive polymer film (ICPF), electrochemical, and electrowetting (EO) actuation mechanisms. In dynamic microactuators, on the other hand, energy is continuously applied to the working fluid in a manner that increases either its pressure directly or its momentum that is subsequently converted into pressure by the action of an external fluid resistance [17]. Electrohydrodynamic (EHD)/electroosmotic (EO), magnetohydrodynamic (MHD), and acoustic/ultrasonic are dynamic actuation mechanisms. In the following, a brief description of each of these actuation methods is provided (Table 7.1) along with examples of their implementation in drug delivery micropumps.

Displacement Micropumps

Piezoelectric

Piezoelectric actuation involves applying a piezoelectric material to the actuator's movable membrane and inducing a transverse piezoelectric strain by an applied electric field. This results in bending deformation in the membrane that is directed to expel the fluid out of the chamber of the micropump. High stress, fast response times, and operation at relatively high frequency are advantages of piezoelectric micropumps, however, they require high driving voltage (~200 V) to generate a useful deformation, and fabrication can be complicated, especially in cases where reduced dimensions require direct deposition thin film piezoelectric materials onto the movable membrane [18,20]. A piezoelectric drug delivery device reported by Junwu et al. is capable of delivering 3.5 mL/min at 27 kPa backpressure. The 11-mm diameter micropump is intended for site-specific drug delivery (Figure 7.4) [37]. Evans et al. also developed a piezoelectric micropump with low power flow regulating check-valves, designed for intrathecal chronic pain management (Figure 7.5) [38]. Their design includes embedded sensors for closed-loop control and error monitoring of the drug pumping, and it delivers at rates of 2.30 to 0.51 mL/h. To create a completely implantable system, electronics and 3.3-V batteries are added. The overall system size is 5.08 cm × 9 cm × 3 cm, which is considerably smaller than commercially available intrathecal pumps that do not employ MEMS [8,39,40].

TABLE 7.1
Schematic Diagram of Active MEMS Micropumps Based on Actuation Mechanism

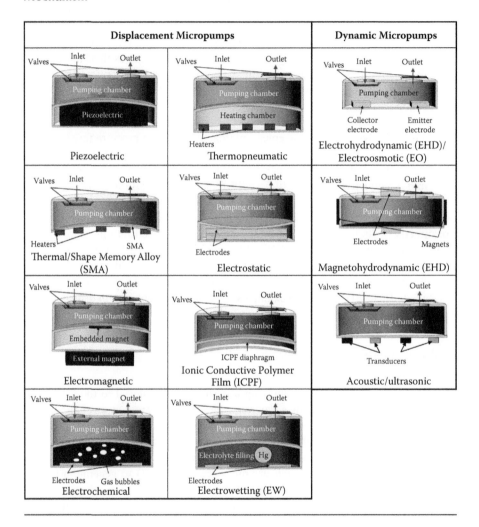

Displacement Micropumps		Dynamic Micropumps
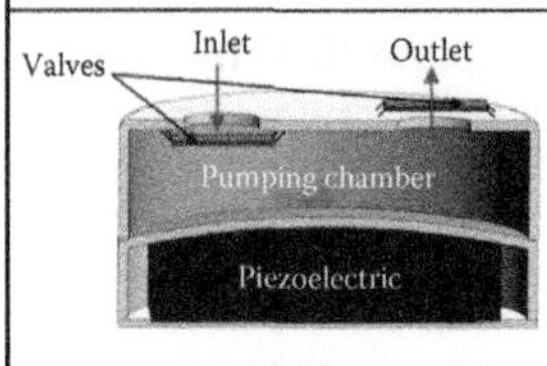 Piezoelectric	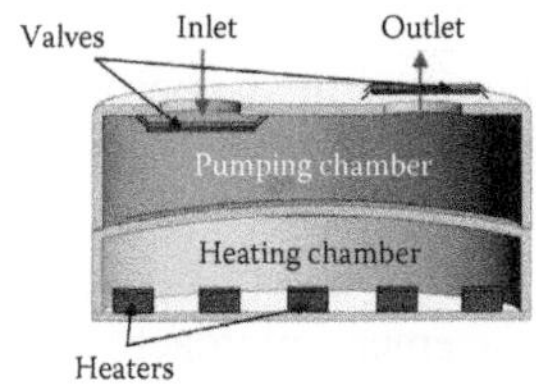 Thermopneumatic	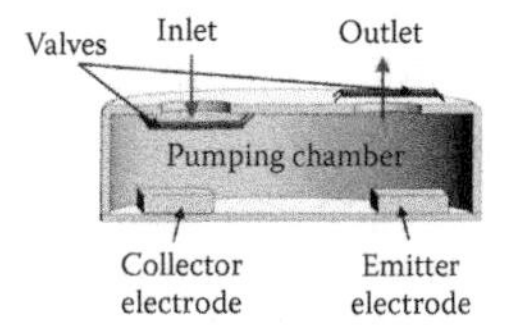 Electrohydrodynamic (EHD)/ Electroosmotic (EO)
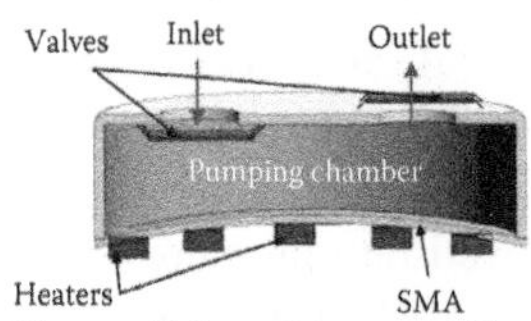 Thermal/Shape Memory Alloy (SMA)	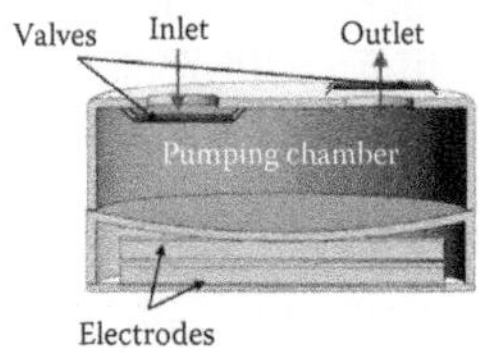 Electrostatic	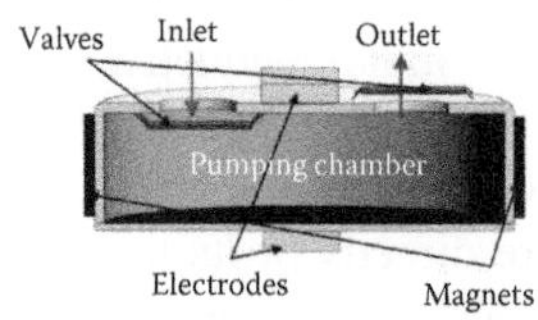 Magnetohydrodynamic (EHD)
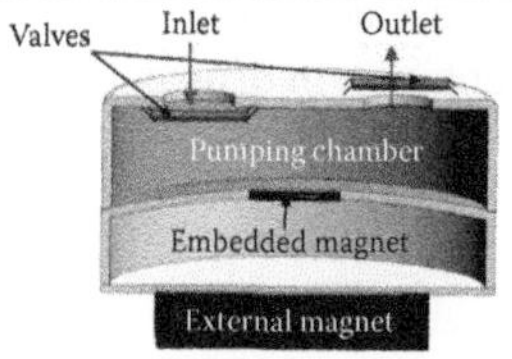 Electromagnetic	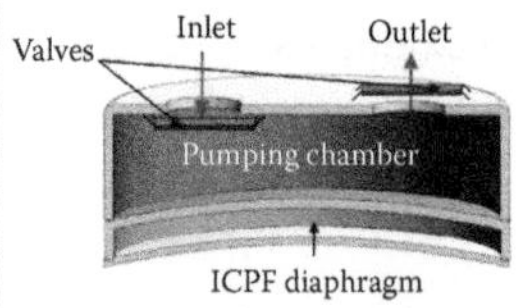 Ionic Conductive Polymer Film (ICPF)	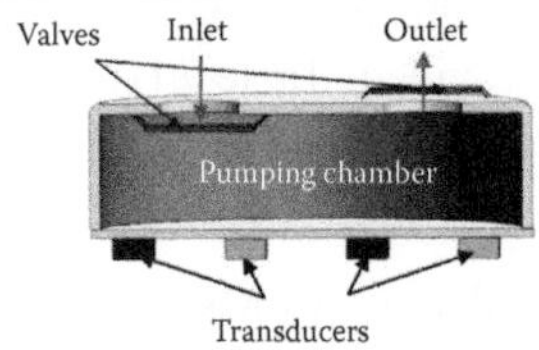 Acoustic/ultrasonic
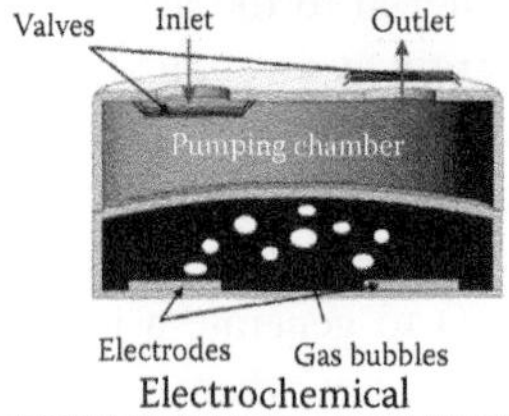 Electrochemical	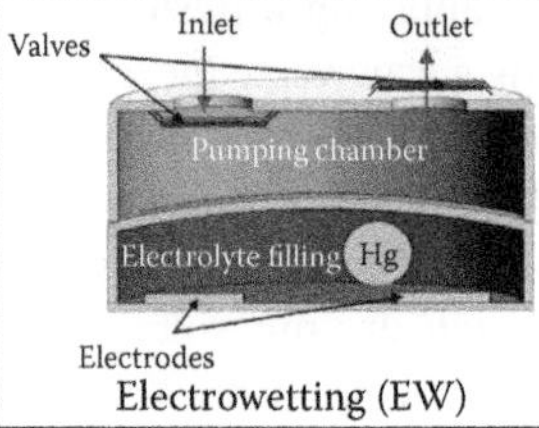 Electrowetting (EW)	

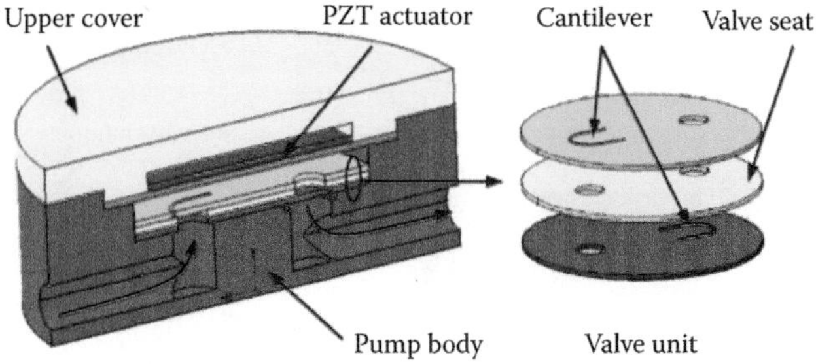

FIGURE 7.4 Schematic of piezoelectric micropump developed by Junwu et al. (Reprinted from K. Junwu et al., *Sensors and Actuators A (Physical)*, 121, 156–161, 2005, with permission Elsevier.)

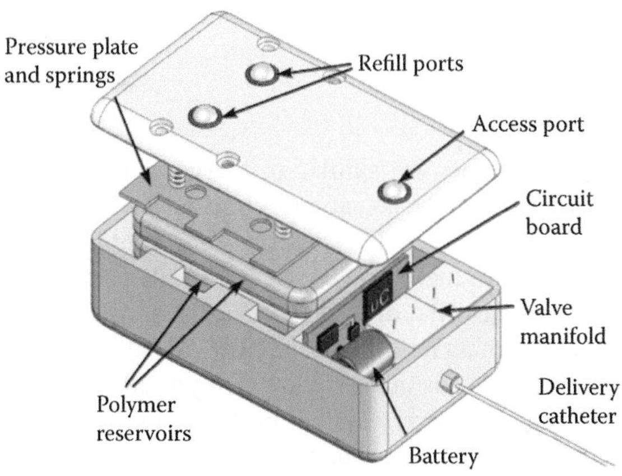

FIGURE 7.5 Conceptual drawing of piezoelectric drug delivery device by Evans et al. (Reprinted from T. Li et al., *Advanced Drug Delivery Reviews*, 2012, with permission Elsevier.)

Thermopneumatic

Thermopneumatic actuation involves the use of a heater to periodically expand a fluid-filled chamber to expel drug from an adjacent reservoir. Thermopneumatic micropumps generate relatively large induced pressure and membrane displacement; however, their structure can be complicated, and they suffer from slow response and low efficiency because cooling times can be significant [20]. Ochoa and Ziaie developed a transdermal fermentation-powered thermopneumatic micropump capable of delivering <0.23 μL/min while continuously pumping for over 2 hours (Figure 7.6) [41]. The device includes a thermally conductive silicon substrate that transfers body heat to a yeast-filled compartment to initiate the fermentation process. The resulting CO_2 gas by-product deflects a polydimethylsiloxane (PDMS) membrane and displaces the drug from an adjacent reservoir. However, irregularities in flow were reported and attributed to the CO_2 permeability of PDMS, which may be mitigated in part by coating with Parylene [42].

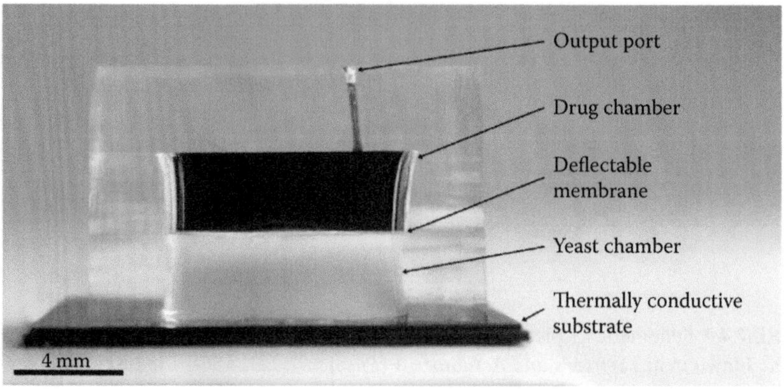

FIGURE 7.6 Photograph of thermopneumatic drug delivery device by Ochoa and Ziaie. (Reprinted from M. Ochoa and B. Ziaie, *Lab on a Chip*, 12, 4044–4048, 2012, with permission Royal Society of Chemistry.)

Thermal/Shape Memory Alloy

Shape memory alloy actuators are similar to thermopnuematic actuators in that heating/cooling is used to drive the actuation. A bimetallic diaphragm typically constructed of titanium–nickel alloy (TiNi) deforms following heat application and is capable of returning to its original shape upon cooling. Shape deformation is utilized as the actuating force to eject the drug. SMA micropumps retain linearity during deflection of the diaphragm, attain high stress (>200 MPa), and achieve long operation cycles. However, power consumption may be high [20]. Spieth et al. developed a thermal intracerebral drug delivery system for freely moving animals suitable for preclinical research (Figure 7.7). The actuator, made of thermally expandable microspheres (Expancel® 820 DU 40), is capable of delivering sixteen 0.25 μL metered doses. The device is low power (each dosage requiring 3.375 Ws of electrical power) allowing for future wireless integration [43]. Heat can also be used to boil water

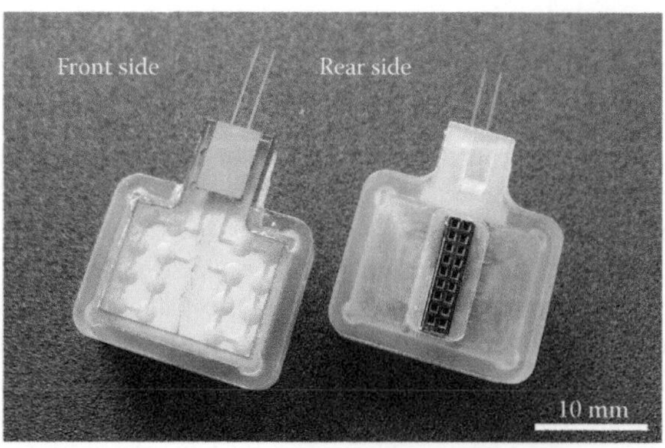

FIGURE 7.7 Photograph of SMA drug delivery device by Spieth et al. (Reprinted from S. Spieth et al., *Biomedical Microdevices*, 14, 799–809, Oct 2012, with permission Springer.)

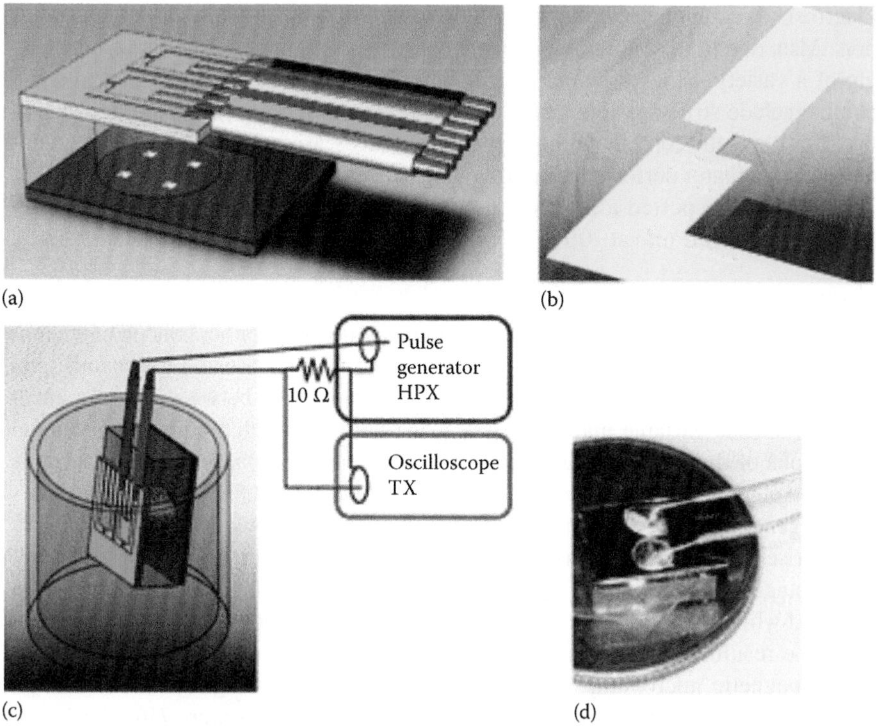

FIGURE 7.8 Thermally actuated device. (a) Conceptual drawing, (b) close-up of the fuse device (the fuse is the thin gold strip that bridges the larger gold strips over the membrane), (c) experimental setup for activation and controlled release, and (d) photograph of the device. (Reprinted from N. Elman et al., *Lab on a Chip*, 10, 2796–2804, 2010, with permission Royal Society of Chemistry.)

to increase pressure in a hermetically sealed drug reservoir. A small (~38 μm × 385 μm × 2.25 mm) implantable MEMS drug delivery device for rapid delivery in ambulatory emergency care utilizes the boiling concept to deliver 20 μL of vasopressin (a commonly used drug for cardiac resuscitation) in 45 s (Figure 7.8) [44]. This device may be implanted with and support the function of current cardiac devices, such as pacemakers and defibrillators; however, vasopressin currently is only stable for 5 days within the reservoir and heating limits release of the active drug to only 85% of that originally loaded [45].

Electrostatic

An electrostatic microactuator consists of two opposite metallic plates that are displaced as a result of electrically induced Coloumbic attraction [18]. If one of these plates is a movable membrane, then the membrane deforms when an appropriate control voltage is applied to the plates. When the applied voltage is shut off, the membrane returns to its original position. Thus, periodic switching of applied voltage will lead to alternating changes in the chamber volume and pressure that pumps fluid.

Electrostatic actuation offers operation up to several kHz and low power consumption. Also, due to the bidirectional movement of the membrane, simultaneous missing of a variety of doses before delivery is possible. Shortcomings of electrostatic pumps include structure complexity, high applied voltages, small membrane deflection (~5 μm with corresponding actuation voltages around 200 V), and degradation of the actuator performance during long-term high-voltage operation [18,20,34]. Zengerle et al. reported a bidirectional electrostatic micropump with a maximum flow rate of 850 μL/min at 200 V applied voltage for fluid handling applications [46].

Electromagnetic

In an electromagnetic microactuator, a permanent magnet is either bonded or embedded in the membrane. An external magnetic field is created using microcoils, and movement of the membrane is achieved through interaction between the permanent magnet and the variable magnetic field generated by the microcoils. Bidirectional deflections of the membrane are possible by switching the phases of input currents since magnetic actuation forces can be either attractive or repulsive [18]. Large forces can be generated, the membrane frequency is highly tunable, and electromagnetic fields arise and disappear rapidly, allowing for very fast operation speed. However, electromagnetic micropumps have high power consumption and heat dissipation [18], and while modular optimization of the micropump and actuation unit are possible, the resulting micropump is often bulky [34]. Pirmoradi et al. developed an electromagnetic micropump for controlled delivery of anti-angiogenic drugs (e.g., docetaxel [DTX]) to the posterior segment of the human eye (Figure 7.9). The device uses iron oxide as the magnetic core embedded in a PDMS membrane and is curved to match the eye. Drug is expelled from the reservoir on demand at the exterior eye wall but must rely on diffusion to reach the interior of the eye, which may not be practical for all drug formulations. The group reports 73% uptake of the dispensed DTX 2 hours after actuation [47,48]. Electromagnetic actuation was also used for an

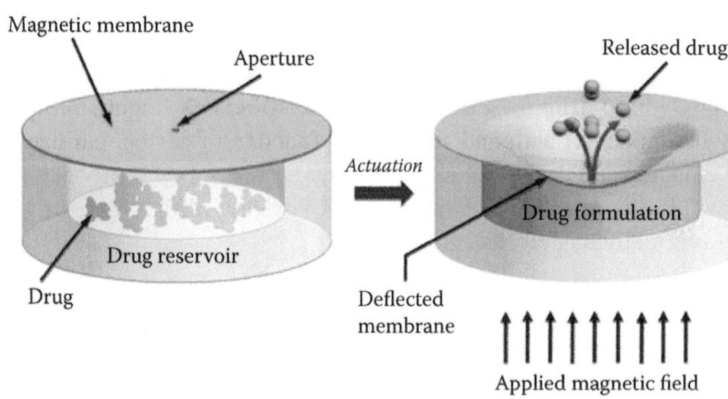

FIGURE 7.9 Conceptual drawing of electromagnetic drug delivery device by Pirmoradi et al. (Reprinted from F. N. Pirmoradi et al., *Lab on a Chip*, 11, 2744–2752, 2011, with permission Royal Society of Chemistry.)

application in increasing and regulating the flow and pressure of blood in pulmonary arteries. This microactuator is capable of delivering flow rates up to 1.98 mL/s [49].

Ionic Conductive Polymer Film

Ionic conductive polymer films are composed of a layer of perfluorosulfonic acid polymer or Nafion/silica with both sides chemically plated with materials having high electrical conductivity, such as gold or platinum, as electrodes. When an alternating voltage is applied across these electrodes, the electroactive polymer diaphragm can be controlled to bend bidirectionally [18]. ICPF microactuators require a low driving voltage, have quick response, are biocompatible, and are capable of working in aqueous environments. However, they suffer from low repeatability of material properties in batch fabrication processes [20]. Hiraoka et al. have utilized polypyrrole and gold to fabricate a miniaturized ICPF micropump for lab on a chip and chemical analysis applications (Figure 7.10) [50]. Their 25 mm × 15 mm device is capable of delivering 1.5 μL/min [51].

Electrochemical

In electrochemical micropumps, the large volume expansion resulting from electrolysis of water into hydrogen and oxygen gases is used to exert force on the membrane and subsequently force the fluid out of the chamber [52]. These micropumps are relatively simple in structure, can be constructed from biocompatible materials, and are easily integrated with other microfluidic devices. In some cases, however, depending on bubble generation rate, bubbles might partially collapse and recombine prematurely, affecting the stability of drug release [20]. Electrolysis, the oldest example of direct conversion of electrical energy to pressure–volume changes [53,54], has been explored by several groups for implantable pump applications [55–60]. Meng et al. have developed a low-power (0.66–51.31 mW) electrolysis-based

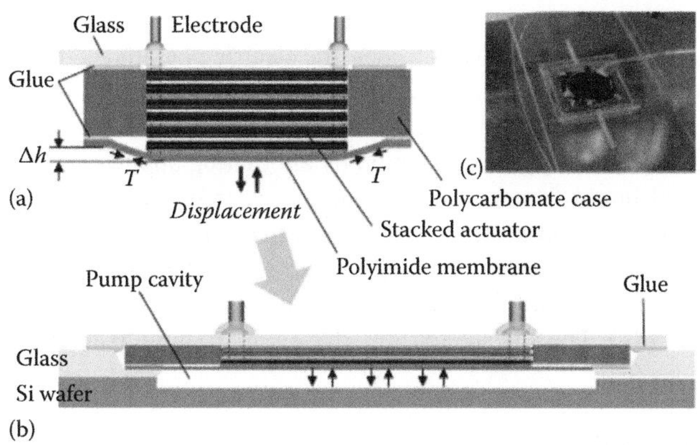

FIGURE 7.10 ICPF microactuator by Hiraoka et al. (a) Schematic of the packaged actuator; (b) packaged actuator glued to a micro-fluidic system; (c) photograph of the packaged actuator mounted on a fluidic structure. (Reprinted from M. Hiraoka et al., *Sensors and Actuators A: Physical*, 177, 23–29, 2012, with permission Elsevier.)

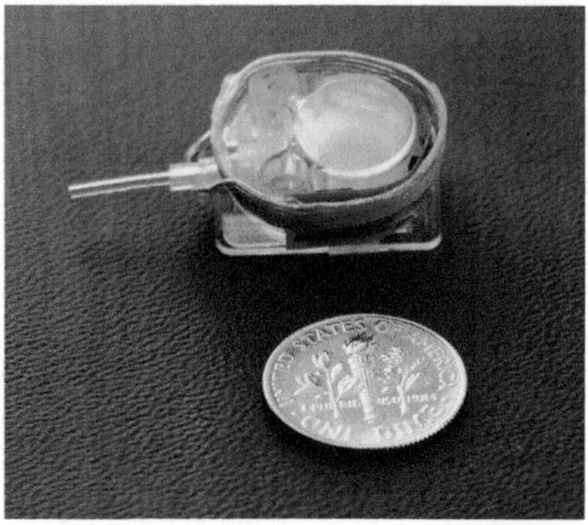

FIGURE 7.11 Photograph of electrochemical drug delivery device by Meng et al.

micropump capable of accurate delivery of a diverse assortment of liquid drug formulations within a wide dynamic range of flow rates (0.33–141.9 μL/min). This system incorporates an electrochemically based dose tracking system that is capable of real-time tracking and confirmation of delivery of doses as small as 0.004% of the reservoir (Figure 7.11) [52,61,62].

Electrowetting

Electrowetting actuation involves the electrically induced change of a surface's wettability, which is achieved by exerting electrostatic force to control the surface tension between two layers of material that could be solid–liquid or liquid–liquid as long as they are immiscible and explicitly two-phased [20]. Without bias voltage, a liquid metal (typically mercury, gallium, and low-melting-temperature alloys) placed in a capillary filled with an electrolyte has a uniformly distributed charge density. If a voltage is applied between two electrodes, the electric potential difference between the metal and the electrolyte varies, causing charge redistribution and altering surface tension around the metal. This gradient in surface tension induces motion of the liquid metal. Oscillating metal motion by alternating applied signals can generate a net flow of liquid from the inlet to the outlet [63]. EW micropumps require low operating voltages and low power; however, they suffer from irreproducible and unreliable fabrication and low biocompatibility. A MEMS micropump developed by Yun et al. utilizes electrowetting to achieve 70 μL/min fluid flow at 2.3 V applied voltage (Figure 7.12). The surface tension–driven micropump is intended for lab on chip applications [63].

Dynamic Micropumps

Electrohydrodynamic/Electroosmotic

In these microactuators, the driving momentum produced arises from a combination of the electrical field, dielectrophoretic force, dielectric force, and electrostrictive force. Flow of the electrically conductive working fluid is achieved by appropriately

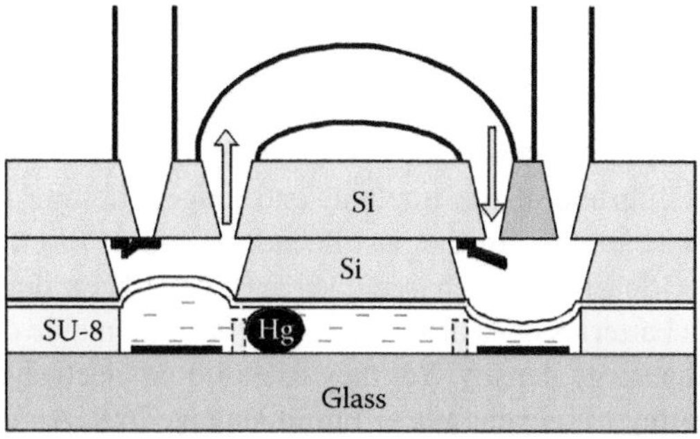

FIGURE 7.12 Conceptual drawing of electrowetting (EW) microactuator by Yun et al.

exerting an external electrical field upon the channel walls that are naturally charged. These pumps require high voltages, a relatively complicated 3-D overall geometry to ensure sufficient electrochemical reactions [20], and a well-prepared solution with specific electrical properties (permittivity and conductivity) and pH [18]. An electroosmotic micropump was developed for high-concentration insulin delivery and is capable of delivering 0.15–0.60 μL/min at 2.5–10 mA applied current [64].

Magnetohydrodynamic

In MHD microactuators, fluid flow is achieved when current-carrying ions in aqueous solutions are subjected to a magnetic field [17]. While flow in MHD microactuators can be bidirectional, the working fluid must have conductivity 1 S/m or higher, in addition to external electric and magnetic fields. Their performance is typically limited by the magnetic flux density and thermal effects restricting current density. An uncommon drawback is that significant bubbles, due to ionization, might be generated [20]. These bubbles change the pressure difference between the inlet and outlet and disrupt the flow. This problem may be alleviated by choosing an appropriate selection of electrolytes and electrode material that yield a nongaseous product in the electrode reaction [65]. Lemoff and Lee created an MHD micropump for biological lab on chip applications capable of delivering 18.3 μl/min [66].

Acoustic/Ultrasonic

In radio frequency (RF) and ultrasonic micropumps, actuation is achieved by exploiting the dragging force of a progressive mechanical wave. These operate at frequencies from the ultrasonic range up to several 10 MHz. Such microactuators suffer from a very small pump outlet pressure. Therefore, they are more suited for micromixing than fluid transport [34]. Several examples of ultrasonic drug delivery devices are reviewed [67].

Powering of Active Microactuators

As previously mentioned, active microactuators require power for their operation. This chapter focuses on implantable or wearable/ambulatory systems for which wireless operation is desired. The conventional method of supplying electrical power to implantable devices is to utilize internal microbatteries. These batteries are hardwired at the time of manufacturing before they are hermetically sealed with the implant. As a result, they cannot be replaced and are meant to power the device during final testing at the factory, during shelf storage, and throughout the useful life of the device while it is implanted [68]. Therefore, unless the battery is rechargeable, it dictates the lifetime of the implant, and longer lifetime typically requires larger, high-capacity batteries. In the past decade, compact thin-film Li-ion batteries with long cycle life and high charge/discharge have been developed. Lithium/polycarbon fluoride batteries have also been used for implantable drug pumps. They offer relatively high energy density. Yet they use a liquid electrolyte, requiring special attention to sealing to prevent gas or liquid leakage [69]. An overview of available implantable battery technologies can be found [70].

Another approach is to obtain electrical power from external sources [71,72], for example, power transmitted wirelessly to the device through inductive transmission. These wirelessly powered devices have significantly increased the operating time of the device. However, since the communication range is limited, devices that are implanted deep within the body may not be able to receive the telemetric signal due to the attenuation of the signal in tissue [4].

SUITABLE MATERIALS

One of the important requirements for an implantable device is biocompatibility. In this regard, several factors need to be considered when designing the device: impact of the implantable device on the immune response, physical effect of the implant on the surrounding tissues, biofouling of implanted device surfaces, and integration of the implanted device with tissue [4]. The intensity of the inflammatory response caused by the tissue injury that results from surgical implantation of the device as well as the continual presence of the device in the body depends on the properties of the device, such as shape, size, surface chemistry and roughness, design, morphology and porosity, composition, sterility issues, contact duration, and degradation [19,73]. Various natural, synthetic, and semisynthetic materials are currently utilized in the fabrication and packaging of implantable devices. Naturally occurring materials include silicon, glass, and various metals as well as collagen, chitosan, alginate, hyaluronan, and dextran. Commonly used synthetic polymers include poly(lactic acid) (PLA) and poly(lactic-co-glycolic acid) (PLGA), poly(ethylene glycol) (PEG), poly (2-hydroxyethyl methacrylate) (pHEMA), poly(vinyl alcohol) (PVA), polyetheretherketone (PEEK), polyimide (PL), polydimethylsiloxane (PDMS), poly(tetramethylene oxide) (PTMO), and Parylene (poly[p-xylylene]) [4,17,73]. Harder materials, such as hermetically welded titanium canisters and glass, are used to prevent any moisture ingress from damaging the electronic components [4]. An important factor when choosing device materials for implantation is their stability during and after sterilization; sterilization methods must also be carefully selected so as not to affect the device performance [4].

To prevent biofouling, various coatings in addition to the device packaging are used. Materials such as gold, silicon nitride, silicon dioxide, and silicon carbide have been shown to reduce biofouling [4]. Research has also focused on the release of growth factors and/or anti-inflammatory agents at the implantation site to minimize negative responses [73].

In the United States, the FDA has adopted the ISO-10993 standard table of tests as its criteria for guiding the selection of biocompatibility testing for a given type of device [74]. Biocompatibility testing must be conducted on the finished device, and the FDA generally does not accept demonstration of biocompatibility of each individual material component alone. However, device manufacturers are encouraged to use raw materials that have a proven track record of biocompatibility. U.S. Pharmacopeia (USP) is a private (nongovernmental) organization that establishes standards to ensure the quality of medicines and other health care technologies. USP defines a set of *in vivo* biological reactivity tests to conduct biocompatibility screening of plastics. Six classes of plastics are defined based on the application and duration (similar to ISO-10993), and each class has a different set of testing requirements. Class VI is the most stringent and requires three types of tests: systemic injection test, intracutaneous test, and implantation test [75]. It is recommended to use Class VI products and materials that have been used in previously FDA-approved devices for implants whenever possible.

EXAMPLES OF COMMERCIALLY AVAILABLE DRUG DELIVERY DEVICES THAT UTILIZE MEMS

Several companies are actively commercializing miniature or MEMS-based drug delivery devices. Durect Corporation developed a mini osmotic pump suitable for subcutaneous systematic drug delivery. The Duros® pump measures 3.8 mm in diameter and 44 mm long (Figure 7.13). It can deliver up to 1000 mg of concentrated drug for up to a year at a constant rate (±10%), ultimately releasing greater than 95% of its drug content. The device was FDA approved for prostate cancer treatment in 2000; however, clinical trials for new indications have been suspended pending redesign of the delivery system in order to address performance issues caused by premature shutdown of devices [76,77].

Debiotech's JewelPump™ containing a piezoelectric actuator is currently in the final stage of development in Europe. This insulin delivery system is worn as a patch on the skin and can be wirelessly programmed and monitored using a personal handheld device, such as a cell phone. Each disposable reservoir is used for 7 days. However, wireless technology is only used for communication, and the device still

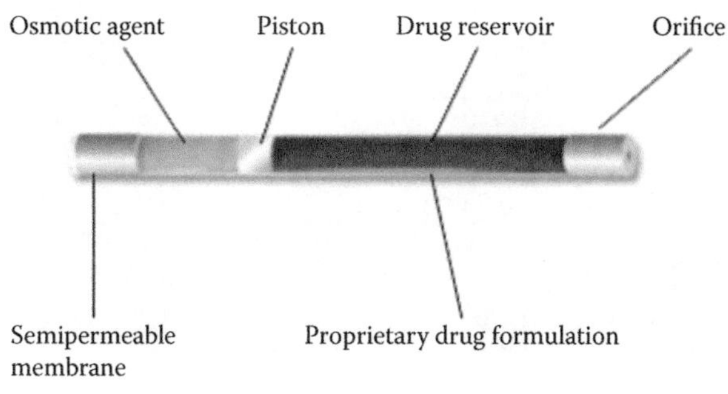

FIGURE 7.13 Conceptual drawing of the Duros® pump. (Courtesy of DURECT Corporation.)

requires a battery for operation [78]. Debiotech is in the process of further miniaturizing the device so that it can be completely implantable inside the body [79].

The implantable MicroCHIPS® microreservoir device utilizes thermal actuation to initiate the onset of drug release [77]. An array of 100 tiny reservoirs, each capable of holding 300 nl drug formulation per reservoir, store the drug until it is ready to be released into the body (Figure 7.14). Individual reservoirs are wirelessly activated to thermally open a membrane seal and initiate drug release, thereby precisely controlling the dose delivered in single-reservoir increments. Dosing can be terminated without the need for device extraction [80,81].

An SMA actuated minipump, OmniPod®, developed by Insulet Corp., stores 2000 μL of insulin, which can be delivered in 0.5 μL boluses continuously for about 72 hours (Figure 7.15) [42]. Replenish has developed an electrochemically driven,

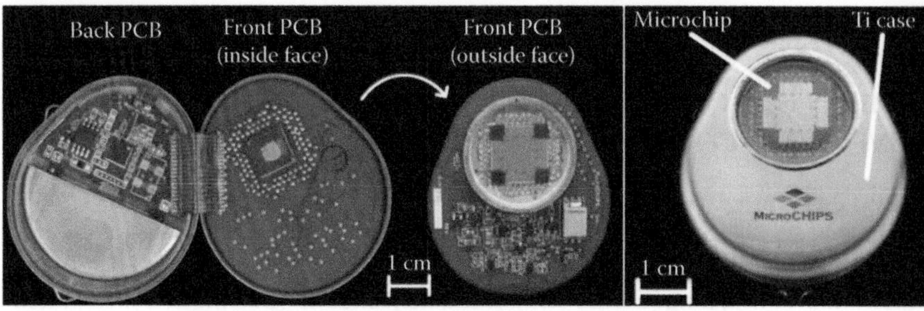

FIGURE 7.14 Photograph of MicroCHIPS® micro-reservoir device. (Reprinted from J. H. Prescott et al., *Nature Biotechnology*, 24, 437–438, 2006, with permission *Nature Publishing Group*.)

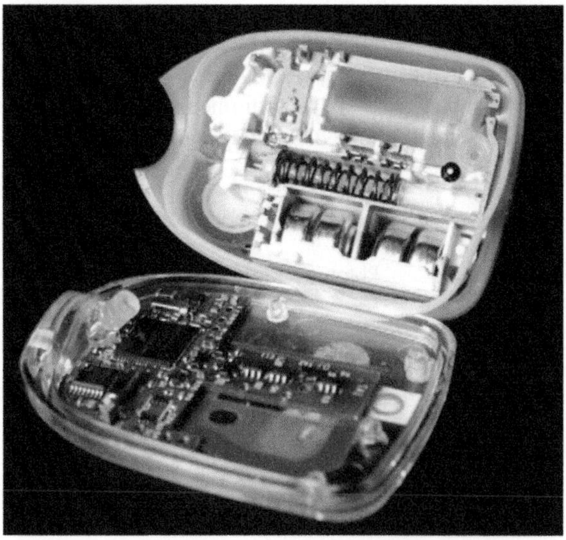

FIGURE 7.15 Photograph of OmniPod® insulin delivery device. (Reprinted from M. Ochoa et al., *Advanced Drug Delivery Reviews*, 2012, with permission Elsevier.)

refillable ophthalmic micropump designed to allow variable nanoliter drug delivery rates along with an external wireless programmer/charger for bidirectional communication [77,82].

PRECLINICAL AND CLINICAL DATA TO FURTHER ENHANCE DRUG DELIVERY

Most implantable drug delivery devices fall within FDA's Class III classification as they are intended to be used in supporting or sustaining human life or preventing impairment of human health. For these devices, the manufacturer needs to prove device safety and efficacy in order to obtain FDA premarket notification or approval. Safety and efficacy are first shown in preclinical animal studies and later in clinical trials [83].

Preclinical data gathered using implantable tether-free devices is important in evaluating drugs and devices [61]. Rodents comprise an estimated 95% of laboratory animals used in research [84], and many disease models have been developed in rats and mice to better understand human diseases and the effects of drug treatments [85,86]. These preclinical studies are the cornerstone of drug and device development and determine whether a product advances to further clinical testing or further development is required.

Fluid Synchrony is developing wirelessly controlled micropumps for tether-free administration in freely moving laboratory animals. The low-power electrochemically actuated micropump is capable of accurate delivery of a diverse assortment of liquid drug formulations within a wide dynamic range of flow rates (0.33–141.9 μL/min) (Figure 7.16) [52,62]. The group has used the device to gather preclinical data for several applications. Ocular drug delivery was first demonstrated in enucleated porcine eyes prior to acute drug pumping performed in rabbits [87,88]. Another application was to study drug self-administration in animal models of drug addiction. Preliminary results demonstrated the micropumps capability of rapid and repeatable delivery of precise boluses (up to 40 boluses of 19.12 ± 0.73 μL in 15 s bursts within

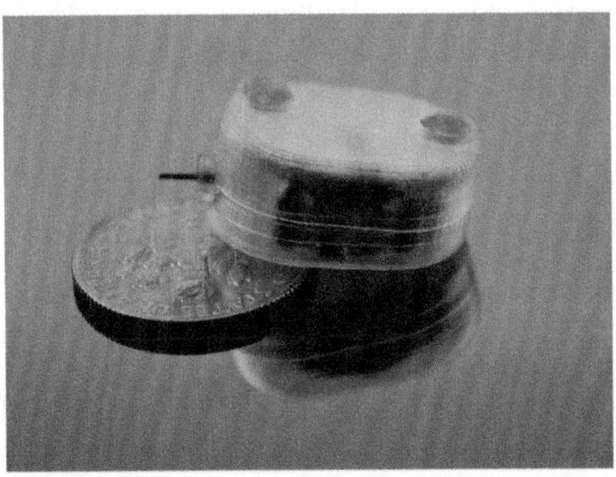

FIGURE 7.16 Photograph of FluidSync® electrochemically actuated micropump.

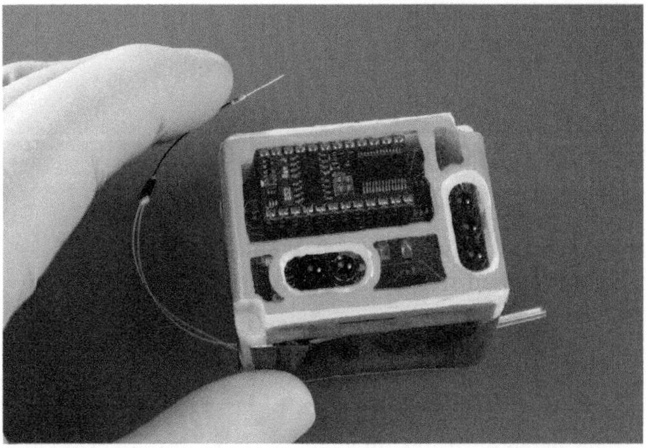

FIGURE 7.17 Photograph of intracochlear drug delivery device developed by Fiering et al.

a time span of 50 min) suitable for this self-administration paradigm [5]. Currently, the device is being used to deliver chemotherapy drugs to the intrathecal space of the mouse model for leptomeningeal metastases.

A group from Draper Laboratory and Massachusetts Eye and Ear is developing a wearable reciprocating delivery system for direct intracochlear delivery and has published preclinical results from acute delivery of DNQX, a glutamate receptor blocker, to guinea pigs (Figure 7.17). The device operation consists of repeatedly injecting a small volume (0.2 to a few μl) of fluid into the cochlea over a short (1–10 s) time, and then withdrawing the lower concentrated perilymph into the device over a period of several minutes [89].

In February 2012, MicroCHIPS published its results on the first-in-human testing of their wirelessly controlled drug delivery microchip (Figure 7.14). The device was implanted in eight osteoporotic postmenopausal women for 4 months and wirelessly programmed to release human parathyroid hormone fragment (hPTH) doses from the device once daily for up to 20 days. Their results showed that device dosing produced similar pharmacokinetics to multiple injections and had lower coefficients of variation. There were no toxic or adverse events due to the device or drug, and patients stated that the implant did not affect their quality of life [90].

SHORTCOMINGS OF AVAILABLE TECHNOLOGY AND FUTURE TRENDS

Advances in implantable drug delivery pumps are poised to offer greater freedom and improved quality of life to patients [5]. However, despite their numerous advantages, there are many challenges facing the implementation of these devices for the treatment of any specific disease. For each case, these devices must be specially optimized with regard to their drug reservoir size, relative size, operation lifetime, controllability, and biocompatibility [4]. Moreover, in order for true effective patient tailored therapies to become a reality, implantable pumps need to move beyond simple open loop systems to enable physiological feedback to the pump to confirm that the drug action has produced the desired therapeutic effect. This can be achieved through the incorporation of physical sensors that provide information on pressure, flow rate, or otherwise report to the user the state of the pump and confirm delivery volumes. Various sensors that are suitable for direct integration into MEMS pumps are currently under development. Sensors may be implanted along with the pump either locally or in a remote location [5].

It is also important to note that drug delivery technology can bring both therapeutic and commercial value to health care products. Big pharmaceutical companies have recently started losing their market share to generic competitors after their patents expired, and therefore, they have started recognizing the importance of drug delivery companies. Pharmaceutical companies are looking to extend their patents' lifetimes by making strategic alliances with drug delivery technology companies, by presenting old drugs in new forms as well as gaining the ability to market novel pharmaceutical agents, including biologics, biosimilars, and other small molecules, that are not suitable for administration through conventional routes of drug delivery. Most of the drug delivery products therefore reach the market as a result of a strategic alliance between drug delivery companies and pharmaceutical companies [3].

ACKNOWLEDGMENT

This work was supported by Wallace H. Coulter Foundation Early Career Translational Research Award, Coulter Translational Research Partnership award and National Institutes of Health under award number R21 GM104583.

REFERENCES

1. K. Menehan, "Partnership for Solutions: Better Lives for People with Chronic Conditions," Robert Wood Johnson Foundation, 2006.
2. The Council of State Governments, "Costs of Chronic Diseases: What Are States Facing?," 2006.
3. D. Paolino et al., "Drug delivery systems," *Encyclopedia of Medical Devices and Instrumentation*, 2006.
4. D. J. H. Tng et al., "Approaches and challenges of engineering implantable microelectromechanical systems (mems) drug delivery systems for in vitro and in vivo applications," *Micromachines*, vol. 3, pp. 615–631, 2012.
5. E. Meng and T. Hoang, "MEMS-enabled implantable drug infusion pumps for laboratory animal research, preclinical, and clinical applications," *Advanced Drug Delivery Reviews*, 2012.
6. M. Ferrari, "Cancer nanotechnology: Opportunities and challenges," *Nature Reviews Cancer*, vol. 5, pp. 161–171, 2005.
7. E. Meng et al., "Implantable Infusion Pumps Incorporating Nanotechnology," in *The Textbook of Nanoneuroscience and Nanoneurosurgery*, B. Kateb and J. D. Heiss, Eds., ed: CRC Press, pp. 211–225, 2013.
8. E. F. Lawson and M. S. Wallace, "Current developments in intraspinal agents for cancer and noncancer pain," *Current Pain and Headache Reports*, vol. 14, pp. 8–16, 2010.
9. FDA: US Food and Drug Administration. (2012, 3/25/2012). *Medtronic SynchroMed II Implantable Drug Infusion Pump and SynchroMed EL Implantable Drug Infusion Pump*. Available: http://www.fda.gov/MedicalDevices/Safety/ListofRecalls/ucm333231.htm

10. J. Fiering et al., "Local drug delivery with a self-contained, programmable, microfluidic system," *Biomedical Microdevices*, vol. 11, pp. 571–578, 2009.
11. B. Bruguerolle and G. Labrecque, "Rhythmic pattern in pain and their chronotherapy," *Advanced Drug Delivery Reviews*, vol. 59, pp. 883–895, 2007.
12. B.-B. C. Youan, "Chronopharmaceutics: Gimmick or clinically relevant approach to drug delivery?," *Journal of Controlled Release*, vol. 98, pp. 337–353, 2004.
13. W. Hrushesky, "Cancer chronotherapy: A drug delivery challenge," *Progress in Clinical and Biological Research A*, vol. 341, pp. 1–10, 1990.
14. F. Halberg et al., "Toward a chronotherapy of neoplasia: Tolerance of treatment depends upon host rhythms," *Cellular and Molecular Life Sciences*, vol. 29, pp. 909–934, 1973.
15. C. G. Lis et al., "Circadian timing in cancer treatment: The biological foundation for an integrative approach," *Integrative Cancer Therapies*, vol. 2, pp. 105–111, 2003.
16. J. Urquhart et al., "Rate-controlled delivery systems in drug and hormone research," *Annual Review of Pharmacology and Toxicology*, vol. 24, pp. 199–236, 1984.
17. D. Laser and J. Santiago, "A review of micropumps," *Journal of Micromechanics and Microengineering*, vol. 14, p. R35, 2004.
18. F. Amirouche et al., "Current micropump technologies and their biomedical applications," *Microsystem Technologies*, vol. 15, pp. 647–666, 2009.
19. V. V. Ranade, "Drug delivery systems. 4. Implants in drug delivery," *The Journal of Clinical Pharmacology*, vol. 30, pp. 871–889, 1990.
20. N.-C. Tsai and C. Y. Sue, "Review of MEMS-based drug delivery and dosing systems," *Sensors and Actuators A (Physical)*, vol. 134, pp. 555–564, 2007.
21. N.-T. Nguyen and S. T. Wereley, *Fundamentals and applications of microfluidics*, 2nd ed. Boston: Artech House, 2006.
22. T. A. Desai et al., "Microfabricated immunoisolating biocapsules," *Biotechnology and Bioengineering*, vol. 57, pp. 118–120, 1998.
23. F. Martin et al., "Tailoring width of microfabricated nanochannels to solute size can be used to control diffusion kinetics," *Journal of Controlled Release*, vol. 102, pp. 123–133, 2005.
24. T. A. Desai et al., "Microfabricated biocapsules provide short-term immunoisolation of insulinoma xenografts," *Biomedical Microdevices*, vol. 1, pp. 131–138, 1999.
25. Drugs.com. (2000–2013, 4/6/2013). *Abraxane Approval History* Available: http://www.drugs.com/history/abraxane.html
26. C. G. Keller, Ferrari, Mauro, "Microfabricated particle filter," US Patent 5,651,900, 1997.
27. J. Lewis and M. Ferrari, "BioMEMS for drug delivery applications," in *Lab-on-a-Chip: Miniaturized Systems for (Bio) Chemical Analysis and Synthesis*, p. 373, 2003.
28. B. Smith et al., "A biological perspective of particulate nanoporous silicon," *Materials Technology (UK)*, vol. 19, pp. 16–20, 2004.
29. J. G. Smits, "Piezoelectric micropump with microvalves," in *Proceedings of the Eighth Biennial University/Government/Industry Microelectronics Symposium*, Westborough, MA, USA, pp. 92–94, 1989.
30. S. Herrlich et al., "Osmotic micropumps for drug delivery," *Advanced Drug Delivery Reviews*, 2012.
31. W. H. Ryu et al., "Biodegradable micro-osmotic pump for long-term and controlled release of basic fibroblast growth factor," *Journal of Controlled Release*, vol. 124, pp. 98–105, 2007.
32. J. Urquhart, "Controlled drug delivery: Therapeutic and pharmacological aspects," *Journal of Internal Medicine*, vol. 249, pp. 75–94, 2001.
33. Y.-H. Li and Y.-C. Su, "Miniature osmotic actuators for controlled maxillofacial distraction osteogenesis," *Journal of Micromechanics and Microengineering*, vol. 20, p. 065013, 2010.

34. P. Woias, "Micropumps—Past, progress and future prospects," *Sensors and Actuators B: Chemical*, vol. 105, pp. 28–38, 2005.
35. A. K. Au et al., "Microvalves and micropumps for biomems," *Micromachines*, vol. 2, pp. 179–220, 2011.
36. K. W. Oh and C. H. Ahn, "A review of microvalves," *Journal of Micromechanics and Microengineering*, vol. 16, p. R13, 2006.
37. K. Junwu et al., "Design and test of a high-performance piezoelectric micropump for drug delivery," *Sensors and Actuators A (Physical)*, vol. 121, pp. 156–161, 2005.
38. T. Li et al., "Compact, power-efficient architectures using microvalves and microsensors, for intrathecal, insulin, and other drug delivery systems," *Advanced Drug Delivery Reviews*, 2012.
39. A. T. Evans et al., "Dual drug delivery device for chronic pain management using micromachined elastic metal structures and silicon microvalves," in *Micro Electro Mechanical Systems, 2008. MEMS 2008. IEEE 21st International Conference on*, pp. 252–255, 2008.
40. A. T. Evans et al., "A multidrug delivery system using a piezoelectrically actuated silicon valve manifold with embedded sensors," *Journal of Microelectromechanical Systems*, vol. 20, pp. 231–238, 2011.
41. M. Ochoa and B. Ziaie, "A fermentation-powered thermopneumatic pump for biomedical applications," *Lab on a Chip*, vol. 12, pp. 4044–4048, 2012.
42. M. Ochoa et al., "Polymeric microdevices for transdermal and subcutaneous drug delivery," *Advanced Drug Delivery Reviews*, 2012.
43. S. Spieth et al., "An intra-cerebral drug delivery system for freely moving animals," *Biomedical Microdevices*, vol. 14, pp. 799–809, 2012.
44. N. Elman et al., "Electro-thermally induced structural failure actuator (ETISFA) for implantable controlled drug delivery devices based on Micro-Electro-Mechanical-Systems," *Lab on a Chip*, vol. 10, pp. 2796–2804, 2010.
45. N. Elman et al., "An implantable MEMS drug delivery device for rapid delivery in ambulatory emergency care," *Biomedical Microdevices*, vol. 11, pp. 625–631, 2009.
46. R. Zengerle et al., "A bidirectional silicon micropump," *Sensors and Actuators A: Physical*, vol. 50, pp. 81–86, 1995.
47. F. N. Pirmoradi et al., "On-demand controlled release of docetaxel from a battery-less MEMS drug delivery device," *Lab on a Chip*, vol. 11, pp. 2744–2752, 2011.
48. Fatemeh Nazly Pirmoradi et al., "Controlled Delivery of Antiangiogenic Drug to Human Eye Tissue Using MEMS Device" presented at the The 26th IEEE International Conference on Micro Electro Mechanical Systems (IEEE MEMS 2013) Taipei, Taiwan, 2013.
49. J. O. Kwon et al., "A Novel Drug Delivery Method by using a Microrobot Incorporated with an Acoustically Oscillating Bubble," presented at the The 26th IEEE International Conference on Micro Electro Mechanical Systems (IEEE MEMS 2013), Taipei, Taiwan, 2013.
50. M. Hiraoka et al., "Miniature conductive polymer actuators for high pressure generation in lab on chip systems," *Sensors and Actuators A: Physical*, vol. 177, pp. 23–29, 2012.
51. M. Hiraoka et al., "Miniaturized Pumps and Valves, Based on Conductive Polymer Actuators, for Lab-On-Chip Application," presented at the The 26th IEEE International Conference on Micro Electro Mechanical Systems (IEEE MEMS 2013) Taipei, Taiwan, 2013.
52. R. Sheybani et al., "A MEMS electrochemical bellows actuator for fluid metering applications," *Biomedical Microdevices*, pp. 1–12, 2012/07/01, 2012.
53. M. Faraday, "Proceedings of the Royal Society of London," *Philosophical Transactions of the Royal Society of London*, vol. 124, pp. 77–122, 1834.

54. W. Nicholson, *A Journal of natural philosophy, chemistry and the arts*. G. G. and J. Robinson, 1800.
55. B. Cordovez et al., "A novel polymer microneedle fabrication process for active fluidic delivery," *Microfluidics and Nanofluidics*, vol. 10, pp. 785–791, 2011.
56. A. Kabata et al., "Prototype micropump for insulin administration based on electrochemical bubble formation," *Journal of Pharmaceutical Sciences*, vol. 97, pp. 5037–5045, 2008.
57. D. B. Young et al., "A portable infusion pump for use on large laboratory animals," *Biomedical Engineering, IEEE Transactions on*, pp. 543–545, 1977.
58. S.-C. Chan et al., "A bubble-activated micropump with high-frequency flow reversal," *Sensors and Actuators A: Physical*, vol. 163, pp. 501–509, 2010.
59. M. Nałęcz et al., "Bioengineering aspects of the artificial pancreas," *Artificial Organs*, vol. 2, pp. 305–309, 1978.
60. J. Marcial Portilla and U. Kim, "Low-Power, Self-Contained, Reciprocating Micropump through Electrolysis and Catalyst-Driven Recombination toward Drug Delivery Applications," presented at the 26th IEEE International Conference on Micro Electro Mechanical Systems (IEEE MEMS 2013) Taipei, Taiwan, 2013.
61. H. Gensler et al., "An implantable MEMS micropump system for drug delivery in small animals," *Biomedical Microdevices*, vol. 14, pp. 483–496, 2012.
62. R. Sheybani et al., "Design, fabrication, and characterization of an electrochemically-based dose tracking system for closed-loop drug delivery," in *Engineering in Medicine and Biology Society (EMBC), 2012 Annual International Conference of the IEEE*, pp. 519–522, 2012.
63. K.-S. Yun et al., "A surface-tension driven micropump for low-voltage and low-power operations," *Journal of Microelctromechanical Systems*, vol. 11, pp. 454–461, 2002.
64. E. Uhlig et al., "The electro-osmotic actuation of implantable insulin micropumps," *Journal of Biomedical Materials Research*, vol. 17, pp. 931–943, 1983.
65. A. Homsy, "Design, Microfabrication, and Characterization of MHD Pumps and Their Applications in NMR Environments," University of Neuchâtel, 2006.
66. A. V. Lemoff and A. P. Lee, "An AC magnetohydrodynamic micropump," *Sensors and Actuators B: Chemical*, vol. 63, pp. 178–185, 2000.
67. S. Mitragotri, "Devices for overcoming biological barriers: The use of physical forces to disrupt the barriers," *Advanced Drug Delivery Reviews*, 2012.
68. O. Soykan, "Power sources for implantable medical devices," *Medical Device Manufacturing and Technology*, pp. 76–79, 2002.
69. J. Kraska. (2008–2012), Battery Technology for Implants Is Overcoming Technological Hurdles. *Nerac*.
70. C. F. Holmes and B. B. Owens, "Batteries for implantable biomedical applications," *Wiley Encyclopedia of Biomedical Engineering*, 2006.
71. D. Panescu, "Wireless communication systems for implantable medical devices," *IEEE Engineering in Medicine and Biology Magazine*, vol. 27, pp. 96–101, 2008.
72. B. Lenaerts, *Omnidirectional inductive powering for biomedical implants*, 1st ed. New York: Springer, 2008.
73. Y. Onuki et al., "A review of the biocompatibility of implantable devices: Current challenges to overcome foreign body response," *Journal of Diabetes Science and Technology* vol. 2, pp. 1003–1015, 2008.
74. E. Meng, *Biomedical microsystems*: CRC Press, 2011.
75. Biomerics, "Quadrathane™ and Quadraflex™ Biocompatibility Guide," Biomerics, Ed., ed, 2011.
76. DURECT Corporation. (2013, 2/28/2013). *Duros System*. Available: http://www.durect.com/wt/durect/page_name/duros

77. C. L. Stevenson et al., "Reservoir-based drug delivery systems utilizing microtechnology," *Advanced Drug Delivery Reviews*, 2012.
78. Debiotech S. A. Switzerland. (2013, *Debiotech Jewel Pump*. Available: http://www.jewelpump.com/standard.html
79. Debiotech S. A. Switzerland. (2013, 2/28/2013). *MIP implantable: The new generation of implantable pumps*. Available: http://www.debiotech.com/
80. J. H. Prescott et al., "Chronic, programmed polypeptide delivery from an implanted, multireservoir microchip device," *Nature Biotechnology*, vol. 24, pp. 437–438, 2006.
81. MicroCHIPS Inc. (2011, *MicroCHIPS platform*. Available: http://www.mchips.com/technology.html
82. Replenish Inc. (2010–2013, 2/28/2013). *Replenish, Inc. ophthalmic Micropumps*. Available: http://replenishinc.com/our-technology/product-description
83. US Food and Drug Administration. (2013, 4/15/2013). *Overview of Medical Device Regulation: Regulatory Controls*. Available: http://www.fda.gov/MedicalDevices/DeviceRegulationandGuidance/Overview/GeneralandSpecialControls/default.htm
84. F. L. Trull and B. A. Rich, "More regulation of rodents," *Science (New York)*, vol. 284, p. 1463, 1999.
85. E. Benedikz et al., "The rat as an animal model of Alzheimer's disease," *Journal of Cellular and Molecular Medicine*, vol. 13, pp. 1034–1042, 2009.
86. K. C. Worley et al., "Rats in the genomic era," *Physiological Genomics*, vol. 32, pp. 273–282, 2008.
87. R. Lo et al., "A refillable microfabricated drug delivery device for treatment of ocular diseases," *Lab on a Chip*, vol. 8, pp. 1027–1030, 2008.
88. R. Lo et al., "A passive MEMS drug delivery pump for treatment of ocular diseases," *Biomedical Microdevices*, vol. 11, pp. 959–970, 2009.
89. Z. Chen et al., "Inner ear drug delivery via a reciprocating perfusion system in the guinea pig," *Journal of Controlled Release*, vol. 110, pp. 1–19, 2005.
90. R. Farra et al., "First-in-human testing of a wirelessly controlled drug delivery microchip," *Science Translational Medicine*, vol. 4, p. 122ra21, February 22, 2012.

8 Microneedle-Mediated Vaccines

Ryan F. Donnelly, Maelíosa T. C. McCrudden, Sharifa Al-Zahrani, and Steven J. Fallows

CONTENTS

VACCINE DELIVERY

Vaccination

Vaccination, or immunization, is the most cost-effective public health measure to protect against infectious disease-related morbidity and mortality. A vaccine is a biological preparation that improves immunity to a particular disease. A vaccine typically contains an agent that resembles a disease-causing microorganism and is often made from weakened or killed forms of the microorganism or its toxins. The agent stimulates the body's immune system to recognize the agent as foreign, destroy it, and "remember" it so that the immune system can more easily recognize and destroy any of these microorganisms that it later encounters.

An ideal vaccine is safe, cost-effective, and efficient after a single dose. The route by which a vaccine is delivered can have considerable bearing on these factors through its influence on the efficiency of the procedure, the dose required, compliance, and safety. For vaccination to succeed holistically in contributing to public health, vaccine delivery systems must allow efficient delivery without compromising product stability during storage and transport and without negatively influencing patient perception [1]. To be considered safe, new delivery systems should reduce the risk of injury and infection of health care workers and prevent illicit reuse. A delivery system combining all these qualities would facilitate vaccination of greater proportions of the population [1–3].

Currently licensed vaccines are delivered via one of five main administration routes: intramuscular for the majority of vaccines, including hepatitis A and B, rabies, influenza, and diphtheria–tetanus–pertussis–based combination vaccines; subcutaneous for vaccines such as measles, mumps, and rubella and yellow fever; intradermal for BCG and rabies; intranasal for live attenuated influenza vaccine; and oral for poliomyelitis, cholera, rotavirus, and typhoid fever [1,3,4]. With the rare exception of jet injectors (devices that use a coiled spring or compressed gas to propel liquid or powder jets through the *stratum corneum* into the skin), intramuscular, subcutaneous, and intradermal delivery are all affected using needles. In fact, of the more than 5 billion human vaccine doses given each year, 3 billion are delivered using needles [1,5]. These techniques, while having proven efficacy in terms of achieving the required immune responses, have significant drawbacks relating to safety and patient compliance. The invasive nature of the parenteral injection procedure and the potential for inappropriate reuse of equipment, particularly in developing countries, exposes patients to the risk of transmission of blood-borne pathogens. A study by the World Health Organization (WHO) estimated that at least 50% of childhood vaccinations were unsafe in 14 countries located in five different developing world regions [1,5]. Moreover, and critically, the use and disposal of equipment is associated with the risk of needle-stick injury. Estimates of occupational injuries due to a sharp object, the most common of which are needle-stick injuries, vary from a low of 0.18 sharps injuries per health care worker per year in the United States and Canada to around 4.7 sharps injuries per health care worker per year in Egypt and Pakistan. An estimated 3 million health care workers worldwide are injured annually with a sharp object contaminated with hepatitis C virus, hepatitis B virus, or human immunodeficiency virus [1,5].

The introduction of safer devices engineered to prevent needle reuse and reduce the risk of needle-stick infections is likely to lessen these concerns. However, the perceived or real pain and trauma sometimes associated with needle-based vaccination can be barriers to vaccination uptake, particularly by needle-phobic patients, who constitute at least 10% of the population [4,6]. These drawbacks and the development of new types of vaccines are some of the reasons driving the pharmaceutical industry and public health organizations to search for new delivery methods that are safe, cost-effective, and efficient. While the majority of vaccines in clinical development are envisioned as needle and syringe products, a number of research groups and vaccine manufacturers are exploring the advantages of new parenteral delivery systems as well as of mucosal and transcutaneous delivery [7]. Mucosal delivery is currently only used for live attenuated vaccines against poliomyelitis [1–3], typhoid fever (oral), rotavirus, and influenza (nasal). Mucosally administered vaccines have a number of benefits. They eliminate the risk of transmission of blood-borne diseases and needle-stick injury. They can potentially be given by personnel with little medical training, which provides significant practical and cost benefits, particularly in the context of large-scale immunization programs in the developing world. This route can also, in theory, elicit both mucosal and humoral immunity, offering advantages against diseases contracted via mucosal surfaces. However, there are also a number of drawbacks. The live attenuated viruses in oral poliomyelitis vaccine (OPV) can revert to virulence, causing vaccine-associated paralytic poliomyelitis (VAPP) in the vaccinated child or their close contacts, particularly in the immunodepressed patients. This has resulted in a shift from the use of OPV to the use of injectable poliomyelitis vaccine containing inactivated virus, especially in countries that have eliminated naturally occurring polio [3,7]. Oral vaccines have to overcome problems associated with poor absorption or degradation within the digestive system that may require the concomitant administration of antacids. Finally, to date no mucosal vaccine adjuvant (an agent that enhances the immune response to an antigen) is available with the required safety and efficacy. Such safety issues were encountered with an intranasal adjuvant-containing influenza vaccine that was associated with the occurrence of facial palsy [1–4,7].

New vaccines to be developed should, ideally, have an additional level of safety. They should be needle-free or, if needle-based administration is unavoidable, the needle should be retractable or otherwise self-disabling to prevent reuse and reduce the risk of needle-stick injuries. Reducing or eliminating pain during vaccination is likely to improve uptake of vaccines by both needle-phobic individuals and parents concerned about the pain endured by their child during multiple-injection vaccination schedules [4,6]. Administering vaccines without the use of a needle and syringe would mean that less health care training would be required by vaccinators. This would be especially helpful should mass vaccination be required in the case of, for example, a natural pandemic or bioterrorism attack. Improved ease of delivery would also be of great benefit in the developing world, where there is often a shortage of trained health care workers. Increasing the speed of vaccine delivery, while not compromising on safety, has obvious advantages. Decreasing the time required for each individual to be vaccinated means less time is required to complete vaccination of the same number of people. New vaccines should not be more costly to make, transport, store, or administer than their currently available counterparts. This is especially true considering the limited resources for vaccination in the developing world.

Many of the vaccines currently in use worldwide must be maintained within a specific temperature range (often 2°C to 8°C) to maintain potency. Some vaccines, such as oral polio vaccine, MMR, varicella, and yellow fever, are sensitive to heat, and others, such as diphtheria and tetanus toxoids, pertussis vaccine, and hepatitis B vaccine, are sensitive to freezing [1–6]. The "cold chain" refers to the materials, equipment, and procedures required to maintain vaccines within this temperature range from the time that they are manufactured until they are given to patients. Due to the expense of maintaining cold storage facilities, cold transportation, and cold boxes that preserve vaccines at the proper temperature, the cold chain is estimated to cost vaccine programs worldwide $200–$300 million annually. New vaccine strategies that avoid the necessity of the cold chain should further decrease the cost of vaccine delivery.

No cold chain would also make delivering vaccine to more remote locations more straightforward. The savings could make it possible to vaccinate millions more people worldwide.

In considering alternate methods for vaccine delivery that do not involve a syringe and needle, it is important that once the vaccine is delivered it must reach the immune system and elicit a protective response. Parenteral administration of vaccines by needle and syringe has proven success in reaching immune effectors and protecting those vaccinated from infection. Alternate methods of vaccine delivery must prove to be at least equally immunogenic and protective. Recently, the intradermal route of vaccine delivery has attracted great interests in both industry and academia.

INTRADERMAL VACCINATION

In the past, the skin was seen as a barrier through which vaccines could not be easily delivered. More recently, the skin, a highly immune-competent organ and often the first line of defense against entry of an array of different pathogens, has been recognized as an excellent site for vaccine administration.

Skin Structure

Human skin is composed of a number of functional layers (Figure 8.1). The outermost layer and the principal barrier to transdermal/intradermal administration, the *stratum corneum* is composed of dead, cornified keratinocytes. The viable epidermis is composed of keratinocytes and immunocompetent cells [2,7]. The dermis supports the epidermis with collagen fibers and also contains a dense network of capillary blood vessels and lymphatics in which dermal dendritic cells, monocytes, polymorphonuclear lymphocytes, and mast cells circulate. Lymphatic vessels drain

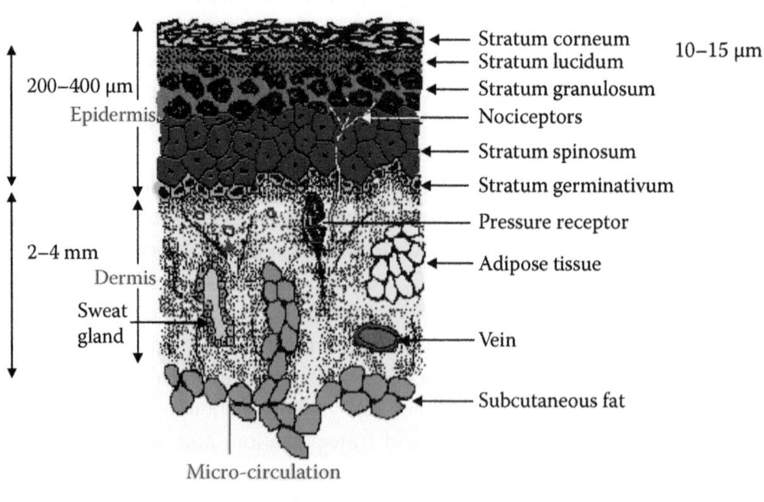

FIGURE 8.1 Diagrammatic representation of the basic anatomy of human skin.

the dermis to satellite lymph nodes, and fibroblasts are the most abundant cell type. The subcutaneous layer consists of loose connective tissue and elastin located immediately beneath the dermis. The arteries and veins that drain the skin dermis issue from the vascular plexus located in subcutaneous tissue. When entering the skin, dermal arteries form a dense network of capillary loops in the papillary dermis layer. Numerous lymphatic vessels draining the skin dermis pass through the hypodermis before reaching draining lymph nodes. While skin thickness can vary significantly between different parts of the body, a number of recent studies have shown consistency in skin thickness across people with different ethnic backgrounds at deltoid and suprascapular body sites—likely sites for intradermal vaccine administration [8]. This consistency in skin thickness across people with different demographic profiles represents a major advantage over classic intramuscular vaccination as, to correctly perform an intramuscular vaccination, it is important to select the appropriate needle length based on considerations of the muscle mass of the injection site, the amount of subcutaneous fat, and the weight of the patient.

Skin Immune Response

The skin generates both innate (antigen nonspecific response without immunological memory) and adaptive immune responses (antigen specific response with immunological memory). While the adaptive response is primordial in generating a response to vaccination and generally becomes more effective with each successive encounter with an antigen, innate immune mechanisms also play a key role as they are activated first in response to pathogen invasion or contact with foreign antigens. The key group of immune cells involved in the skin's innate immune response is bone marrow–derived dendritic leukocytes, namely Langerhans cells in the epidermis and dermal dendritic cells in the dermis [2,3,7]. Langerhan's cells are efficient antigen-presenting cells (APCs). While only constituting around 1% of the cells in the epidermis, they occupy 20%–25% of its entire surface area. Langerhans cells take up and process antigens entering the skin. During their migration via the local lymphatics to the paracortical T cell areas of the draining lymph nodes, they mature and present antigenic peptides to naïve T cells [3].

Activated Langerhans cells produce inflammatory cytokines and costimulatory molecules that induce strong antigen-specific responses by B- and T-lymphocytes. This occurs in an antigen-specific fashion and, therefore, results in expansion in numbers of potent immune-stimulatory cells that control the development of adaptive immunity. It appears that nonactivated dermal dendritic cells can downregulate potentially harmful immune responses. Importantly for intradermal vaccine delivery, it has been reported that excessive UVB exposure can affect immune responses by depletion of Langerhans cells, increased dermal recruitment of macrophages, and release of proinflammatory cytokines [2,3,7].

Conventional Strategies for Intradermal Vaccine Delivery

It has been widely reported that intradermal vaccine delivery very often results in more potent immune responses than vaccines administered by intramuscular or subcutaneous routes. This has been attributed to the superior collection of immune components in the skin compared to in the subcutaneous or muscular compartments [3,8]. The skin also appears to behave as mucosal tissue, since intradermal vaccine delivery results in immune responses at mucosal sites, such as those in the gastrointestinal tract, a feature common to mucosal vaccine administration at other body sites. This could be important in generation of protective vaginal mucosal immunity to sexually transmitted infections, such as HIV. Importantly for widespread vaccination in the cases of pandemic and bioterrorism and for cost reduction in developing countries, intradermal administration of vaccines appears to be dose-sparing with similar immune responses often achieved with lower vaccine doses than those administered via conventional routes [2,3,5,8].

A number of methods for intradermal vaccine delivery have been developed. The standard intradermal injection technique, developed a century ago by Mantoux, consists of stretching the surface of the skin and inserting the tip of a 27-gauge, 3/8-inch bevel needle attached to a 1-ml syringe [3]. The needle is inserted bevel upward, almost parallel to the skin surface, and vaccine is injected slowly into the uppermost layer of the skin. If placed properly, there is considerable resistance to injection and a raised papule immediately appears. This can cause pain during injection. The correct placing of the needle tip in the dermis is critical to avoid fluid injection difficulties. This technique is associated with inconsistency in injection volume, partly due to the difficulty of performing it correctly, but also to the unavoidable leakage of vaccine from the injection site, fluid wastage when filling disposable syringes and when purging the needle of air, and the large dead volume of the assembled needle and syringe. Bifurcated needles can accommodate around 2 μl of vaccine solution between their prongs. However, only part of this volume is capable of introduction into the skin, and precise control of dosing accuracy is not possible. The needle is jabbed into the papillary dermis, yielding a spot of blood, meaning the device has had to be redesigned somewhat to help protect health care workers. The multipuncture unit is a cylinder-like device with small needles, around 1 mm in length, which should be pressed firmly against the skin within the area where the vaccine dose is spread on the skin surface. In contrast with the intradermal technique, this percutaneous method does not allow a precise estimation of the dose injected into the epidermis or dermis skin layers. Needle-free jet injectors deliver vaccine to the dermis, subcutaneous tissue, and muscle with some vaccine also deposited in the epidermis [2,4]. This means precise control over intradermal dosing is unachievable. Studies have shown that vaccination via jet injection can elicit an immune response comparable to or better than other delivery methods. This may possibly be due to increased inflammation with jet injectors, leading to the recruitment of more immune cells to the injection site. Indeed jet injection causes at least as much pain, bruising, swelling, and induration as needle-mediated vaccine delivery. While jet injection requires little medical training and enables rapid vaccination of multiple subjects and new versions of multidose jet injectors don't allow infection transmission in the way their 1940s progenitors did, they have yet to replace conventional needle-and-syringe–based methods.

ALTERNATIVE VACCINATION METHODS

Abrasion and Stripping Methods

These methods employ simple tools such as Cellotape®, a razor, toothbrush, or abrasive paper to slowly remove each successive layer of cells of the *stratum corneum*. Methods such as these are inexpensive yet are very slow and can be painful to the patient. Moreover, the long-term effects of continual trauma to the stratum corneum and the effects these may have on its ability to recover, the potential for abrasion-site inflammatory reactions, and the potential for infection have yet to be established. Application of tumor epitope peptides to tape-stripped mouse skin primed tumor-specific cytotoxic T cells in the spleen and lymph nodes, protecting mice against a subsequent challenge with the same tumor cells. Established tumors' growth was also suppressed [9]. Pretreatment of skin in humans with a razor and toothbrush followed by application of adenoviral vectors has produced interesting results in humans [10]. Removal of the *stratum corneum* using abrasive paper is the most common method used within the literature prior to vaccination. Following skin hydration, the use of emery paper allowed for deep penetration of anthrax vaccine [11] and influenza virus vaccine [12]. The Skin Prep System (SPS®) currently under development by Intercell provides a controlled means of *stratum corneum* disruption for transcutaneous immunization [13]. It consists of a mild abrasive affixed to a pressure-sensitive device, which lightly scratches the surface of the skin, after which a patch containing the vaccine is applied. The system is single use and disposable. In one study following skin abrasion with SPS®, a patch containing a vaccine against traveler's diarrhea (LT patch) was applied to the scratched area and worn for 6 h before removal and being discarded by the patient. Fifty-nine LT patch recipients were protected against moderate-to-severe diarrhea (protective efficacy of 75%) and severe diarrhea (protective efficacy of 84%). LT patch recipients who became ill had shorter periods of diarrhea (0.5 days versus 2.1 days) and with fewer loose stools relative to placebo [14]. Another study used a similar technique to boost the response against an influenza vaccine. However, skin pretreatment was achieved using ECG-grade emery paper on skin wetted with 10% glycerol/70% alcohol, which disrupts the tight lipidic nature of the *stratum corneum*. Several weeks following vaccination, hemagglutination inhibition (HAI) responses in LT patch recipients were higher in those who received the vaccine alone [15]. Microdermabrasion has been adapted to remove layers of skin of defined thicknesses, allowing selective removal of the *stratum corneum*. This approach increases skin permeability to immunostimulatory molecules and has enabled the topical application of live attenuated vaccinia virus on microdermabraded skin to generate virus-specific antibodies in blood [16].

Ultrasound

Low-frequency ultrasound waves are very effective in increasing the permeability of skin to a range of low molecular weight drugs and macromolecules, including vaccines [17]. Permeability enhancement is achieved through acoustic cavitation, which is the formation, pulsation, and collapse of gas bubbles under the oscillating pressure field of ultrasound. It is estimated that 10 bubbles collapses/s/cm^2 in the form of symmetric collapses (generating shockwaves) or asymmetric collapses (producing microjets) near the surface of the skin are required to explain the skin permeabilizing effects of ultrasound [18]. Studies in mice have shown that the immune response generated by ultrasonically delivered vaccine was approximately tenfold greater relative to SC injection per unit dose of vaccine that entered the skin (about 1% of the topically applied dose entered the skin). Moreover ultrasound activated skin Langerhans cells by a yet unknown mechanism [19]. Another study found that pretreating skin with ultrasound followed by application of tetanus toxoid generated antitetanus IgG and neutralizing antibody titers [20].

Electroporation

This electrical method involves the application of short-duration, high-voltage electrical pulses, which disrupt the lipidic *stratum corneum* allowing vaccine to be delivered into the skin. Most uses of electroporation within vaccine delivery have been for DNA vaccine uptake into skin epidermal and dermal cells [21]. However many of these studies involve insertion of electrodes into the skin, akin to needles, thereby causing pain to patients, infection potential, and local electrode-insertion site inflammation. A few studies though have examined the technique's use for topical vaccine delivery. One study by Zhao et al. found that electroporation stimulates the exit of Langerhans cells from the skin, giving an adjuvant-like effect. In the same study, efficacy of peptide delivery was similar to intradermal injection with Freund's complete adjuvant, and the subsequent peptide-specific CTL response of the vaccine delivered by electroporation was equivalent to the vaccine given by intradermal injection [22]. Studies indicate that electroporation is effective in stimulating an immune response after DNA delivery [23–25] and that in vivo electroporation can be used to increase transgene expression relative to naked DNA injection [26]. Transfected cells were mainly located in the dermis and included endothelial cells, adipocytes, fibroblasts, and mononuclear cells with dendritic processes in a porcine model. Transfected cells also were found in lymph nodes that drained the electroporated sites. To test skin electroporation-mediated nucleic acid vaccination in a murine model, a HBsAg-coding plasmid was used. Potential use of these findings include modulation of immune responses to pathogens, allergens, tumor-specific antigens, and tolerance modification. Protection against avian influenza achieved by electroporation has been demonstrated in nonhuman primates [27]. A number of clinical trials are currently underway testing electroporation-enhanced vaccine delivery in humans.

As a result of the great potential of the intradermal route for immunization and the largely unsatisfactory nature of conventional methods of administration, it is unsurprising that newfound expertise in microneedle manufacture has been focused intently on vaccine delivery. Microneedles (Figure 8.2) are minimally invasive devices that, upon insertion, bypass the skin's *stratum corneum* barrier. Microneedles (50–900 μm in height, up to 2000 microneedles cm^{-2}), produced by microfabrication in various geometries and materials, have recently been extensively investigated for enhanced transdermal drug and vaccine delivery [1,2]. Microneedles painlessly pierce the epidermis, creating microscopic holes through which drugs diffuse to the dermal microcirculation. Importantly, microneedles do not penetrate deeply enough to damage nerves or blood vessels. Delivery of antigens, adjuvants, inactivated and

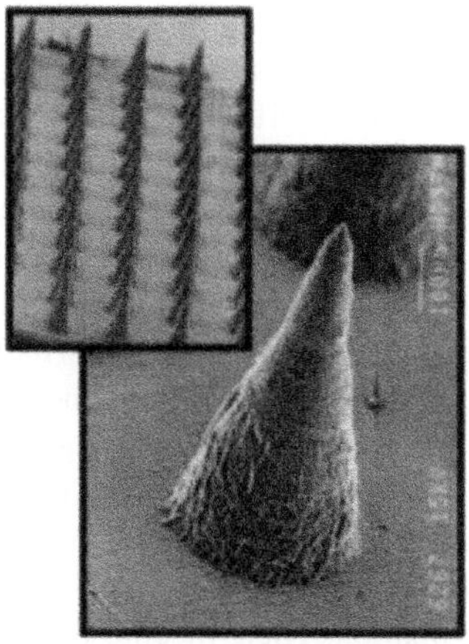

FIGURE 8.2 Scanning electron micrograph of 600-µm polymeric microneedles prepared from aqueous blends of poly(methlyvinylether-***co***-maleic acid). Light micrograph of the same microneedles and 300-µm silicon microneedles prepared by wet etching beside a BIC Biro® pen.

attenuated infectious agents, and genes encoding antigen production has been investigated in vitro and in vivo using a wide range of microneedle designs. The most common approaches have been coating of microneedles, poke-and-patch delivery, and, importantly, dissolving/biodegrading microneedles.

Coated Microneedles

The Group of Prausnitz at Georgia Tech in Atlanta have carried out extensive and innovative immunization studies based on stainless steel monument-shaped arrays of five microneedles dip-coated with vaccine. The microneedles were fabricated by laser-cutting stainless steel sheets and were designed to be long enough to penetrate through the *stratum corneum* and viable epidermis and into the superficial dermis by gentle manual insertion but short enough to avoid pain [28]. The length of the microneedles was approximately 700 µm, which is similar to the depth of the outer layers of skin including the *stratum corneum*, epidermis, and the upper part of the dermis. The coating solution typically contained the film-forming polymer sodium carboxymethyl cellulose and the surfactant Lutrol F-68 NF.

Recognizing that dip-coating microneedles with vaccine-containing solutions or suspensions can reduce antigen activity, the group sought to determine the experimental factors and mechanistic pathways by which inactivated influenza vaccine can lose activity as well as develop and assess improved microneedle coating formulations that protect the antigen from activity loss [28]. After coating their stainless steel microneedles using a standard vaccine formulation, the stability of influenza vaccine was reduced to 2% as measured by hemagglutination activity. The presence of carboxymethyl cellulose, which was added to increase viscosity of the coating formulation, was shown to contribute to vaccine activity loss. After screening a panel of candidate stabilizers, the addition of trehalose to the coating formulation was found to protect the antigen and retain 48%–82% antigen activity for all three major strains of seasonal influenza: H1N1, H3N2, and B. Influenza vaccine coated in this way also exhibited thermal stability, such that activity loss was independent of temperature over the range of 4°C–37°C for 24 h. Dynamic light scattering measurements showed that antigen activity loss was associated with virus particle aggregation and that stabilization using trehalose largely blocked this aggregation. Finally, microneedles using an optimized vaccine coating formulation were applied to the skin to vaccinate mice. Microneedle vaccination induced robust systemic and functional antibodies and provided complete protection against lethal challenge infection similar to conventional intramuscular injection. The group concluded that their results showed that antigen activity loss during microneedle coating can be largely prevented through optimized formulation and that stabilized microneedle patches can be used for effective vaccination. Their vaccine-containing coating formulations have typically contained trehalose in ensuing studies.

They carried out a detailed study of protective immune responses after a single influenza vaccination to the skin of mice with their microneedle patch [29]. Skin vaccination with inactivated virus-coated microneedles provided superior protection against lethal challenge compared to intramuscular injection as evidenced by effective virus clearance in lungs. Detailed immunologic analysis suggested that induction of virus neutralizing antibodies as well as enhanced anamnestic humoral and cellular responses contributed to improved protection by microneedle vaccination to the skin.

The same system was coated with inactivated influenza virus [30]. As much as 10 μg of viral proteins could be coated onto an array of five microneedles, and the coating was delivered into the skin at high efficiency within minutes. The coated microneedles were used to immunize mice in comparison with conventional intramuscular injection at the same dose. Analysis of immune responses showed that a single immunization with coated microneedles induced strong antibody responses against influenza virus with significant levels of hemagglutination inhibition activities (>1:40), which were comparable to those induced by conventional intramuscular immunization. Moreover, mice immunized by a single dose of inactivated influenza virus coated on microneedles were effectively protected against lethal challenge by a high dose of mouse-adapted influenza virus.

These microneedles were coated with influenza virus-like particles (VLP) [31] and reproducibly penetrated freshly excised human skin, depositing 80% of the coating within 60 seconds of insertion. Human skin experiments showed that H1 and H5 VLPs, delivered via microneedles, stimulated Langerhans cells, resulting in changes in cell morphology and a reduction in cell number in epidermal sheets. Langerhans cell response was significantly more pronounced in skin treated with H1 VLPs compared with H5 VLPs. This data provided some evidence that microneedle-facilitated delivery of influenza VLP vaccines initiates a stimulatory response in Langerhans cells in human skin. The group concluded that their results supported and validated animal data, suggesting that dendritic cells targeted through deposition of vaccines in skin generate immune responses.

The group then investigated the immunogenicity and protective efficacy of influenza H5 VLPs containing the hemagglutinin (HA) of A/Vietnam/1203/04 (H5N1) virus delivered into the skin of mice using the metal microneedle patches and also studied the response of Langerhans cells in a human skin model [32]. Prime-boost microneedle vaccinations with H5 VLPs elicited higher levels of virus-specific IgG1 and IgG2a antibodies, virus-specific antibody-secreting cells, and cytokine-producing cells up to 8 months after vaccination, compared to the same antigen delivered intramuscularly. Both prime-boost microneedle and intramuscular vaccinations with H5 VLPs induced similar hemagglutination inhibition titers and conferred 100% protection against lethal challenge with the wild-type A/Vietnam/1203/04 virus 16 weeks after vaccination. Microneedle delivery of influenza VLPs to viable human skin using microneedles induced the movement of CD207(+) Langerhans cells toward the basement membrane.

They then demonstrated enhanced memory responses to seasonal H1N1 influenza following intradermal vaccination using their coated microneedles [33]. Mice vaccinated with a single microneedle dose of trehalose-stabilized influenza vaccine developed strong antibody responses that were long-lived. Compared with traditional intramuscular vaccination, stabilized microneedle vaccination was superior in inducing protective immunity as was evidenced by efficient clearance of virus from the lung and enhanced humoral and antibody-secreting cell immune responses after 100% survival from lethal challenge. Vaccine stabilization was found to be important because mice vaccinated with an unstabilized microneedle vaccine elicited a weaker immunoglobulin IgG2a antibody response compared with the stabilized microneedle vaccine and were only partially protected against viral challenge. The group suggested that improved trafficking of dendritic cells to regional lymph nodes as a result of microneedle delivery to the skin may possibly play a role in contributing to improved protective immunity.

The same group examined the immunogenicity and protective efficacy of influenza VLPs (H1N1 A/PR/8/34) after skin vaccination using vaccine dried onto their solid microneedle arrays [34]. Coating of microneedles with influenza VLPs using an unstabilized formulation was found to decrease hemagglutinin (HA) activity whereas inclusion of trehalose disaccharide preserved the HA activity of influenza VLP vaccines after microneedles were coated. Microneedle vaccination of mice in the skin with a single dose of stabilized influenza VLPs induced 100% protection against challenge infection with a high lethal dose. In contrast, unstabilized influenza VLPs as well as intramuscularly injected vaccines provided inferior immunity and only partial protection (≤40%). The stabilized microneedle vaccination group showed IgG2a levels that were one order of magnitude higher than those of other groups and had the lowest lung viral titers after challenge. Also, levels of recall immune responses, including hemagglutination inhibition titers, neutralizing antibodies, and antibody-secreting plasma cells, were significantly higher after skin vaccination with stabilized formulations. The group stated that their results indicated that HA stabilization, combined with vaccination via the skin using a vaccine formulated as a solid microneedle patch, confers protection superior to that with intramuscular injection and enables potential dose-sparing effects, which are reflected by pronounced increases in rapid recall immune responses against influenza virus.

The group stated that while intradermal immunization using microneedles can enhance immune responses and provide antigen sparing and potentially offer improved shelf-life, the approach is not fully compatible with many vaccine adjuvants. This includes alum, the most common adjuvant used in the vaccine market globally. They studied a polyphosphazene immunoadjuvant to investigate its potential as a synergistic constituent of microneedle-based intradermal immunization systems [35]. Polyphosphazenes are synthetic macromolecules with a phosphorous-nitrogen backbone and organic side groups. They can be rendered water-soluble and are known to possess potent immune-stimulating properties. Poly[di(carboxylatophenoxy)phosphazene] (PCPP) is the most advanced member of this group and has a history of use in clinical trials. The group used it here in coating formulations for an amended version of their metal microneedle system with titanium arrays composed of 50 600-μm needles. PCPP was used to replace both sodium carboxymethyl cellulose and surfactant. This may be important due to potential effects on vaccine stability from polymers and surfactants typically used to enhance the efficiency of the coating process. When used as part of an intradermal delivery system for hepatitis B surface antigen, PCPP demonstrated superior activity in pigs compared to intramuscular administration and significant antigen sparing potential. It also accelerated the microneedle fabrication process and reduced its dependence on the use of surfactants. In this way, PCPP-coated microneedles may enable effective intradermal vaccination from an adjuvanted patch delivery system.

Han et al. [36] presented a new fabrication method for grooves-embedded microneedle arrays composed of the biocompatible polymer poly-L-lactic acid. The microneedles, fabricated using a hot embossing process, had three-dimensional sharp tips, smooth or grooves-embedded shafts, and large bases. The height, base width, and thickness were 880 ± 20 μm, 710 ± 15 μm, and 145 ± 15 μm, respectively. To perform an immune response test, the ovalbumin-coated microneedle arrays were inserted into mouse skin and then, the titer of antibody to ovalbumin was analyzed. Increasing the number of grooves and making them deeper induced higher antibody responses. The results suggested that such grooves-embedded microneedle arrays may be loaded with more antigen than their smooth counterparts and that the antigens are efficiently delivered into the skin although they are located on the deep grooves of the microneedles.

Widera et al. investigated immunization to the model antigen ovalbumin using antigen dip-coated onto titanium microneedle arrays which varied in height from 100 μm to 600 μm and in density from 280 to 1314 microneedles per array [37]. The authors studied the influence of depth of vaccine delivery, dose of vaccine delivered, density of microneedles on the array, and area of application on the resulting immune responses. The immune response was found to be dose-dependent and mostly independent of depth of delivery, density of microneedles, or area of application. The authors concluded that the shortest, most tolerable microneedle arrays can be used for achieving consistent and high antibody titers.

The Kendall Group at The University of Queensland in Queensland, Australia, have carried out a significant body of work using miniaturized needle arrays, termed

Nanopatches™. They used Nanopatches™ to target intradermal vaccination against West Nile Virus and Chikungunya virus in mice [38]. These miniaturized arrays are two orders of magnitude smaller than standard needles and are also much smaller than typical microneedle arrays. Nanopatches™ (NP) are fabricated from silicon using a process of deep reactive ion etching. The projections are solid silicon, sputter-coated with a thin (~100 nm) layer of gold. An individual NP is 5 × 5 mm in size and the central 4 × 4 mm area contains 3364 densely packed projections. The distance between the centers of adjacent projections is 70 mm. NPs have 65 mm long micro-nanoprojections. NPs were dry-coated with antigen, adjuvant, and/or DNA payloads. After the NP was pressed onto mouse skin, a protein payload colocalized with 91.4 ± 4.1 antigen-presenting cells mm^{-2} (or 2925 in total) representing 52% of the delivery sites within the NP contact area, agreeing well with a probability-based model used to guide the device design; it then substantially increases as the antigen diffuses in the skin to many more cells. Antigen-presenting cells (APC) colocalizing with protein payloads rapidly disappear from the application area, suggesting APC migration. The NP also delivered DNA payloads, leading to cutaneous expression of encoded proteins within 24 h. The efficiency of NP immunization was demonstrated using an inactivated whole Chikungunya virus vaccine and a DNA-delivered attenuated West Nile Virus vaccine.

In another study, the group investigated dry-coated NPs as an alternate delivery system to intramuscular injection for delivering the alum-adjuvanted human papillomavirus (HPV) vaccine Gardasil®, now commonly used as a prophylactic vaccine against cervical cancer [39]. NPs delivered vaccine to mouse ear skin within 5 minutes. To assess vaccine immunogenicity, doses corresponding to the HPV-16 component of the vaccine between 0.43 ± 0.084 ng and 300 ± 120 ng were administered to mice at day 0 and day 14. A dose of 55 ± 6.0 ng delivered intracutaneously by NPs was sufficient to produce a maximal virus neutralizing serum antibody response at day 28 postvaccination. Neutralizing antibody titers were sustained up to 16 weeks postvaccination and, for comparable doses of vaccine, somewhat higher titers were observed with intracutaneous patch delivery than with intramuscular delivery with the needle and syringe at this time point.

The group then used a probability-based theoretical approach for targeting skin APCs [40]. NPs comprised of 21,025 needles per cm^2 and 110 μm in length, tapering to tips with a sharpness of <1000 nm were dry-coated with vaccine and applied to mouse skin in vivo for 2 minutes. In this study, the group showed that NPs deliver a seasonal influenza vaccine Fluvax® 2008 to directly contact thousands of APCs, in excellent agreement with theoretical prediction. By physically targeting vaccine directly to these cells, they induced protective levels of functional antibody responses in mice and also protection against an influenza virus challenge that are comparable to the vaccine delivered intramuscularly with the needle and syringe but with less than 1/100th of the delivered antigen. They concluded that this study provided a proven mathematical/engineering delivery device template for extension into human studies and speculated that successful translation of these findings into humans could assist with problems of vaccine shortages and distribution together with alleviating fear of the needle and the need for trained practitioners to administer vaccine during an influenza pandemic.

"Poke and Patch" Approaches

The Bouwstra Group in Leiden, The Netherlands, have done considerable work using "poke and patch" approaches, where microneedles are applied and removed prior to topical vaccine application. They investigated mouse immune responses after intradermal immunization using two model antigens, diphtheria toxoid (DT) and influenza subunit vaccine [41]. Three types of microneedle arrays were used in this study. First, "assembled" microneedle arrays were manufactured from commercially available 30G hypodermic needles. The needles were assembled as a 4 × 4 array on a polymer plate with the surface area of around 0.5 cm^2. Serials of assembled microneedle arrays were fabricated with needle lengths of 300, 550, 700, and 900 μm. The second type was made of stainless steel wire with a diameter of about 200 μm and a length of 300 μm with a tangentially cut tip. The third one was silicon hollow microneedle arrays with a length of 245 μm, available as 4 × 4 and 9 × 9 arrays. A custom-designed electric applicator enabled shorter microneedles (300 μm) to pierce mouse skin effectively as shown by Trypan blue staining and trans-epidermal water loss measurements. The vaccines were topically applied with and without cholera toxin (CT) on microneedle-treated skin. In DT intradermal immunization, microneedle array pretreatment of the skin was essential to achieve substantial IgG and toxin-neutralizing antibody titers. Addition of CT further boosted the immune response to similar levels as observed after subcutaneous injection of AlPO4-adsorbed DT (DT-alum). In contrast, microneedle array pretreatment showed no effect on the immune response to plain influenza vaccine. This response was strongly improved by inclusion of CT, independent of microneedle treatment. The authors concluded that their study indicated that intradermal immunization of DT and CT following microneedle treatment results in comparable protection to injection of DT-alum, and intradermal immunization of influenza vaccine adjuvanted with CT is superior to the injection of plain vaccine.

In another study, this group looked at modulation of the immune response against DT by various adjuvants in intradermal immunization with microneedle array pretreatment [42]. Intradermal immunization was performed on BALB/c mice with or without microneedle array pretreatment using DT as a model antigen coadministrated with lipopolysaccharide (LPS), Quil A, CpG oligo deoxynucleotide (CpG), or CT as adjuvant. The immunogenicity was evaluated by measuring serum IgG subtype titers and neutralizing antibody titers. Intradermal immunization with microneedle array pretreatment resulted in a thousandfold increase of DT-specific serum IgG levels. The immune response was further improved by coadministration of adjuvants, showing a progressive increase in serum IgG titers when adjuvanted with LPS, Quil A, CpG, and CT. IgG titers of the CT-adjuvanted group reached levels comparable to those obtained after DT-alum subcutaneous injection. The group concluded that the potency and quality of the immune response against DT mediated by microneedle arrays can be modulated by coadministration of adjuvants.

The same group aimed to gain insight into the delivery and immunogenicity of N-trimethyl chitosan (TMC) adjuvanted diphtheria toxoid (DT) formulations applied transcutaneously with microneedles [43]. Mice were vaccinated with DT-loaded TMC nanoparticles, a solution of TMC and DT (TMC/DT), or DT alone. The formulations were applied onto the skin before or after microneedle treatment with two different 300 μm long microneedle arrays and also injected intradermally (ID). As a positive control, alum-adjuvanted DT (DT-alum) was injected subcutaneously (SC). Ex vivo confocal microscopy studies were performed with rhodamine-labeled TMC. Independent of the microneedle array used and the sequence of microneedle treatment and vaccine application, intradermal immunization with the TMC/DT mixture elicited eightfold higher IgG titers compared to the TMC nanoparticles or DT solution. The toxin-neutralizing antibody titers from this group were similar to those elicited by SC DT-alum. After ID immunization, both TMC-containing formulations induced enhanced titers compared to a DT solution. Confocal microscopy studies revealed that transport of the TMC nanoparticles across the microneedle conduits was limited compared to a TMC solution. They concluded that TMC has an adjuvant function in transcutaneous immunization with microneedles but only if applied in solution.

Hollow Microneedles

Hollow microneedles (Figure 8.3) have a central or off-center bore that allows liquids to be pumped into the skin using a suitable device.

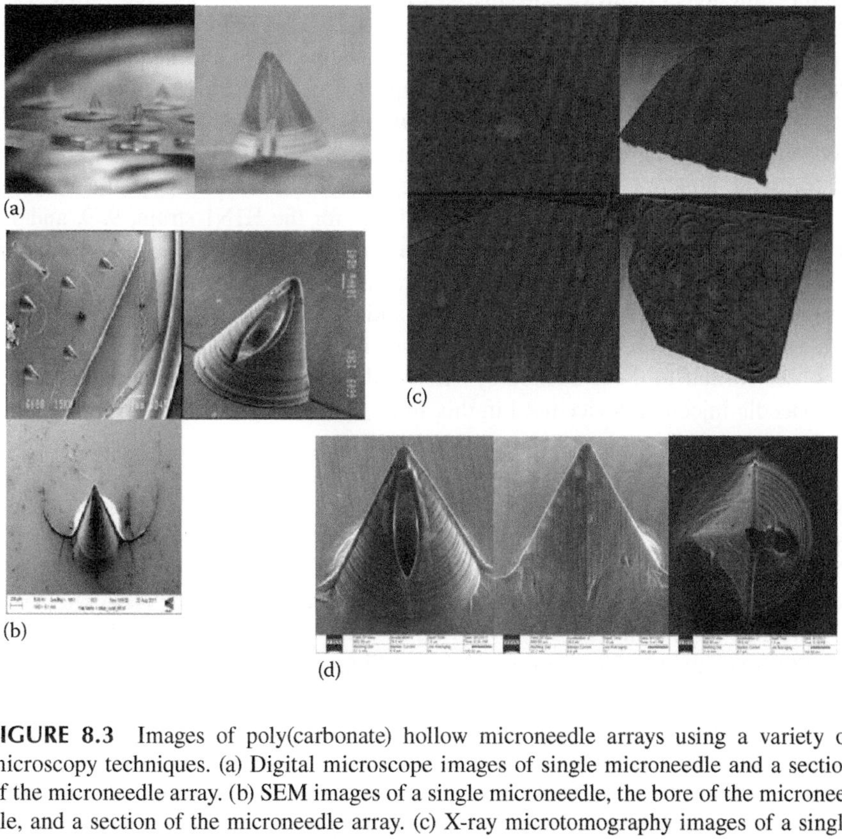

FIGURE 8.3 Images of poly(carbonate) hollow microneedle arrays using a variety of microscopy techniques. (a) Digital microscope images of single microneedle and a section of the microneedle array. (b) SEM images of a single microneedle, the bore of the microneedle, and a section of the microneedle array. (c) X-ray microtomography images of a single microneedle, the bore of the microneedle, and the microneedle array. (d) He-ion images of a single microneedle, illustrating the bore of the needle and a radial view of the microneedle.

Van Damme et al. (2009) investigated safety and efficacy of a novel microneedle device for dose-sparing intradermal influenza vaccination in healthy adults [44]. They conducted a prospective, randomized trial in 180 intended-to-treat healthy adults. Study objectives were to evaluate the safety and immunogenicity of low-dose intradermal (ID) influenza vaccines delivered using a novel microneedle device (Micronjet®). This device replaces a conventional needle and is designed specifically for intradermal delivery. The microneedle device used in this study comprised an array of four microneedles, each 0.45 mm in length. The needles were made of silicon crystal and were bonded to the tip of a plastic adapter, which can be mounted on any standard syringe. The device could be used, in theory, in the same way as any other needle except that the needles can be used for intradermal delivery only due to the limited length of the microneedles.

Subjects were randomly assigned to receive either the full dose standard flu vaccine (containing 15 μg hemagglutinin per strain) delivered intramuscularly using a conventional needle (IM group), a medium dose intradermal injection (6 μg hemagglutinin per strain) delivered with the Micronjet® (ID2 group), or a low-dose intradermal injection (3 μg hemagglutinin per strain) delivered with the Micronjet® (ID1 group). A marketed influenza vaccine for the 2006/2007 influenza season (α-RIX®, GSK Biologicals) was used for all injections. Adverse events were recorded over a 42-day period. Immunogenicity was evaluated by changes in hemagglutination inhibition (HAI) antibody titer and by comparing geometric mean titers (GMTs), seroconversion, and seroprotection rates between the study groups. Local reactions were significantly more frequent following intradermal vaccination but were mild and transient in nature. At 21 days after injection, GMT fold increase was 22.18 and 22 in the ID1, ID2, and IM groups, respectively, for the H1N1 strain; 9, 9, and 16 for the H3N2 strain; and 9, 13, and 11 for strain B. The Committee for Proprietary Medicinal Products (CPMP) criteria for relicensure of seasonal influenza vaccines were met in full for all study groups. The authors concluded that low-dose influenza vaccines delivered intradermally using microneedles elicited immunogenic responses similar to those elicited by the full-dose intramuscular vaccination. The microneedle injection device used in this study was found to be effective, safe, and reliable.

The group at BD Technologies, led by John Mikszta, has carried out a series of investigations using single hollow microneedles to inject vaccine solutions or suspensions. They described the first preclinical use of microneedle technology for ID administration of three different types of influenza vaccines: a whole inactivated influenza virus, a trivalent split-virion human vaccine, and a plasmid DNA encoding the influenza virus hemagglutinin [45]. In this study, a 34G stainless steel microneedle with inner diameter of 76 μm, an outer diameter of 178 μm, and an exposed length of 1 mm was used. The microneedle was inserted perpendicularly to the skin surface to its full exposed length in order to control the dermal penetration depth. In a rat model, ID delivery of the whole inactivated virus provided up to a hundredfold dose sparing compared to IM injection. In addition, ID delivery of the trivalent human vaccine enabled at least tenfold dose sparing for the H1N1 strain and elicited levels of response across the dose range similar to those of IM injection for the H3N2 and B strains. Furthermore, at least fivefold dose sparing from ID delivery was evident in animals treated with multiple doses of DNA plasmid vaccine although such effects were not apparent after the first immunization. The group concluded that their results demonstrated that microneedle-based ID delivery elicits antibody responses that are at least as strong as via IM injection and that, in many cases, dose sparing can be achieved by this new immunization method.

In a pilot study, the same group investigated intradermal delivery systems with a BD microneedle from 1 to 3 mm in length and epidermal delivery (BD skin abrader) through an abraded skin surface relative to standard intramuscular injection [46]. The prototype skin-microabrader, known as Onvax™, consists of an array of plastic microprojections with a height of approximately 200 μm from the base to the top and spacing between projections of twice the height. Rubbing the skin surface with Onvax™ results in *stratum corneum* disruption with possible antigen delivery as close as possible to Langerhans cells distributed in the germinative layer of the epidermis. The group emphasized the fact that rabies vaccination by the ID route is widely promoted by the World Health Organization (WHO). However, well-designed studies to formally demonstrate the degree of dose sparing and to determine whether there are real differences between the ID and IM routes are currently lacking and would be valuable. Rabies represents a good model vaccine for evaluating novel ID devices in naïve recipients. In this study, circulating neutralizing antibodies were measured against the rabies virus after the Vero cells rabies vaccine was administered at Day 0, Day 7, Day 21, and Day 49. This clinical evaluation in 66 healthy volunteers showed that ID delivery using BD microneedle technology of one fourth the IM antigen dose is safe, efficient, and reliable, resulting in a protective seroconversion rate. In contrast, the epidermal delivery route did not produce an immune response against the rabies vaccine.

The recombinant protective antigen (rPA) of *Bacillus anthracis* is a promising anthrax vaccine [47]. The Mikszta Group compared serum IgG levels and toxin-neutralizing antibody titers in rabbits following delivery of various doses of vaccine by microneedle-based ID delivery or IM injection using conventional needles. ID required less antigen to induce levels of antibody similar to those produced via ID injection during the first 2 weeks following primary and booster inoculation. This dose-sparing effect was less evident at the later stages of the immune response. Rabbits immunized ID with 10 μg of rPA displayed 100% protection from aerosol spore challenge while IM injection of the same dose provided slightly lower protection (71%). Groups immunized with lower antigen doses were partially protected (13% to 29%) regardless of the mode of administration. Overall, the group suggested that rPA formulated with aluminum adjuvant and administered to the skin by a microneedle-based device is as efficacious as IM vaccination.

Dissolving/Biodegrading Polymeric Microneedles

Recently, a number of research groups have considered self-disabling microneedles, prepared from dissolving or biodegradable polymeric or carbohydrate materials, as an innovative approach to vaccine delivery. The premise here is that the microneedles rapidly dissolve in skin interstitial fluid in the viable epidermis and/or dermis, releasing their payload (Figure 8.4). This approach holds great promise

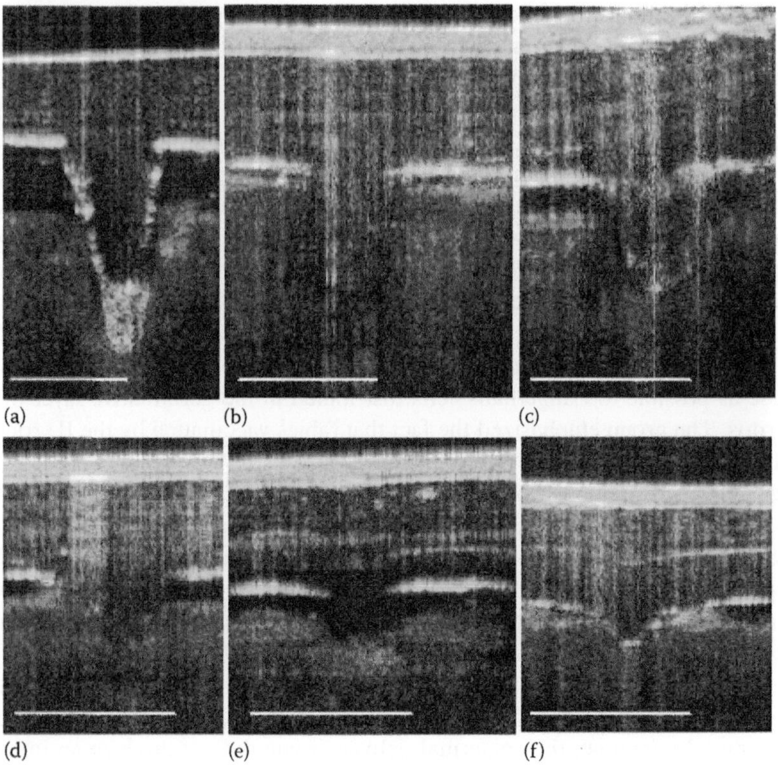

FIGURE 8.4 In-skin dissolution of microneedles prepared from aqueous blends of poly(methylvinylether-co-maleic acid) following application to rat skin in vivo. (a) time = 0 min, (b) time = 3 min, (c) time = 5 min, (d) time = 7 min, (e) time = 10 min, (f) time = 15 min. Scale bar represents a length of 300 μm.

since the microneedles would be unusable after removal from a patient's skin, meaning insertion into the skin of another person would not be possible. This should greatly reduce any risk of infection transmission. In addition, no special disposal mechanism will be required since no "sharp" exists. The solid-state nature of the contained/encapsulated vaccine should also reduce the need for cold chain storage and transport. Successful optimization and commercialization of such systems will be of undoubted benefit to patients, especially those in the developing world.

The Prausnitz Group introduced, for the first time, dissolving microneedle patches for influenza vaccination using a simple patch-based system fabricated at room temperature by photopolymerization of liquid vinyl pyrrolidone monomer within microneedle molds to form poly(vinyl pyrrolidone) microneedles 650 μm in height and encapsulating 3 μg of lyophilized inactivated influenza virus vaccine [48]. Microneedles were inserted into mouse skin in vivo by gentle hand pressure and dissolved within minutes. Microneedle vaccination generated robust antibody and cellular immune responses that provided complete protection against lethal challenge. Compared to conventional intramuscular injection, microneedle vaccination resulted in more efficient lung virus clearance and enhanced cellular recall responses after challenge. The group stated that their results suggest that dissolving microneedle patches can provide a new technology for simpler and safer vaccination with improved immunogenicity that could facilitate increased vaccination coverage.

The Kendall Group described the micromolding of dissolving microneedle arrays from master templates of one of their Nanopatch™ designs [49]. Replica microneedles were formed from carboxymethyl cellulose by multiple castings into poly(dimethylsiloxane) molds. The microneedles were 88 μm in height with base diameters of 17 μm, showing slight shrinkage from the master templates. Microneedles dissolved in mouse ear skin within 5 minutes and successfully delivered model dyes. Importantly, enhanced diffusion of the dye payloads was observed in the dermis compared to the skin layers above. The group suggested that this was due to the known higher hydration levels in the skin's deeper layers. Dual-layer microneedles containing the model antigen ovalbumin, along with the adjuvant Quil-A, elicited post-immunization schedule antibody levels in mice that were comparable to an IM ovalbumin/Quil-A immunization group at day 28 and superior to the IM group at day 102, despite using a lower antigen dose in the microneedles. Similar results were seen using influenza vaccine.

In a slight variation on this theme, the Banga Group at Mercer University, Atlanta investigated the microneedle-mediated in vitro transdermal delivery of human IgG and demonstrated the applicability of microneedles in delivery of a monoclonal antibody [50]. Microchannels created by the treatment of maltose microneedles in full thickness hairless rat skin were visualized using methylene blue staining. Cryostat sections were prepared and stained using hematoxylin and eosin to locate the depth of penetration. In vitro penetration studies were conducted using freshly excised full thickness hairless rat skin. Microneedles were applied and allowed to dissolve in skin before adding an antibody solution to the skin surface. Various parameters, such as needle length, number of needles, and effect of donor concentration were examined. The pathway of IgG transport across skin was confirmed by immunohistochemical studies. The monoclonal antibody was then delivered under optimized conditions. Methylene blue was taken up by microchannels, indicating disruption of the *stratum corneum*, and cryosections showed that microneedles just reached the dermis. Human IgG delivery increased with increase in numbers of microneedles, IgG concentration, and length of microneedles. IHC studies demonstrated that IgG moved through microchannels for transport across the skin. Transdermal delivery was also demonstrated for the monoclonal antibody.

Epidermal Gene Delivery

Gene therapy may be defined as the insertion, alteration, or removal of genes from an individual's cells and biological tissues to treat disease. The most common form of gene therapy involves the insertion of functional genes into an unspecified genomic location in order to replace a mutated gene, but other forms involve directly correcting the mutation or modifying normal genes. Although the technology is still in its infancy, it has been used with some success. The most common form of genetic engineering involves insertion of a functional gene into host cells. This is accomplished by isolating and copying the gene of interest, generating a construct containing all the genetic elements for correct expression, and then inserting this construct into the host organism. Localized delivery and expression of gene therapeutics within the skin may provide novel treatment options for a number of pathological conditions, including correction of genetic skin disorders and the nonsurgical management of malignancy. If epidermal cells could be induced by genetic manipulation to produce and secrete antigenic molecules, then the potent immunostimulatory properties of the skin should ensure efficient protection from the disease of interest.

The Birchall Group at Cardiff University in Wales have pioneered epidermal gene delivery using microneedle arrays of varying designs to bypass the *stratum corneum* barrier, which would otherwise prevent intradermal delivery of genetic constructs. In their initial studies, the group aimed to determine whether silicon-based microneedles (150 μm in height, base width 45–50 μm), microfabricated via an isotropic etching/BOSCH reaction process, could generate microchannels in the skin of sufficient dimensions to facilitate access of lipid:polycation:plasmid DNA (LPD) nonviral gene therapy vectors [51]. Scanning electron microscopy was used to visualize the microconduits created in heat-separated human epidermal sheets after application of the microneedles. Following confirmation of particle size and particle surface charge by photon correlation spectrocopy and microelectrophoresis, respectively, the diffusion of fluorescent polystyrene nanospheres and LPD complexes through heat-separated human epidermal sheets was determined in vitro using a Franz-type diffusion cell. In vitro cell culture with quantification by flow cytometry was used to determine gene expression in human keratinocytes (HaCaT cells). The diffusion of 100 nm diameter fluorescent polystyrene nanospheres, used as a readily quantifiable predictive model for LPD complexes, through epidermal sheets was significantly enhanced following membrane treatment with microneedles. The delivery of LPD complexes either into or through the membrane microchannels was also demonstrated. In both cases, considerable interaction between the particles and the epidermal sheet was observed. In vitro cell culture was used to confirm that LPD complexes mediated efficient reporter gene expression in human keratinocytes in culture when formulated at the appropriate surface charge.

In their next study, they used platinum-coated silicon microneedles to create microconduits approximately 50 μm in diameter and extending through the *stratum corneum* and viable epidermis [52]. Following optimization of skin explant culturing techniques and confirmation of tissue viability, the ability of the microneedles to mediate gene expression was demonstrated using the beta-galactosidase reporter gene. Preliminary studies confirmed localized delivery, cellular internalization and subsequent gene expression of pDNA following microneedle disruption of skin.

They followed this by investigating the ability of a microfabricated silicon microneedle arrays to facilitate localized delivery of charged macromolecules and plasmid DNA (pDNA) [53]. Microscopic studies of microneedle-treated human epidermal membrane revealed the presence of microconduits (10–20 μm diameter). The delivery of the marker biomolecule beta-galactosidase and of a "nonviral gene vector mimicking" charged fluorescent nanoparticle to the viable epidermis of microneedle-treated tissue was demonstrated using light and fluorescent microscopy. Track-etched permeation profiles, generated using "Franz-type" diffusion cell methodology and a model synthetic membrane showed that >50% of a colloidal particle suspension permeated through membrane pores in approximately 2 hours. The group suggested that, on the basis of their results, it is probable that microneedle treatment of the skin surface would facilitate cutaneous delivery of lipid:polycation:pDNA (LPD) gene vectors and other related vectors to the viable epidermis. Preliminary gene expression studies confirmed that naked pDNA can be expressed in excised human skin following microneedle disruption of the SC barrier. The presence of a limited number of microchannels, positive for gene expression, indicates that further studies to optimize the microneedle device morphology, its method of application, and the pDNA formulation are warranted to facilitate more reproducible cutaneous gene delivery.

Realizing that aqueous solutions loaded with gene delivery vehicles would be impractical in the clinic due to their inability to remain in place on the skin surface, the group then investigated the potential for improved delivery of plasmid DNA (pDNA) in skin by combining their microneedle delivery system with sustained release pDNA hydrogel formulations [54]. Microneedles were again fabricated by wet etching silicon in potassium hydroxide. Hydrogels based on Carbopol® polymers and thermosensitive PLGA-PEG-PLGA triblock copolymers were prepared. Freshly excised human skin was used to characterize microneedle penetration (microscopy and skin water loss), gel residence in microchannels, pDNA diffusion and reporter gene (beta-galactosidase) expression. Following microneedle treatment, channels of approximately 150–200 μm depth increased trans-epidermal water loss in skin. pDNA hydrogels were shown to harbor and gradually release pDNA. Following microneedle-assisted delivery of pDNA hydrogels to human skin, expression of the pCMV beta reporter gene was demonstrated in the viable epidermis proximal to microchannels. The group concluded that pDNA hydrogels can be successfully targeted to the viable epidermis to potentially provide sustained gene expression therein.

The Prausnitz Group has also recently investigated microneedle-mediated intradermal gene delivery [55]. Vaccination with a plasmid encoding hepatitis C virus nonstructural 3/4A protein using coated microneedles effectively primed specific cytotoxic T lymphocytes (CTLs). Importantly, the minimally invasive microneedles were as efficient in priming CTLs as more complicated or invasive delivery techniques, such as gene guns and hypodermic needles. The Kendall Group has also investigated gene delivery using coated Nanopatches™ [39] as described above.

The idea of using microneedles in combination with electroporation was first proposed by Prausnitz in 2005 [56]. However, it was not realized in skin until 2007, when Hooper and colleagues reported that an experimental smallpox DNA vaccine comprised of four vaccinia virus genes (4pox) can be efficiently delivered by a novel method involving skin electroporation using plasmid DNA-coated microneedle arrays [57]. Electroporation is a process where cells are transiently permeabilized using high-intensity electric field pulses. The Easy Vax™ delivery system employed consisted of 80 electrically conducting microneedles around 1 mm in height coated with dried vaccine DNA. The pulse protocol consisted of six pulses of 100 V, 100 μS pulse duration, and 125 mS pulse interval. Mice vaccinated with the 4pox DNA vaccine were administered four arrays, each coated with 30 μg of a separate plasmid (four total). Each array was administered to a separate site (inner and outer right and left thigh). Mice vaccinated with the negative controls plasmids were administered using one array to an inner thigh. Mice vaccinated with the smallpox DNA vaccine mounted robust antibody responses against the four immunogens of interest, including neutralizing antibody titers that were greater than those elicited by the traditional live virus vaccine administered by scarification. Moreover, vaccinated mice were completely protected against a lethal intranasal challenge with vaccinia virus strain IHD-J. This study represented the first demonstration of a protective immune response being elicited by microneedle-mediated skin electroporation, thus opening up a new area worthy of investigation. Indeed, Daugimont et al. [58] followed up on this by studying hollow conductive microneedles for needle-free intradermal injection and electric pulse application in order to generate an electric field in the superficial layers of the skin sufficient for electroporation. Microneedle arrays were used in combination with a vibratory inserter to disrupt the *stratum corneum*, thus piercing the skin. Effective injection of proteins into the skin was achieved, resulting in an immune response directed to the model antigen ovalbumin. However, when used both as microneedles to inject and as electrodes to apply the electric pulses, the setup showed several limitations for DNA electrotransfer. This could be due to the distribution of the electric field in the skin as shown by numerical calculations and/or the low dose of DNA injected. The authors concluded that further investigation of these parameters is needed in order to optimize minimally invasive DNA electrotransfer in the skin.

INTRADERMAL DELIVERY OF NANOPARTICLES

Nanoparticles administered into the skin using microneedles have a number of potential uses. They could be employed in order to prolong drug release in the skin for local or systemic action. Alternatively, they could be used to enhance "visibility" of a vaccine antigen to the Langerhans and dendritic cells. Topically applied nanoparticles deposit within the *stratum corneum* layers or in hair follicles and sweat glands [59].

Zhang et al. [60] investigated the penetration and the distribution of coumarin 6-loaded fluorescent poly(d,l-lactic-co-glycolic acid) (PLGA) nanoparticles in human skin pretreated with silicon microneedles (200 μm in height, 10 × 10 arrays). Fluorescent nanoparticles were prepared to indicate their transdermal transport. Permeation studies were performed on Franz-type diffusion cells in vitro, and nanoparticle distribution was visualized by confocal laser scanning microscopy (CLSM) and quantified by high-performance liquid chromatography (HPLC). CLSM images showed that nanoparticles were delivered into the microconduits created by microneedles and permeated into the epidermis and the dermis. Quantitative determination showed that permeation of nanoparticles into skin was enhanced by microneedles, but nanoparticles did not reach the receptor solution. Much greater numbers of nanoparticles deposited in the epidermis than in the dermis. Permeation was found to occur in a particle size–dependent manner, and permeation increased with nanoparticle concentration until a plateau was reached. These results suggested that microneedles could enhance intradermal delivery of PLGA nanoparticles.

Coulman et al. [61] studied delivery of fluorescent yellow/green polystyrene amine-modified nanospheres across human epidermal membranes following treatment with platinum-coated silicon microneedle arrays (arrays were approximately 0.5 cm^2 and consisted of 16 individual microneedles, approximately 280 μm in length and with base diameters of up to 200 μm). The work demonstrated the significant impact of surface charge and pore size on the permeation characteristics of a nanoparticle formulation through microchannels. Maximizing the diameter of such conduits in the skin surface facilitated more rapid and complete nanoparticle permeation. However, the authors cautioned that the maximum dimensions of conduits would also be governed by the desire for limited invasiveness from a pain and safety perspective. Electrostatic interaction of the nanoparticle formulation with the skin surface or microchannel inner surface was also found to influence permeation characteristics, and the authors therefore advised that surface charge of particles within a colloidal formulation must be carefully controlled to optimize delivery.

While the microneedle device employed demonstrated utility in localized nanoparticulate delivery into human epidermis, results showed considerable variability. High-resolution scanning electron microscopy (SEM) images illustrated some of the complexities that are associated with microneedle-mediated delivery of a nanoparticle formulation across a multilayered tissue structure. Inconsistencies in microneedle penetration of the skin, the unpredictable stability of the colloidal formulation in the extracellular milieu, and direct interaction of nanoparticles with the exposed tissue were identified as key determinants of nanoparticle permeation. The authors concluded that further work will be required to characterize the physicochemical and biological barriers that influence both the permeation properties and, importantly for cutaneous delivery, the distribution of nanoparticle therapeutics within the skin strata. Recently, Kissenpfennig et al. [62] highlighted the potential of dissolving microneedle arrays laden with nano-encapsulated antigen to increase vaccine immunogenicity by targeting antigen delivery specifically to skin dendritic cells (DCs). Following in situ uptake in a murine model in vivo, skin resident DCs were able to deliver polymeric nanoparticles to cutaneous draining lymph nodes where they subsequently induced significant expansion of antigen specific T cells. Moreover, the authors showed that antigen encapsulated nanoparticle vaccination via microneedles generated robust antigen-specific cellular immune responses in mice, providing complete protection against both the development of antigen-expressing melanoma tumors in vivo and a murine model of para-influenza through the activation of antigen-specific cytotoxic CD8 T cells that resulted in efficient clearance of tumors and virus, respectively. In addition, they also demonstrated promising findings that nano-encapsulation facilitates antigen retention in skin layers and provides antigen stability in microneedles. Therefore, the use of biodegradable polymeric nanoparticles for selective targeting of antigen to the skin DCs subsets through dissolvable microneedles can provide a promising technology for improved vaccination efficacy.

CONCLUSION

Dendritic cells (DCs), as key regulators of immune responses, play a critical role in the design of modern vaccines. The skin harbors a network of these cells and, for that reason, is recognized as an attractive target for immunization. However, one important element that has not been dealt with successfully yet is the functional heterogeneity of DC subsets. Researchers are now trying to improve intracutaneous vaccination by harnessing specific properties of particular DC subsets as they became known. In the future, it might be possible to deliver antigen alongside a specific adjuvant to a particular DC subpopulation while avoiding others with opposite effects. Targeting of antigen to the specific, functionally defined subsets of skin DCs is a promising strategy to further develop not only protective, but also therapeutic vaccines.

Given the ever-increasing evidence available within the academic and patent literature that microneedles of a wide variety of designs are capable of achieving successful intradermal and transdermal delivery of vaccines, it is envisaged that the already concerted industrial effort into development of microneedle devices will now intensify. Furthermore, novel applications of microneedle technology are likely to come to the forefront. The ability of MN arrays to extract bodily fluids for determination of efficacy of vaccination is particularly interesting. As technological advances continue, microneedle arrays may well become the pharmaceutical dosage forms and monitoring devices of the near future. However, there are a number of barriers that will first need to be addressed in order for microneedle technology to progress.

The ultimate commercial success of microneedle-based delivery and monitoring devices will depend upon not only the ability of the devices to perform their intended function, but also their overall acceptability by both health care professionals (e.g., doctors, nurses, and pharmacists) and patients. Accordingly, efforts to ascertain the views of these end users will be essential moving forward. The seminal study by the Birchall Group [63] in this regard was highly informative. The majority of health care professionals and members of the public recruited into this focus group–centered study were able to appreciate the potential advantage of using microneedles, including reduced pain, tissue damage, risk of transmitting infections, and needle-stick injuries and feasibility for self-administration and use in children, needlephobes, and/or diabetics. However, some concerns regarding effectiveness, means to confirm successful drug delivery (such as a visual dose indicator), delayed onset of action, cost of the delivery system, possible accidental use, and misuse or abuse were also raised. Health care professionals were also concerned about interindividual variation in skin thickness, problems associated with injecting small volumes, and risk of infection. Several other possible issues (accidental or error-based) and interesting doubts regarding microneedle use were discussed in this study. Overall, the group reported that 100% of the public participants and 74% of the health care professional participants were optimistic about the future of microneedle technology. Such studies, when appropriately planned to capture the necessary demographics, will undoubtedly aid industry in taking necessary action to address concerns and develop informative labeling and patient counseling strategies to ensure safe and effective use of microneedle-based devices. Marketing strategies will, obviously, also be vitally important in achieving maximum market shares relative to existing and widely used conventional delivery systems.

In order to gain acceptance from health care professionals, patients, and, importantly, regulatory authorities (e.g., the U.S. FDA and the MHRA in the UK), it appears a strong possibility that an applicator aid and a "dosing indicator" be included within the overall microneedle "package" with the microneedle array itself being disposable and the applicator/dosing indicator reusable. While a wide variety of applicator designs have been disclosed within the patent literature, only a few, relatively crude, designs based upon high-impact/-velocity insertion or rotary devices have been described. Application force has a significant role to play in microneedle insertion depth. Clearly, patients cannot "calibrate" their hands and so will apply microneedles with different forces. Unless a large-scale study can be done showing consistent rates and extents of microneedle-mediated drug delivery when the microneedles have been inserted by hand, then, for consistent dosing across the population, applicator devices will need to be supplied. Moreover, patients will need a level of assurance that the microneedle device has actually been inserted properly into their skin. This would be especially true in cases of global pandemics or bioterrorism incidents where self-administration of microneedle-based vaccines becomes a necessity. Accordingly, a suitable means of confirming that skin puncture has taken place may need to be included within an applicator device or the microneedle product itself.

From a regulatory point of view, currently little is known about the safety aspects that would be involved with long-term usage of microneedle devices. In particular, studies will need to be conducted to assess the effect that repeated microporation has upon recovery of skin barrier function. However, given the minimally invasive nature of the micropores created within the skin following microneedle application, especially in comparison to the use of a hypodermic needle, and the fact that statistically it is highly unlikely that microneedles would be inserted at exactly the same sites more than once in a patient's lifetime, it is envisaged that microneedle technology will be shown to have a favorable safety profile. Indeed, skin barrier function is known to completely recover within a few hours of microneedle removal regardless of how long the microneedles were in place. Local irritation or erythema (reddening) of the skin may be an issue for some patients. Since the skin is a potent immunostimulatory organ, it would be interesting to know whether repeated microneedle use would ever cause an immune reaction to the drug or excipients of microneedle materials and whether such an effect would be so significant as to cause problems for patients.

Infection is an issue that has long been discussed in relation to use of microneedle-based systems since they, by necessity, puncture the skin's protective *stratum corneum* barrier. However, as we have shown [64], microbial penetration through microneedle-induced holes is minimal. Indeed, there have never been any reports of microneedles causing skin or systemic infections. This may be because of the abovementioned immune component of the skin or the skin's inherent nonimmune, enzyme-based defenses. Alternatively, since the micropores are aqueous in nature, microorganisms may be more inclined to remain on the more hydrophobic *stratum corneum*. Whether skin cleansing before microneedle application is necessary remains to be seen and is a vital question. Ideally, this would not have to be done so as to avoid unnecessarily inconveniencing patients and making the use of the product in the domiciliary setting appear more akin to a self-administered injection than application of a conventional transdermal patch. Regulators will ultimately make the key decisions based on the weight of available evidence. Depending upon the application (e.g., drug/vaccine/active cosmeceutical ingredient delivery or minimally invasive monitoring), microneedle-based devices may be classed as drug delivery systems, consumer products, or medical devices. From a delivery perspective, it will be important if microneedles are considered as injections rather than topical/transdermal/intradermal delivery systems since this will determine whether the final product will need to be sterilized, prepared under aseptic conditions, or simply host a low bioburden. Any contained microorganisms may need to be identified and quantified as may the pyrogen content. Should sterilization be required, then the method chosen will be crucial since the most commonly employed approaches (moist heat, gamma or microwave radiation, ethylene oxide) may adversely affect the microneedles themselves and/or any contained active ingredient (e.g., biomolecules). Importantly, the first two microneedle-based products have now received FDA approval and have recently been marketed. These products, namely Soluvia® and Micronjet® (both hollow microneedle devices, made from metal and silicon, respectively, for intradermal vaccine delivery), are likely to pave the way for ever-more sophisticated microneedle devices for delivery of vaccines as well as a wide range of other therapeutic agents to the benefit of patients worldwide.

REFERENCES

1. Kersten, G., and H. Hirschberg. 2007. Needle-free vaccine delivery. *Expert Opinion on Drug Delivery* 4 (5):459–474.
2. Kendall, M. 2006. Engineering of needle-free physical methods to target epidermal cells for DNA vaccination. *Vaccine* 24 (21):4651–4656.
3. Lambert, P. H., and P. E. Laurent. 2008. Intradermal vaccine delivery: Will new delivery systems transform vaccine administration? *Vaccine* 26 (26):3197–3208.
4. Giudice, E. L., and J. D. Campbell. 2006. Needle-free vaccine delivery. *Advanced Drug Delivery Reviews* 58 (1):68–89.
5. Simonsen, L., A. Kane, J. Lloyd, M. Zaffran, and M. Kane. 1999. Unsafe injections in the developing world and transmission of blood borne pathogens: A review. *Bulletin of the World Health Organization* 77 (10):789–800.
6. Hamilton, J. G. 1995. Needle phobia—A neglected diagnosis. *Journal of Family Practice* 41 (2):169–175.
7. Huang, C. M. 2007. Topical vaccination: The skin as a unique portal to adaptive immune responses. *Seminars in Immunopathology* 29 (1):71–80.
8. Laurent, A., F. Mistretta, D. Bottigioli, K. Dahel, C. Goujon, J. F. Nicolas, A. Hennino, and P. E. Laurent. 2007. Echographic measurement of skin thickness in adults by high frequency ultrasound to assess the appropriate microneedle length for intradermal delivery of vaccines. *Vaccine* 25 (34):6423–6430.
9. Takigawa, M., Y. Tokura, H. Hashizume, H. Yagi, and N. Seo. 2001. Percutaneous peptide immunization via corneum barrier-disrupted murine skin for experimental tumor immunoprophylaxis. In *Cutaneous T Cell Lymphoma: Basic and Clinically Relevant Biology*, edited by R. L. Edelson and V. T. DeVita, 139–146.
10. Van Kampen, K. R., Z. K. Shi, P. Gao, J. F. Zhang, K. W. Foster, D. T. Chen, D. Marks, C. A. Elmets, and D. C. C. Tang. 2005. Safety and immunogenicity of adenovirus-vectored nasal and epicutaneous influenza vaccines in humans. *Vaccine* 23 (8):1029–1036. doi: 10.1016/j.vaccine.2004.07.043.

11. Matyas, G. R., J. M. Yu, G. M. Glenn, A. M. Friedlander, S. F. Little, and C. R. Alving. 2004. A needle-free skin patch vaccination method for protection against anthrax. *Faseb Journal* 18 (5):A820–A821.
12. Guebre-Xabier, M., S. A. Hammond, D. E. Epperson, J. M. Yu, L. Ellingsworth, and G. M. Glenn. 2003. Immunostimulant patch containing heat-labile enterotoxin from *Escherichia coli* enhances immune responses to injected influenza virus vaccine through activation of skin dendritic cells. *Journal of Virology* 77 (9):5218–5225. doi: 10.1128/jvi.77.9.5218-5225.2003.
13. Frerichs, D. M., L. R. Ellingsworth, S. A. Frech, D. C. Flyer, C. P. Villar, J. M. Yu, and G. M. Glenn. 2008. Controlled, single-step, stratum corneum disruption as a pretreatment for immunization via a patch. *Vaccine* 26 (22):2782–2787. doi: 10.1016/j.vaccine.2008.02.070.
14. Frech, S. A., H. L. DuPont, A. L. Bourgeois, R. McKenzie, J. Belkind-Gerson, J. F. Figueroa, P. C. Okhuysen et al. 2008. Use of a patch containing heat-labile toxin from *Escherichia coli* against travellers' diarrhoea: A phase II, randomised, double-blind, placebo-controlled field trial. *Lancet* 371 (9629):2019–2025. doi: 10.1016/s0140-6736(08)60839-9.
15. Frech, S. A., R. T. Kenney, C. A. Spyr, H. Lazar, J. F. Viret, C. Herzog, R. Gluck, and G. M. Glenn. 2005. Improved immune responses to influenza vaccination in the elderly using an immunostimulant patch. *Vaccine* 23 (7):946–950. doi: 10.1016/j.vaccine.2004.06.036.
16. Gill, H. S., S. N. Andrews, S. K. Sakthivel, A. Fedanov, I. R. Williams, D. A. Garber, F. H. Priddy et al. 2009. Selective removal of stratum corneum by microdermabrasion to increase skin permeability. *European Journal of Pharmaceutical Sciences* 38 (2):95–103. doi: 10.1016/j.ejps.2009.06.004.
17. Ogura, M., S. Pahwal, and S. Mitragotri. 2008. Low-frequency sonophoresis: Current status and future prospects. *Advanced Drug Delivery Reviews* 60 (10):1218–1223. doi: 10.1016/j.addr.2008.03.006.
18. Tezel, A., A. Sens, and S. Mitragotri. 2003. Description of transdermal transport of hydrophilic solutes during low-frequency sonophoresis based on a modified porous pathway model. *Journal of Pharmaceutical Sciences* 92 (2):381–393. doi: 10.1002/jps.10299.
19. Tezel, A., S. Paliwal, Z. C. Shen, and S. Mitragotri. 2005. Low-frequency ultrasound as a transcutaneous immunization adjuvant. *Vaccine* 23 (29):3800–3807. doi: 10.1016/j.vaccine.2005.02.027.
20. Dahlan, A., H. O. Alpar, P. Stickings, D. Sesardic, and S. Murdan. 2009. Transcutaneous immunisation assisted by low-frequency ultrasound. *International Journal of Pharmaceutics* 368 (1–2):123–128. doi: 10.1016/j.ijpharm.2008.10.014.
21. Luxembourg, A., C. F. Evans, and D. Hannaman. 2007. Electroporation-based DNA immunisation: Translation to the clinic. *Expert Opinion on Biological Therapy* 7 (11):1647–1664. doi: 10.1517/14712598.7.11.1647.
22. Zhao, Y. L., S. N. Murthy, M. H. Manjili, L. J. Guan, A. Sen, and S. W. Hui. 2006. Induction of cytotoxic T-lymphocytes by electroporation-enhanced needle-free skin immunization. *Vaccine* 24 (9):1282–1290. doi: 10.1016/j.vaccine.2005.09.035.
23. Medi, B. M., and J. Singh. 2008. Delivery of DNA into skin via electroporation. *Methods in Molecular Biology* 423:225–232. doi: 10.1007/978-1-59745-194-9_16.
24. Peachman, K. K., M. Rao, and C. R. Alving. 2003. Immunization with DNA through the skin. *Methods* 31 (3):232–242. doi: 10.1016/s1046-2023(03)00137-3.
25. Vandermeulen, G., L. Daugimont, H. Richiardi, M. L. Vanderhaeghen, N. Lecouturier, B. Ucakar, and V. Preat. 2009. Effect of tape stripping and adjuvants on immune response after intradermal DNA electroporation. *Pharmaceutical Research* 26 (7):1745–1751. doi: 10.1007/s11095-009-9885-3.

26. Drabick, J. J., J. Glasspool-Malone, A. King, and R. W. Malone. 2001. Cutaneous transfection and immune responses to intradermal nucleic acid vaccination are significantly enhanced by in vivo electropermeabilization. *Molecular Therapy* 3 (2):249–255. doi: 10.1006/mthe.2000.0257.
27. Laddy, D. J., J. Yan, A. S. Khan, H. Andersen, A. Cohn, J. Greenhouse, M. Lewis et al. 2009. Electroporation of synthetic DNA antigens offers protection in nonhuman primates challenged with highly pathogenic avian influenza virus. *Journal of Virology* 83 (9):4624–4630. doi: 10.1128/jvi.02335-08.
28. Kim, Y. C., F. S. Quan, R. W. Compans, S. M. Kang, and M. R. Prausnitz. 2010. Formulation and coating of microneedles with inactivated influenza virus to improve vaccine stability and immunogenicity. *Journal of Controlled Release* 142 (2):187–195.
29. Kim, Y. C., F. S. Quan, D. G. Yoo, R. W. Compans, S. M. Kang, and M. R. Prausnitz. 2009. Improved influenza vaccination in the skin using vaccine coated microneedles. *Vaccine* 27 (49):6932–6938.
30. Zhu, Q. Y., V. G. Zarnitsyn, L. Ye, Z. Y. Wen, Y. L. Gao, L. Pan, I. Skountzou et al. 2009. Immunization by vaccine-coated microneedle arrays protects against lethal influenza virus challenge. *Proceedings of the National Academy of Sciences of the United States of America* 106 (19):7968–7973.
31. Pearton, M., S. M. Kang, J. M. Song, Y. C. Kim, F. S. Quan, A. Anstey, M. Ivory, M. R. Prausnitz, R. W. Compans, and J. C. Birchall. 2010. Influenza virus-like particles coated onto microneedles can elicit stimulatory effects on Langerhans cells in human skin. *Vaccine* 28 (37):6104–6113.
32. Song, J. M., Y. C. Kim, A. S. Lipatov, M. Pearton, C. T. Davis, D. G. Yoo, K. M. Park et al. 2010. Microneedle Delivery of H5N1 influenza virus-like particles to the skin induces long-lasting B- and T-Cell responses in mice. *Clinical and Vaccine Immunology* 17 (9):1381–1389.
33. Kim, Y. C., F. S. Quan, D. G. Yoo, R. W. Compans, S. M. Kang, and M. R. Prausnitz. 2010. Enhanced memory responses to seasonal H1N1 influenza vaccination of the skin with the use of vaccine-coated microneedles. *Journal of Infectious Diseases* 201 (2):190–198.
34. Quan, F. S., Y. C. Kim, A. Vunnava, D. G. Yoo, J. M. Song, M. R. Prausnitz, R. W. Compans, and S. M. Kang. 2010. Intradermal vaccination with influenza virus-like particles by using microneedles induces protection superior to that with intramuscular immunization. *Journal of Virology* 84 (15):7760–7769.
35. Andrianov, A. K., D. P. DeCollibus, H. A. Gillis, H. H. Kha, A. Marin, M. R. Prausnitz, L. A. Babiuk, H. Townsend, and G. Mutwiri. 2009. Poly di(carboxylatophenoxy) phosphazene is a potent adjuvant for intradermal immunization. *Proceedings of the National Academy of Sciences of the United States of America* 106 (45):18936–18941.
36. Han, M., D. K. Kim, S. H. Kang, H. R. Yoon, B. Y. Kim, S. S. Lee, K. D. Kim, and H. G. Lee. 2009. Improvement in antigen-delivery using fabrication of a grooves-embedded microneedle array. *Sensors and Actuators B-Chemical* 137 (1):274–280.
37. Widera, G., J. Johnson, L. Kim, L. Libiran, K. Nyam, P. E. Daddona, and M. Cormier. 2006. Effect of delivery parameters on immunization to ovalbumin following intracutaneous administration by a coated microneedle array patch system. *Vaccine* 24 (10):1653–1664.
38. Prow, T. W., X. F. Chen, N. A. Prow, G. J. P. Fernando, C. S. E. Tan, A. P. Raphael, D. Chang et al. 2010. Nanopatch-targeted skin vaccination against west nile virus and chikungunya virus in mice. *Small* 6 (16):1776–1784.
39. Corbett, H. J., G. J. P. Fernando, X. F. Chen, I. H. Frazer, and M. A. F. Kendall. 2010. Skin vaccination against cervical cancer associated human papillomavirus with a novel micro-projection array in a mouse model. *Plos One* 5 (10).

40. Fernando, G. J. P., X. F. Chen, T. W. Prow, M. L. Crichton, E. J. Fairmaid, M. S. Roberts, I. H. Frazer, L. E. Brown, and M. A. F. Kendall. 2010. Potent immunity to low doses of influenza vaccine by probabilistic guided micro-targeted skin delivery in a mouse model. *Plos One* 5 (4).
41. Ding, Z., F. J. Verbaan, M. Bivas-Benita, L. Bungener, A. Huckriede, D. J. van den Berg, G. Kersten, and J. A. Bouwstra. 2009. Microneedle arrays for the transcutaneous immunization of diphtheria and influenza in BALB/c mice. *Journal of Controlled Release* 136 (1):71–78.
42. Ding, Z., E. Van Riet, S. Romeijn, G. F. A. Kersten, W. Jiskoot, and J. A. Bouwstra. 2009. Immune modulation by adjuvants combined with wiphtheria toxoid administered topically in BALB/c mice after microneedle array pretreatment. *Pharmaceutical Research (Dordrecht)* 26 (7):1635–1643.
43. Bal, S. M., Z. Ding, G. F. A. Kersten, W. Jiskoot, and J. A. Bouwstra. 2010. Microneedle-based transcutaneous immunisation in mice with N-trimethyl chitosan adjuvanted diphtheria toxoid formulations. *Pharmaceutical Research* 27 (9):1837–1847.
44. Van Damme, P., F. Oosterhuis-Kafeja, M. Van der Wielen, Y. Almagor, O. Sharon, and Y. Levin. 2009. Safety and efficacy of a novel microneedle device for dose sparing intradermal influenza vaccination in healthy adults. *Vaccine* 27 (3):454–459.
45. Alarcon, J. B., A. W. Hartley, N. G. Harvey, and J. A. Mikszta. 2007. Preclinical evaluation of microneedle technology for intradermal delivery of influenza vaccines. *Clinical and Vaccine Immunology* 14 (4):375–381.
46. Laurent, P. E., H. Bourhy, M. Fantino, P. Alchas, and J. A. Mikszta. 2010. Safety and efficacy of novel dermal and epidermal microneedle delivery systems for rabies vaccination in healthy adults. *Vaccine* 28 (36):5850–5856.
47. Mikszta, J. A., J. P. Dekker, N. G. Harvey, C. H. Dean, J. M. Brittingham, J. Huang, V. J. Sullivan, B. Dyas, C. J. Roy, and R. G. Ulrich. 2006. Microneedle-based intradermal delivery of the anthrax recombinant protective antigen vaccine. *Infection and Immunity* 74 (12):6806–6810.
48. Sullivan, S. P., D. G. Koutsonanos, M. D. Martin, J. W. Lee, V. Zarnitsyn, S. O. Choi, N. Murthy, R. W. Compans, I. Skountzou, and M. R. Prausnitz. 2010. Dissolving polymer microneedle patches for influenza vaccination. *Nature Medicine* 16 (8):915–920.
49. Raphael, A. P., T. W. Prow, M. L. Crichton, X. F. Chen, G. I. P. Fernando, and M. A. F. Kendall. 2010. Targeted, needle-free vaccinations in skin using multi layered, densely-packed dissolving microprojection arrays. *Small* 6 (16):1785–1793.
50. Li, G. H., A. Badkar, S. Nema, C. S. Kolli, and A. K. Banga. 2009. In vitro transdermal delivery of therapeutic antibodies using maltose microneedles. *International Journal of Pharmaceutics* 368 (1–2):109–115.
51. Chabri, F., K. Bouris, T. Jones, D. Barrow, A. Hann, C. Allender, K. Brain, and J. Birchall. 2004. Microfabricated silicon microneedles for nonviral cutaneous gene delivery. *British Journal of Dermatology* 150 (5):869–877.
52. Birchall, J., S. Coulman, M. Pearton, C. Allender, K. Brain, A. Anstey, C. Gateley, N. Wilke, and A. Morrissey. 2005. Cutaneous DNA delivery and gene expression in ex vivo human skin explants via wet-etch microfabricated microneedles. *Journal of Drug Targeting* 13 (7):415–421.
53. Coulman, S., D. Barrow, A. Anstey, C. Gateley, A. Morrissey, N. Wilke, K. Brain, and J. Birchall. 2006. Minimally invasive cutaneous delivey of macromolecules and plasmid DNA via microneedles. *Current Drug Delivery* 3:65–75.
54. Pearton, M., C. Allender, K. Brain, A. Anstey, C. Gateley, N. Wilke, A. Morrissey, and J. Birchall. 2008. Gene delivery to the epidermal cells of human skin explants using microfabricated microneedles and hydrogel formulations. *Pharmaceutical Research* 25 (2):407–416.

55. Gill, H. S., J. Soderholm, M. R. Prausnitz, and M. Sallberg. 2010. Cutaneous vaccination using microneedles coated with hepatitis C DNA vaccine. *Gene Therapy* 17 (6):811–814.
56. Choi, S. O., J. H. Park, H. S. Gill, Y. Choi, M. G. Allen, and M. R. Prausnitz. 2005. Microneedle electrode array for electroporation of skin for gene therapy. *Controlled Release Society 32nd Annual Meeting & Exposition Transactions*: 318.
57. Hooper, J. W., J. W. Golden, A. M. Ferro, and A. D. King. 2007. Smallpox DNA vaccine delivered by novel skin electroporation device protects mice against intranasal poxvirus challenge. *Vaccine* 25 (10):1814–1823.
58. Daugimont, L., N. Baron, G. Vandermeulen, N. Pavselj, D. Miklavcic, M. C. Jullien, G. Cabodevila, L. M. Mir, and V. Preat. 2010. Hollow microneedle arrays for intradermal drug delivery and DNA electroporation. *Journal of Membrane Biology* 236 (1):117–125.
59. Donnelly, R. F., D. I. J. Morrow, F. Fay, C. J. Scott, S. Abdelghany, T. R. R. Singh, M. J. Garland, and A. D. Woolfson. 2010. Microneedle-mediated intradermal nanoparticle delivery: Potential for enhanced local administration of hydrophobic pre-formed photosensitisers. *Photodiagnosis and Photodynamic Therapy* 7:222–231.
60. Zhang, W., J. Gao, Q. Zhu, M. Zhang, X. Ding, X. Wang, X. Hou et al. 2010. Penetration and distribution of PLGA nanoparticles in the human skin treated with microneedles. *International Journal of Pharmaceutics* 402 (1–2):205–212.
61. Coulman, S. A., A. Anstey, C. Gateley, A. Morrissey, P. McLoughlin, C. Allender, and J. C. Birchall. 2009. Microneedle mediated delivery of nanoparticles into human skin. *International Journal of Pharmaceutics* 366 (1–2):190–200.
62. Zaric, M., O. Lyubomska, O. Touzelet, C. Poux, S. Al-Zahrani, F. Fay, L. Wallace et al. 2013. Targeting of skin dendritic cells via microneedle arrays laden with antigen encapsulated PLGA nanoparticles induces efficient anti-tumour and anti-viral immune responses. *ACS Nano.* 7:2042–2055.
63. Birchall J., R. Clemo, A, Anstey, D. John. 2011. Microneedles in clinical practice—An explanatory study into the views and opinions of healthcare professionals and the public. *Pharmaceutical Research* 28:95–106.
64. Donnelly R. F., R. R. S. Thakur, M. M. Tunney, D. I. J. Morrow, P. A. McCarron, C. O'Mahony, and A. D. Woolfson. 2009. Microneedle arrays allow lower microbial penetration than hypodermic needles *in vitro. Pharmaceutical Research* 26:2513–2522.

9 Application of Nanoparticle Tracking Analysis in Drug Delivery

Matthew Wright

CONTENTS

As the use of nanoscale materials in the field of medicine and drug delivery continues to grow, so does the need for methodology to effectively characterize these materials. At this scale, small changes in properties, such as size, zeta potential, aggregation state, and concentration of materials, can have a large impact on the effectiveness, bioavailability, and even toxicology of a product. This chapter discusses the use of a technique known as nanoparticle tracking analysis (NTA) for the characterization of nanoscale drug delivery systems. An explanation of the principles of the technique is followed by a brief discussion of comparable technologies and then a review of the literature in which NTA has been utilized in order to characterize drug delivery and nanomedicine products.

NANOPARTICLE TRACKING ANALYSIS: PRINCIPLES OF OPERATION

NTA allows the direct and real-time visualization, sizing, and counting of materials between 10 nm and 1000 nm in liquid suspension. Information is recorded on a particle-by-particle basis allowing analysis of polydisperse systems resulting in high-resolution particle size distributions for samples of organic and inorganic origin.

NTA utilizes the principles of light scattering and Brownian motion in order to characterize materials. In order to do this, the user injects a small amount of sample (0.3 ml) of liquid containing nanomaterial into a sample chamber. A finely focused laser beam (typically of wavelength 635 nm, 532 nm, 488 nm, or 405 nm) is passed through a prism-edged glass flat beneath the sample chamber. The angle at which this laser enters the prism, along with a refractive index difference between the glass and the fluid containing the nanomaterial above it, causes this beam to refract to an intense low profile as it passes from the glass to the sample. This compression of the profile results in a high power density within the laser. The particles suspended in the liquid through which this beam now passes scatter light in all directions (through Rayleigh scattering) allowing them to be visualized using a long working distance, ×20 magnification microscope objective fitted to an otherwise conventional microscope configuration. A schematic of this configuration can be seen in Figure 9.1.

After the illumination of materials previously outlined, the particles can now be visualized either by eye using microscope oculars or via a camera output fitted to the microscope. This arrangement includes either a charged coupled device (CCD),

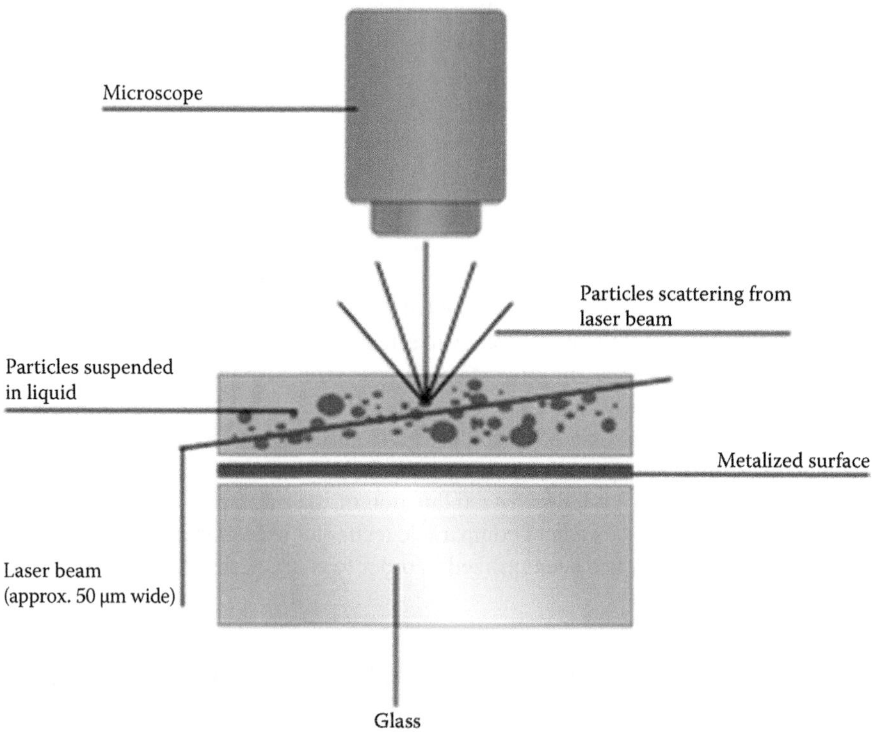

FIGURE 9.1 A schematic showing the laser configuration utilized by NTA. (From Malvern 2015 Nanoparticle Tracking Analysis—A review of the first 1000 reports of applications and usage of NTA.)

electron multiplied charged coupled device (EMCCD), or high-sensitivity complementary metal-oxide semiconductor (CMOS) camera, capturing a video file of the particles moving under Brownian motion within a field of view of approximately 100 μm × 80 μm × 10 μm at 30 frames per second. The NTA software captures a (typically) 60-second video of particles moving under Brownian motion, and once recorded, this video is then analyzed as the software identifies and tracks the center of each particle on a frame-by-frame basis. The average distance moved in the x and y planes is determined for each particle, allowing the diffusion coefficient (D_t) to be calculated. The system also records the temperature (T) of the medium, so as long as the viscosity (η) of the material is known, then the Stokes-Einstein equation (Equation 9.1) can be used in order to determine the sphere-equivalent hydrodynamic diameter (d) of each of the particles within the field of view.

$$D_t = \frac{K_B T}{3\pi\eta d_h} \tag{9.1}$$

where K_B is the Boltzmann's constant.

Clearly Brownian motion occurs in three dimensions; however, the fact that NTA only measures the displacement in two dimensions is accounted for by using a variation of the Stokes-Einstein equation. In fact, particle size can be calculated using the displacement in one, two, or three dimensions (Equation 9.2a through c, respectively).

$$\overline{(x^2)} = \frac{2TK_B t}{3\pi\eta d} \qquad \overline{(x,y)}^2 = \frac{4TK_B t}{3\pi\eta d} \qquad \overline{(x,y,z)}^2 = \frac{2TK_B t}{\pi\eta d} \tag{9.2}$$

a b c

Therefore, Equation 9.3 is used to calculate the diffusion coefficient from two-dimensional movements and relate this to particle size.

$$\frac{\overline{(x,y)}^2}{4} = D_t = \frac{TK_B}{3\pi\eta d} \tag{9.3}$$

Technique Limitations

Two factors affect the lower limit of detection of NTA. The first of these is the efficiency with which light scattered from the particles can be collected. It is clear that as the effectiveness of a camera to pick up light decreases, the potential for the system to visualize the smallest, dimmest particles also decreases. The second factor contributing to the lower limit of detection of the technique is the amount of light scattered by a particle. This is a function of many contributing factors, including the particle size, material, illumination power, wavelength, and polarization.

Light scattering theory is well established, and the formula for Rayleigh scattering of small particles of radius a, refractive index n_1 in a liquid of refractive index n_2 can be given using Equation 9.4 [1].

$$\frac{I}{I_{in}} = \frac{16\pi^4 a^6}{r^2\lambda^4}\left(\frac{n^2-1}{n^2+2}\right)\sin^2\psi, \tag{9.4}$$

where λ is the wavelength of the incident beam, n the relative refractive index (n_2/n_1), I_{in} is incident power per unit area, I the scattered power per unit area *(a)*. r is the distance from the scattering region, and ψ is the angle between the input polarization and the scattering direction.

To determine the total scattering (P_{scat}) into an aperture of collection angle θ, the following is used:

$$P_{scat} = \frac{64\pi^4 a^6}{\lambda^4}\left(\frac{n^2-1}{n^2+2}\right)\eta_o I_{in}$$

where

$$\eta_o = \frac{(1-\cos\theta)}{4} + \frac{(1-\cos^3\theta)}{12} \tag{9.5}$$

The NTA instrumentation has fixed incident laser power and wavelength, numerical aperture, and detection angle. This results in particle size and the refractive index difference between the particles and the solvent in which they are suspended being the only variables limiting the detection of small materials through NTA. As a result, it is possible to see materials of very high refractive index difference to water, such as colloidal gold or silver, down to around 10 nm and to size them accurately. However, for materials where the refractive index is more closely matched with the solvent, such as those of biological origin, the lower limit of detection may only reach 25–35 nm.

The upper limit of detection is not affected by the amount of light scattered to such an extent (however, once particles reach a certain size, they will fill the field of view blocking others from being seen), but rather, as particles reach 1–2 μm, the rate of Brownian motion becomes so low that it can be negated by the small centering errors present in the software. As a result of this, sizing becomes inaccurate, which is why systems are stated as having an upper limit of detection of around 1 μm.

As well as having a fixed set of sizes through which the system can operate, NTA can also only work through a specific range of concentrations of particles. As the technique tracks and analyzes each particle on an individual basis, rather than relying on the average results from many particles at once, it is important that the sample contains a sufficient number of particles so that the data produced is statistically viable. Typically, this value is in the region of 10^7 to 10^9 particles per ml, with 10^8 particles per ml being the ideal concentration for analysis. Below this value, there are so few particles within the system that only one or two will be seen in the field of view, leading to poor statistics and decreased reproducibility. Above 10^9 particles per ml, the field of view becomes crowded with particles. As the technique relies on tracking the random movement of individual particles, when they become close to one another, the software must stop tracking them to avoid crossover events. If the field of view is very crowded, the chances of tracking a particle for any length of time before it becomes proximate to another particle and therefore must stop being tracked is negligible.

As the system operates in a fixed field of view, several steps can be taken to try and reduce the risk of sample bias. The first of these is the combining of repeat measurements. The effect of averaging out several readings means any small anomalies in a single reading that come about as a result of sample bias become negligible when amalgamated into a large data set. The second step that can be taken to avoid possible inaccuracies due to sample bias is to use a flowing sample rather than a static one. When a static sample is analyzed, even though the materials are moving under Brownian motion, the likelihood of a significant number of new materials entering the field of view is minimal. However, if a slow flow is applied to the system, new materials are forced into the field of view, effectively presenting the system with the equivalent of several repeat experiments in one analysis. As the software is able to remove any external movement from the overall Brownian motion of a particle, the use of a syringe pump to flow the system does not present a problem with accuracy when sizing particles.

Sample Preparation

The technique requires a minimal amount of sample preparation with most instances simply requiring a dilution of raw material to a suitable concentration (as described above) using an applicable solvent. When samples require dilution, it is always recommended that the solvent used for this is tested before dilution of the sample in order to test for the possible presence of contaminating nanoparticles. Finding and keeping a particle-free solvent for analysis can sometimes be a difficult task; however, it is clear that this is an important step in the analysis to ensure that the results obtained by NTA represent only the materials of interest rather than a combination of the materials of interest and contaminant particles from the solvent.

If a sample contains a large amount of sediment, this is an indication that the original sample contains a population of materials that are, by definition, not freely diffusing nanoparticles. In these circumstances, it is wise to avoid the resuspension of any sediment as it is more than likely that materials of this size will scatter so much light that they will fill a field of view and make the analysis of other materials difficult or impossible. Instead, it is recommended that a sample of the supernatant is taken for sample analysis. If necessary it is recommended that particles >2 µm are removed from samples using either centrifugation, filtration, or sample settling.

Additional Measurable Parameters

Although the intensity of light scattered by a material is not required by this technique in order to produce a particle size distribution, the relative amount of light scattered by particles (I_{scat}) is measured as an additional parameter in order to try and differentiate between similarly sized particles of differing material/refractive index. For example, a sample analysis of a mixture of 92-nm polystyrene particles and 90-nm gold particles would give a single peak when particle size is plotted against number of particles. However, when the relative amount of light scattered by the particles is added as a third variable, it is possible to differentiate the two populations owing to the huge differences in the amount of light scattered between gold and polystyrene particles of similar sizes. Figure 9.2 shows the separation possible when a mixture of 30-nm and 60-nm gold is analyzed alongside 100-nm polystyrene.

Originally, the technique of NTA was developed around a laser of wavelength 638 nm; however, in recent years, further wavelengths of 532 nm, 488 nm, and 405 nm have been introduced. The combination of these wavelengths allow the excitation of many fluorescent or fluorescently labeled particles and when used in conjunction with appropriate optical filters allow the user to selectively identify and track only those materials showing fluorescent properties. This leads to the possibility of selectively identifying, sizing, and counting specific subpopulations in complex backgrounds through the use of fluorescent labeling. This may be achieved through the use of antibody-mediated fluorophores, giving rise to the phenotyping of a particular species of nanoparticles [2]. It is also possible to use fluorescent stains and reagents that are specific to certain components, such as proteins, lipids, or nucleic acid, to distinguish particle populations from one another.

More complications arise when using fluorescent or fluorescently labeled materials than would be apparent when analyzing nanoparticles under light scatter. The ability for NTA to visualize and track materials depends on the fluorescent signal being sufficiently intense for long enough for particle movement to be tracked. The strength of the fluorescent signal is determined by a combination of various factors. First of these is the choice of excitation laser wavelength. This must be sufficiently well matched to the excitation profile of the fluorophore in question in order to ensure a sufficient amount of fluorescence is emitted from the material. Along with this, the

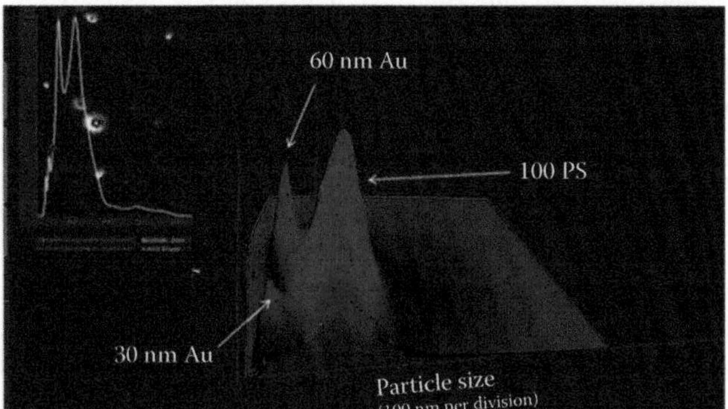

FIGURE 9.2 Separation by particle size and relative refractive index. (From Malvern 2015 Nanoparticle Tracking Analysis—A review of the first 1000 reports of applications and usage of NTA.)

extinction coefficient and the quantum yield of the fluorophores are also important parameters for a successful fluorescent analysis. The optical filters used in the instrumentation must also be compatible with the excitation and emission profiles of the fluorophore in question so that the filter used removes the maximum possible amount of the excitation wavelength while removing the minimal amount of the emission wavelength. Stable fluorophores must be used in order to operate NTA in fluorescent mode as readings are required in the time domain. Therefore, rapidly bleaching fluorophores cannot be used in a static system. However, if a flow is placed across the sample chamber by a syringe pump as described earlier when discussing reducing sample bias, fresh material is constantly moved into the laser beam, allowing the analysis of rapidly bleaching materials.

By utilizing electrodes immersed in the sample, it is possible to apply an electrical field across the sample chamber. This causes electrophoresis in charged particles from which zeta potential can be calculated. Zeta potential is central to colloidal stability and performance, and as such, a measure of zeta potential determines the tendency for materials to aggregate over time. This value not only varies between different particle types, but also pH, temperature, concentration of particles, and particle size, so it is important to see how changes in any of these variables have an effect on the overall result.

As NTA works on a particle-by-particle basis, it is possible to determine the electrophoretic velocity and polarity of each particle within the field of view under an applied electrical field. However, as this technique works in the time domain, it is not possible to apply the high-frequency change in polarity utilized in other zeta potential analysis instruments as changing the polarity so often would result in no discernible electophoretic movement being tracked by the software. As a result, a constant field is applied, resulting in not only electrophoretic movement of the particles in the solution, but also a parabolic flow profile of solvent in the sample chamber as a result of electro-osmosis occurring independently of particle motion. Therefore, the motion of a particle observed at any point will be an amalgamation of Brownian motion, electro-osmosis, and particle electrophoresis. Figure 9.3 shows

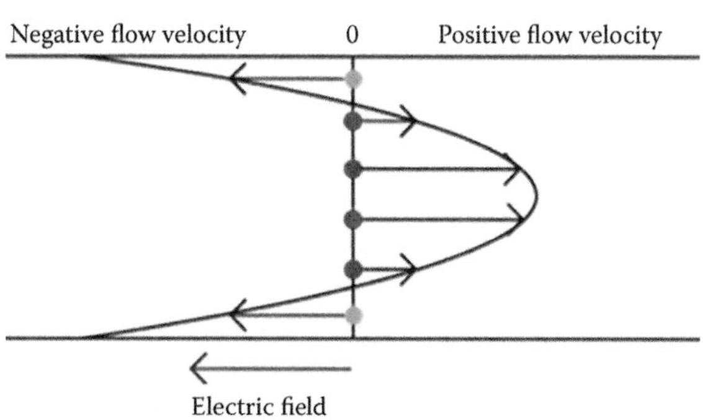

FIGURE 9.3 Flow profile observed when electrical field is applied along a sample cell. (From Malvern 2015 Nanoparticle Tracking Analysis—A review of the first 1000 reports of applications and usage of NTA.)

the flow profile created when an electrical field is applied along a sample chamber used for NTA with the upper and lower boundaries representing the top and bottom of the cell.

The NTA software allows the removal of external forces from the movement of particles under Brownian motion; however, in order to separate the two forces of electro-osmosis and electrophoresis (the parameter of interest), it is required to take multiple measurements through the depth of the flow profile in order to map the electro-osmotic profile. Once this has been obtained, the software is then able to deduct this component from the observed velocities of the charged particles in order to obtain the electrophoretic mobility and zeta potential for each particle tracked. This whole process takes around 15–20 minutes as opposed to the 60 seconds or so for a regular analysis; however, this process is fully automated and controlled by the system software, requiring minimal input from the operator, and gives a particle-by-particle zeta potential profile rather than an average reading.

Given knowledge of the solvent viscosity is a prerequisite for the accurate measurement of nanoparticle size; it is axiomatic that nanoparticles of known size (perhaps fluorescently labeled to improve visibility in high background matrices) can be used to probe changes in the nano-rheology of a nanoparticle's immediate micro-environment and changes therein (e.g., on gelling or melting).

ASSESSMENT OF NTA

NTA has been thoroughly assessed in a number of recent studies as a technique for nanoscale analysis in a variety of different applications. Saveyn et al. [3] conducted a study into accurate particle size distribution determination using NTA. During this investigation, they illustrated that simulation of step length distribution within analysis allowed more accurate and reliable estimation of particle size distribution to be determined, leading to a reduction in the artificial broadening seen when step length is directly converted to particle size data. A variation of this type of modeling is included in the processing software of NTA as a "finite track length adjustment," allowing users to obtain the true distribution widths of narrow distributions of calibration quality nanoparticles.

An investigation into the analysis of mixtures of calibration standard polystyrene nanoparticles of varying sizes from 60 nm to 1000 nm was conducted by Filipe et al. [4]. The study also looked at heat-induced protein aggregates and showed that the presence of small amounts of large particles (1000 nm) generally did not have a great bearing on the accuracy of NTA measurements. NTA was shown to be a complementary technique to dynamic light scattering (DLS) and suitable for the characterization of both drug delivery particles and protein aggregates.

Mahl et al. [5] looked at a variety of different analytical methodologies (including scanning electron microscopy [SEM], DLS, NTA, and analytical disc centrifugation) and compared their benefits and limitations while assessing a bimodal population of metallic nanoparticles. During the analysis of 15-nm gold particles (approaching the lower limit of detection by NTA) mixed with 70-nm silver particles, it was found that the presence of the larger particles tended to mask that of the smaller particles in both DLS and NTA. While electron microscopy methods were found to be suitable for sizing particle populations, difficulty was encountered when trying to accurately detect aggregates. It was stated for NTA, "The inspection of a large number of particles also permits the analysis of mixtures of small and large particles. For both pure silver or gold nanoparticle dispersions the analysis gave very satisfactory results. However, the particle size distribution was broader than obtained by other methods, and a clear differentiation between silver and gold nanoparticles was not possible."

Boyd et al. [6] have compared atomic force microscopy (AFM), NTA, and DLS for nanoparticle size measurements. They concluded that the different techniques gave different results, but these are all consistent considering the exact nature of each measurand and its physical condition. They showed that while AFM analyzed individual particles with agglomerates not being detected, NTA detected both, and combining the two techniques allowed the effect of agglomerates on DLS to be quantified.

Van der Meeren et al. [7] have discussed the relevance of two-dimensional Brownian motion dynamics in applying NTA, emphasizing that an understanding of the basic principles underlying the technique helps avoid incorrect analyses. In more general terms, Gayatri et al. [8] and Liu [9] have assessed the preparation and characterization of nanoparticles and, more specifically, Du et al. [10] have used NTA and DLS to measure aggregation and adhesion of gold nanoparticles in phosphate-buffered saline. Troiber et al. [11] have recently undertaken a comparison of four different particle-sizing methods (DLS, AFM, NTA, and fluorescence correlation spectroscopy [FCS]) for siRNA polyplex 26 characterization, pointing out that while NTA was unable to measure the smaller 40-nm primary particles, it alone could analyze the larger polydisperse 120-nm aggregates. It was concluded that a comprehensive analysis by more than one method is of particular importance.

The advantages and limitations of NTA for the analysis and characterization of low-concentration particle populations in complex matrixes, such as environmental, biological, and food samples, were discussed by Gallego-Urrea et al. [12]. In a discussion on the requirement to produce stable reference materials and prevention of agglomeration Dean [13] cited NTA as a suitable method for the visualization and analysis of particle size distributions.

Given protein-conjugated gold nanoparticles (AuNPs) have been extensively explored for the development of many novel protein assays, James and Driskell [14] demonstrated that NTA can be used as a rapid and simple analytical tool to monitor bioconjugation and to study protein–protein interactions. First, the adsorption of protein A onto gold nanoparticles was analyzed using NTA, resulting in a measureable increase in hydrodynamic radius that correlated with protein A concentration. NTA was then used to investigate the binding of mouse IgG to Protein A–conjugated AuNPs, and the Ka was measured as 2×10^7 M-1. Furthermore, an assay for the detection of mouse IgG was developed using NTA to detect the binding to antibody-AuNP conjugates exhibiting a detection limit of 3.2 ng/mL; however, the formation of aggregates resulting from the use of a polyclonal antibody and multiple binding sites on the antigen prevented the determination of binding affinity for this antibody–antigen system. To measure the binding affinity for this antibody–antigen system, the IgG antigen was conjugated to the AuNPs and NTA was used to monitor the binding of the antibody. In this configuration, aggregation of conjugates was not detected, and a binding affinity constant of 2.80×10^8 M-1 was measured. NTA results obtained in this work were validated by comparison to DLS. This work represented the first evaluation of NTA as an analytical tool for characterizing AuNP bioconjugates, investigating protein–protein binding, and detecting low levels of antigen in a bioassay.

The American Society for Testing and Materials (ASTM) have recently published a standard guide for the measurement of particle size distribution of 27 nanomaterials in suspension by NTA through adoption of which users of the technique can achieve standardization of results [15].

Other Techniques for Characterization of Materials on the Nanoscale

While much of this chapter is on the application and use of NTA for the assessment of nanoscale materials in drug delivery, it is also important to consider some of the other characterization equipment used for this type of work. These techniques include dynamic light scattering, also known as photon correlation spectroscopy (PCS), disk centrifuge, flow cytometry, transmission electron microscopy (TEM), and scanning electron microscopy (SEM). However, this is by no means an exhaustive list. NTA is most commonly compared to DLS as it also utilizes the properties of light scattering and Brownian motion in order to obtain a particle size. Although it utilizes some of the same phenomena in order to obtain a particle size, the way in which this is achieved is very different, which can lead to differing results. DLS relies on analysis of intensity fluctuations in a coherent light source having been passed through a solution containing particles. These fluctuations are a result of interference of scattered light caused by Brownian motion of the particles in solution with the speed of the fluctuation being directly linked to the size of the materials present. This technique has the benefits of being widely used and being very fast, reproducible, and accurate for a monodispersed system. Problems can arise however when performing DLS analysis on polydisperse systems owing to the fact that the relationship between the size of a particle and the amount of light that it scatters varies as a function of radius^6, resulting in a significant bias toward the larger particles in the distribution, which is observed as the technique relies on analyzing the intensity of light scattered. Similarly, if particles of high refractive index are introduced to a system of weakly scattering particles, they will dominate the signal observed. The methodology also requires that the user inputs the refractive index of both the particles and the solvent used into the software in order to relate the intensity fluctuations to the volume and then number of particles in solution. This parameter can prove difficult to characterize, especially in the field of drug delivery where newly created particles and preparations will have unknown characteristics.

Analytical ultracentrifugation is a high-resolution technique allowing the analysis of polydisperse systems. In this technique, the sample is introduced to a spinning disk rotating at high RPM. The *g* force that this applies to the particles causes them to separate as a function of their size as they pass from the center to the outer edge of the spinning disk. The particles pass through a counter as they reach the end of the system, meaning that not only size, but also count can be determined. Although this technique offers high-resolution separation of particles, the system does require calibration and knowledge of the density of the material. As a result of this, it is not possible to analyze mixtures of differing materials due to their different specific densities.

Various types of electron microscopy offer users the ability to see, count, and size their materials in minute detail with sizes in the picometer range achievable for resolution. These microscopes use a beam of electrons (in much the same way light is used in optical microscopy) to give high-resolution images of materials. Once visualized, users can use scales to obtain information on size and can count the number of particles present. Although this technique offers users a high degree of detail, it can be both expensive and time-consuming to size and count each particle manually. Also, as these systems work in a vacuum, samples must be prepared and "fixed" before analysis. The user has no way of knowing the effect that the fixing process and exposure to vacuum has on the sample if the technique is used in isolation.

APPLICATION OF NANOPARTICLE TRACKING ANALYSIS IN THE FIELD OF NANOMEDICINE

The use of nanotechnology in the field of medicine and drug delivery is growing rapidly. This is partially driven by a decrease in the rate of discovery of new biologically active compounds to be therapeutically exploited. Therefore, interest in the use of nanoparticles as versatile and multifunctional vectors for drug delivery has grown rapidly in recent years. Among the desirable properties of nanomaterials are better pharmacokinetic properties, controlled and sustained release, and targeting of specific cells, tissues, or organs (for example, developing new ways of crossing the blood–brain barrier). These features are all believed to improve the efficacy of existing drugs [16].

In the field of drug delivery, common nanoscale vectors for drug delivery include liposomes, micelles, dendrimers, solid lipid nanoparticles, metallic nanoparticles, semiconductor nanoparticles, and polymeric nanoparticles. These materials have been commonly used to deliver drugs, genes, vaccines, and diagnostics to specific cells and/or tissues [17].

Properties that make the use of nanoscale drug delivery vectors attractive are reduced toxicity and side effects owing to the fact a small dose of drug can be delivered to a specific site. However, it has recently been recognized that patients may be put at risk by the carrier systems themselves. A variety of different substances are currently under investigation for the preparation of nanoparticles for drug delivery, varying from chemical systems, such as polymers and solid metals containing nanoparticles, to more biological substances, for example, albumin, gelatin, and phospholipids. As these materials are small enough to cross barriers previously impenetrable to drugs it has been recognized that the potential interaction with tissues and cells, and therefore the potential toxicity, greatly depends on the actual composition of the nanoparticles in question [18,19].

This being the case, it is unsurprising that the characterization of drug delivery nanoparticles has been the subject of a recent review by McNeil [20] in which the benefits of nanotechnology have been described but with warnings concerning the fact that the physical nature of the nanoparticles can interfere with conventional and standardized biocompatibility and immunotoxicity testing protocols. A further review of the subject led the same author to describe the physical and chemical property testing assays currently available, including batch-mode DLS, MALDI-TOF, zeta potential measurement, AFM, TEM, and SEM X-ray microanalysis of nanoparticles present in tissue or cultured cell thin sections [21]. NTA, being a recently developed technique, was not considered in this review but is, however, gaining use in the characterization of nanoparticulate suspensions being developed for drug delivery usage as is described below.

NTA in Nanomedicine

NTA has been applied to many areas of investigation within the field of drug delivery. Early work in this application looked at the characterization of casein micelles [22,23], the dispersion of poly(3,4-ethylenedioxythiophene) in organic liquids [24], and sodium caproate-mediated promotion of oral drug absorption [25]. Furthermore, recent work in nanomedicine, including NTA, has included the study of magnetic particles for use as magnetic resonance contrast agents [26] and holonium particles for use in radio ablation [27].

Jensen et al. [28] recently used NTA in their work on dendrimer structures being utilized as vehicles for the delivery of siRNA. They were able to show that an increase in dendrimer concentration resulted in changes in both modal size and particle size distribution. This indicated that electrostatic complexation results in an equilibrium between differently sized complex aggregates and allowed the optimum dendrimer structure for nucleic acid delivery to be determined. Further work on the analysis of polyamidoamine dendrimers included the work of Ciolkowski et al. [29], who utilized NTA to look at self-aggregation processes. Clementi et al. [30] worked on developing dendritic pol(ethylene glycol) (PEG)-bearing paclitaxel (PTX) and alendronate (ALN) for the targeted treatment of bone tumors. They were able to determine an average hydrodynamic diameter of 200 nm and the particle size distribution of their PTX-PEG-ALN and PTX-PEG conjugates through the use of NTA.

While working on the development of nanoparticles for use as gene delivery vehicles, Ghonaim and his coworkers [31–37] have reported extensively on the use of NTA to characterize physical changes in various nonviral plasmid DNA and siRNA delivery systems, brought about by chemical modifications to the lipopolamines and spermines contained within.

In a similar study, Ofek et al. [38] also characterized dendritic nanocarriers for the delivery of siRNA using NTA, and while investigating the application of gene delivery polymers in cell culture, Bhise et al. [39] measured particle size distribution through NTA. This work was then further extended into the development of an assay for quantitating plasmids encapsulated by polymer nanoparticles. In this instance, NTA was used to determine the number density of plasmids per 100 nm particle.

NTA has been used in the development of nonviral gene delivery systems based on a lipophilic plasmid DNA condensate [40] and poly(β-amino esters) [41].

Sunshine et al. [42] looked at the development of poly(beta-amino ester) (PBAEs) as a safe and effective means of gene delivery and concluded that they showed great potential owing to the fact that synthesis is simple and they are able to transfect a variety of cell types with high efficacy in vitro. Immediately prior to subretinal injection, NTA was used to characterize particle size. The successful transfection of the RPE in vivo suggested that these nanoparticles could be used to study a number of genetic diseases in the laboratory with the potential to treat debilitating eye diseases.

A field of constant development in the field of nanomedicine is the investigation into new imaging agents for cancer therapy. Plasmonic gold nanostars have been shown to exhibit tunable plasmons in the near infrared tissue optic window, generating intense two-photon photoluminescence capable of in vitro cell labeling and in vivo particle tracking. The multiparameter analysis capability of NTA not only allowed Yuan et al. [43] to determine the size of these nanostars before investigation, but also the concentration and zeta-potential.

An investigation into the reduction of toxic effects of the common clinical immunosuppressant mycophenolic acid (MPA) allowed Shirali et al. [44] to utilize NTA for checking particle size in the development of poly(lactic-co-glycolic acid) (PLGA) nanoparticle formulations.

The use of sustained release of encapsulated itraconazole from PGLA has been shown to be of use for the treatment of the endemic disease Paracoccidioidomycosis. Cunha-Azevedo [45] investigated this effect and, after characterizing the average size of the PGLA as 174 nm using NTA, found that the encapsulated delivery system exhibited improved performance along with a reduction in the cytotoxic effects.

Dimitrova [46] has recently described NTA in a discussion on the applications of subvisible particle analysis in the development of protein therapeutics, and Jouffray [47] has addressed the growing concern over the unexpected interactions of highly sensitive biotech drugs with the silicone oil that is commonly used as a lubricant coating in prefilled syringes. He was working on the production of an innovative immobilized cross-linked silicone coating, which significantly reduced subvisible particles while retaining lubrication performance, using NTA to show the reduction in numbers of 200- to 1000-nm particles between the novel silicone formulation and baked silicone and conventionally lubricated syringes. Similarly, Kumru et al. [48] studied the compatibility, physical stability, and characterization of an IgG4 monoclonal antibody after dilution into different intravenous administration bags using a combination of SE-HPLC, NTA, microflow digital imaging (MFI), and turbidity measurements to follow the formation of soluble aggregates and particulates. He noted, however, that NTA quantification results were interfered with by the presence of polysorbate 20.

An exploration into the challenges and opportunities in the advancement of nanomedicines carried out by Wei et al. [49] identified numerous needs, including that for robust and general methods for accurately characterizing nanoparticle shape, size, and composition and methodologies in engineering that allow the maintenance of low levels of nonspecific cytotoxicity and good levels of stability during storage. NTA and DLS were compared when carrying out size analysis of nanocarriers composed of (a) trimethyl chitosan (TMC), (b) 50:50 (PLGA), and (c) commercial liposomes showing that DLS rarely reported accurate data except in the more monodisperse sample types.

Photoactive drug carriers were studied by Reshetov [50] when NTA was used to show that liposomes with added mTHPC showed increases in structural stability of carriers in serum compared to un-PEGylated liposomes, which were shown to have faster kinetics of degradation.

Finally, Smith et al. [51] have used NTA to show that the change in flux was not a result of a change in size due to aggregation of the hemoglobin at the different pHs tested when confirming that alginate hydrogel has a negative impact on in vitro collagen 1 deposition by fibroblasts.

Encapsulation and Nanocarrier Production

Some of the earliest studies incorporating NTA in the field of nanocarrier production included investigations into cholesteric and nematic emulsions [52] and binary microgel thin films [53]. This led to further work where NTA was used to follow changes in size of nanocapsules for intestinal delivery and enhanced oral bioavailability of tacrolimus (a P-gp substrate) [54] as well as a range of other carriers [55–57].

As described in the methodology section of this chapter, the lower limit of detection of NTA is often reached when materials with low light-scattering properties are characterized. However, in spite of this property being present in micellar systems, Vakurov et al. [58] successfully used the technology to characterize this type of structure. This work was then built on as researchers looked at drug delivery micellar formulations for controlled release of covalently entrapped doxorubicin [59] and the encapsulation of mithramycin [60,61]. These later studies demonstrated that microfluidics is a powerful technology for nanoprecipitation-based production of drug-loaded polymeric micelles as compared to batch systems since it enabled better control, reproducibility, and homogeneity of the size characteristics of the produced micelles.

The work by Pazik et al. [62] looking at $BaTiO_3$ explored the surface functionalization of the metal oxide nanoparticles with biologically active molecules containing phosphonate moieties. A wealth of techniques were employed in the investigation, including SEM/energy dispersive spectroscopy, pH-metric titration, nuclear magnetic resonance (NMR) and infrared (IR) spectroscopy, dynamic light scattering, zeta potential, thermogravimetric analysis, and radiometric measurements with NTA aiding them to come to the conclusion that the application of amino phosphonic acids as surface ligands provided nanoparticles with considerable solution stability in an aqueous medium at neutral pH and especially in the presence of electrolytes, thus opening the broad prospect of applications for the thus produced nanoparticle dispersions in the domains of nano-optics and nanomagnetism.

Biosilicate nanoparticles formed by mimicking peptides using polyethyleneimine were fabricated and characterized by Neville et al. [63]. Using a combination of NTA and TEM, they characterized for the first time nanoparticles made from tetramethyl orthosilicate to entrap enzymes. This work was built on and explained further in a recent report on the production and characterization of bioactive thiol-silicate nanoparticles [64]. Zu et al. [65] have also described the preparation of ultrafine polyethylene-silica composite particles with a core-shell structure using SEM observation and NTA to determine particle sphericity and a mean size of 160 nm, respectively.

Sokolova et al. [66] used the respective benefits of SEM, DLS, analytical ultracentrifugation, and NTA to analyze size, surface charge, and morphology of nanoparticles in their investigation into the dendritic cell maturation and T cell activation through the application of calcium phosphate nanoparticles encapsulating toll-like receptor ligands and the antigen hemagglutinin. Similarly, recent developments of a nanoparticulate formulation of retinoic acid that suppresses Th17 cells and upregulates regulatory T cells employed NTA to measure particle size [67], and the stability of nanometer-sized prodrug (nanoprodrug) production by a spontaneous emulsification mechanism was confirmed by NTA to be constant at 120–140 nm in diameter [68].

Geng et al. [69] used NTA to establish that the development and characterizations of maleimide-functionalized biopolymer (Mal-PGA-Asp) as an effective targeted drug delivery carrier synthesized from an amidation reaction between aspartylated PGA (PGA-Asp) and N-(maleimidohexanoyl)-ethylenediamine (NME) led to significantly enhanced cellular uptake of TP13-Mal-PGA-Asp3-Pt in the human hepatoma cell line SMMC-7721 as shown by fluorescence imaging and flow cytometry. NTA was used to show the biopolymer had an average size 87 ± 28 nm.

During attempts to improve the homogeneity of nanosized lipid vesicles made by constant pressure-controlled extrusion processes for use as drug delivery vehicles, NTA, DLS, and EM were all used to characterize the degree of polydispersity within the product [70]. NTA was also used in determining the optimum formulation of albumin based theragnostic nanoparticles as a potential delivery system for tumor targeting, and when used in conjunction with DLS confirmed that the optimized nanoparticle formulation had a modal size of 125 nm [71].

The counting capability of NTA was put to use in the study by Wrenn et al. [72] as they looked at the number and size of liposomes when exposed to ultrasound in an initial attempt to distinguish mechanisms and quantify the relative contributions of liposome destruction versus diffusion through the bilayer. It was shown that the overall number of liposomes decreased with an increase in ultrasound exposure time with nearly 50% of the reduction occurring within the first 4 minutes of exposure. This result strongly implied that some vesicle destruction occurs as a result of exposure, a view that is consistent with prior studies by the group.

Yandrapu et al. [73] used NTA to characterize dendrimer conjugates in their study for the development of novel thiolated dendrimers for mucoadhesive drug delivery. The study showed that their developed particles exhibited sustained release of acyclovir and higher levels of mucoadhesion.

In a study to develop curcumin-loaded lipid-core nanocapsules (C-LNC), in an attempt to improve the antiglioma activity of this polyphenol, visualization of the C-LNC was carried out by NTA. The data obtained suggested that the nanoencapsulation of curcumin in LNC is an important strategy to improve its pharmacological efficacy in the treatment of gliomas [74].

A recent set of experiments explored the effect of different relative humidity conditions on the stability of freeze-dried formulations containing trehalose or melibiose. NTA was used to determine there to be a huge range polydisperisty with particle sizes starting at 50 nm and going up to 1000 nm [75].

Using DLS and NTA to confirm formulation unimodal size distribution (with polydispersity value <0.1 from DLS) at the nanoemulsion as well as the multiunit pellet system (MUPS) stage, Sangwai et al. [76] reported a nanoemulsified poorly water-soluble antiobesity drug *Orlistat*-embedded MUPS with improved dissolution and pancreatic lipase inhibition.

Targeting and Delivery

In order to target drug delivery nanoparticles to specific sites, the addition of molecular structures with an affinity for specific cell surface biomarkers is frequently required. This allows the drug-containing nanoparticle to be accumulated by the target cell types presenting such biomarker structures. The addition of such capture molecules (frequently antibodies) to the surface of the drug delivery nanoparticle structure can be problematic, retention of activity, sufficient loading, and minimization of aggregation being necessary for optimum performance. Similarly, addition of other biochemical species designed to stabilize the functional structures added to the nanoparticles or which act to reduce the immunogenicity of the nanoparticle may result in similar deleterious effects. NTA is capable of detecting small changes in hydrodynamic diameter following the addition of layers of macromolecules to nanoparticles and can both detect and enumerate any aggregates that may form during such modifications.

As a result of this ability to see small differences in hydrodynamic diameter, NTA has been used in a number of studies of this nature, including the work by Miller et al. [77] looking at the effect of conjugating polymer-alendronate-taxane complexes for use in targeting bone metastases. This work was continued, and the group showed, through the use of NTA, that successful conjugation for the targeting of angiogenesis-dependent calcified neoplasms using different polymers resulted in very much smaller sizes and narrower polydispersities and that together with a cathepsin-K-cleavable system they achieved a more specific drug release and therefore focused the toxicity of the free drugs to the bone tumor.

In the development of novel nanoscale immunization vector modules (Ag, adjuvant and carrier), which were assembled into units that were optimized for stimulating immune responses to specific pathogens, including the Dengue and West Nile (WN) flaviviruses, Demento et al. [78] used NTA to help optimize immune responses in mice.

Inclusion of affinity tags has greatly facilitated process development for protein antigens, primarily for their recovery from complex mixtures, and although generally viewed as supportive of product development, affinity tags may have unintended consequences on protein solubility, susceptibility to aggregation, and immunogenicity. Accordingly, Khan et al. [79] employed NTA to establish particle sizes and, importantly, concentrations, showing the influence of His-affinity tags on protein expression levels, solubility, secondary structure, thermal denaturation, aggregation, and the impact on humoral and cellular immune responses in mice, the results of which suggested the usefulness of affinity tags may be outweighed by their potential impact on structure and function, stressing the need for caution in their use.

Moddaresi et al. [80] monitored the rate of Browning motion and showed that semisolid gel hyaluronic acid matrices, used for the application of drug delivery nanovesicles (in this case Tocopheryl acetate [TA] lipid nanoparticles), inhibited the mobility. However, varying the particle mobility within the gel by changing the concentration of hyaluronic acid used had little effect on the TA delivery. This suggested that the limiting step within the drug delivery process was not the nanoparticle vehicle–skin interaction, but rather the drug release from the lipid nanoparticles.

Bhuiyan [81] used NTA to characterize liposome preparations and showed that localized drug release from thermosensitive liposomes could be induced by hypothermia.

Mazzarino et al. [82] developed a chitosan-coated nanoparticle loaded with curcuma for mucoadhesive applications when working on designing drug delivery vehicles capable of buccal delivery. This was created by the nanoprecipitation methodology using different molar masses and concentrations of chitosan and concentrations of triblock surfactant poloxamer (PEO–PPO–PEO) in order to optimize the preparation conditions. Studies using DLS at different angles suggested that the preparations were fairly monodispersed with polydispersity indices of lower that 0.3 being reported. These same systems were also analyzed by NTA, which produced values in accordance with those that would be expected given the DLS data. Colloidal systems showed mean drug content about 460 μg/mL and encapsulation efficiency higher than 99%. When coated with chitosan, these nanoparticles show a great ability to interact with mucin, indicating also their suitability for mucoadhesive applications.

Thermosensitive hydrogels were the subject of another study by de Graaf et al. [83] in which they developed a micelle-shedding thermosensitive hydrogel based on poly(N-isopropylacrylamide)-poly(ethylene glycol)-poly(N-isopropylacrylamide) (pNIPAm-PEG-pNIPAm), a sustained-release formulation for the delivery of the cytostatic agent paclitaxel (PTX). They showed that, at the highest dose, PTX completely inhibited tumor growth for at least 3 weeks with a single hydrogel injection. This promising concept may find application as a depot formulation for sustained, metronomic dosing of chemotherapeutics.

Corradetti et al. [84] used affinity targeted biodegradable nanoparticles to mediate paracrine stimulation as an alternative approach to sustain the growth and pluripotency of mouse embryonic stem cells. They showed sustained release of leukaemia inhibitory factor (LIF) from nanoparticles composed of a solid poly(lactide-co-glycolic acid) polyester or a hydrogel-based liposomal system, which they termed Nanolipogel, replenished once after each cell passage.

Other examples of the importance of sizing and enumerating nanoparticulate drug delivery systems by NTA have been reported [85–87]. In a study involving dissolution measurements of polydisperse smoke particles in a liquid-based suspension, Cabot et al. [88] used NTA to measure changes in tobacco smoke particle size over a series of different time points, providing an input into residence time estimates, thus aiding dose calculations to the lower airways.

As well as being used for delivery and treatment, nanoparticles have also found use in certain areas as aides for detection. An example of this is the work of Wang and Vo-Dinh [89], who used plasmonic coupling interference (PCI) nanoprobes for the detection of nucleic acid using surface-enhanced Raman scattering (SERS). NTA was required in this investigation to show the potential of these nucleic acid diagnostic tools for biomedical diagnostics and biosensing applications. Similarly, Kell et al. [90] developed a silica nanoparticle-based DNA biosensor capable of detecting *Bacillus anthracis* bacteria through the use of unlabeled ss-oligonucleotides. The biosensor makes use of the optical changes that accompany a nanoparticle-immobilized cationic conjugated polymer (polythiophene) interacting with single-stranded versus hybridized oligonucleotides, where a fluorescence signal appears only when hybridized DNA is present (i.e., only when the ss-oligonucleotide interacting with the polymer has hybridized with its complement). NTA was used to show that the silica nanoparticle scaffold employed in this investigation was 196 ± 36 nm in diameter in close correlation to the 188 ± 30 nm in diameter as measured by TEM.

The delivery of siRNA to cell systems has been the subject of much recent work as a way to enhance human mesenchymal stem cell (hMSC) differentiation via RNA interference (RNAi), which could provide an effective way of controlling cell fate for tissue engineering, but a safe and effective delivery vehicle must first be developed. Tzeng et al. [91] employed cystamine-terminated poly (beta-amino ester) to this end, using NTA to follow size and concentration of different polymer formulations of nanoparticle production. Tzeng and Green [92] then extended this work to explore subtle changes to the polymer structure and degradation mechanisms of such structures for the highly effective siRNA and DNA delivery to human brain tumors.

SiRNA delivery has also been studied through the use of cell-penetrating peptides (CPPs), which are short cationic peptides that have been extensively studied as drug delivery vehicles for proteins, nucleic acids, and nanoparticles. A newly developed CPP, PepFect 14 (PF14), which forms noncovalent nanocomplexes with short interfering RNA (siRNA), was shown to elicit efficient RNA-interference (RNAi) response in different cell lines. NTA was used to demonstrate stability of the nanoparticles on drying and resuspension [93].

As no standard technique for the size measurement of siRNA polyplexes was currently available, Troiber et al. [94] compared four different particle-sizing techniques. The four analytical techniques compared and evaluated for their suitability to analyze the characteristics of homogeneous and heterogeneous siRNA polyplexes were DLS, AFM, NTA, and FCS. The results showed that while some of the smallest 40-nm particles were of too low a refractive index to be visualized and tracked using NTA, the larger particles within the sample (those around 120 nm) could be sized using all of the methods that were assessed.

A key point in biology and medicine is the successful transportation of molecules across the cell membrane. In most cases, an efficient carrier is required as molecules cannot penetrate the cell membrane alone. Sokolova et al. [95] investigated calcium phosphate nanoparticles as a versatile carrier for small and large molecules across cell membranes. They characterized their material with a variety of techniques, including EM, DLS, and NTA, and found the particles to vary in size from 100 nm to 250 nm in diameter dependent on the functionalization. Ohlsson et al. [96] used NTA to check the stability and integrity of liposomes when looking into solute transport on the sub 100 ms scale across the lipid bilayer membrane.

Brinkhuis et al. [97] utilized the ability of NTA to determine the zeta potential of particle populations to establish this value for polymersomes, self-assembled from the block copolymer polybutadiene-block-poly(ethylene glycol), in investigating of the size-dependent biodistribution and single-photon emission computed tomography imaging of 111In-labeled polymersomes. The results showed that size will influence the pharmacokinetics, much more so than for liposomes, and as a result, long circulating preparations should be kept well below 100 nm.

Chitosan-based nanoparticles were also studied using NTA for gene and siRNA delivery [98] and as permeating vectors for the blood–brain barrier when functionalized with alkylglyceryl [99].

Exosomes and Microvesicles

The recent and very rapid growth of interest in and research on exosomes and microvesicles and their therapeutic potential has already resulted in the use of NTA to both detect and size these structures. Thus, van Dommelen et al. [100] has reviewed the potential for microvesicles and exosomes to be used in drug delivery given they would appear to be capable of delivering lipids, proteins, mRNA, and microRNA to change the phenotype of the receiving cells. They concluded that although a number of limiting factors in the clinical translation of the exciting research findings so far exist, it is promising for the development of a potentially novel generation of drug carriers.

Zhu et al. [101] employed a quartz crystal microbalance with the dissipation monitor method in their study of lipid exchange between membranes and the effects of membrane surface charge, composition, and curvature on the exchange. They showed that vesicle adsorption rate, membrane lateral pressure gradient, and lipid lateral diffusion coefficient are critical in deciding the lipid exchange kinetics between membranes. NTA was used in order to determine that vesicle size was inversely proportional to the membrane contact area, which directly affected the intermembrane lipid exchange rate.

Both membrane curvature and lipid composition have roles in regulating important biological processes within a cell. At present, several proteins have been reported in the literature to sense and/or induce membrane curvatures, for example, synaptotagmin-1 and amphiphysin. Morton et al. [102] identified a 25-mer peptide, MARCKS-ED, based on the effector domain sequence of the intracellular membrane protein myristoylated alanine-rich C-kinase substrate that can recognize plasma serum with preferences for highly curved vesicles in a sequence-specific manner. These studies further contribute to the understanding of how proteins and peptides sense membrane curvature as well as providing potential probes for membrane shape and lipid composition with NTA being used to monitor vesicle size.

Calò et al. [103] recognized the potential of natural vesicles produced from genetically engineered cells with tailored membrane receptor composition as building blocks for sensing biodevices. NTA was used in order to establish vesicle size in liquid suspension while AFM was used to show that nanovesicles deposit and flatten without rupturing on glass substrates. It has been claimed that this is an important step in the practical realization of biosensor devices based on natural nanovesicles integrating G-protein coupled membrane receptors.

Vallhov et al. [104] used a number of sophisticated techniques in an investigation into the potential of exosomes for use in vaccine and immune therapeutic strategies. These techniques included flow cytometry, confocal laser scanning microscopy, and multispectral imaging flow cytometry for characterizing interactions with other cell types, while EM and NTA proved to be useful in discrimination between exosomes and virions in exosome preparations.

Recent investigations into prostasomes (microvesicles shed from the prostate gland) as mediators of intracellular communication and their potential to provide new therapeutic and diagnostic strategies allowed NTA to be used to confirm prostasome size as being 143 nm [105].

Simonsson et al. [106] presented an amperometric study of content release from individual vesicles in an artificial secretory cell, designed with the minimal components required to carry out exocytosis using NTA, to measure catechol-filled large unilamellar vesicles at an average diameter of ~200 nm. In fact, using NTA, they observed that catechol filled vesicles are larger (mean diameter ≈200 nm) than vesicles typically obtained from extrusion though a 100 nm pore–sized polycarbonate filter.

CONCLUSION

NTA is a technique for the direct and real-time visualization, sizing, and counting of nanoscale materials in liquid suspension. It is based on the well-understood principles of light scattering and the relationship between the rate of Brownian motion and the sphere equivalent hydrodynamic diameters of particles in suspension. The nature in which particles are tracked on an individual basis allows high-resolution particle size distributions to be obtained along with information on the concentration of materials.

The ability for the technique to measure simultaneously more than one parameter, such as zeta potential, fluorescent properties, or amount of light scattered, allows users to obtain an unprecedentedly rich profile of nanoparticle properties. This along with the unique visual validation available to users has proved useful in a variety of nanomedical applications, ranging from encapsulation and nanocarrier production to targeting and delivery.

REFERENCES

1. Bohren C. F., and Huffman D. R. 1983. *Absorption and Scattering of Light by Small Particles*, John Wiley & Sons. ISBN: 9780471293408.
2. Dragovic R. A., Gardiner C., Brooks A. S., Tannetta D. S., Ferguson D. J. P., Hole P., Carr B. et al. 2011. Sizing and phenotyping of cellular vesicles using nanoparticle tracking analysis, *Nanomedicine: Nanotechnology, Biology and Medicine*, Volume 7, Issue 6, December 2011, Pages 780–788.
3. Saveyn H., De Baets B., Thas O., Hole P., Smith J., and Van der Meeren P. 2010. Accurate particle size distribution determination by nanoparticle tracking analysis based on 2-D Brownian dynamics simulation, *Journal of Colloid and Interface Science*, Volume 352, Pages 593–600.

4. Filipe V., Hawe A., and Jiskoot W. 2010. Critical evaluation of nanoparticle tracking analysis (NTA) by NanoSight for the measurement of nanoparticles and protein aggregates, *Pharmaceutical Research*, Volume 27, Number 5, Pages 796–810.
5. Mahl D., Diendorf J., Meyer-Zaika W., and Epple M. 2011. Possibilities and limitations of different analytical methods for the size determination of a bimodal dispersion of metallic nanoparticles, *Colloids and Surfaces A: Physicochemical and Engineering Aspects*, Volume 377, Issues 1–3, 5 March 2011, Pages 386–392.
6. Boyd R. D., Pichaimuthu S. K., and Cuenat A. 2011. New approach to inter-technique comparisons for nanoparticle size measurements; using atomic force microscopy, nanoparticle tracking analysis and dynamic light scattering, *Colloids and Surfaces A: Physicochemical and Engineering Aspects*, Volume 387, Issues 1–3, 20 August 2011, Pages 35–42.
7. Van der Meeren P., Kasinos M., and Saveyn H. 2012. Relevance of two-dimensional Brownian motion dynamics in applying nanoparticle tracking analysis, *Nanoparticles in Biology and Medicine, Methods in Molecular Biology*, 2012, Volume 906, Pages 525–534.
8. Gayatri K., Lakshmi G., and Preeti K. 2012. Nanoparticles—An overview of preparation and characterization, *Novel Science International Journal of Pharmaceutical Science*, Volume 1, Issue 8, Pages 557–562.
9. Liu J. 2012. Nanoparticle Size Measurement by Nanoparticle Tracking Analysis (NTA) Method, *Metrology for Green Growth*, September 9–14, 2012, Busan, Republic of Korea.
10. Du S., Kendall K., Toloueinia P., Mehrabadi Y., Gupta G., and Newton J. 2012. Aggregation and adhesion of gold nanoparticles in phosphate buffered saline, *Journal of Nanoparticle Research*, Volume 14, Number 3, Page 758.
11. Troiber C., Kasper J. C., Milani S., Scheible M., Martin I., Schaubhut F., Küchler S. et al. 2012. Comparison of four different particle sizing methods for siRNA polyplex characterization, *European Journal of Pharmaceutics and Biopharmaceutics*, Volume 84, Issue 2, June 2013, Pages 255–264.
12. Gallego-Urrea J. A., Tuoriniemi J., and Hassellöv M. 2011. Applications of particle-tracking analysis to the determination of size distributions and concentrations of nanoparticles in environmental, biological and food samples, *TrAC Trends in Analytical Chemistry*, Volume 30, Issue 3, Pages 473–483.
13. Dean L. 2012. Size Matters, *Chemistry International*, July–August 2012, Pages 6–9.
14. James A. E., and Driskell J. 2012. Monitoring Gold Nanoparticle Conjugation and Analysis of Biomolecular Binding with Nanoparticle Tracking Analysis (NTA) and Dynamic Light Scattering (DLS), *Analyst*, 2012, Issue 4, Pages 1212–1218.
15. ASTM E2834 – 12. 2012. *Standard Guide for Measurement of Particle Size Distribution of Nanomaterials in Suspension by Nanoparticle Tracking Analysis (NTA)*, Active Standard ASTM E2834 Developed by Subcommittee: E56.02|Book of Standards Volume: 14.02.
16. Malam Y., Lim E., and Seifalian A. 2011. Current Trends in the Application of Nanoparticles in Drug Delivery, *Current Medicinal Chemistry*, Volume 18, Number 7, March 2011, Pages 1067–1078.
17. Ram M., Yaduvanshi K. S., Yadav H., Singh N., Mangla G., and Shivakumar H. 2011. Nanoparticles, Promising Carriers in Drug Targeting: A Review, *Current Drug Therapy*, Volume 6, Number 2, May 2011, Pages 87–96.
18. De Jong W. H., and Borm P. J. 2008. Drug delivery and nanoparticles: Applications and hazards, *International Journal of Nanomedicine*, Volume 3, Issue 2, Pages 133–149.
19. Moquin A., and Winnik F. M. 2012. The Use of FieldFlow Fractionation for the Analysis of Drug and Gene Delivery Systems, *Field-Flow Fractionation in Biopolymer Analysis* (eds. S. Kim R. Williams, K. D. Caldwell). ISBN3709101530, Chapter 13, Pages 187–207.

20. McNeil S. E. 2011. Unique Benefits of Nanotechnology to Drug Delivery and Diagnostics, Characterization of Nanoparticles Intended for Drug Delivery (ed. S. E. McNeil), *Methods in Molecular Biology*, 2011, Volume 697, Part 1, Pages 3–8, doi: 10.1007/978-1-60327-198-1_1
21. McNeil S. E. 2011. Challenges for Nanoparticle Characterization, Characterization of Nanoparticles Intended for Drug Delivery (ed. S. E. McNeil), *Methods in Molecular Biology*, 2011, Volume 697, Part 1, Pages 3–8, doi: 10.1007/978-1-60327-198-1_1
22. Thu T. L., Saveyn P., Hoa H. D., and Van der Meeren P. 2007. A nanoparticle tracking analysis study of size distributions of casein micelle dispersions, *International Dairy Journal*, 20th Asian Food Conference, Malaysia.
23. Thu T. L., Saveyn P., Hoa H. D., and Van der Meeren P. 2008. Determination of heat-induced effects on the particle size distribution of casein micelles by dynamic light scattering and nanoparticle tracking analysis, *International Dairy Journal*, Volume 18, Issue 12, Pages 1090–1096.
24. Kim T. Y., Lee T. H., Kim J. E., Kasi R. M., Sung C. S. P., and Suh K. S. 2008. Organic solvent dispersion of poly(3,4-ethylenedioxythiophene) with the use of polymeric ionic liquid, *Journal of Polymer Science Part A: Polymer Chemistry*, Volume 46, Pages 6872–6879.
25. Maher S., Leonard T. W., Jacobsen J., and Brayden D. J. 2009. Safety and efficacy of sodium caprate in promoting oral drug absorption: From in vitro to the clinic, *Advanced Drug Delivery Reviews*, Volume 61, Issue 15, Pages 1427–1449.
26. Banerjee R., Katsenovich Y., Lagos L., McIintosh M., Zhang X., and Li C.-Z. 2010. Nanomedicine: Magnetic nanoparticles and their biomedical applications, *Current Medicinal Chemistry*, Volume 17, Number 27, September 2010, Pages 3120–3141.
27. Bult W., Varkevisser R., Soulimani F., Seevinck P. R., de Leeuw H., Bakker C. J. G., Luijten P. R., van het Schip A. D., Hennink W. E., and Nijsen J. F. W. 2010. Holmium nanoparticles: Preparation and in vitro characterization of a new device for radioablation of solid malignancies, *Pharmaceutical Research*, Volume 27, Issue 10, Pages 2205–2212.
28. Jensen L. B., Pavan G. M., Kasimova M. R., Rutherford S., Danani A., Nielsen H. M., and Foged C. 2011. Elucidating the molecular mechanism of PAMAM-siRNA dendriplex self-assembly: Effect of dendrimer charge density, *International Journal of Pharmaceutics*, Volume 416, Issue 2, Pages 410–418.
29. Ciolkowski M., Rozanek M., Szewczyk M., Klajnert B., and Bryszewska M. 2011. The influence of PAMAM-OH dendrimers on the activity of human erythrocytes ATPases, *Biochimica et Biophysica Acta (BBA)—Biomembranes*, Volume 1808, Issue 11, Pages 2714–2723.
30. Clementi C., Miller K., Mero A., Satchi-Fainaro R., and Pasut G. 2011. Dendritic Poly(ethylene glycol) Bearing Paclitaxel and Alendronate for Targeting Bone Neoplasms, *Molecular Pharmaceutics*, Volume 8, Issue 4, Pages 1063–1072.
31. Ghonaim H. M., Li S., Soltan M. K., Pourzand C., and Blagbrough I. S. 2007. *Chain Length Modulation in Symmetrical Lipopolyamines and the effect on Nanoparticle Formulations for Gene Delivery*, British Pharmaceutical Conference BPC2007, Manchester, 10 Sept.
32. Ghonaim H., Li S., and Blagbrough I. S., 2009. Very long chain N4, N9-diacyl spermines: Non-viral lipopolyamine vectors for efficient plasmid DNA and siRNA delivery, *Pharmaceutical Research*, Volume 26, Number 1, Pages 19–31.
33. Ghonaim H. M. 2008. *Design and Development of Pharmaceutical Dosage Forms for Gene and siRNA Delivery*, PhD Thesis University of Bath, Department of Pharmacy and Pharmacology, September 2008.
34. Ghonaim H. M., Li S., Pourzand C., and Blagbrough I. S. 2007. *Efficient Novel Unsymmetrical Lipopolyamine Formulations for Gene Delivery*, British Pharmaceutical Conference BPC2007, Manchester, 10 Sept.

35. Ghonaim H. M., Li S., Pourzand C., and Blagbrough I. S. 2007. *Formulation and Delivery of Fluorescent siRNA by Lipospermine Nanoparticle Complex Formation*, British Pharmaceutical Conference BPC2007, Manchester, 10 Sept.
36. Soltan M. K., Ghonaim H. M., El Sadek M., Kull M. A., El-aziz L. A., and Blagbrough I. S. 2009. Design and synthesis of N4, N9-disubstituted spermines for non-viral siRNA delivery—Structure-activity relationship studies of siFection efficiency versus toxicity, *Pharmaceutical Research*, Volume 26, Number 2, Pages 286–295.
37. Ghonaim H. M., Li S., and Blagbrough I. S. 2010. N1,N12-Diacyl spermines: SAR studies on non-viral lipopolyamine vectors for plasmid DNA and siRNA formulation, *Pharmaceutical Research*, Volume 27, Issue 1, Pages 17–29.
38. Ofek P., Fischer W., Calderón M., Haag R., and Satchi-Fainaro R. 2010. In vivo delivery of small interfering RNA to tumors and their vasculature by novel dendritic nanocarriers, *The FASEB Journal*, Volume 24, Issue 9, Pages 3122–3134.
39. Bhise N. S., Gray R. S., Sunshine J. C., Htet S., Ewald A. J., and Green J. J. 2010. The relationship between terminal functionalization and molecular weight of a gene delivery polymer and transfection efficacy in mammary epithelial 2-D cultures and 3-D organotypic cultures, *Biomaterials*, Volume 31, Issue 31, November 2010, Pages 8088–8096.
40. Do T. T., Tang V. J., Aguilera J. A., Perry C. C., and Milligan J. R. 2011. Characterization of a lipophilic plasmid DNA condensate formed with a cationic peptide fatty acid conjugate, *Biomacromolecules*, Volume 12, Issue 5, Pages 1731–1737.
41. Tzeng S. Y., Guerrero-Cázares H., Martinez E. E., Sunshine J. C., Quiñones-Hinojosa A., and Green J. J. 2011. Non-viral gene delivery nanoparticles based on Poly(β-amino esters) for treatment of glioblastoma, *Biomaterials*, Volume 32, Issue 23, Pages 5402–5410.
42. Sunshine J. C., Sunshine S. B., Bhutto I., Handa J. T., and Green J. J. 2012. Poly(β-amino ester)-nanoparticle mediated transfection of retinal pigment epithelial cells in vitro and in vivo, *PLoS One*, Volume 7, Issue 5, Page 1.
43. Yuan H., Khoury C., Fales A., Wilson C., Grant G., and Vo-Dinh T. 2012. Plasmonic gold nanostars: A potential agent for molecular imaging and cancer therapy, *Biomedical Optics*, Miami Florida, April 28–May 2, 2012.
44. Shirali A. C., Look M., Du W., Kassis E., Stout-Delgado H. W., Fahmy T. M., and Goldstein D. R. 2011. Nanoparticle delivery of mycophenolic acid upregulates PD-L1 on dendritic cells to prolong murine allograft survival, *American Journal of Transplantation*, Volume 11, Issue 12, Pages 2582–2592.
45. Cunha-Azevedo E. P. 2011. *Biodegradable nanoparticles of PLGA, covered with DMSA, containing itraconazole for treatment of Paracoccidioidomycosis*, PhD Thesis (PhD in health sciences)—University of Brasília, Brasília, 2011.
46. Dimitrova M. 2011. *Applications of sub-visible particle analysis in the development of protein therapeutics*, Proc FIP Pharmaceutical Sciences 2010 World Congress, November 14–18, 2010, Morial Convention Center, New Orleans, Louisiana.
47. Jouffray S. 2012. *Advancements in prefilled syringe technology: Improving compatibility with biologics with a novel cross-linked silicone coating*, http://www.ondrugdelivery.com/publications/Injectable%20Devices%202012/BD.pdf, Frederick Furness Publishing.
48. Kumru O. S., Liu J., Ji J. A., Cheng W., Wang Y. J., Wang T., Joshi S. B., Middaugh C. R., and Volkin D. B. 2012. Compatibility, physical stability, and characterization of an IgG4 monoclonal antibody after dilution into different intravenous administration bags, *Journal of Pharmaceutical Sciences*, Volume 101, Issue 10, Pages 3636–3650.
49. Wei A., Mehtala J. G., and Patri A. K. 2012. Challenges and opportunities in the advancement of nanomedicines, *Journal of Controlled Release*, Volume 164, Issue 2, 10 December 2012, Pages 236–246.

50. Reshetov L. 2012. *Photobiological properties of photoactive nanoparticles for the treatment of Cancer*, Ecole Doctorale BioSE (Biologie-Santé-Environnement) UThèse, http://tel.archives-ouvertes.fr/docs/00/76/13/00/PDF/Thesis_Vadim_RESHETOV_FINAL.pdf
51. Smith A., Hunt N. C., Shelton R. M., Birdi G., and Grover L. M. 2012. Alginate hydrogel has a negative impact on in vitro collagen 1 deposition by fibroblasts, *Biomacromolecules*, Volume 13, Issue 12, Pages 4032–4038.
52. Tixier T., Heppenstall-Butler M., and Terentjev E. M. 2006. Spontaneous size selection in cholesteric and nematic emulsions, *Langmuir*, Volume 22, Issue 5, Pages 2365–2370.
53. Sorrell C. D., and Lyon L. A. 2008. Deformation controlled assembly of binary microgel thin films, *Langmuir*, 2008, Volume 24, Issue 14, Pages 7216–7222.
54. Nyska A., and Benita S. 2009. Novel double coated nanocapsules for intestinal delivery and enhanced oral bioavailability of tacrolimus, a P-gp substrate drug, *Journal of Controlled Release*, Volume 133, Issue 1, Pages 77–84.
55. Debotton N., Harush-Frenkel O., Gofrit O., and Benita S. 2010. *Antibody-nanocarrier conjugates for drug targeting and improved cancer therapy*, Unither Nanomedical & Telemedical Technology Conference—The Future's Approach to Medicine, Hotel Manoir Des Sables, Orford (Quebec), Canada, 23–26 February, 2010.
56. Sundar S., Kundu J., and Kundu S. C. 2010. Biopolymeric nanoparticles, *Science and Technology of Advanced Materials*, Volume 11, Issue 1.
57. Smith M. H., South A. B., Gaulding J. C., and Lyon L. A. 2010. Monitoring the erosion of hydrolytically-degradable nanogels via multiangle light scattering coupled to asymmetrical flow field-flow fractionation, *Analytical Chemistry*, Volume 82, Issue 2, Pages 523–530.
58. Vakurov A., Pchelintsev N. A., Forde J., Ó'Fágáin C., Gibson T., and Millner P. 2009. The preparation of size-controlled functionalized polymeric nanoparticles in micelles, *Nanotechnology*, Volume 20, Issue 29, Page 7.
59. Talelli M., Iman M., Varkouhi A. K., Rijcken C. J. F., Schiffelers R. M., Etrych T., Ulbrich K. et al. 2010. Core-crosslinked polymeric micelles with controlled release of covalently entrapped doxorubicin, *Biomaterials*, Volume 31, Issue 30, Pages 7797–7804.
60. Capretto L., Hill M., Zhang X., Mazzitelli S., and Nastruzzi C. 2010. *Microfluidic production of polymeric micelles for mithramycin encapsulation*, XVIII International Conference on Bioencapsulation—Porto, Portugal—October 1–2, 2010, Abstract No. O2-3.
61. Capretto L., Carugo D., Cheng W., Hill M., and Zhang X. 2011. Continuous-flow production of polymeric micelles in microreactors: Experimental and computational analysis, *Journal of Colloid and Interface Science*, Volume 357, Issue 1, Pages 243–251.
62. Pazik R., Andersson R., Kepinski L., Nedelec J.-M., Kessler V. G., and Seisenbaeva G. A. 2011. Surface Functionalization of the Metal Oxide Nanoparticles with Biologically Active Molecules Containing Phosphonate Moieties. Case Study of $BaTiO_3$, *Journal of Biomedical Materials Research*, Volume 115, Issue 20, Pages 9850–9860.
63. Neville F., Broderick M. J. F., Gibson T., and Millner P. A. 2010. Fabrication and activity of silicate nanoparticles and nanosilicate-entrapped enzymes using polyethyleneimine as a biomimetic polymer, *Langmuir*, Volume 27, Issue 1, Pages 279–285.
64. Neville F. and Millner P. 2011. Fabrication and characterization of bioactive thiol-silicate nanoparticles, *Methods in Molecular Biology, Nanoscale Biocatalysis*, Volume 743, Pages 131–145.
65. Zu L., Han S. Y., Gu K., and Cui X. G. 2012. Preparation of ultrafine polyethylene-silica composite particle with core-shell structure, *Advanced Materials Research*, Volumes 557–559, Pages 554–557.

66. Sokolova V., Knuschke T., Kovtun A., Buer J., Epple M., and Westendorf A. M. 2010. The use of calcium phosphate nanoparticles encapsulating Toll-like receptor ligands and the antigen hemagglutinin to induce dendritic cell maturation and T cell activation, *Biomaterials*, Volume 31, Issue 21, Pages 5627–5633.
67. Capurso N. A., Look M., Jeanbart L., Nowyhed H., Abraham C., Craft J., and Fahmy T. M. 2010. Development of a nanoparticulate formulation of retinoic acid that suppresses Th17 cells and upregulates regulatory T cells, *Self/Nonself*, Volume 1, Issue 4, Pages 1–6.
68. Lee B.-S., Yoon C., Osipov A., Moghavem N., Nwachokor D., Amatya R., Na R. et al. 2011. Nanoprodrugs of NSAIDs: Preparation and characterization of flufenamic acid nanoprodrugs, *Journal of Drug Delivery*, Volume 2011, Article ID 980720, doi: 10.1155/2011/980720
69. Geng X., Ye H., Feng Z., Lao X., Zhang L., Huang J., Wu Z.-R. 2012. Synthesis and characterization of cisplatinloaded, EGFR-targeted biopolymer and in vitro evaluation for targeted delivery, *Journal of Biomedical Materials Research Part A*, Volume 100, Issue 10, Pages 2839–2848.
70. Morton L. A., Saludes J. P., and Yin H. 2012. Constant pressure-controlled extrusion method for the preparation of nano-sized lipid vesicles, *Journal of Visualized Experiments (JoVE)*, Volume 64, e4151, doi: 10.3791/4151 (2012).
71. Kolluru L. P., Syed A., Rizvi A., D'Souza M., and D'Souza M. J. 2012. Formulation development of albumin based theragnostic nanoparticles as a potential delivery system for tumor targeting, *Journal of Drug Targeting*, Volume 21, Issue 1, Pages 77–86.
72. Wrenn S. P., Dicker S. M., Small E. F., Dan N. R., Mleczko M., Schmitz G., and Lewin P. A. 2012. Bursting bubbles and bilayers, *Theranostics*, ISSN: 1838-7640 http://www.thno.org/ms/doc/1514/epub/4305t2.pdf
73. Yandrapu S. K., Kanujia P., Chalasani K., Mangamoori L., Kolapalli R. V., and Chauhan A. 2012. Development and optimization of thiolated dendrimer as a viable mucoadhesive excipient for the controlled drug delivery: An acyclovir model formulation, *Nanomedicine: Nanotechnology, Biology and Medicine*, Volume 9, Issue 4, Pages 514–522.
74. Zanotto-Filho A., Coradini K., Braganhol E., Schröder R., Melo de Oliveira C., Simões-Pires A., Battastini A. M. O. et al. 2012. Curcumin-loaded lipid-core nanocapsules as a strategy to improve pharmacological efficacy of curcumin in glioma treatment, *European Journal of Pharmaceutics and Biopharmaceutics*, Volume 83, Issue 2, Pages 156–167.
75. Heljo V. P., Filipe V., Romeijn S., Jiskoot W., and Juppo A. M. 2012. Stability of rituximab in freeze-dried formulations containing trehalose or melibiose under different relative humidity atmospheres, *Journal of Pharmaceutical Sciences*, Volume 102, Issue 2, Pages 401–414.
76. Sangwai M., Sardar S., and Vavia P. 2012. Nanoemulsified orlistat-embedded multi-unit pellet system (MUPS) with improved dissolution and pancreatic lipase inhibition, *Pharmaceutical Development and Technology*, Posted online on December 24, 2012.
77. Miller K., Erez R., Segal E., Shabat D., and Satchi-Fainaro R. 2009. Targeting bone metastases with a bispecific anticancer and antiangiogenic polymer-alendronate-taxane conjugate, *Angewandte Chemie International Edition*, Volume 48, Issue 16, Pages 2949–2954.
78. Demento S. L., Bonafé N., Cui W., Kaech S. M., Caplan M. J., Fikrig E., Ledizet M., and Fahmy T. M. 2010. TLR9-targeted biodegradable nanoparticles as immunization vectors protect against West Nile encephalitis, *The Journal of Immunology*, Volume 185, Issue 5, Pages 2989–2997.
79. Khan F., Legler P. M., Mease R. M., Duncan E. H., Bergmann-Leitner E. S., and Angov E. 2011. Histidine affinity tags affect MSP142 structural stability and immunodominance in mice, *Biotechnology Journal*, Volume 7, Issue 1, Pages 133–147.

80. Moddaresi M., Brown M. B., Zhao Y., Tamburic S., and Jones S. A. 2010. The role of vehicle–nanoparticle interactions in topical drug delivery, *International Journal of Pharmaceutics*, Volume 400, Issues 1–2, Pages 176–182.
81. Bhuiyan D. B. 2010 *Application of hyperthermia for localized drug release from thermosensitive liposomes*, Master's Thesis in Biomedical Engineering, Chalmers University of Technology, Goteborg, Sweden 2010.
82. Mazzarino L., Traveleta C., Ortega-Murilloa S., Otsukaa I., Pignot-Paintranda I., Lemos-Sennab E., and Borsalia R. 2012. Elaboration of chitosan-coated nanoparticles loaded with curcumin for mucoadhesive applications, *Journal of Colloid and Interface Science*, Volume 370, Issue 1, Pages 58–66.
83. de Graaf A., I Próspero dos Santos I. I. A., Pieters E. H. E., Rijkers D. T. S., van Nostrum C. F., Vermonden T., Kok R. J., Hennink W. E., Mastrobattista E. 2012. A micelle-shedding thermosensitive hydrogel as sustained release formulation, *Journal of Controlled Release*, Volume 162, Issue 3, Pages 582–590.
84. Corradetti B., Freile P., Pells S., Bagnaninchi P., Park J., Fahmy T. M., and de Sousa P. A. 2012. Paracrine signalling events in embryonic stem cell renewal mediated by affinity targeted nanoparticles, *Biomaterials*, Volume 33, Issue 28, Pages 6634–6643.
85. Hsu J., Serrano D., Bhowmick T., Kumar K., Shen Y., Kuo Y. C., Garnacho C., and Muro S. 2010. Enhanced endothelial delivery and biochemical effects of α-galactosidase by ICAM-1-targeted nanocarriers for Fabry disease, *Journal of Controlled Release*, Volume 149, Issue 3, Pages 323–331.
86. Park J., Gao W., Whiston R., Strom T., Metcalfe S., and Fahmy T. M. 2010. Modulation of CD4+ T Lymphocyte Lineage Outcomes with Targeted, Nanoparticle-Mediated Cytokine Delivery, *Molecular Pharmaceutics*, Volume 8, Issue 1, Pages 143–152.
87. Tagalakis A. D., Grosse S. M., Meng Q.-H., Mustapa M. F. M., Kwok A., Salehi S. E., Tabor A. B., Hailes H. C., and Hart S. L. 2010. Integrin-targeted nanocomplexes for tumour specific delivery and therapy by systemic administration, *Biomaterials*, Volume 32, Issue 5, Pages 1370–1376.
88. Cabot R., Hawke J., McAughey J., Dickens C. 2012. *Dissolution Measurements of Smoke Particles in a Liquid Based Suspension*, Poster V13, Drug Delivery to the Lungs 22, Edinburgh, 7–9 December 2011.
89. Wang H. N and Vo-Dinh T. 2011. Plasmonic coupling interference (PCI) nanoprobes for nucleic acid detection, *Small*, Volume 7, Issue 21, Pages 3067–3074.
90. Kell A. J., Pagé L., Tan S., Charlebois I., Boissinot M., LeClerc M., and Simard B. 2011. The development of a silica nanoparticle-based label-free DNA biosensor, *Nanoscale*, Volume 3, Issue 9, Pages 3747–3754.
91. Tzeng S. Y., Hung B. P., Grayson W. L., and Green J. J. 2012. Cystamine-terminated poly (beta-amino ester)s for siRNA delivery to human mesenchymal stem cells and enhancement of osteogenic differentiation, *Biomaterials*, Volume 33, Issue 32, Pages 8142–8151.
92. Tzeng S. Y., and Green J. J. 2012. Subtle changes to polymer structure and degradation mechanism enable highly effective nanoparticles for siRNA and DNA delivery to human brain cancer, *Advanced Healthcare Materials*, Volume 2, Issue 3, Pages 468–480.
93. Ezzat K., Zaghloul E. M., Andaloussi S. E. L., Lehto T., El-Sayed R., Magdy T., Smith C. I. E., and Langel U. 2012. Solid formulation of cell-penetrating peptide nanocomplexes with siRNA and their stability in simulated gastric conditions, *Journal of Controlled Release*, Volume 162, Issue 1, Pages 1–8.
94. Troiber C., Kasper J. C., Milani S., Scheible M., Martin I., Schaubhut F., Küchler S. et al. 2012. Comparison of four different particle sizing methods for siRNA polyplex characterization, *European Journal of Pharmaceutics and Biopharmaceutics*, Volume 84, Issue 2, Pages 255–264.

95. Sokolova V., Ludwig A.-K., Hornung S., Rotan O., Horn P. A., Epple M., and Giebel B., 2011. Characterization of exosomes derived from human cells by Nanoparticle Tracking Analysis and scanning electron microscopy, *Colloids and Surfaces, B: Biointerfaces*, Volume 87, Issue 1, Pages 146–150.
96. Ohlsson G., Tabaei S., Beech J. P., Kvassman J., Johansson U., Kjellbom P., Tegenfeldt J. O., and Höök F. 2012. Solute transport on the sub 100 ms scale across the lipid bilayer membrane of individual proteoliposomes, *Lab Chip*, Volume 12, Issue 22, Pages 4635–4643.
97. Brinkhuis R. P., Stojanov K., Laverman P., Eilander J., Zuhorn I. S., Floris P. J., Rutjes T., and van Hest J. C. M. 2012. Size dependent biodistribution and SPECT imaging of 111In-labeled polymersomes, *Bioconjugate Chemistry*, Volume 23, Issue 5, Pages 958–965.
98. Malmo J. 2012. *Chitosan-based nanocarriers for gene-and siRNA-delivery*, PhD Thesis, Norwegian University of Science and Technology, Faculty of Natural Sciences and Technology, Department of Biotechnology, ISBN 978-82-471-3748-2.
99. Lien C.-F., Molnár E., Toman P., Tsibouklis J., Pilkington G. J., Górecki D. C., and Barbu E. 2012. In vitro assessment of alkylglyceryl-functionalized chitosan nanoparticles as permeating vectors for the blood–brain barrier, *Biomacromolecules*, Volume 13, Issue 4, Pages 1067–1073.
100. van Dommelen S. M., Vader P., Lakhal S., van Solinge W. W., Wood M. J. A., and Schiffelers R. M. 2011. Microvesicles and exosomes: Opportunities for cell-derived membrane vesicles in drug delivery, *Journal of Controlled Release*, Volume 161, Issue 2, Pages 635–644.
101. Zhu T., Jiang Z., and Ma Y. 2012. Lipid Exchange between Membranes: Effects of Membrane Surface Charge, Composition, and Curvature, *Colloids and Surfaces B: Biointerfaces*, Volume 97, Pages 155–161.
102. Morton L., Saludes J., Beninson L., Chapman E., Fleshner M., and Hang Y. 2012. *Marcks Peptide As A Probe To Target Microvesicles*, International Society for Extracellular Vesicles meeting—ISEV 2012, Gothenburg, Sweden, 18–21 April 2012.
103. Calò A., Sanmartí-Espinal M., Lavicoli P., Persuy M. A., Pajot-Augy E., Gomila G., and Samitier J. 2012. Diffusion-controlled deposition of natural nanovesicles containing G-protein coupled receptors for biosensing platforms, *Soft Matter*, Volume 8, Issue 46, Pages 11632–11643.
104. Vallhov H., Gutzeit C., Johansson S. M., Nagy N., Paul M., Li Q., Friend S. et al. 2010. Exosomes Containing Glycoprotein 350 Released by EBV-Transformed B Cells Selectively Target B Cells through CD21 and Block EBV Infection In vitro, *The Journal of Immunology*, Volume 186, Issue 1, Pages 73–82.
105. Ronquist G. 2011 Prostasomes are mediators of intercellular communication: From basic research to clinical implications, *Journal of Internal Medicine*, Volume 271, Issue 4, Pages 400–413.
106. Simonsson L., Kurczy M. E., Trouillon R., Hook F., and Cans A.-S. 2012. A functioning artificial secretory cell, *Scientific Reports*, 2012 Volume 2, Page 824. Published online 2012 November 8. doi: 10.1038/srep00824

10 Microsponges for Drug Delivery

Rishabh Srivastava

CONTENTS

OVERVIEW

The drug delivery technology landscape has become highly competitive and rapidly evolving to develop new generation drug delivery systems. These developments in delivery systems are being integrated to optimize the clinical outcomes—that is, efficacy, safety, and cost-effectiveness of the therapy [1]. The new generation pharmaceuticals and biopharmaceuticals (peptides, proteins, and DNA-based therapeutics) are also fueling such advancement of drug delivery technology as these new drugs cannot be effectively delivered by conventional means. Thus, the targeted and localized delivery of therapeutic agents is the need of the hour. These attempts for development of novel drug carrier systems led to the development of a microparticulate drug carrier approach, which offers an intelligent approach by coupling the drug to a carrier particle that modulates the release and absorption characteristics of the drug [2]. In such attempts to develop next-generation carriers, Won (1987) developed the porous particles [3] that provided various advantages, such as ease of fabrication, better drug loading, and rate control over other microparticulate systems. The fundamental appeal of the microsponge technology stems from the difficulty experienced with conventional formulations in releasing active ingredients over an extended period of time.

Microsponge technology was introduced to facilitate the controlled release of active drug into the skin in order to reduce systemic exposure and minimize local cutaneous reactions to active drugs. Consequently, this carrier system has been commercially utilized for chronotherapeutic topical drug delivery but has also been studied for oral, pulmonary, and parenteral drug delivery. Although this carrier system has a range of advantages over other microparticulate systems, its commercial application for oral drug delivery is still in its infancy.

MICROSPONGE

The microsponge delivery system (MDS) or solid phase porous microsphere (SPPM) (Figure 10.1) is a patented microparticulate system [4] comprised of interconnected voids with polymeric, porous, and collapsible structures [5]. It has a large porous surface to entrap active agents efficiently that can be released at the desired site of absorption. The porous structure forms a continuous arrangement open to the exterior surface of particles, which permits the outward diffusion of the entrapped drug molecule at a controlled rate, depending on the pore size [6]. These microparticles were once supposed to consist of several nanoparticles under a porous polymeric outer surface [7]. These microparticles have the capacity to adsorb on its surface and/or load into the bulk of the particle high quantities of the active ingredient [8]. Microsponge systems are based on microscopic, polymer-based microspheres that can entrap a

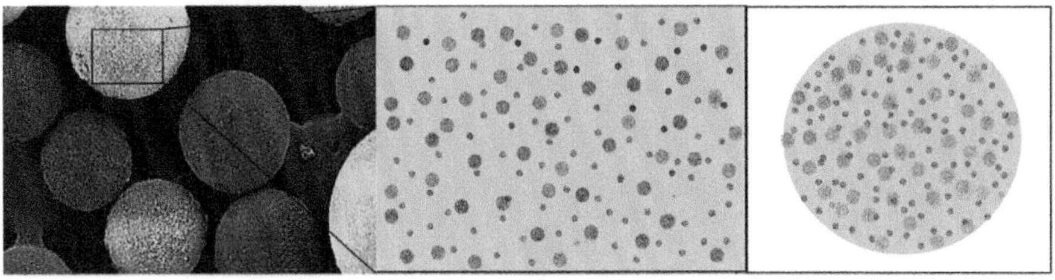

FIGURE 10.1 Microsponge and its matrix character. (a) Microsponges, (b) artwork showing the presence of pores and drug molecules on the surface of microsponges, and (c) artwork showing the presence of pores and drug molecules in the cross-section of the microsponges.

wide variety of active ingredients and then incorporated them into a commercially viable formulation, such as gels, creams, liquids, or solid dosage forms.

The rate of release of the active ingredients from the formulation is an influential factor for determining the severity of the skin irritation; however, this rate cannot be controlled with the microcapsules and vesicular drug carriers as once their wall is ruptured, the contents are released. On the other hand, these drug carriers have some other limitations, such as being relatively expensive and difficult to manufacture with low drug entrapment efficacy. The rate of release associated with MDS provides more control, which potentially has an impact on the intensity of skin irritancy provoked by the topical agent.

The microsponge delivery system provides the following:

- Sustained release technology for reducing irritation of a wide range of APIs and other skin care actives thereby increasing patient/client compliance and results.
- Enhanced formulation stability, ensuring long-term product efficacy and extended shelf life.
- Superior skin feel and exceptional product esthetics.
- Microsponges are also found to control the release of a water-soluble drug, such as hydrquinone, for sustained activity.

PREPARATION OF MICROSPONGES

Microsponges are most commonly prepared by two methods—that is, liquid–liquid suspension polymerization and quasiemulsion solvent diffusion—but some novel techniques were recently developed.

Proposed Mechanism of Microsponge Preparation

Liquid–Liquid Suspension Polymerization

In this method, microsponges are generated through a free radical suspension polymerization reaction where the reaction is carried out in a reaction flask fitted

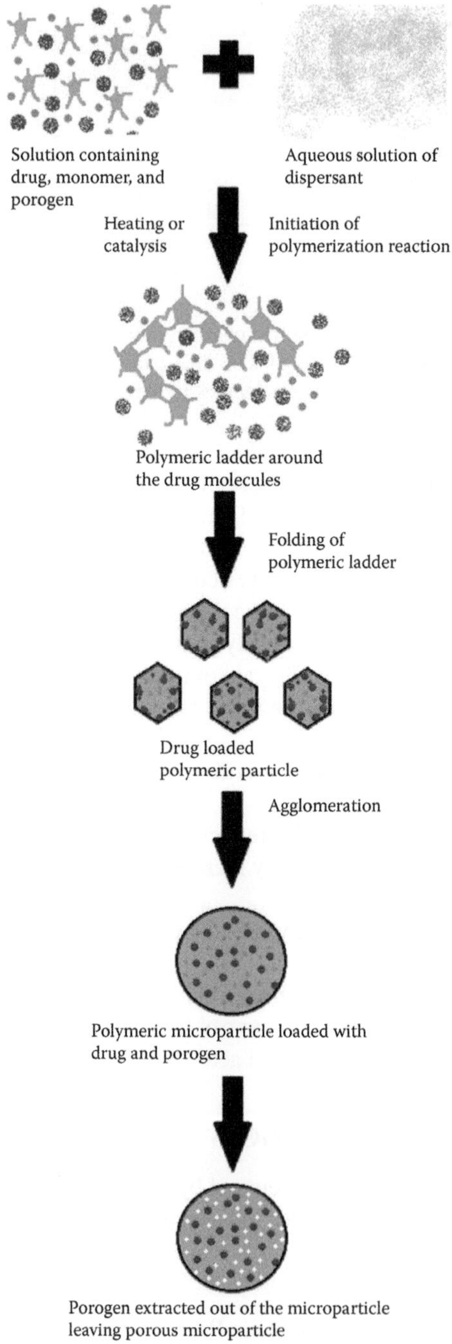

FIGURE 10.2 Mechanism of microsponge formation through liquid–liquid suspension polymerization.

with a stirrer, a water condenser, and a thermometer [9]. A solution of nonpolar drug, monomer(s), and water-insoluble porogen is prepared, to which aqueous phase is added containing surfactant and dispersant. Polymerization, initiated by activating the monomers, leads to the formation of a ladder structure (Figure 10.2) as a result of cross-linking between monomers. Folding of this ladder leads to the formation of spherical particles, and their agglomeration results in formation of bunches of microspheres. Binding of these bunches forms the microsponge. After polymerization, the liquid is diffused out, leaving microsponges. Microsponges can be prepared by one-step or two-step synthesis. When the drug is sensitive to the polymerization conditions, two-step synthesis is used. In the two-step method, blank microsponges are generated by polymerization and then drug loading is performed by an active method but gives lower loading efficacy. Although a convenient method, a major disadvantage of this process is probable entrapment of unreacted monomeric residues and failure to use it to get high drug entrapment for thermolabile drugs.

Quasiemulsion Solvent Diffusion

The mechanism involved in the generation of microsponges by this method involves counter diffusion of the two phases of quasiemulsion along with continuous stirring. Stirring leads to the formation of emulsion globules called quasiemulsion globules. The finely dispersed droplets of the polymeric solution of the drug (dispersed phase) get solidified in aqueous phase via counter diffusion of organic solvent and water out of and into the droplets [10]. The continued diffusion of water within the droplets decreases the solubility of the drug and polymer while the counter diffusion of organic solvent results in the coprecipitation of the components of internal phase and solidification, producing porous microspheres. In comparison with the liquid–liquid suspension polymerization method, this method offers the advantage of less exposure of the drug to the ambient conditions and low solvent residues in the product because the solvent gets extracted out due to its solubility in aqueous media or due to its volatile nature.

It can be assumed that the coprecipitation of the drug and polymers first occurs on the surface of the quasiemulsion droplets and forms the film-like shell on the outer surface of the droplets. Further diffusion of the organic solvents out of the droplets results in the cavity and micropores being left inside of the microsponge.

Some other novel methods include water in oil in water (w/o/w) emulsion solvent diffusion, oil in oil (o/o) emulsion solvent diffusion, lyophilization, the vibrating orifice aerosol generator method, addition of porogen, ultrasound-assisted production, and the electrohydrodynamic atomization method. These methods were developed by modifying the quasiemulsion solvent diffusion or the liquid–liquid suspension polymerization method.

PHARMACEUTICAL CHARACTERISTICS, THEIR DETERMINATION AND INFLUENCES

Particle Size

Particle size of the microsponges can be measured by the optical method (microscopy) or instrumental method (Coulter counter method). Various factors, such as temperature during preparation, viscosity of the organic phase, viscosity of the aqueous phase, and drug polymer ratio, have an effect on the particle size. Increasing the temperature during preparation of the microsponges results in abrupt sized particles as the organic phase would easily get evaporated from the emulsion. Increasing in the drug:polymer ratio results in small particles to combat the better entrapment of the drug by microparticles. On the other hand, increasing the viscosity of the aqueous phase by increasing the emulsifying agent (PVA), leads to the formation of large-sized microsponges [8]. Large particles are also produced if the viscosity of the organic phase is increased [11]. It can be interpreted that the high viscosity of phases leads to an increase in surface tension, producing larger globules for solidification [12]. Particle size has its impact on drug loading and drug release profile. Smaller particles have better drug entrapment ability and have good control over drug release.

Morphology and Surface Topography

The surface morphological study performed by scanning electron microscopy with the microsponges established the existence of a porous surface structure on the particle. In a similar way, its internal morphology showed cross-linking pores throughout the matrix. Its morphology is influenced by the temperature maintained during the preparation and the selection of solvent system for the inner phase. The presence of environmental conditions that caused quick precipitation of the organic phase—that is, polymer—results in a nonporous or less porous surface. Similarly, if the organic solvent is highly water-miscible, the organic phase would easily be mixed with the aqueous phase, resulting in a nonporous surface [13]. Thus, during the preparation of microsponges, controlled temperature and a solvent that is not miscible in aqueous phase is required. The porous nature of the microsponges results in better penetration of the release media deep into the particle, which leads to the improved drug release character. This porous surface also results in the roughness that leads to the easy attachment of the microsponges to the surface. Thus, microsponges are also used in bone regeneration therapy.

It was also observed that the surface of the microsponges became rough after the drug release as the drug molecules attached to the external surface are released first. As the molecules on the surface released, the smooth surface became rough [11].

Rheological Properties

Good rheological properties are among the most required properties for product development as it helps in better die or capsule filling and compression. Tablets and capsules constitute the most feasible dosage form for oral use, and their formulation requires good flow properties of the material to be compressed or encapsulated. As microsponges are spherical, they have good flow properties, and their microstructure helps in better compression. Good rheological properties also constitute an essential requirement for the better spreading of a formulation on the skin. If the formulation does not possess the spreading property, it will form a clump and result in irritation. Rheological properties that are to be determined for the microsponges are Hausner's ratio, Carr's compressibility index, and angle of repose.

True Density

The true density of microparticles was measured using an ultra-pycnometer under helium gas and was calculated from a mean of repeated determinations. Determination of this parameter helps in determining the porous character of the microsponge. Highly porous particles have low true density as maximum volume is covered by the pores. Such systems have higher release rates but are fragile; such particles are preferred for topical drug delivery while microsponges with high true density have a collapsible structure and permit slower drug release. Such carrier particles are preferred for tableting as they easily regain their shape on contact with dissolution fluid.

Pore Structure

Pore volume and diameter are vital in controlling the intensity and duration of effectiveness of the active ingredient. Pore diameter also affects the migration of active ingredients from microsponges into the vehicle in which the material is dispersed. Mercury intrusion porosimetry can be employed to study the effect of pore diameter and volume with rate of drug release from microsponges. Microsponges prepared by the suspension polymerization method have been reported to have smaller pore size as compared with that of the microsponges prepared by the quasiemulsion solvent diffusion method [14]; thus, the microsponges by the former method release drug slowly. It was observed that the pore diameter of the microsponges after the drug release is more than the pore diameter of the microsponges before drug release [11]. This change in the pore diameter is caused as the release of the drug molecule from the pore surfaces leads to the increased pore diameter.

Porosity parameters of microsponges, such as intrusion–extrusion isotherms, pore size distribution, total pore surface area, average pore diameters, shape and morphology of the pores, bulk, and apparent density, can be determined by using mercury intrusion porosimetry [15]. Incremental intrusion volumes can be plotted against pore diameters that represented pore size distributions. The pore diameter of microsponges can be calculated by using the Washburn equation [16].

$$D = \frac{-4y\cos\theta}{P}, \tag{10.1}$$

where D is the pore diameter (μm), γ the surface tension of mercury (485 dyncm^{-1}), θ the contact angle (130°), and P is the pressure (psig).

Total pore area (Atot) was calculated by using following equation:

$$Atot = \frac{1}{\gamma\cos\theta}\int_{0}^{Vtot} P.dv, \tag{10.2}$$

where P is the pressure (psia), V the intrusion volume (mL g^{-1}), and Vtot is the total specific intrusion volume (mL g^{-1}).

The average pore diameter (Dm) was calculated by using the following equation:

$$Dm = \frac{4Vtot}{Atot}. \tag{10.3}$$

Envelope (bulk) density (ρse) of the microsponges was calculated by using the following equation:

$$\rho se = \frac{Ws}{Vp - VHg}, \tag{10.4}$$

where Ws is the weight of the microsponge sample (g), Vp the empty penetrometer (mL), and VHg is the volume of mercury (mL).

Absolute (skeletal) density (ρsa) of microsponges was calculated by using the following equation:

$$\rho sa = \frac{Ws}{Vse - Vtot}, \tag{10.5}$$

where Vse is the volume of the penetrometer minus the volume of the mercury (mL).

Finally, the percentage porosity of the sample was found from the following equation:

$$Porosity\ (\%) = \left(1 - \frac{\rho se}{\rho sa}\right) \times 100. \tag{10.6}$$

Pore morphology can be characterized from the intrusion–extrusion profiles of mercury in the microsponges as described by Orr [17].

Resiliency

Resiliency (viscoelastic properties) of microsponges is used to define the firmness of the final formulation (either soft or firm). This property influences the collapsible characteristic as well as drug release of the microsponges. It is very necessary to optimize the firmness of the microsponges, which can be done by optimizing the cross-linking and observing the drug release behavior [18], but unfortunately no validated and optimized method has been developed to determine the resiliency of microsponges. To increase the resilient character of the microsponges the addition of a water-insoluble plasticizer like triethyl phthalate is suggested.

Internal Porosity

The internal porosity of the microsponges can be easily controlled by changing the content of the drug and the polymer in the emulsion droplet. At lower drug:polymer ratios, the microspheres with higher porosity are obtained while increasing the drug:polymer ratio results in low internal porosity. The internal porosity of microsponges significantly influences the characteristics of microsponges [19]. The drug release profile from these carrier particles best fits the Higuchi model that indicates its dependency on the internal porosity. Particles with similar internal texture showed almost the same tortuosity irrespective of their surface porosity.

Surface Retentive Ability

Microsponges have a rough surface that results in the surface retentive ability [11] (Figure 10.3). This adherence takes place due to the fact that the body accepts a rough material more easily than a smoother one. By virtue of this property, microsponges get attached to the surface of the targeted organ. This property enables them to prevent the washout of the drug carrier from the site of action, and thus, the drug is present on that surface for a longer time period. This property also results in the absorption of the maximum part of the entrapped drug, and if the delivery is aimed for a local therapy, the drug is present at the site of action for a longer period.

Release Mechanism and Character

Microsponge drug carrier systems show the matrix type of drug release with an initial burst release that helps in attainment of minimum effective concentration while the further controlled release due to the release of entrapped drug molecules from the

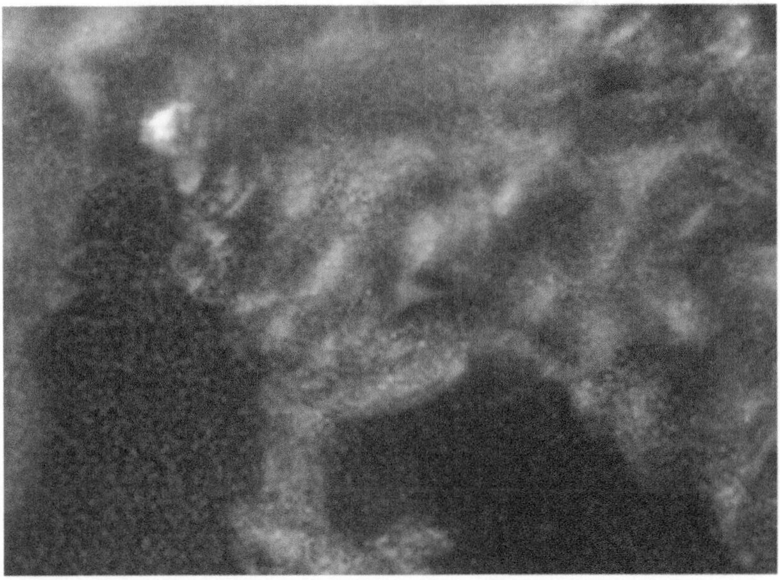

FIGURE 10.3 CLSM image depicting the presence of Rhodamine on the surface, thus showing the surface retentive ability of the microsponge.

bulk maintain the concentration of the drug above effective concentration. Such type of release character helps in better clinical effects as easy attainment of the minimum effective concentration (MEC) results in improved efficacy while further controlled release to maintain the drug concentration results in maintenance of the therapeutic level. Also, due to such release character, drug concentration does not exceed the maximum safe concentration (MSC), resulting in low occurrence of side effects.

PROPOSED MECHANISM OF DRUG RELEASE FROM MICROSPONGES

On the basis of these properties, a mechanism for the drug release from the microsponge is proposed (Figure 10.4). Microsponges, due to their rough surface, get attached to the surface of application, administration, or absorption. The initial burst release from the microsponges is due to the drug molecules present on the surface of the particle. This removal of the drug molecules from the surface causes

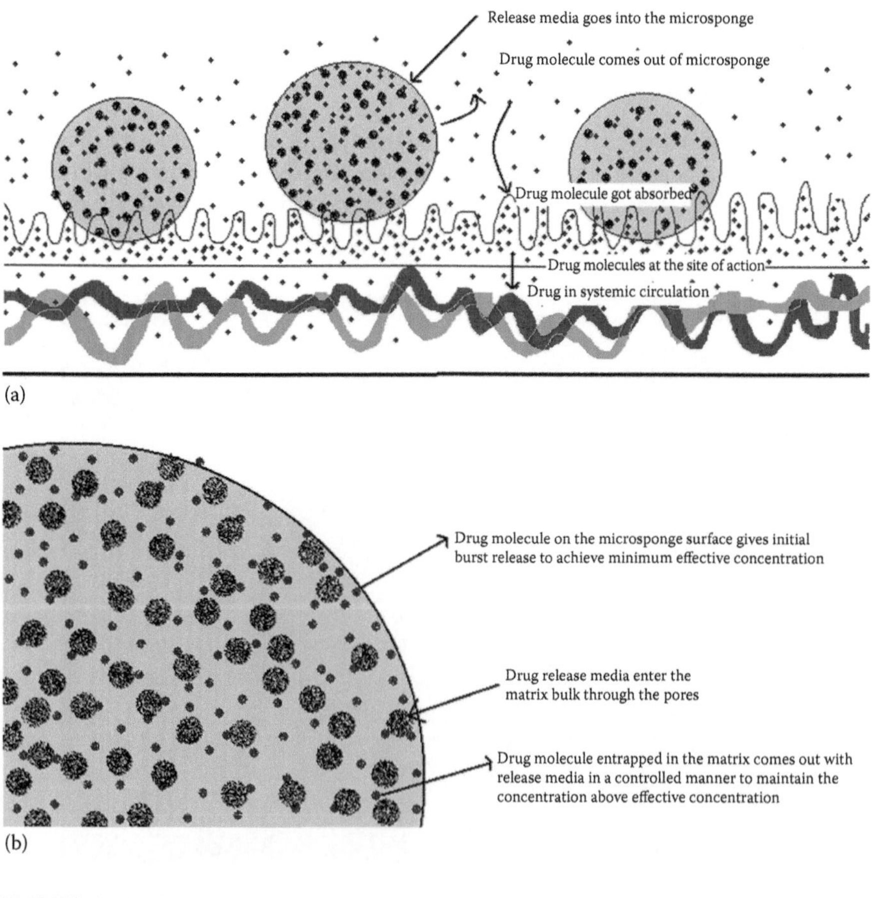

FIGURE 10.4 Drug release from the microsponges. (a) Drug release and absorption from the microsponges. (b) Mechanism of drug release from microsponge.

the increased pore size that results in easy penetration of release media to the matrix. The diffusion of the drug release media from the external environment into the bulk of the microsponge matrix through pores leads to the release of the drug molecules to the release media. As the microsponges have an open structure, the active is free to move in and out of the matrix until equilibrium is attained. Thereafter, the diffused drug molecules get absorbed through the biological membrane to maintain the sink condition in the release media. This sink condition further leads to the release of the active ingredient from the bulk matrix. The adherence of the microsponge to the surface causes the retention of the drug at the site of action for a longer duration; thus, the drug is available for a longer period. There are some other factors or triggers that have influence over the release from the microsponges.

While the active payload is protected in the formulation by the microsponge particle, it is delivered to the skin via controlled diffusion. This sustained release of actives to skin over time is an extremely valuable tool to extend the efficacy and lessen the irritation commonly associated with powerful therapeutic agents [4].

Pressure

Rubbing or pressure applied can release the active ingredient from SPMs onto skin. The SPM system releases the entrapped material when pressurized; the amount released depends upon various characteristics of the sponge. By varying the type of material and different process variables, the SPM best suited for a given application may be optimized. When compared with mineral oil–containing microcapsules, mineral oil–containing SPMs showed a much more softening effect. The duration of emolliency was also much longer for the SPM systems.

Temperature Change

Some entrapped actives can be too viscous at room temperature to flow spontaneously from SPMs onto the skin. An increase in skin temperature can result in an increased flow rate and hence release. So it is possible to modulate the release of substances from the SPM by modulation of temperature. For example, viscous sunscreens were found to show a higher release from SPMs when exposed to higher temperatures; thus, a sunscreen would be released from a SPM only upon exposure to the heat from the sun.

Solubility

SPMs loaded with water-soluble ingredients, such as antiperspirants and antiseptics, will release the ingredient in the presence of water. The release can also be activated by diffusion, taking into consideration the partition coefficient of the ingredient between the SPMs and the outside system and the ability to swell the microspore network.

Drug Polymer Content

The drug release from microsponges decreases as the total amount of polymer increases. Theoretically, the drug release should be slower as the amount of polymer is increased because of an increase in the path length through which the drug has to diffuse. The dissolution behavior is greatly influenced by the surface area and particle size distribution

ADVANTAGES AND LIMITATIONS OF MICROSPONGES OVER OTHER MICROPARTICLES

Microsponges were found to have improved thermal, physical, and chemical stability over other microparticulate and vesicular systems. Microsponges also provide better entrapment efficiency when compared with other carrier systems. Using microsponge carrier systems, liquids can be converted into powders, leading to improved material processing. Microsponges are flexible for the development of novel dosage forms. The system is free-flowing and cost-effective and thus can be used at commercial level. A generally accepted view is that multiparticulate systems perform better in vivo than single unit systems as they spread throughout the GIT, causing less irritation, enjoying a slower transit and extended retention, and giving a more reproducible drug release. Microsponges have shown a better compressibility for tableting when compared with the other microparticulate systems or the physical mixture of the drug and the polymer. An added benefit is that the time it takes the microsponge system to traverse the small and large intestine is significantly increased, thus maximizing the amount of drug that is absorbed. In addition, the entrapment process in the microsponge allows for both coloading and subsequent loading steps, including coatings.

But irrespective of their various advantages, microsponges also suffer from some barriers that limit their applications. These barriers include the uncertainty in the production techniques and no efforts for a pilot plant on a commercial level. Various methods that were developed for their production are not reproducible. Research has shown the efficacy of microsponges toward protein delivery, but after release, microsponges cannot protect them from microbial flora at the site of release. Although smaller pores of microsponges limit the entry of microorganisms to the bulk, they can grow on the surface of microsponges. Similarly, the use of biodegradable polymers for the delivery of amino acids and proteins leads to the generation of monomers at the site, which may cause harm to the physiology of the human body. Another such barrier includes the development of a suitable dosage form for their targeted delivery. Microsponges can be suitably converted to a colon-targeted tablet by using pectin for compression coating or calcium pectinate as a matrix former, but these microsponges on their own cannot protect the active ingredient from release in the upper part of the GIT.

FORMULATION CONSIDERATIONS

When formulating the microsponge, certain considerations are taken into account in order to achieve the desired product characteristics. The aqueous solubility of the active agent must be limited; otherwise, the continuous phase will deplete the microsponges during formulation, and polymer design and payload of the microsponges for the active must be optimized for required release after given time period.

Actives entrapped in MDS can then be incorporated into many products, such as creams, lotions, powders, and soaps. When formulating the vehicle, certain considerations are taken into account in order to achieve the desired product characteristics. The solubility of actives in the vehicle must be limited. Otherwise, the vehicle will deplete the microsponges before the application. To avoid cosmetic problems, not more than 10% to 12% w/w microsponges must be incorporated into the vehicle. Polymer design and payload of the microsponges for the active must be optimized for required release rate for a given time period.

There remains equilibrium between the microsponge and vehicle, and the microsponge releases the drug in response to the depletion of drug concentration in the vehicle. Drug concentration in the vehicle is depleted by absorption of the drug into the skin. Hence, continuous and steady release of actives onto the skin is accomplished with this system. Drug release from the topical semisolid formulation can be studied by using Franz-type static diffusion cells.

POLYMERS AND FORMULATION AIDS IN MICROSPONGES

Various polymers and formulation aids were reported to form a microsponge "cage." Polymers studied for the preparation of microsponges for oral purposes include Eudragit RS-100, Eudragit RSPO, Eudragit S-100, polylactide-co-glycolic acid, polylactic acid, polydivinyl benzene, and polyhydroxyl butyrate. Eudragit RS-100 formed the most widely studied polymer due to its versatility, enabling the researchers to employ it in various ways. It was mostly exploited for the development of colon-targeted microsponges due to its high transition pH (above 7), which enabled the protection of the release in lower pH. Eudragit RSPO also modulated the drug release along with enhancing the solubility of the drug by forming a solid dispersion-like structure. Polylactide-co-glycolic acid and polylactic acid were studied for delivering proteins and peptides. Microsponges fabricated with these polymers also possessed a floating ability due to the hydrophobicity of the polymer, which limited the wetting of the particles with aqueous media; thus, these microparticles can be employed for fabricating floating microsponges. Polydivinyl benzene was studied for fabricating porous microparticles by the polymerization technique using divinyl benzene as a monomer, but entrapping the drug with this process may cause alteration in the structure of the drug molecule or conjugation of the drug with the monomer. The use of such a large variety of polymers for the fabrication of the microsponges showed that the method of preparation of microsponges can be modified as per the requirement. In addition to polymers and active ingredients, some researchers also used triethylcitrate as a plasticizer that helps to stabilize the resilient property of the microsponges. During the preparation of microsponges by the quasiemulsion solvent diffusion method, it is reported that the presence of an emulsifier having a tendency to maintain the viscosity of the aqueous phase is compulsory. Researchers attempted the use of cellulose ethers and PVA for such a role and found the use of PVA to be a better emulsifier. Some researchers also used some porogens as the pore forming agents, such as sodium bicarbonate and sodium chloride.

THE CLINICAL UNMET NEEDS IT MAY ADDRESS

Conventional formulations, such as gels and immediate-release oral formulations, are intended to release the active ingredient at the site of absorption, the outer layers of the skin, or the gastrointestinal tract. Typically, such products release their active ingredients on administration, producing a highly concentrated layer or solution of active ingredient, which is supposed to be rapidly absorbed.

On oral administration, this quick release of the active ingredient may also lead to the degradation of the active ingredient due to enzymatic activity or pH in the gastrointestinal tract. This degradation would reduce the efficacy of the formulation as it will reduce the bioavailability. Also the accumulation of some active ingredients due to the immediate release may lead to site-specific side effects, such as G.I. disturbances. Conventional topical formulations require high concentrations of active agents for effective therapy because of the low efficiency of their delivery system, resulting in excessive accumulation of active ingredients on the skin that would lead to topical side effects, such as irritation and inflammation.

Microsponge technology is believed to contribute toward enhanced clinical efficacy with reduced side effects, improved stability, elegance, and enhanced formulation flexibility. While the active payload is protected in the formulation by the microsponge particle, it is delivered to the site of action via controlled diffusion [11]. This sustained release of actives over time is an extremely valuable tool to extend the efficacy and lessen the irritation commonly associated with powerful therapeutic agents, such as retinoids or benzoyl peroxide [6]. Microsponge polymers possess the versatility to load a wide range of actives, providing the benefits of enhanced product efficacy, mildness, tolerability, and extended wear to a wide range of skin therapies. The spherical nature of the microsponge particle, combined with its rigidity, enhances the skin feel and elegance of creams and lotions, resulting in uncompromising performance [18].

For better efficacy, the drug carrier should remain at the site of action and release the medicament slowly. Microsponges maintain the equilibrium between the drug-loaded matrix and site of release. As the microsponge releases the drug in response to the depletion of drug concentration at the desired site, drug concentration in the vehicle is depleted by absorption. Hence a continuous and steady release of actives can be easily achieved with this system. As the steady release of the active ingredient maintains the concentration above the minimum effective concentration, thus the microsponge delivery system provides better and sustained efficacy.

In addition, studies have found that microsponge systems provide surface retentive ability [11], thus the presence of the active ingredient is observed only at the desired site, thus reducing the systemic side effects. The surface retentive ability of the microsponges leads to the retention of drug at the site, and thus, efficacious concentration can be easily attained. In this way, with the help of microsponge technology, a quick and sustained action can be achieved. As the drug will be concentrated at the site of action, its systemic side effects would not be observed. Second, as the drug release is controlled by the absorption of the drug from the site of release, the site-specific side effect would also not be observed.

The microsponge system maximizes the amount of time that an active ingredient is present either on the skin surface or within the epidermis while minimizing its transdermal penetration into the body. In addition to the above properties, during application of the microsponge delivery system to the skin, the release of the drug can be controlled through diffusion or a variety of other triggers, including rubbing, moisture, pH, friction, or ambient skin temperature. The microsponge system can prevent excessive accumulation of ingredients within the epidermis and the dermis. Potentially, the microsponge system can significantly reduce the irritation of the skin due to drugs without reducing their efficacy. Due to these attributes, the microsponge delivery system is regarded as a leading technology for addressing skin conditions, such as acne, hyperpigmentation, actinic keratosis, aging, and photo damage.

Results from various human clinical studies have proven that the technology offers the potential to reduce the drug side effects, maintain the therapeutic efficacy, and potentially increase patient compliance with the treatment regimen. During the clinical studies, tretinoin formulations demonstrated efficacy but also resulted in significant irritation, erythema, and peeling. But the clinical study for the microsponge gel showed improved tolerability. During a clinical trial assessing the safety of the tretinoin formulations on 48 individuals having both an atopic background and a tendency toward rosacea, it was shown that, although the tretinoin 0.1% microsponge slowed the rate of subjects discontinuing topical retinoid therapy due to irritation compared with tretinoin 0.1% cream, it did not prevent all patients from eventually discontinuing. Thus, it may be considered that microsponges have the tendency to reduce topical irritation. The drug retention and sustained release property can be considered as the main reason behind this.

Another clinical study proved that the microsponge delivery system is efficacious in minimizing the appearance of fine lines, wrinkles, surface roughness, and age spots to give the skin a youthful glow. This study also proved that the irritation reduction benefit of the microsponge delivery system is unique. This gave the system a market leveragability aspect. While known for its high level of performance in skincare products, concerns over the irritation potential of Retinol are ever-present. The microsponge-based system, containing 50% more Retinol, exhibited half the irritation potential compared to the leading brand. Another clinical study showed that products containing a benzoyl peroxide formulation comprising a microsponge-based delivery system are significantly less irritating than existing commercial products while providing the desired efficacy. As an added benefit, microsponges adsorb excess skin oil, thereby enhancing the antiacne performance of the product and enabling a fresh, nonshiny appearance.

Microsponge-based salicylic acid products are clinically proven to increase the rate of clearance of existing blemishes and prevent new acne pimples and blackheads by exfoliating and preventing clogged pores. The microsponge delivery system provides a sustained release of the active ingredient allowing for both an extended wear and a reduced irritation/mildness claim.

The topical antihistaminic effect of the microsponge-based Hydroxizine formulation was assessed by the determination of the onset and extent of wheal suppression. For dosing, an amount of powder microsponges containing 10 mg of drug was applied by rubbing to the defined area on a rabbit's back. The rabbit was placed in a wooden cage with an approved collar allowing the head out during the 5-h study to prevent it from licking its back. After topical application of the chosen microsponge preparations on the inflamed back of rabbits, the mean wheal areas obtained at different time intervals were calculated in each group of rabbit. It was observed that the wheal disappeared completely in the group treated with medicated microsponges. A study on the topical delivery with microsponges suggested the passage of the drug at higher concentrations to the first skin layers to an occlusive effect exerted by microsponges. That effect produced a film on the skin surface, which reduced the transepidermal water loss and favored drug penetration into the skin.

The histopathological patterns of the inflamed and treated skin varied greatly according to the type of the applied formula. A focal area of mild acanthosis was observed in the prickle cell layer of the epidermis of the skin of rabbits treated with the microsponge formulation. The study demonstrated that invaginated acanthosis of the prickle area of the skin was associated with blood cell infiltration in the dermal layer in the case of skin treated with a plain formulation. It was obvious that an antihistaminic effect was exerted from the medicated formulae. Hydroquinone, despite its ionic properties, succeeded in passing through the stratum corneum to reach the lower epidermal layers, inhibiting the action of histamine. Such passage could be realized through channels in protein molecules embedded in the lipid bilayer of the cell membrane.

Due to their clinical superiority over other carrier systems, they were approved for the treatment of dermatomycosis, acne, and actinic keratosis. Various performed clinical studies suggested that entrapping any active agent in microsponges or nanosponges would increase their efficacy and safety. In such effort, hydroquinone and retinol were entrapped in microsponges and studied clinically in an open-label study for the treatment of hyperpigmentation, and the developed system was compared against an unentrapped drug. The study concluded that the disease severity and pigmentation intensity was statistically improved compared with baseline. Microentrapped drug components were well tolerated, safe, and effective. In the same perspective, while studying the in vitro efficacy of such carriers to treat cancer, the study showed that the efficacy of tamoxifen and paclitaxel were improved by entrapping them in the nanosponges.

CLINICAL APPLICATIONS

Microsponges are designed to deliver the pharmaceutical active ingredient efficiently at the minimum dose and also to enhance stability, reduce side effects, and modify drug release. Microsponges are porous, polymeric microspheres that are used mostly for topical drug delivery, but due to their versatile character were highly explored for various other clinical applications, including oral drug delivery and bone and tissue engineering. These were also studied as culture media as they provide large surface for growth.

Microsponges for Topical Delivery

Benzoyl peroxide is mainly used in the treatment of mild-to-moderate acne and athlete's foot, and the most common side effect associated with benzoyl peroxide is skin irritation. It has been shown that controlled release of benzoyl peroxide from a delivery system to the skin could lessen the side effect while reducing percutaneous absorption. A topical delivery system with reduced irritancy was successfully developed [20]. Jelvehgari et al. developed benzoyl peroxide microsponges by using the emulsion solvent diffusion method and investigated the parameters affecting the morphology and other characteristics by using scanning electron microscopy (SEM). The morphology and particle size of microsponges were affected by the drug:polymer ratio, amount of emulsifier used, and stirring rate. The results showed that with an increase in the ratio of drug to polymer resulted in a reduction in the rate of release of benzoyl peroxide from the microsponges. The release data showed that the highest and the lowest release rates were obtained from lotions containing plain benzoyl peroxide particles and benzoyl peroxide microsponges with the drug:polymer ratio at 13:1, respectively [10]. Amrutiya et al. developed a microsponge-based topical delivery system of mupirocin by using the emulsion solvent diffusion method for sustained release and enhanced drug deposition in the skin. In vitro drug release, ex vivo drug deposition, and in vivo antibacterial activity of mupirocin-loaded formulations were studied. Microsponges were spherical and porous, and there was no interaction between drug and polymer molecules. Emulgels containing microsponges showed desired physical properties. Drug release through a cellulose dialysis membrane showed a diffusion controlled release pattern, and drug deposition studies using rat abdominal skin exhibited significant retention of active in skin from microsponge-based formulations by 24 h [21]. D'souza et al. developed topical anti-inflammatory gels of fluocinolone acetonide entrapped in Eudragit-based microsponge delivery system. FA is a corticosteroid chiefly used in dermatology to lessen skin inflammation and relieve itching. The percutaneous absorption increases the risk related to systemic absorption of the topically applied formulation. Thus, the goal of the study was to produce FA entrapped microsponges, which were prepared by the quasiemulsion solvent diffusion method in order to control release of the drug to the skin, which, in turn, lessens the side effect while also reducing percutaneous absorption. FTIR and DSC studies showed that there is no incompatibility between formulation adjuvant and process parameters. Surface morphology can be done by SEM, which showed the microporous nature of microsponges. Drug release was also observed to be controlled with comparative anti-inflammatory activity with the gels that contain free drug [14]. Grimes et al. developed microsponge-based delivery of hydroquinone 4% and retinol 0.15% for the treatment of melasma and postinflammatory hyperpigmentation and also to minimize skin irritation. Hydroquinone (HQ) bleaching creams are generally considered as the gold standard for treating hyperpigmentation. The formulation was evaluated in a 12-week open-label study for safety and efficacy. The study included pigmentation intensity, disease severity, lesion area, and colorimetry assessments. Adverse events were also recorded. Patients were applied the microsponge formulation entrapped HQ 4% to the full face in the morning and evening (twice) daily. After 15 minutes of application, of the test product, a broad-spectrum sunscreen was applied once in the morning. Then, patients were evaluated at baseline and at 4, 8, and 12 weeks. The study showed that the micro-entrapped HQ 4% with retinol 0.15% formulation produced improvement at all study end points. The open-label study concluded that micro-entrapped HQ 4% with retinol 0.15% was safe and effective [22].

Some of the topical products comprised of microsponges dispersed in a cream base showed the ability to reduce the duration of therapy, dosing frequency, and skin irritation. These products are approved by the FDA to be used for the treatment of acne (retinol) and actinic and solar keratoses (5-fluorouracil). Gel comprising microsponges loaded with fluconazole showed sustained drug release to reduce the dosing frequency. Studies were also performed to prepare the nail lacquer comprised of ketoconazole-loaded microsponges to treat the fungal infection of nails (onchomycosis). Microsponges loaded with retinoic acid were observed to improve the anti-acne efficacy. Reduction in inflammatory and noninflammatory lesions was observed when tretinoin was loaded in microsponges.

Genetically engineered melanin incorporated in microsponges provided the ease to spread it evenly and hence give protection against UV-A and UV-B radiation. Other over-the-counter products incorporated with microsponges include moisturizers, specialized rejuvenative products, and sunscreens. Currently, prescription products employing this technology are indicated for acne vulgaris, actinic keratoses (AK), and pigmentary changes.

Microsponges for Oral Drug Delivery

An SPM system offers the potential to hold active ingredients in a protected environment and provide controlled delivery of oral medication to the lower gastrointestinal (GI) tract, where it will be released upon exposure to specific enzymes in the colon. In oral applications, the SPM system has been shown to increase the rate of solubilization of poorly water-soluble drugs by entrapping such drugs in the SPM system's pores. Because these pores are very small, the drug is in effect reduced to microscopic particles, and the significantly increased surface area thus greatly increases the rate of solubilization. Also the time taken by the SPMs to traverse the large and small intestine is also increased; therefore, the amount of the drug that is absorbed is also increased. In SPMs prepared using ethanol to dissolve the drug and polymer, variation in the ratios of drug and polymer gave control over the porosity of the particle, and drug release properties are fitted to Higuchi model 48. Ketoprofen and flurbiprofen SPMs produce mechanically strong tablets due to plastic deformation of the sponge-like structure.

Baykara and collaborators formulated the ketoprofen microsponges for oral use and observed that the release of ketoprofen was modified with the formulation following the Higuchi model [23]. They also studied the effect of pressure for compression for tableting of ketoprofen microsponges and demonstrated that microsponges have better compressibility, owing to the plastic deformation of the sponge-like structure, and produced mechanically strong tablets [24]. They also proved that tablets comprising microsponges improved bioavailability, but these tablets showed delayed drug release and absorption. This led to the conclusion that tableting of the microsponges increases the lag time for drug appearance in plasma and maintains the drug concentration for a longer period [25].

Cui et al. designed microsponges for nitrendipine, which behaved like a solid dispersion, by modifying the quasiemulsion solvent diffusion method. Hydroxypropyl methyl cellulose (HPMC) phthalate was used as solid dispersion carrier, Eudragit RS-100 and ethyl cellulose as retarding agents, and anhydrous silicic acid as a dispersing agent to increase the release rate. Oral administration of microsponges in male dogs demonstrated threefold increase in relative bioavailability when compared with a conventional dosage form [26]. Graves et al. formulated biodegradable microsponges of polylactide glycolic acid (PLGA) for the delivery of proteins and peptides [27]. In another report, Gao and collaborators prepared porous polylactide microspheres by emulsion solvent evaporation based on solution–induced phase separation. They revealed that particles with larger pores enabled the porous microspheres to float, and these can also be used to develop microsponge-based novel gastroretentive drug delivery systems [28].

Preliminary studies as performed by A. P. Pharma, Inc. (Redwood City, CA, USA) indicated that the microsponge particles bind to the rough surface of the intestinal mucosa; thus these carrier systems have the potential to increase bioavailability by the combination of the enhanced rate of adsorption and dissolution [29]. A microsponge system offers the potential to hold active ingredients in a protected environment and provide controlled delivery to the lower GIT. The reason for selection of microsponges as a colonic delivery system is due to the fact that a drug carrier system has a size less than 200 ìm that can be efficiently taken up by the macrophages present in colonic tissue, thus exhibiting effective localized drug action at the desired site [30]. To determine if coated microsponges form a viable option for sustained release of chlorpheniramine maleate, drug-loaded cellulose microparticles were coated with Eudragit RS-100 to form powder-coated microsponges. The researchers observed that the powder-coated granules demonstrated lower Cmax (maximum plasma drug concentration) and longer Tmax (time for maximum plasma drug concentration) than the powder chlorpheniramine maleate, following oral administration in dogs [31]. Orlu et al. made an approach for the colon targeting of flurbiprofen by preparing pectin-coated tablets containing microsponges as the core. Additionally, they studied the active drug-loading method with the commercially available Microsponge 5640 system and determined that active loading in the case of microsponges reduced the drug content and encapsulation efficiency while the microsponges prepared by quasiemulsion solvent diffusion possessed spherical pores with larger diameter. Their study also revealed that a very high drug:polymer ratio failed to prepare microsponges while by reducing the drug:polymer ratio highly porous spherical microsponges were obtained. Microsponges on compression gave mechanically strong core tablets, which provided sustained drug release. They also prepared a colon-specific tablet by the pore-plugged method using the same polymeric mixture. Tablets prepared by the pore-plugged method showed zero-order release kinetics [8].

Devrim and Canefe in 2006 prepared microsponges for the delivery of ibuprofen and also studied the effect of polymers (Eudragit RS-100, Eudragit RS PM, and Eudragit RL 100) on various characteristics of the microsponges, including rheological properties along with the particle size and release characteristics, and concluded that all the microsponges possessed good flow properties required for the maintenance of the dose and weight uniformity during tablet compression or capsule filling. They also observed that smaller particles with better control over drug release were obtained with Eudragit RS-100 when compared with that formed with other grades of Eudragit [32].

Jain and Singh prepared dicyclomine-loaded microsponges for colonic delivery by the quasiemulsion solvent diffusion method to study the effect of process variables and analyzed in vitro drug release data. This research illustrated that increasing the quantity of the emulsifying agent increases the particle size of the microsponges. Another observation related to the drug:polymer ratio showed that increasing the drug:polymer ratio resulted in reduced production yield and smaller particles but increased drug content. The drug release profile of the microsponges showed the best fit for the Higuchi model. The researchers also observed that increasing the polymeric content resulted in better control over drug release [33]. The authors had also developed and characterized the paracetamol-loaded colon-targeted drug delivery system employing microsponges by coating them with natural polysaccharides, such as citrus pectin, which enabled it to inhibit the drug release for an initial 8 h while releasing the drug after adding the enzyme pectinex. This study also revealed the capability of the microsponges to load the drugs that are required to be used in the high dose, thus proving that the microsponges have better loading efficiency than other microparticulate (microballoons, microcapsules, and microspheres) systems. They observed a decrease in drug release rate with the increase in drug:polymer ratio following a biphasic release [34]. The authors performed in vitro release studies and observed that the main mechanism of drug release was diffusion [35]. Kadam et al. developed microsponge-based drug delivery system for the delivery of aceclofenac and observed that such systems reduced the crystallinity of the drug particles, and their compressed tablets can be used for chronic purposes [36]. Jain et al. revealed the capability of Eudragit S-100 for the development of microsponges for colon targeting [30].

Dhawale et al. prepared the percentage fluorouracil-loaded porous microspheres and observed that drug release showed generally similar behavior at different pH. These carriers were efficient enough to retain the drug inside the microspheres during the in vitro drug release study in simulated gastric and intestinal fluids while a fast release was observed in the colonic range, which delivered about 100% of the incorporated drug within 60 min [37]. Srivastava et al. developed microsponges by using sodium chloride as porogen and observed that the use of porogen led to the uniform porous outer surface with an interlinked porous internal structure. They also observed that structural integrity was not lost during drug release, but the surface got eroded as a phase transition of surface occurred by the release of drug molecules adsorbed on the surface. Their research showed compression to a matrix tablet fabricated with microsponges did not cause any disruption in the integrity of microsponges. Their experiment also revealed the surface retentive ability of the microsponges, leading to the reduced systemic exposure of the active ingredient [11].

Grafts and Implants

Biodegradable materials with autologous cell seeding have attracted much interest as potential cardiovascular grafts. However, pretreatment of these materials requires a complicated and invasive procedure that carries the risk of infection. To avoid these problems, biodegradable graft material containing collagen SPM was developed that would permit the regeneration of autologous vessel tissue. Poly (lactic-coglycolic acid) as a biodegradable scaffold was compounded with collagen SPM to form a vascular patch material. It showed good histologic findings and durability with and without pre-cellularization. This patch shows promise as a bioengineered material for promoting in situ cellularization and the regeneration of autologous tissue in cardiovascular surgery [38,39]. A thin biodegradable hybrid mesh of synthetic poly (DL-lactic-co-glycolic acid) (PLGA) and naturally derived collagen was used for three-dimensional culture of human skin fibroblasts. The hybrid mesh was constructed by forming web-like collagen SPMs in the openings of a PLGA knitted mesh. The behaviors of the fibroblasts on the hybrid mesh and PLGA knitted mesh were compared. The efficiency of cell seeding was much higher, and the cells grew more quickly in the hybrid mesh than in the PLGA mesh. The fibroblasts in the PLGA mesh grew from the peripheral PLGA fibers toward the centers of the openings while those in the hybrid mesh also grew from the collagen SPMs in the openings of the mesh resulting in a more homogenous growth. The proliferated cells and secreted extracellular matrices were more uniformly distributed in the hybrid mesh than in the PLGA mesh. Histological staining of in vitro cultured fibroblast/mesh implants indicated that the fibroblasts were distributed throughout the hybrid mesh and formed a uniform layer of dermal tissue having almost the same thickness as that of the hybrid mesh. However, the tissue formed in the PLGA mesh was thick adjacent to the PLGA fibers and thin in the center of the openings. Fibroblasts cultured in the hybrid mesh were implanted in the back of a nude mouse. Dermal tissues were formed after 2 weeks and became epithelialized after 4 weeks. The results indicate that the web-like collagen SPMs formed in the openings of the PLGA knitted mesh increased the efficiency of cell seeding, improved cell distribution, and therefore facilitated rapid formation of dermal tissue having a uniform thickness. PLGA–collagen hybrid mesh may be useful for skin tissue engineering. Human skin fibroblasts were cultured in a thin biodegradable mesh having a hybrid structure with web-like collagen SPMs formed in the openings of a PLGA knitted mesh. More fibroblasts adhered and proliferated more quickly in the hybrid mesh than in the PLGA knitted mesh. The collagen SPMs in the hybrid meshes facilitated cell seeding, uniform cell distribution, and, therefore, the formation of homogenous dermis tissue. The PLGA knitted mesh served as a skeleton, reinforced the hybrid mesh, maintained the integrity of the forming tissue, and resulted in easy handling. PLGA–collagen hybrid mesh could be a useful candidate as a porous scaffold for skin tissue engineering [40–42].

Bone Substitutes

Bone substitute compounds were obtained by mixing prepolymerized powders of polymethylmethacrylate and liquid methylmethacrylate monomer with two aqueous dispersions of a-tricalcium phosphate (a-TCP) grains and calcium-deficient hydroxyapatite (CDHA) powders. The final composites appeared to be porous. Osteoconductivity and osteoinductivity of the final composites were tested in vivo by implantation in rabbits. Formation of new trabecular bone was observed inside the pores where the inorganic powders had been placed. The material produced shows a good level of biocompatibility, good osteointegration rate, and osteogenetic properties.

Pulmonary Route

Sun et al. also investigated the potential of porous microspheres as an injectable drug delivery system for controlled protein delivery using human serum albumin as a model drug [43]. Giovagnoli et al. studied the potential of the porous microspheres of capreomycin sulfate for pulmonary use [44].

CLINICAL PERSPECTIVE

Due to their clinical superiority over other carrier systems, they were approved for the treatment of dermatomycosis, acne, and actinic keratosis. Various performed clinical studies suggested that entrapping any active agent in microsponges or nanosponges would increase their efficacy and safety. In such effort, hydroquinone and retinol were entrapped in microsponges and studied clinically in an open-label study for the treatment of hyperpigmentation, and the developed system was compared against unentrapped drug. The study concluded that the disease severity and pigmentation intensity was statistically improved compared with baseline. Microentrapped drug components were well tolerated, safe, and effective. In the same perspective, while studying the in vitro efficacy of such carriers to treat cancer, the study showed that efficacy of tamoxifen and paclitaxel was improved by entrapping them in the nanosponges.

RECENT ADVANCES IN MICROSPONGE DRUG DELIVERY SYSTEM

Various advances were made by modifying the methods to form nanosponges, nanoferrosponges, and porous microbeads. Nanosponges were used for the passive targeting of cosmetic agents to the skin, thereby reducing the total dose, avoiding systemic absorption, and extending retention of dosage form on the skin [45]. These were developed by modifying various parameters of the quasiemulsion solvent diffusion method, such as agitation rate, amount of polymer, amount of emulsifying agent, and volume of inner phase and continuous phase. Decreasing the amount of the polymer or increasing the drug:polymer ratio resulted in decreased particle size [46]. b-CD nanosponges were also developed that can be used for hydrophobic as well as hydrophilic drugs in contrast to polymeric micro or nanosponges [47–49]. These advanced systems were studied for oral administration of dexamethasone, flurbiprofen, doxorubicin hydrochloride, itraconazole, and serum albumin as a model drug. These nanosponges were developed by cross-linking the b-CD molecule by reacting the b-CD with diphenylcarbonate. The pore size of these cross-linked, nanoporous materials can be modulated by varying the CD/PMA molar ratio. In the presence of aqueous solutions, they can show gel-like behavior [47]. b-CD nanosponges were observed to increase the drug release rate of a practically insoluble drug, itraconazole, by forming a ternary complex using copovidone [48]. Swellable nanosponges of b-CD were developed by crosslinking b-CD with 2, 2-bisacrylamido acetic acid in aqueous solution. Homogenized nanosponges showed stability as these did not undergo aggregation during storage [49]. Some researchers also observed the nanosponges as good carriers for the delivery of gases [50]. Researchers also observed that incorporating a cytotoxic in a nanosponge carrier system can increase the potency of the drug, suggesting that these carriers can be potentially used for targeting of cancerous cells [51,52].

The nanoferrosponge, a novel approach, constituted the self pore-forming carriers having better penetration to the targeted site due to the external magnetic trigger, which forces the carriers to penetrate to the deeper tissue and then causes the removal of magnetic material from the particle, leaving a porous system. These were prepared by coprecipitating the polymer and magnetite. The ferrosponges showed high swelling ratios together with excellent elasticity, hydrophilicity, and rapid response to an external magnetic stimulation for fast and repeatable swelling–deswelling (or expansion–contractile) operations [53]. Due to the improved characteristics of porous microspheres, a process was developed to produce porous microbeads. This method (high internal phase emulsion, HIPE) consisted of the monomer containing continuous oil phase, cross-linking agent, and aqueous internal phase. Polymerization and cross-linking was activated by heating them to convert the liquid HIPE microdroplets to solid microbeads [38]. Some authors also described the addition of magnesium stearate to the dispersed phase to prevent flocculation of the Eudragit RS-100 microsponges when preparing these particles by oil in an oil emulsion solvent diffusion method. Pore inducers, such as sucrose and pregelatinized starch, were also reported to enhance the rate of drug release [40]. Some researchers also performed the accumulation study with resveratrol-loaded nanosponges in rabbit mucosa and observed that nanosponges have better accumulation than plain drug. These results signify that nanosponge formulations can be used for buccal delivery and topical application [41]. Some other researchers also observed the effect of nanosponge formulations to protect the lactone ring of camptothecin after their incubation in physiological conditions at 37°C for 24 h. Their study showed that nanosponge formulations are able to enhance the stability of the labile drug compounds [54]. Lee et al. developed a self-assembled microsponge system for the delivery of short interfering RNA (siRNA). They reported the synthesis of a delivery vehicle that combines carrier and cargo: RNA interference (RNAi) polymers that self assemble into nanoscale pleated sheets of hairpin RNA, which, in turn, form sponge-like microspheres consisting entirely of cleavable RNA strands, and are processed by the cell's RNA machinery to convert the stable hairpin RNA to siRNA only after cellular uptake, thus inherently providing protection for siRNA during delivery and transport to the cytoplasm. They also observed an improved stability of RNA and the relatively effective encapsulation process of siRNA. The approach could lead to novel therapeutic routes for siRNA delivery [42]. In an attempt to determine the influence of microsponge formulation on the flux for percutaneous drug delivery, Maiti et al. developed a diclofenac sodium-loaded ethyl cellulose microsponge-loaded gel through the w/o/w emulsion technique. They reported that microsponge formulation reduced the flux of drug across the skin and thus can retain the drug at the delivery site. These formulations reduced the drug permeation through skin and maintained the required concentration of drug at the desired site [55].

INTELLECTUAL PROSPECT OF MICROSPONGES

Various patents were reported on microsponge drug delivery systems, but none of them deals with oral drug delivery. Advanced Polymer Systems, Inc., and subsidiaries (APS or the Co.) were using patented MDS and related proprietary technologies to enhance the safety, effectiveness, and aesthetic quality of topical prescription, over-the-counter, and personal care products, such as tretinoin, 5-fluorouracil (5-FU), vitamin A, and so on. As of July 2006, the company had a total of 10 issued U.S. patents and an additional 92 issued foreign patents; 21 patent applications were pending worldwide. Dean et al. in 1989 disclosed the preparation of weighted collagen microsponges for immobilizing microorganisms. This patent was assigned to Verax Corp. (Germany). The disclosed invention permitted the continuous growth of entrapped microbes and was formed of highly cross-linked collagen. Other such disclosed patents include a microsponge-impregnated nonwoven towel assigned to the Millikan and Co. (Spartanburg, South Carolina) and invented by Love et al. in 2008. A. P. Pharma developed the proprietary technology for oral controlled delivery using porous alginate microspheres as an effective carrier for delivery of hydrophilic molecules in addition to macromolecules, such as vaccines and peptides, orally. The company investigated and conducted clinical studies for these carriers as vehicle to deliver agents to the lower GIT, specifically the colon, by developing a composite tablet designed with the active agent loaded into the microsponge system. Human proof-of-principle studies demonstrated the ability of the tablet design to bypass degradation in the stomach and small intestine to deliver drugs to the colon; thus, this system is potentially applicable to a large group of chemically diverse agents for selective delivery to the colon, including laxatives, steroids, amino salicylic acids, and so on. The company is trying to deliver corticosteroids by appropriately modifying the microsponge system due to its ability to entrap and release the water-insoluble drugs at rates several times higher than the conventional micronized versions of the drugs. At present, this technology is patented to Cardinal Health, Inc. (Dublin, Ohio) for topical use.

FUTURE PROSPECTS

The microsponge drug delivery system holds a promising opportunity in various pharmaceutical applications in the future as it has unique properties, such as enhanced product performance and elegance; extended release; improved drug release profile; reduced irritation; and improved physical, chemical, and thermal stability, which makes it flexible to develop novel product forms. The real challenge of MDS in the future is the development of the delivery system for oral peptide delivery by varying the ratio of polymers. The use of bioerodible and biodegradable polymers for drug delivery is enabling it for the safe delivery of the active material. As these porous systems have also been studied for drug delivery through the pulmonary route, this shows that these systems can show effective drug release even in the scarcity of the dissolution fluid; thus, the colon is an effective site for targeting drug release. These carriers are also required to be developed for alternative drug administration routes, such as the parenteral and pulmonary routes. These particles can also be used as cell culture media and thus can also be employed for stem cell culture and cellular regeneration in the body. Due to their elegance, these carrier systems have also found their application in cosmetics. These characteristic features of porous microspheres motivated researchers to develop other such particles, including nanosponges, nanoferrosponges, and porous microbeads. These developments enabled researchers to utilize them variably. These novelties in formulation also open new ways for drug delivery.

REFERENCES

1. Patel A, Upahyay P, Trivedi J, Shah S, Patel J. Microsponges as the versatile tool for topical tool. *Int J Pharm Sci Res* 2012; 3(9): 2926–37.
2. Srivastava R, Pathak K. Microsponges: A futuristic approach for oral drug delivery. *Expert Opin Drug Deliv* 2012; 9(7): 863–78.
3. Won R. Two step method for preparation of controlled release formulation. United States patent number. US5145675; 1992.
4. Microsponge technology, AMCOL health and beauty solutions. Inc. http://www.amcolhpc.com/Product/SkinCare//MDS/Microsponge.aspx.
5. Embil K, Nacht S. The microsponge delivery system (MDS): A topical delivery system with reduced irritancy incorporating multiple triggering mechanisms for the release of actives. *J Microencapsul* 1996; 13: 575–88.
6. Katz MA, Cheng CH, Nacht S. Methods and composition for topical delivery of benzoyl peroxide. United States patent number. US5879716; 1999.
7. Gans EH. Polymer Developments of cosmetic interest. *Cosmet Toilet* 1999; 114: 53–60.
8. Orlu M, Cevher E, Araman A. Design and evaluation of colon specific drug delivery system containing flurbiprofen microsponges. *Int J Pharm* 2006; 318: 103–17.
9. Grochowicz M, Bartnicki A, Gawdzik B. Preparation and characterization of porous polymeric microspheres obtained from multifunctional methacrylate monomers. *J Polymer Sci* 2008; 46: 6165–74.
10. Jelvehgari MR, Siahi-Shadbad S, Azarmi GP et al. The microsponge delivery system of benzoyl peroxide: Preparation, characterization and release studies. *Int J Pharm* 2006; 308: 124–32.
11. Srivastava R, Kumar D, Pathak K. Colonic luminal surface retention of meloxicam microsponges delivered by erosion based colon targeted matrix tablet. *Int J Pharm* 2012; 427(2): 153–62.
12. Nokhodchi A, Jelveghari M, Siahi M, Dastmalchi S. The effect of formulation type on the release of benzoyl peroxide from microsponges. *Iran J Pharm Sci* 2005; 1: 131–42.
13. Hong Y, Gao C, Shi Y et al. Preparation of porous polylactide microsphere by emulsion solvent evaporation based on solution induced phase separation. *Polym Adv Technol* 2005; 16: 622–7.
14. D'souza JI, More HN. Topical anti-inflammatory gels of flucinolone acetonide entrapped in eudragit based microsponge delivery system. *Res J Pharm Technol* 2008; 1(4): 502–6.
15. Poresizer Model No. 9310, Micromeritics Instrument Corp., Norcross, Georgia. http://www.micromeritics.com.
16. Washburn EW. Note on a method of determining the distribution of pore sizes in a porous material. *Proc Natl Acad Sci U.S.A.* 1921; 7: 115–6.

17. Orr Jr. C. Application of mercury penetration to material analysis. *Powder Technol* 1969; 3: 117–23.
18. Nacht S, Kantz M. The microsponge: A novel topical programmable delivery system. In: David WO, Anfon HA, editors. *Topical drug delivery systems.* Marcel Dekker; New York: 1992. Vol. 42, pp. 299–325.
19. Kawashima Y, Niwa T, Takeuchi H et al. Control of prolonged drug release and compression properties of ibuprofen microspheres with acrylic polymer, eudragit RS, by changing their intraparticle porosity. *Chem Pharm Bull (Tokyo)* 1992; 40(1): 196–201.
20. D'souza JI, Jagdish K, Saboji, Suresh G, Killedar, Harinath N. Design and evaluation of benzoyl peroxide microsponges to enhance therapeutic efficacy in acne treatment, in 20th FAPA congress, Bangkok, 2004.
21. Amrutiya N, Bajaj A, Madan M. Development of microsponges for topical delivery of mupirocin. *AAPS PharmSciTech* 2009; 10(2): 402–9.
22. Grimes PE, A microsponge formulation of hydroquinone 4% and retinol 0.15% in the treatment of melasma and post-inflammatory hyper-pigmentation. Cutis, Vitiligo and Pigmentation Institute of Southern California, Los Angeles, 2004; 74(6): 362–8.
23. Comoglu T, Gonul N, Baykara T. Preparation and in vitro evaluation of modified release ketoprofen microsponges. *Il Farmaco* 2003; 58: 101–6.
24. Comoglu T, Gonul N, Baykara T. The effects of pressure and direct compression on tabletting of microsponges. *Int J Pharm* 2002; 242: 191–5.
25. Comoglu T, Savaser A, Ozkan Y et al. Enhancement of ketoprofen bioavailability by formation of microsponge tablets. *Pharmazie* 2007; 62(1): 51–4.
26. Cui F, Yang M, Jiang Y et al. Design of sustained release nitrendipine microspheres having solid dispersion by quasi emulsion solvent method. *J Control Release* 2003; 91: 375–84.
27. Graves R, Moiseyev R, Pamujula S et al. Spherical biodegradable microsponge particle for drug delivery. *Am Assoc Pharm Sci J* 2005; 7(S2).
28. Hong Y, Gao C, Shi Y et al. Preparation of porous polylactide microsphere by emulsion solvent evaporation based on solution induced phase separation. *Polym Adv Technol* 2005; 16: 622–7.
29. Product information sheet. Oral technology. A. P. Pharma, Inc., Redwood City, California, United States. http://appharma.com.
30. Jain V, Jain D, Singh R. Factors affecting the morphology of eudragit s-100 based microsponges bearing dicyclomine for colonic delivery. *J Pharm Sci* 2010; 100(4): 1–8.
31. Aritomi H, Yamasaki Y, Yamada K et al. Development of sustained release formulation of chlorpheniramine maleate using powder coated microsponges prepared by dry impact blending method. *J Pharm Sci Technol* 1996; 56(1): 49–56.
32. Devrim B, Canefe K. Preparation and evaluation of modified release ibuprofen microspheres with acrylic polymers (Eudragit) by quasi emulsion solvent diffusion method: Effect of variables. *Acta Pol Pharm Drug Res* 2006; 63(6): 521–34.
33. Jain V, Singh R. Dicyclomine-loaded Eudragit-based microsponge with potential for colonic delivery: Preparation and characterization. *Trop J Pharm Res* 2010; 9(1): 67–72.
34. Jain V, Singh R. Development and characterization of eudragit RS 100 loaded microsponges and its colonic delivery using natural polysaccharides. *Acta Pol Pharm Drug Res* 2010; 67(4): 407–15.
35. Jain V, Singh R. Design and characterization of colon-specific drug delivery system containing paracetamol microsponges. *Arch Pharm Res* 2011; 34(5): 733–40.
36. Kadam HM, Disouja JI, Yadav SB. Development of microsponge formulations of aceclofenac for chronotherapy of rheumatoid arthritis. *Am Assoc Pharm Sci J* 2010.
37. Dhawale SC, Bankar AS, Patro MN. Formulation and evaluation porous microspheres of 5- Fluorouracil for colon targeting. *Int J PharmTech Res* 2010; 2(2): 1112–8.

38. LI NH, Benson JR, Kitagawa N. Polymeric microbeads and method of preparation. International publication number. WO1995033553; 2003.
39. Iwai S, Sawa Y, Ichikawa H, Taketani S, Uchimura E, Chen G, Hara M, Miyake J, Matsuda H. Biodegradable polymer with collagen microsponge serves as a new bioengineered cardiovascular prosthesis. *J Thorac Cardiovasc Surg* 2004; 128(3): 472–79.
40. Zaki Rizkalla CM, Latif Aziz R, Soliman II. In vitro and in vivo evaluation of hydroxyzine hydrochloride microsponges for topical delivery. *AAPS PharmSciTech* 2011; 12(3): 989–1001.
41. Ansari KA, Vavia PR, Trotta F et al. Cyclodextrin-based nanosponges for delivery of resveratrol: In vitro characterisation, stability, cytotoxicity and permeation study. *AAPS PharmSciTech* 2011; 12(1): 279–86.
42. Lee JB, Hong J, Bonner DK et al. Self-assembled RNA interference microsponges for efficient siRNA delivery. *Nat Mater* 2012; 11(4): 316–22.
43. Sun L, Zhou S, Wang W et al. Preparation and characterization of porous biodegradable microspheres used for controlled protein delivery. *Colloids Surf A Physicochem Eng Aspects* 2009; 345(1–3): 173–81.
44. Giovagnoli S, Blasi P, Schoubben A et al. Preparation of large porous biodegradable microspheres by using a simple double-emulsion method for capreomycin sulfate pulmonary delivery. *Int J Pharm* 2007; 333: 103–11.
45. Sharma R, Pathak K. Polymeric nanosponges as an alternative carrier for improved retention of Econazole nitrate onto the skin through topical hydrogel formulation. *Pharm Dev Technol* 2011; 16(4): 367–76.
46. Emanuele AD, Dinarvand R. Preparation, characterization and drug release from thermoresponsive microsphere. *Int J Pharm* 1995; 118(2): 237–42.
47. Trotta F, Cavalli R, Tumiatti W. Cyclodextrin-based nanosponges for drug delivery. *J Incl Phenom Macrocyclic Chem* 2006; 56: 209–13.
48. Swaminathan S, Vavia PR, Trotta F et al. Formulation of betacyclodextrin based nanosponges of itraconazole. *J Incl Phenom Macrocyclic Chem* 2007; 57: 89–94.
49. Swaminathan S, Cavalli R, Trotta F et al. In vitro release modulation and conformational stabilization of a model protein using swellable polyamidoamine nanosponges of beta-cyclodextrin. *J Incl Phenom Macrocyclic Chem* 2010; 68: 183–91.
50. Cavalli R, Akhter AK, Bisazza A et al. Nanosponge formulations as oxygen delivery systems. *Int J Pharm* 2010; 402(1–2): 254–7.
51. Torne S, Darandale S, Vavia P et al. Cyclodextrin-based nanosponges: Effective nanocarrier for Tamoxifen delivery. *Pharm Dev Technol* 2013; 18(3): 619–25.
52. Ansari KA, Torne SJ, Vavia PR et al. Paclitaxel loaded nanosponges: In-vitro characterization and cytotoxicity study on MCF-7 cell line culture. *Curr Drug Deliv* 2011; 8(2): 194–202.
53. Hu SH, Liu TY, Liu DM et al. Nano-ferrosponges for controlled drug release. *J Control Release* 2007; 121(3): 181–9.
54. Swaminathan S, Pastero L, Serpe L et al. Cyclodextrin-based nanosponges encapsulating camptothecin: Physicochemical characterization, stability and cytotoxicity. *Eur J Pharm Biopharm* 2010; 74(2): 193–201.
55. Maiti S, Kaity S, Ray S et al. Development and evaluation of xanthan gum-facilitated ethyl cellulose microsponges for controlled percutaneous delivery of diclofenac sodium. *Acta Pharm* 2011; 61: 257–70.

11 Chitosan for Advancing Drug Delivery

Sanjay K. Jain and Satish Shilpi

CONTENTS

INTRODUCTION

Chitosan is a natural nontoxic biopolymer produced by the deacetylation of chitin, a major component of the shells of crustaceans, such as crab, shrimp, and crawfish. It is a cationic polysaccharide and has received considerable attention as a functional, renewable, nontoxic, and biodegradable biopolymer for diverse applications, especially in commercial applications in the biomedical, pharmaceutics, food, cosmetics, and chemical industries (Knorr, 1984; Razdan & Pettersson, 1994). Chitosan contains three types of reactive functional groups: an amino/acetamido group as well as both primary and secondary hydroxyl groups at the C-2, C-3, and C-6 positions, respectively. The amino contents are the main reason for the differences between their structures and physicochemical properties, which are correlated with their chelation, flocculation, and biological functions. In the medical field, chitosan has been developed not only as artificial skin, absorbable surgical suture, and a wound healing accelerator, but also as a new physiological material due to the antitumor, immunoenhancing, antimicrobial, and hypocholesterolemic properties (Jeon et al., 2000; Shahidi et al., 1999).

These functions have been revealed to be dependent on both their chemical structure and molecular size. As a result, the application of this native polysaccharide is limited by its high molecular weight and highly viscous nature, resulting in its low solubility in acid-free aqueous media. In recent years, studies on the modification of chitosan have intensified since efficient utilization of marine biomass resources has become an environmental priority and for a better use of chitosan. This chapter focuses on the various applications of chitosan in combination with pharmaceutical and biomedical applications, especially in hypocholesterolemic, immunoenhancing, homeostasic, and anticancer functions, based on our current research as well as the recent literature.

SOURCES AND ISOLATION OF CHITOSAN

It is found naturally in the shells of crustaceans, such as crab, shrimp, and lobster, as well as in the exoskeleton of marine zooplankton, including coral and jellyfish. Insects, such as butterflies and ladybugs, have chitin in their wings. And the cell walls of yeast, mushrooms, and other fungi also contain this natural substance. Chitin may be obtained from arthropods/exoskeletons of crustaceans, such as crab, shrimp, lobster, fungi cell wall, and insect shell (scorpions, spiders, cockroaches, and silk worms). Chitin was first found in mushrooms in 1811 by Professor Henri Braconnot while he was professor of natural history and director of the Botanical Gardens at the Academy of Sciences in Nancy, France. In the 1830s, it was isolated from insects and named chitin. Professor C. Rouget discovered chitosan in 1859, and over the next century, much fundamental research took place on these compounds.

An intense interest in new applications grew in the 1930s and early 1940s as evidenced by almost 50 patents; however, the lack of adequate manufacturing facilities and

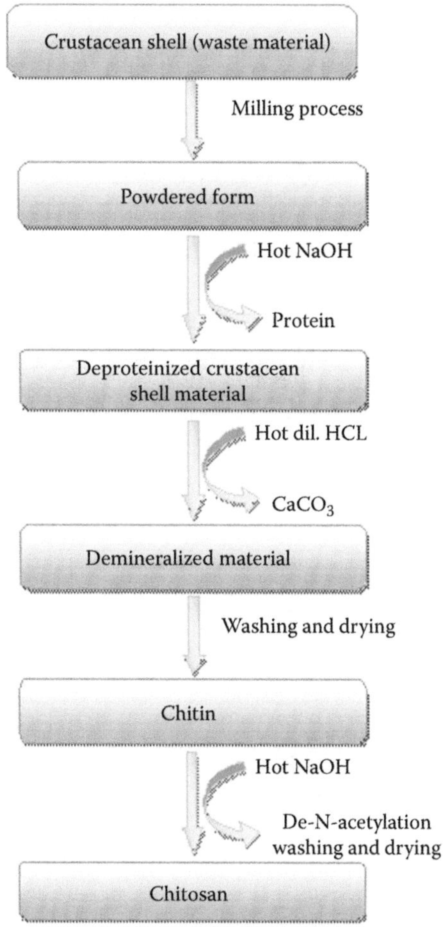

FIGURE 11.1 Schemetic diagram of isolation process of chitosan.

competition from synthetic polymers hampered commercial development. Renewed interest in the 1970s was encouraged by the need to better utilize shellfish shells. Scientists worldwide began to chronicle the more distinct properties of chitin and its derivatives and understand the potential of these natural polymers (Muzzarelli et al., 1988; Jeon et al., 2000; Dutta, 2004; Chung et al., 2006). The isolation process and chemical structure of chitosan is given in Figures 11.1 and 11.2, respectively.

PHYSICOCHEMICAL PROPERTIES OF CHITOSAN

Chitosan (2-amino-2-deoxy-D-glucose) is a polysaccharide and polycationic polymer, which is derived from β linked N-acetyl-D-glucosamine (chitin) after its partial N-deacetylation and hydrolysis, primarily from crustacean and insect shells. It consists of repeating units of glucosamine and N-acetyl-glucosamine; generally, it contains more than 5,000 glucosamine units, the proportions of which determine

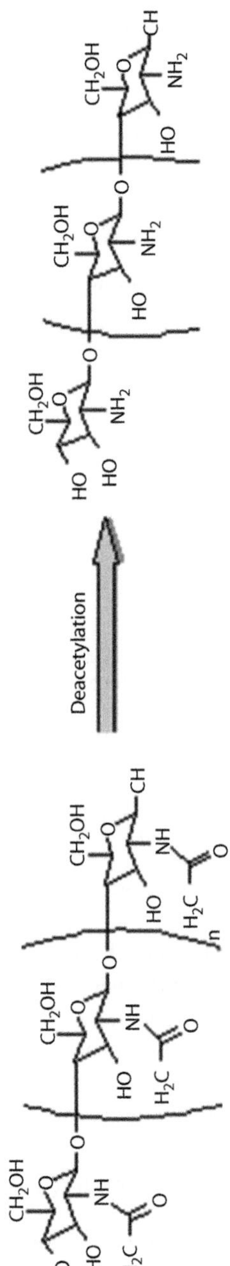

FIGURE 11.2 Chemical structures of chitin and chitosan.

the degree of deacetylation of the polymer. Chitosan has primary and secondary hydroxyl groups along with a free amino group. The chemical structure of chitosan and chitin is shown in Figure 11.2. Chitin is, in fact, the second most abundant polymer on this earth after cellulose (Muzzarelli et al., 1988; Dutta, 2004).

Chitosan possess variety of physicochemical properties. It has a pKa of approximately 6.5. Chitosan is insoluble at neutral pH but is soluble and positively charged at acidic pH. The number of protonatable amine groups along with the degree of deacetylation fundamentally determines the polymer properties, including solubility, hydrophobicity, and its ability to interact electrostatically with polyanions (Hejazi & Amiji, 2003; Huang et al., 2005). The molecular weight of chitosan is also of fundamental importance and exerts its effect on the properties of the chitosan. Commercially available chitosan has an average molecular weight ranging between 3,800 and 20,000 Daltons and is 66% to 95% deacetylated. The molecular weight of chitosan may affect its solubility, viscosity, elasticity, and tear strength. The solubility of chitosan depends on the degree of deacetylation, pH, and on the protonation of free amino groups. Its density is between 1.35 and 1.40 g/cm^3, and its glass transition point temperature is 203°C.

Generally, chitosans, which have lower molecular weights and lower degrees of deacetylation, exhibit greater solubility and faster degradation than their high-molecular-weight counterparts (Mao et al., 2004; Ren et al., 2005). On the other hand, positively charged chitosan will bind to cell membranes and is reported to decrease the transepithelial electrical resistance (TEER) of cell monolayers as well as to increase paracellular permeability. Chitosan solutions have been shown to increase trans- and para-cellular permeability in a reversible, dose-dependent manner that also depends on the molecular weight and degree of deacetylation of the chitosan (Artursson et al., 1994; Schipper et al., 1996). The mechanism of action, which appears to be mediated by the positive charges on the chitosan, includes interactions with the tight junction proteins occludin and ZO-1, redistribution of F-actin, and slight destabilization of the plasma membrane (Deacon et al., 2000; Dodane et al., 1999; Fang et al., 2001). Thus, the ability of chitosan to enhance permeation is influenced by the pH of the environment. As mentioned above, trimethyl chitosan derivatives are soluble at higher pH than unmodified chitosan. Chitosan is also mucoadhesive (Deacon et al., 2000). Mucus is a blend of molecules, including salts, lysozyme, and mucins, which are highly hydrated glycoproteins primarily responsible for the viscoelastic properties of mucus. Sialic acid residues on mucin have a pKa of 2.6, making them negatively charged at physiological pH. Therefore, the presence of mucus affects free drug permeability as well as the uptake of particulates by forming both a physical barrier to diffusion as well as by interacting electrostatically with cationic molecules, such as chitosan. Derivatives of chitosan, such as trimethyl chitosan, retain their mucoadhesive properties although to a lesser extent than unmodified chitosan (Snyman et al., 2003). In addition, formation of chitosan into micro- and nanoparticles also preserves mucoadhesion (Kockisch et al., 2003; Dhawan et al., 2004). Chitosan is generally considered nontoxic and biodegradable with an oral LD_{50} in mice of over 16 g/kg (Hirano, 1996). Antimicrobial, antifungal, and wound-healing properties have also been reported. The safety of chitosan, its ability to prolong residence time in the gastrointestinal tract through mucoadhesion, and its ability to enhance absorption by increasing cellular permeability have all been major factors contributing to its widespread evaluation as a component of oral dosage forms.

SOLUBILITY OF CHITOSAN

The solubility of chitosan depends on the pH and degree of deacetylation of the molecular chain of chitin. Chitosan faces some limitations in its solubility, depending on its molecular structure and pKa. The highly crystalline structure of chitosan enhances inter- and intramolecular hydrogen bonding, which is responsible for limited solubility. The pka solubility of chitosan can be modified by changing the degree of deacetylation or by modifying the pH and ionic strength of the formulation. In neutral pH, chitosan molecules lose their charge and get precipitated from the solution. Solubility of chitosan also depends upon the protonation of the free amino group presence in chitosan molecules, and it does not occur in water or alkaline solution or neutral pH, but in the case of acidic solution, protonation of the free amino group does occur, and this phenomena is responsible for its solubility in acidic conditions as well as for its positively charge nature.

The solubility of chitosan in neutral and basic pH can be improved by quaternization, which forms trimethyl chitosan derivatives. Solubility of chitosan is also dependent upon its molecular weight. Commercially available chitosan has an average molecular weight ranging between 3,800 and 20,000 Daltons and is 66% to 95% deacetylated. Chitosan is readily soluble in dilute solutions of most of the organic acids, such as citric acid and tartaric acid (4% *v/v*) at pH less than 6.5, while soluble to a limited extent in inorganic acids, such as acetic acid (>4% *v/v*). Chitosan can be modified in to N-trimethylene chloride, which is a quaternary derivative of chitosan and has superior aqueous solubility and intestinal permeability as well as higher absorption of neutral and cationic peptide analogue over a wide pH range. However, chemical modifications and derivatization make it soluble in a wide range of pH conditions—that is, derivatives of chitosan exhibit a good solubility profile as compared with its native form (Chung et al., 2006). Modified forms of chitosan, such as chitosan glutamate, chitosan succinate, and chitosan phthalate are esters of chitosan, which have a special solubility profile—that is, they are insoluble in low pH conditions and provide sustained release in higher pH conditions. Figure 11.3 shows some modification techniques for chitosan, which enhance its solubility.

MUCOADHESIVE CHARACTER

CH is a natural bioadhesive polymer having an excellent mucoadhesiveness in its swollen state that can adhere to hard and soft tissues. The adhesive properties of CH in a swollen state might involve some mechanisms, such as adhesion by hydration, hydrogen bonding, and ionic interactions. Effective adhesion has been shown for epithelial tissues and in the mucus coat present on the surface of the tissues. When CH, having a polycationic surface (positively charged amino groups), interacts (electrostatically) with a mucin layer containing residues of sialic acid (negative charged monosaccharide), molecular attractive forces develop that help in the generation of mucoadhesive effect. This property of chitosan is widely utilized in drug delivery. A number of chitosan-based colloidal delivery systems have been developed for the mucosal delivery of polar drugs, peptides, proteins, vaccines, DNA, and other active biomolecules. It has been postulated that residence time of formulations at sites of

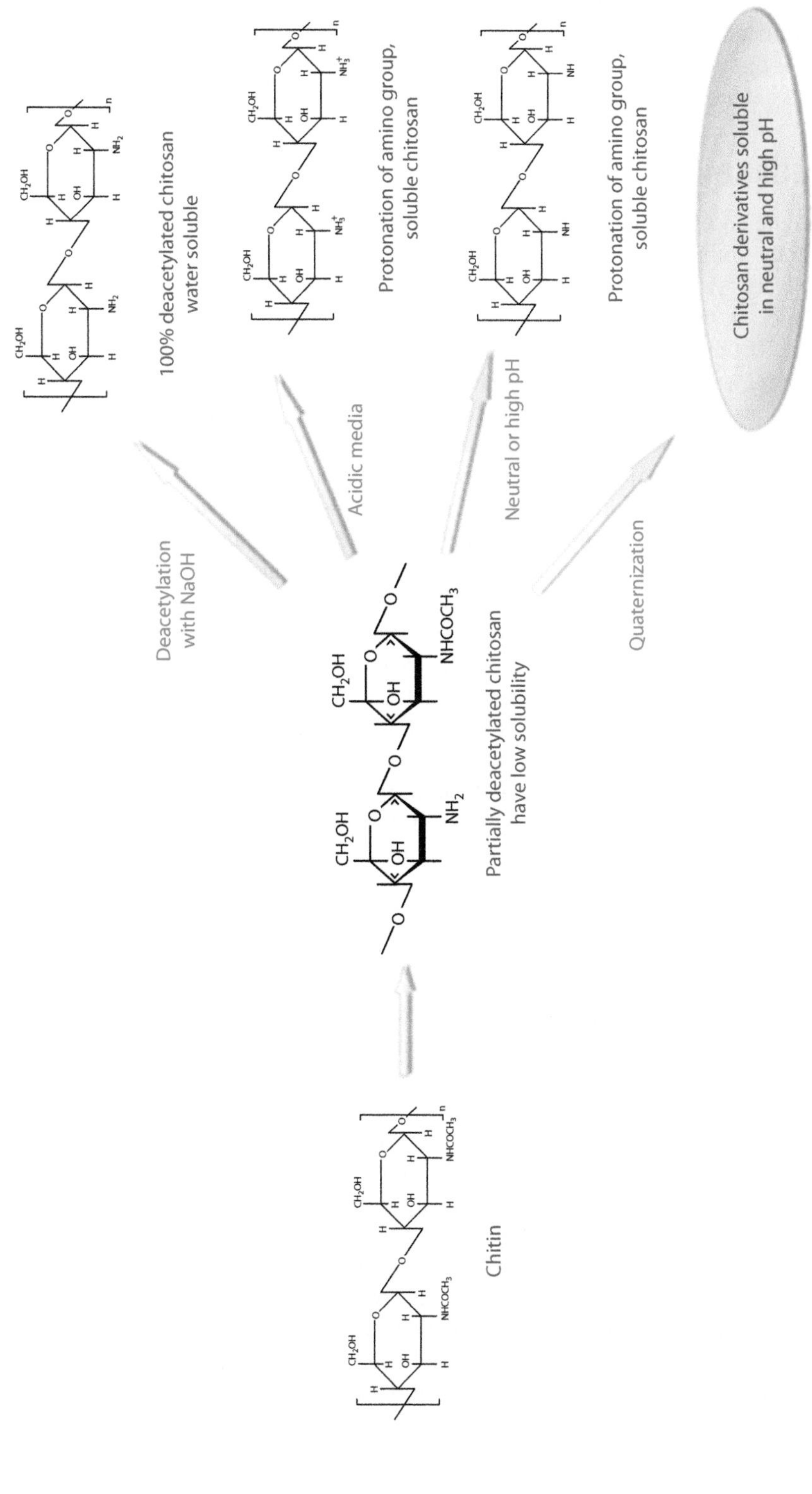

FIGURE 11.3 Techniques for solubility enhancement of chitosan.

drug action or absorption could be prolonged through the use of chitosan. It has also been intimated that CH might be valuable for drug delivery to specific regions of the GIT—that is, buccal mucosa, stomach, small intestine, colon, and nasal route (Miyazaki et al., 1995; Lehr et al., 1992; He et al., 1998).

BIODEGRADATION OF CHITOSAN

It should be necessary that degradation of any polymeric drug carrier occurs in the living body within a period of time. Polymer selection criteria for development of drug delivery systems are dependent on the biometabolism or biodegradation of polymer. Chitosan, with a suitable molecular weight range, can easily excrete by renal clearance. If the high molecular weight chitosan or polymer is administrerd in the form of a nanocarrier, then it may undergo biodegradation (chemical or enzymatic) that would provide fragments suitable for renal clearance. Chemical degradation, in this case, refers to acid-catalyzed degradation *in situ*—that is, in the acidic environment of the stomach, a tumor microenvironment, or in the case of the acidic environment of an endosome—although a peculiar mechanism of *in vivo* degradation like oxidation-reduction depolymerization and free radical degradation have also been reported with chitosan molecules (Hsu et al., 2002, Zoldners et al., 2005). In the case of enzymatic degradation of chitosan, it hydrolyzes in glucosamine–glucosamine, N-acetylglucosamine-N-acetyl-glucosamine, and glucosamine-N-acetyl-glucosamine linkages, which are futher subjected to renal clearance. A study reported that the chitosan is degraded by lysozyme and by bacterial enzymes in vertebrates predominantly in the colon on oral administration (Kean et al., 2009). The rate and amount of chitosan biodegradability in living organisms depend on the degree of deacetylation. The chitosan degradation rate decreases with an increasing degree of deacetylation (Yang et al., 2007; Xu et al., 1996). As the extent of degradation is related to the rate, giving adequate time and appropriate conditions, the CHs would degrade sufficiently for subsequent excretion.

CHITOSAN DERIVATIVES

Chemical modification of chitosan may improve its solubility and widen its applications. Derivatization by introducing small functional groups to the chitosan structure, such as alkyl or carboxymethyl groups, can drastically increase the solubility of chitosan at neutral and alkaline pH values without affecting its cationic character. Substitution with moieties bearing carboxylic groups can yield polymers with polyampholytic properties. Among the various methods of modification, graft copolymerization has been mostly used. Grafting of chitosan allows the formation of functional derivatives by covalent binding of a molecule, the graft, onto the chitosan backbone. Chitosan has two types of reactive groups that can be grafted. First, the free amine groups on deacetylated units and, second, the hydroxyl groups on the C3 and C6 carbons on acetylated or deacetylated units. Recently, researchers have shown that after primary derivation followed by graft modification, chitosan would obtain much improved water solubility, antibacterial and antioxidant properties. Table 11.1 shows different derivatives of chitosan.

TABLE 11.1
Chitosan Derivatives

Chitosan Derivatives							
N-Acyl	**N-Carboxyacyl**	**Sugar Derivatives**	**N-Carboxyalkyl (Aryl)**	**O-Carboxyalkyl**	**Metal Ion Chelates**	**Miscellaneous**	**Natural Polysaccharides**
Octanoyl decanoyl Dodecanoyl Tetradecanoyl Lauroyl Myristroyl Benzoyl Dichloroacetyl Triflouroacetyl Carbamoyl Succinyl Acetoxybenoyl	Maleic, Itaconic, Acetyl-thiosuccinic, Glutaric, Cyclohexane, 1,2-dicarboxylic, Phthalic, cis-tetrahydrophthalic, 5-norbomene-2-3-Dicarboxylic, Diphenic, Salicylic, Tri-mellitic, Pyromellitic anhydride	1-deoxygalactic-1-yl, 1-deoxyglucit-1-yl-, 1-deoxylactit-1-yl-, 1-yl-4 (2, 2, 6, 6-tetramethylpiperidine-1-oxyl)-, 1deoxy-69-aldhydomelibiit-1-yl-, Cellobiit-1-yl-chitosans, product obtained from ascorbic acid	N-Carboxybenzyl, Glycine-glucan (N-Carboxy-methyl chitosan), Alanine glucan, Serine glucan, Glutamic acid glucan, Methionine glucan, Leucine glucan	o-corboxymethyl, Crosslinked o-corboxymethyl	Copper, Palladium, Silver, Iodine	Alkyl chitin, Benzyl chitin, Hydroxyl ethyl glycol, Glutaraldehyde chitosan, Theophylline chitosan, Adenine-chitosan, Chitosansalt and acid polysaccharides, Chitosan streptomycin, 2-amido-2,6-diaminoheptanoic acid chitosan	Chitosan glucagon from various organisms

BIOLOGICAL PROPERTIES

During the last two decades, chitosan has been used as a safe excepient in drug formulations. Due to its bioadhesive property, it can adhere to hard and soft tissues and has been used in dentistry, orthopedics, and ophthalmology and in surgical procedures. It adheres to epithelial tissues and to the mucus coat present on the surface of the tissues. It has also a fungistatic or bacteriostatic, anticancerogen, and anticholestermic action. Clinical tests of chitosan have been carried out in order to promote chitosan-based biomaterials, which do not report any inflammatory or allergic reactions following implantation, injection, topical application, or ingestion in the human body (Tiyaboonchai et al., 2003). The viscosity of chitosan also influences the biological properties, such as wound-healing properties, as well as biodegradation by lysozyme. Since chitosan is hydrophilic in nature, it thereby has the ability to form gels at acidic pH. This type of gel can be used as a slow-release drug-delivery system. The positive charge of chitosan confers to this polymer numerous and unique physiological and biological properties with great potential in a wide range of industries, such as cosmetology, food, biotechnology, pharmacology and medicine, and agriculture. Chitosan and its derivatives may be used as antibacterial, fungistatic, hemostatic, anticancer, bone formation, immunoadjuvant, spermicidal, antioxidant, preservative, metal chelate, artificial organ, tissue engineering, wound-healing, hypocholeteromic, analgesic, anti-inflammatory and immunity-enhancing (immunomodulator) (Figure 11.4).

ANTIFUNGAL ACTIVITY

Activity of chitosan against fungus is assumed to be fungistatic rather than fungicidal with a potential to communicate regulatory changes in both the host and fungus (Miyazaki et al., 1995). Generally, chitosan has been reported very effective in inhibiting spore germination, germ tube elongation, and radial growth. Most of the studies have been done on yeasts and molds associated with food and plant spoilage. For these, in the presence of chitosan, several biological processes are activated in plant tissue, where chitinases are induced with action on biotrophic and necrotrophic mycoparasites, entomopathogenic fungi, and vesicular arbuscular mycorrhizal fungi. The level of inhibition of fungi is highly correlated with chitosan concentration. It is believed that the polycationic nature of this compound is the key to its antifungal properties and that the length of the polymer chain enhances its antifungal activity (Hirano & Nagao, 1989). An additional explanation of the mechanism behind antifugal activity of chitosan involves cell wall morphogenesis with chitosan molecules interfering directly with fungal growth, similar to the effects observed in bacteria cells (Ghaouth et al., 1992). Microscopic observation reported that chitosan oligomers diffuse inside hyphae, interfering with the enzyme activity responsible for the fungus growth (Eweis et al., 2006). The intensity of degradation action of chitosan on fungal cell walls is also dependent upon the concentration, DA, and local pH (Stossel et al., 1984). It is reported that inhibition rates on the order of 80% against plant fungus, such as *Phomopsis asparagi*, and as high as 95% against *Fusarium oxysporum*, *Cucumernum owen*, *Rhizoctonia solani*, and *Fusarium oxysporum* have

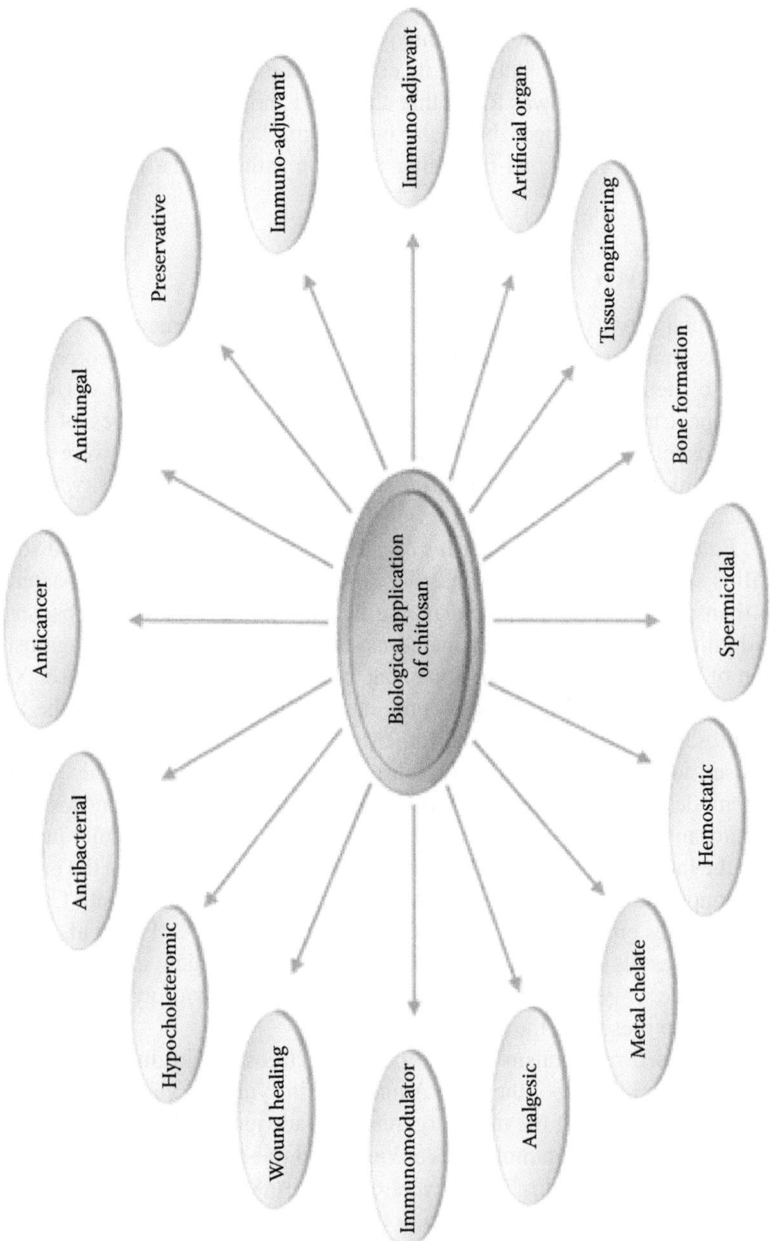

FIGURE 11.4 Some biological properties of chitosan.

been, however, known to occur with low chitosan concentration (20–150 mg.L^{-1}). Zhang et al. (2003) revealed that the percentage of fungus germination decreased with increasing the chitosan concentration in the medium. Generally, the primary observed influence is on the length of the lag phase. As the inhibition process takes place, the medium shifted toward alkalinity, which reduces the effectiveness of the chitosan (Stossel et al., 1984), including its effect on the synthesis of certain fungal enzymes. In another study, it was found that chitosan is not only effective in retardation of the growth of the pathogen, but it also brought marked morphological changes, such as structural alterations and molecular disorganization of the fungal cells (El Ghaouth et al., 1999).

Antimicrobial Activity

The antimicrobial activity of chitosan and its derivatives or oligomers has been recognized and is considered to be one of the most important properties, corresponding directly to their possible biological applications. Chitosan and its derivatives have broad spectrum antimicrobial effects. The antibacterial activities of chitosans and chitosan oligomers with different molecular weights (MV) were examined against some gram-negative bacteria, such as *E. coli*, *Salmonella typhi*, and *Vibrio parahaemolyticus*, and some gram-positive bacteria, such as *Listeria monocytogenes*, *Bacillus megaterium*, *Bacillus cereus*, *Staphylococcus aureus*, and some Lactobacillus species, and it was found that chitosans showed higher antibacterial activities than chitosan oligomers and markedly inhibited the growth of bacteria. Chitin and chitosan have been investigated as an antimicrobial material against a wide range of target organisms, like algae, bacteria, yeasts, and fungi (Wei & Xia, 2003; Xia, 2003; Zhao & Xia, 2006). Coma et al. (2002) have found that the tendency of chitosan is more bacteriostatic rather than bactericidal. Three models have been proposed to explain the antimicrobial activity of chitosan. The ionic surface interaction model is most acceptable, which is the interaction between positively charged chitosan molecules and negatively charged microbial cell membranes. In this model, the interaction is mediated by the electrostatic forces between the protonated NH_3^+ groups and the negative residues, presumably by competing with Ca^{2+} for electronegative sites on the membrane surface (Young et al., 1983; Tsai et al., 1999). This interaction results in a change in cell wall integration, which leads to internal osmotic imbalance, or lyses the bacterial cell wall followed by hydrolysis of peptidoglycans, which are present in the bacterial cell wall.

Another proposed mechanism is the binding of chitosan with microbial DNA, which leads to the inhibition of the mRNA and protein synthesis via the penetration of chitosan into the nuclei of the microorganisms (Hadwiger et al., 1981; Shahidi et al., 1999). In this, the chitosan molecules are assumed to be able to pass through the bacterial cell wall, composed of multilayers of cross-linked murein, and reach the plasma membrane. The third mechanism is the chelation of metals, suppression of spore elements, and binding to essential nutrients for microbial growth (Chen et al., 2002). It is well known that chitosan has excellent metal-binding capacities where the amine groups in the chitosan molecules are responsible for the uptake of metal cations by chelation (Helander et al., 2001). In general, such mechanism is more efficient at high pH where positive ions are bound to chitosan. It is unquestionable that chitosan molecules in bacteria surrounds might complex metals and block some essential nutrients from flowing, contributing to cell death. It is likely that all events occur simultaneously but at different intensities. The molecular weight (MW) and the degree of acetylation (DA) are also important factors in determining such activity. In general, the lower the MW and the DA, the higher will be the effectiveness on reducing microorganism growth and multiplication. It was also found that the higher pH enhances chitosan antibacterial acticity.

Chitosan generally showed stronger bactericidal effects on gram-positive bacteria than gram-negative bacteria at a concentration of 0.1%. The minimum inhibitory concentration (MIC) of chitosans ranged from 0.05% to more than 0.1%, depending on the bacterial species and the MW of the chitosan. The antibacterial activity of chitosan is inversely affected by pH and exerts better effects at a lower pH value.

It has been shown that chitosan derivatives have great potential to be used in other biomedical applications. As a result of the biocompatible properties, such as good blood compatibility and cell growth efficiency, grafted chitosan materials have the potential to be used in cardiovascular applications (Mao et al., 2004; Chung et al., 2006).

Hypocholesterolemic Property

Growing evidence indicates that chitosan can lower plasma and liver triacylglycerol (TG) as well as total cholesterol (TC) levels, hence exhibiting hypocholesterolemic and hypolipidemic effects. It has been reported that chitosan can reduce the risk of cardiovascular diseases (Sugano et al., 1980; Maezaki et al., 1996) and had potent fat-binding capacity *in vitro* (Zhou et al., 2006). In addition, it was shown to increase fecal neutral steroid and bile acid excretion in rats and lower the postprandial plasma TG level in chickens (Razdan & Pettersson, 1996). Among these, Maezaki et al. (1996) reported the hypocholesterolemic effect of chitosan in humans for the first time and found that chitosan effectively decreased plasma lipid levels without side effects. The hypocholesterolemic mechanism of low molecular weight chitosan is dependent upon adsorption, electrostatic force, and entrapment of fatty acids and other lipids.

Although it is not derived from plants, it shares the same characteristics as dietary fiber, which is an indigestible polysaccharide by mammalian digestive enzymes. Several studies showed that chitosan might decrease the level of plasma cholesterol both in animal models and humans (Prashanth et al., 2007; Rha et al., 1984).

The hypocholesterolemic activity of low molecular weight chitosan was higher when its degree of deacetylation was lower (90% deacetylated) at equal MW and particle size; this might be due to the electrostatic attraction between low molecular weight chitosan and anionic substances, such as fatty acids and bile acids. In addition, when fat and low molecular weight chitosan are eaten together, the viscous low molecular weight chitosan will entrap the fat droplets in the stomach. When the complex arrives at the small intestine, chitosan precipitates together with the entrapped fat at neutral pH to prevent the digestion of fat. When the degree of deacetylation and the particle size are comparable, the fat-binding capacity of low molecular weight chitosan is enhanced with increasing MW, suggesting that, during the fat-binding process, the more fat molecules are embedded in the long chain of chitosan (larger molecular weight chitosan). Therefore, the absorption of fat in the diet would reduce due to the fat-binding with various chitosan resulting from electrostatic interactions. The fat-binding capacity of chitosan is better than cellulose. Moreover, at the same molecular weight, powdered chitosan has a smaller particle size, a higher total surface area, and a more open pore structure than flake chitosan for facilitating adsorption. This suggests that the interaction between chitosan and bile salts as well as cholesterol is due to adsorption, which also contributes to its hypocholesterolemic effect. However, this adsorption function is likely weakened *in vivo* as chitosan can be dissolved in the acidic conditions of the stomach. From the above, it is concluded that the combined effects of electrostatic attraction, embedding, adsorption, and entrapment were the probable mechanisms of the hypocholesterolemic effects of chitosan, which was further confirmed by the results of distribution and metabolism of chitosan in rats through measuring the content of fluorescein isothiocyanate labeled chitosan *in vivo*. Therefore, hypocholesterolemic mechanisms of chitosan were identified as the combination of adsorption, electrostatic force, and entrapment.

Hemostasis Effects of Chitosan

Chitosan acts as a hemostatic agent and may be used in various wound-healing applications, such as hemostatic bandages (Jayakumar et al., 2007; Prashanth et al., 2007). However, chitosan, only in its purest form, has an internal hemostatic dressing potentiality. A lot of research has been initiated all over the world into the hemostatic activities of chitin and chitosan (Okamoto et al., 2003; Ishihara et al., 2002; Wang et al., 2006; Gu et al., 2010; Owens et al., 2006). The effects of chitin and chitosan suspensions (0.0001–1.0 mg/mL) on blood coagulation were evaluated by Okamoto et al., and it was found that chitin and chitosan reduced BCT significantly in a dose-dependent manner and enhanced the release of the platelet-derived growth factor-AB (PDGF-AB) and the transforming growth factor-β1 (TGF-β1) from the platelets, particularly with chitosan (Okamoto et al., 2003). Even in a therapeutically anticoagulated (heparinized) rabbit model, chitosan treatment could effectively bring bleeding time within the normal range (Ishihara et al., 2002). The same conclusion was drawn when Wang et al. compared the hemostatic ability of chitosan and collagen sponge. For chitosan and collagen sponges, the total amount of bleeding from the injured veins until hemostasis and the complete hemostasis success rates were similar. But the chitosan sponges strongly adhered to the surface of the rabbit muscles whereas the collagen sponges were easily detached from the muscles (Wang et al., 2006). A fly larva shell–derived chitosan sponge was evaluated as an absorbable surgical hemostatic agent in a rat hepatic hemorrhage model, indicating that chitosan sponge was a suitable implantable hemostatic material when compared to gelatin sponge or oxidized cellulose in both acute and chronic bleeding models. Recently developed internal chitosan bandages have been effective in achieving rapid hemostasis in large surgical and traumatic lacerations of the aorta, liver, lung, kidney, and cardiac ventricles (Gu et al., 2010; Owens et al., 2006). In another study on *in vitro* coagulative activity of chitosan hydrochloride solution with a different degree of deacetylation (DA) and molecular weight (MW) using tube and capillary tube methods indicated that the DA and MW of chitosan had great influence on the hemostasis of chitosan hydrochloride solution. The chitosans with higher DA and MW exhibited better hemostatic activity while the effect of DA and MW was slight on the powder chitosan. From this, it can be deduced that the hemostatic mechanisms of chitosan in powder and hydrochloride solution were different. Meanwhile, organ damage *in vivo* experiments in rabbits showed that chitosan could promote rapid blood clotting at a wound injury in the lung, spleen, and kidney and also reduce the amount of bleeding, exerting a good *in vivo* hemostatic effect. The hemostatic effects of various chitin and chitosan derivatives with different chemical or spatial structures have been studied. It was observed that *N,O*-carboxymethylchitosan (NOCC) could decrease the whole blood clotting time (WHBCT) and lower the plasma recalcification time (PRT) value, similar to that of chitosan and chitin (Janvikul et al., 2006) when used in a hypothermic coagulopathic grade-V liver injury.

Tissue Engineering

Tissue repair requires a complex biological process, where inward cell migration and the proliferation of various types of neighboring cells concertedly restore tissue function. Tissue engineering (TE) is a recent, advanced technology to develop living tissue substitutes and replace diseased or damaged tissues and organs in the human body. Tissue engineering applies the development of polymeric scaffolds that, among other characteristics, are biodegradable and biocompatible. These scaffolds may be used simultaneously as a carrier matrix for bioactive agents and as a support for primary undifferentiated cells *in vitro*. Biological scaffolds are mostly biodegradable and biocompatible and, with the appropriate growth factors, induce cell growth. In addition, a biological scaffold must also fill space with optimal mechanical strength and control the release of bioactive molecules. Current tissue engineered systems cover every tissue and organ with skin and cartilage constructs for repair of skin loss and joints already clinically performed. The present generation of tissue engineering research is based on the seeding of cells onto porous biodegradable polymer matrices. A primary factor is the availability of good biomaterials to serve as the temporary matrix. Recently, chitosan and its derivatives have been reported as attractive candidates for scaffolding materials because they degrade themselves as the new tissues are formed, eventually without inflammatory reactions or toxic degradation (Kim et al., 2001; Tuzlakoglu et al., 2004). In TE applications, the cationic nature of chitosan is primarily responsible for electrostatic interactions with anionic glycosaminoglycans, proteoglycans, and other negatively charged molecules. Very recently, novel PLLA–chitosan hybrid scaffolds were proposed as tissue engineering scaffolds and simultaneously drug release carriers (Prabaharan et al., 2007). In this innovative system, a chitosan porous structure, in which cells and tissues would mostly interact, is created within the pore structure of a stiffer PLLA scaffold. Chitosan-based scaffolds are of current interest for tissue engineering because these natural products are mostly biocompatible and biodegradable. Moreover, the natural components of living structures have biological and chemical similarities to tissues, in which formation of the native extracellular matrix is crucial. One of chitosan's most promising features is its excellent ability to form porous structures for use in tissue transplantation or as a template for tissue regeneration. Chitosan scaffolds are commonly porous-structured by freezing and lyophilizing a chitosan solution or an internal bubbling process. In this process, calcium carbonate ($CaCO_3$) is added to a chitosan solution to generate a chitosan–$CaCO_3$ gel in the specific shape of a mold. The interconnected porous structure is crucial, and numerous cultured cells can be seeded onto it. Cells proliferate and migrate within the scaffold and ultimately form a tissue or organ. For example, a chitosan porous skin regenerating template (CPSRT) that is seeded with skin cells, such as keratinocytes or fibroblasts, may form a skin sheet-like tissue. However, regulation of porosity and pore morphology of a chitosan-based scaffold is particularly important to control angiogenesis, the cellular colonization rate, and organization within an engineered tissue *in vitro*.

It has been shown that thiolated chitosan can provide an adequate scaffold structure: Due to the *in situ* gelling properties, it seems possible to provide a certain shape of the scaffold material by pouring a liquid thiolated chitosan cell suspension into a mold. Furthermore, liquid polymer cell suspensions may be applied by injection, forming semisolid scaffolds at the site of tissue damage. So they seem to be promising candidates for such applications. Another approach regarding the chemical modification of chitosan for TE applications has been to introduce the specific recognition of cells by sugars. A recent example of the synthesis of sugar-bound chitosan can be found in the work of Kim et al. (2001). They prepared mannosylated chitosan, which has the specific recognition to antigen-presenting cells, such as B-cells, dendritic cells, and macrophages. In addition to applications in controlled drug release, poly(N-isopropylacrylamide (PNIPAAm)–grafted chitosan-based materials have been exploited for controlling cell adhesion or detachment by changing the incubation temperature above or below its lower critical solution temperature (LCST). Temperature-responsive chitosan-graft PNIPAAm was applied for the culture of mesenchymal stem cells (MSCs). Chitosan-*g*-PNIPAAm copolymers with chondrogenic MSCs revealed the possibility of clinical applications, particularly as cell therapy technologies for treating vesicoureteral reflux (Gil et al., 2004).

Chitosan in Wound Management

A wound is defined as the disruption of the anatomic structure and function of a body part. This may be the result of a simple cut, burns, and any other injuries. Wounds are generally classified as wounds without tissue loss (e.g., surgical incision) or wounds with tissue loss, such as burn wounds or wounds due to trauma, abrasions, or secondary events to chronic ailments (e.g., venous stasis, diabetic ulcers, and iatrogenic wounds, such as skin graft donor sites and dermabrasions). In contrast, wound healing is a process of restoration by which tissue repair takes place and usually is comprised of a continuous sequence of inflammation and tissue repair during which epithelial, endothelial, inflammatory cells, platelets, and fibroblasts briefly interact to restore normal function. The ordered sequence of healing events is accomplished and regulated by cytokines and growth factors. Soon after the elimination of macrophages, which appear during the inflammatory phase, wound healing is impeded, and the tensile strength of the scar is diminished (Okamoto et al., 1993).

The use of chitosan has advantages due to the biocompatibility and biodegradability of the molecules, which does not harm the environment. When chitosan is applied to the body, besides being biocompatible, it is then slowly biodegraded by lysozymes, chitinase, and chitosanase to harmless oligomers and monomers (amino sugars), which are completely absorbed by the body. Chitosan embodies analgesic, bacteriostatic, and fungistatic properties, which are particularly useful for wound treatment. Additionally, chitosan modulates macrophage function and the secretion of numerous enzymes (e.g., collagenase) and cytokines (e.g., interleukins and tumor necrosis factor) during the wound healing process. The degradation of chitosan into monomers and oligomers at a wound site significantly accelerates the wound-healing process. In addition, clinical studies have shown an absence of scar formation at the wound site in the presence of chitosan (Okamoto et al., 1993).

Chitosan structurally resembles glycosaminoglycans (GAG), which have long-chain, unbranched, repeating disaccharide units and are important for maintaining cell morphology, differentiation, and function. GAG and proteoglycans are widely distributed throughout the human body and may bind and modulate numerous cytokines and growth factors, including heparin and heparan sulfate. Hence, the cell-binding and cell-activating properties of chitosan are crucial for wound healing.

Various chitosan derivatives have been produced for wound management, particularly to enhance wound healing. For example, oligo-chitosan (O-C) and *N, O*-carboxymethylchitosan (NO-CMC) derivatives have been fabricated into films for wound dressing (Lim et al., 2007). *N*-carboxybutyl chitosan has also been used in patients undergoing plastic surgery to promote tissue regeneration. The use of *N*-carboxybutyl chitosan improves cutaneous tissue regeneration with good histoarchitecture and vascularization at the wound site (Biagini et al., 1991). Additionally, 5-methylpyrrolidinone chitosan is compatible with other polymer solutions (e.g., gelatin, polyvinyl alcohol, polyvinyl pyrrolidone, and hyaluronic acid), which are beneficial for the treatment of wounded meniscal tissues, decubitus ulcers, depression of capsule formation around prostheses, scar formation, and retraction during wound healing (Muzzarelli et al., 1995).

Analgesic and Anti-Inflammatory Effects of Chitosan

Chitosan treatment reduces inflammatory pain. Studies suggest that chitosan has potent analgesic actions. Bradykinin is one of the main substances related to pain. Okamoto et al. (2003) reported that the bradykinin concentration during administration of a chitosan–acetic acid solution in the peritoneal lavage fluid was lower than during the administration of a 0.5% acetic acid solution, suggesting that chitosan has analgesic effects. Open wounds are often associated with severe pain in patients. Chitosan that is formulated for wound management may induce analgesia by providing a cool, pleasant, and soothing effect when applied to an open wound. Excellent pain relief is conferred by chitosan when it is applied as a topical agent to open wounds, such as burns, skin abrasions, skin ulcers, and skin-grafted areas. Chitosan has anti-inflammatory effects that are beneficial for the treatment of prolonged inflammation at the wound site. Water-soluble chitosan significantly suppresses the secretion and expression of proinflammatory cytokines (e.g., tumor necrosis factor-α and interleukin-6) and inducible nitric oxide synthase in astrocytes, the predominant neuroglial cells in the central nervous system, and is actively involved in cytokine-mediated inflammatory events (Kim et al., 2002). Moreover, *N*-acetylglucosamine is an anti-inflammatory drug and is synthesized in the human body from glucose. It is incorporated into glycosaminoglycans and glycoproteins. Chito-oligosaccharides, which have a molecular weight of 5 kDa, are better anti-inflammatory agents than indomethacin, a nonsteroidal anti-inflammatory drug. Chitosan exerts anti-inflammatory effects by inhibiting prostaglandin E2 (PGE2) and cyclooxygenase-2 (COX-2) protein expression and attenuating the proinflammatory cytokines (e.g., tumor necrosis factor-α and interleukin-1β).

Immunity-Enhancing (Immunomodulator)

The immunostimulating activity of chitosan and chitosan oligosaccharide has been reported for several decades. Nishimura et al. (1984) first reported that chitosan, especially 70% degree of deactylated chitosan could stimulate rats to produce non-specific host repellence when infected with *E. coli* and *Sendai* virus. They concluded that 70% degree of deactylated chitosan was an immune regulator that can activate macrophages (Mcp) and improve the delayed-type hypersensitive reaction, increase cytotoxicity, and induce mitosis in cells producing interleukins, breeding factors, and interferon. Chitosan has also shown an immunity-enhancing effect by enhancement of antibody response. Later, Suzuki et al. (1986) reported enhanced immune regulation with the increased water-solubility of chitosan. The effect of chitosan as a novel adjuvant to an inactivated influenza vaccine was studied (Chang et al., 2004). Here, BALB/c mice were abdominally inoculated with vaccine and chitosan together twice every 3 weeks. Blood serum was prepared and tested for levels of antibodies IgG, IgG1, and IgG2a as well as IgA antibody in nasal secretions. The results indicated that using chitosan as an adjuvant increased the antibody content in serum remarkably and increased the antiviral defense in the mice, enhancing the immune reaction to the vaccine.

Antitumor and Anticancer Effects

Deactylated (70%) chitosan may help in inducing the natural killer cells (NK). Chitooligosaccharides inhibit tumor growth through an increase in immune effects. The chitooligosaccharides showed strong inhibition of ascites cancer in BALB/c mice while N-acetylglucosamine-6-phosphate (GlcNAC-6-P) and D-glucosamine-6-phosphate (GlcN-6-P) showed very strong inhibiting effects for S-180 and MM156 solid tumor growth in syngenic mice, which was also reported by Tokoro et al. (1988). The antitumor mechanism of these chitooligosaccharides was probably related to their induction of lymphocyte factor, increasing T-cell proliferation to produce the tumor inhibitory effects. Through analysis of the splenic cell, it was found that extreme changes were observed in cancerous mice. Suzuki et al. (1986) proved that the antitumor mechanism of chitooligosaccharides is to enhance acquired immunity by accelerating T-cell differentiation to increase cytotoxicity and maintain T-cell activity. Huang et al. (2005) studied the anticancer activities of differently charged chitooligosaccharide derivatives using three cancer cell lines: HeLa, Hep3B, and SW480. Neutral red and MTT cell-viability studies revealed that highly charged chitooligosaccharide derivatives could significantly reduce cancer cell viability regardless of their positive or negative charge. Furthermore, fluorescence microscopic observations and DNA-fragmentation studies confirmed that the anticancer effect of these highly charged chitooligosaccharide derivatives was due to necrosis.

Antioxidant Activity

Both chitosan and its oligosaccharides showed antioxidant effects. In our recent study, the antioxidant activity of chitosan was studied *in vitro* and *in vivo* (Liu, 2008). The results showed that chitosan at an addition of 0.02% had antioxidant effects in lard and crude rapeseed oil, but the activity was less than ascorbic acid. When the addition was increased, chitosan and ascorbic acid had similar activities; chitosan could significantly reduce serum-free fatty acid and malondialdehyde (MDA) concentrations and elevate sesurm superoxide (SOD), enzyme catalase (CAT), and (GSH-PX) activities, the latter being the major antioxidant enzymes in the body, indicating that chitosan regulated the antioxidant enzyme activities and reduced lipid peroxidation.

The cellular antioxidant effects of chitosan oligosaccharides (MW 229.21-593.12 Da) produced by acidic hydrolysis of crab chitin were also identified by Ngo et al. (2008). Their study showed that chitosan oligosaccharides have free radical scavenging effects in a cellular system. They can inhibit myeloperoxidase activity and decrease free radical oxidation of DNA and membrane proteins. Furthermore, they also stimulate an increase in intracellular GSH levels. Based on the results, they concluded that chitosan oligosaccharides have free radical scavenging effects, acting in both indirect and direct ways to inhibit and prevent biological molecular damage by free radicals in living cells. Hence, chitosan and chitosan oligosaccharides can be used as scavengers to control radical-induced damage to cellular systems and promises further applications in the future.

Chitosan has been modified in variety of forms in accordance with the type of their use or purpose to be served. Various chitosan deriavatives are given in Table 11.1.

CHITOSAN AS A DRUG DELIVERY POLYMER

Chitosans have some special interesting biopharmaceutical characteristics, such as pH sensitivity, biocompatibility, and low toxicity. In addition, chitosan is metabolised by certain human enzymes, especially lysozyme, which makes chitosan biodegradable in nature (Prashanth et al., 2007). Due to these favorable properties, chitosan and its derivatives have been widely used in fabrication of drug delivery systems. It can be used as a carrier for drugs, protein and peptides, enzymes, hormones, gene, vaccines, cells, and other active biomolecules. Moreover, in such applications, it is also extremely important that chitosan is hydrosoluble and positively charged. These properties enable it to interact with negatively charged polymers, macromolecules, and polyanions in an aqueous environment as well as this property helps in targeting of active biomolecules and creating a new concept of targeting delivery systems, such as microspheres, nanoparticles, GIT patches, coated tablets, and so on.

The delivery systems that deploy chitosan can briefly be categorized into conventional, namely matrix tablets and capsules, and novel drug delivery systems, namely microspheres, nanoparticles, and so on. Both categories utilize chitosan in one or the other form for a definite purpose. A brief account of chitosan regarding its use is given below wherein chitosan is used as a constituent of diverse drug delivery systems.

- Chitosan is obtained from a natural source and is the second most abundant polymer on this earth after cellulose as mentioned above. Hence, it is readily available.
- It is cheap, and hence large quantities can be utilized and availed.
- It can be modified in different forms according to need—that is, flexibility of being engineered and developed into carrier system accordingly.
- It is naturally biodegradable and nontoxic in nature.
- It is biosafe and biocompatible and, at the same time, it is also nonimmunogenic. It is compatible with active biomolecules, protein and peptides, genetic materials, and living cells, making it a suitable carrier molecule.
- It increases paracellular permeability across mucosal epithelia and acts as an absorption and permeation enhancer.

On the basis of the delivery systems and the route of administration, different strategies or approaches have been designed using chitosan or chitosan derivatives to achieve a specific goal and achieve maximal therapeutic effectiveness. Some of them are discussed below.

Drug Delivery through Oral Route

The oral administration of therapeutics leads to internalization by the body at the mouth (oral cavity), stomach, small intestine, or colon. The local delivery of therapeutics to the mouth can be used to treat a number of diseases, such as periodontal disease, stomatitis, fungal and viral infections, and oral cavity cancers. In addition, drug administration through the buccal mucosa in the mouth provides some unique advantages, including avoidance of the hepatic first-pass metabolism and the acidity and proteolytic activity of the rest of the GI tract. Oral delivery through the buccal cavity encompasses treatment of local ailments, such as mouth ulcers, stomatitis, and other infections of the cavity along with the delivery of the therapeutic agents, which suffer first-pass metabolism. Chitosan is an example of cationic materials that have been proposed as mucosal-adhesive polymers (Lehr et al., 1992). Chitosan and sodium hyaluronate has been utilized as matrix in some of the buccal adhesive matrix tablet formulations (Takayama et al., 1990). The bioadhesive property of chitosan makes it a suitable candidate for the formulation of buccal delivery systems, which can adhere to the mucosa and release the contents in the buccal cavity for the treatment of local infections. In addition, bioadhesive tablets of nicotine containing 0%–50% w/w glycol chitosan produced good bioadhesion. Due to their mucoadhesive properties, chitosan-based hydrogels have been recognized as excellent candidates for oral drug delivery systems. Indeed, these materials have enhanced drug penetration within the mouth, improving therapeutic efficacy by maintaining high levels of antimicrobial agents in the crevicular fluid with minimal systemic uptake. Another fascinating property of this very interesting polymer is that it acts as permeation enhancer and hence increases the absorption of the molecules across the epithelium. Chitosan hydrogels have led to effective peptide drug transport across a porcine oral mucosa system tested *in vitro*.

Artursson et al. (1994) reported that chitosan can increase the paracellular permeability across caco-2 intestinal epithelia. The findings clearly reflect the permeation enhancement nature of chitosan. Localized administration of a therapeutic drug within the GI tract faces several formidable barriers. A highly acidic environment, destructive enzymes, and low residence times can limit therapeutic efficacy. Targeted drug delivery to the stomach and colon is extremely important for the treatment of local maladies, such as Crohn's disease, inflammation, ulcerative colitis, infection, and carcinomas. Selective drug release reduces the necessary dosage as well as the side effects caused by exposure of drug to nontargeted tissue.

Chitosan hydrogels can be prepared with pH-sensitive or enzyme-specific release triggers (which rapidly swell in acidic environments and release the drug), making their use as oral drug delivery systems. In a similar way, the gastroretentive systems, which stick to the mucosa and release the drug, can also be formulated. Apart from this, delivery of peptides and proteins can be brought about by delivery systems, such as microspheres, nanoparticles to the lower part of the GIT where they are intended to be targeted. Drugs that have absorption windows in the small intestine or the antigen/peptides that are to be targeted to the gut-associated lymphoid tissue (GALT) located mainly in the small intestine can be administered through these carriers. It can be utilized for the delivery of vaccines by targeting the antigen to the GALT tissues for eliciting immune responses (Figure 11.5).

Colon Drug Delivery

Chitosan-based bioadhesive poly electrolyte complex hydrogels have been prepared that can bypass the acidic environment of the stomach and release the drug into the intestine. For example, poly electrolyte complex networks loaded with 5-fluorouracil and insulin showed selective release in the intestine (Bhattarai et al., 2010).

A colon-targeted dosage form and carrier system of chitosan can also be formulated for the delivery of therapeutics to the colon. Lorenzo-Lamosa et al. in 1998 delivered diclofenac sodium to the colon using chitosan microspheres. pH-sensitive polymer Eudragit S-100–coated chitosan microspheres are useful to prevent the release of the drug in the gastric environment and release the drug in the colon. Chitosan-based hydrogels have been utilized for the delivery of therapeutics to the colon wherein the polymer is cleaved due to the presence of enzymes and caecal contents resulting in drug release (Jain et al., 2007, 2008). Chitosan hydrogel loaded with acetaminophen, mesalazine (5-ASA), sodium diclofenac, and insulin showed satisfactory uptake within the colon (Bhattarai et al., 2010). The chitosan itself was found to be degraded by the microflora of the colon, offering a degradation mechanism that leads to controlled drug release.

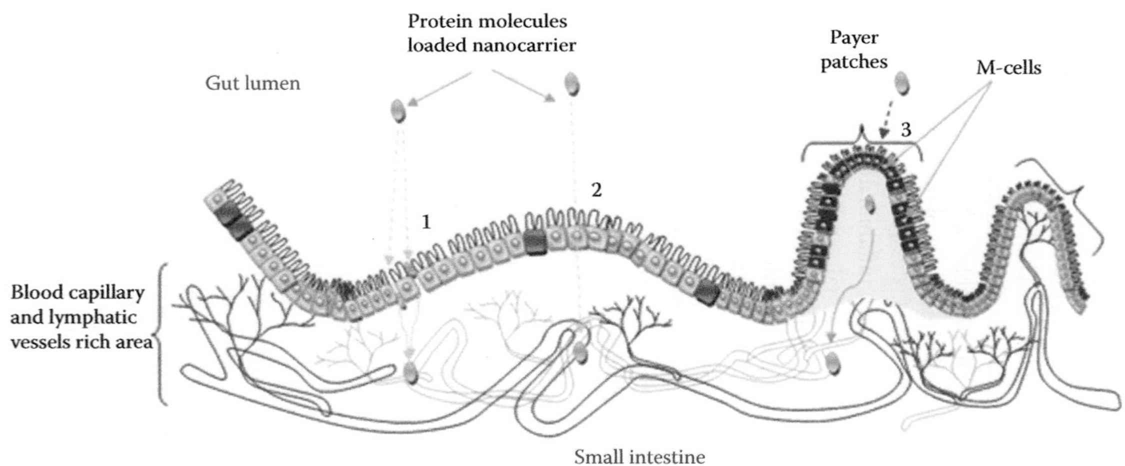

FIGURE 11.5 Schematic representation of strategy to target microparticles to GALT tissue.

Ocular Drug Delivery

Conventional systems tend to be eliminated rapidly from the eye and give limited drug absorption, leading to poor ophthalmic bioavailability. This has initiated the development of new materials that retain and enhance drug penetration using bioadhesive polymers and penetration enhancers. The specific biadhesiveness of chitosan to the ocular surface was first observed in an *ex vivo* study, in which the activity of radiolabeled chitosan was measured by scintillation counting (Henriksen et al., 1996). Chitosan can be utilized for the delivery of drugs, proteins, genes, peptides, and other biological products to the ocular tissues. The polycationic nature of chitosan interacts by hydrogen bonding/ionic interactions with the polyanionic surface of ocular mucosa, which results in mucoadhesivity of chitosan-based formulations. Chitosan has penetration-enhancing properties, which enhance absorption of drug across the mucosal epithelia. Chitosan solutions also exhibit pseudoplastic and viscoelastic nature (Mucha et al., 1997), which is essential for ocular drug delivery since the main aspect of the delivery in ophthalmic therapy centers around the retention time of the delivery system in the eye. Chitosan hydrogels have shown higher corneal residence times when compared with commercial drug solutions as well as sustained and controlled ocular delivery systems, such as micro- and nanoparticle delivery, gels, and chitosan-coated liposome/niosome systems, have been investigated for ocular delivery; *in situ*–forming hydrogels are also an attractive delivery approach because of their ability to be administered as a liquid and their long-term retention after dosing. Chitosan-based carrier systems used in ocular delivery are summarized in Table 11.2.

Transdermal Drug Delivery

In the tactless environment of the GI tract, low-molecular weight drugs can be administered by local transdermal drug delivery systems, which benefit from sustained drug release and easy therapy interruption by removal of the drug delivery systems. As discussed previously, chitosan and its derivatives have the ability to significantly enhance drug absorption across mucosa epithelia, extending a potential approach for transdermal delivery of drugs or biological products. The chitosan interacts with negative charges of the skin to improve diffusion of therapeutic actives to deeper layers of skin (Taveira et al., 2009). He et al. (1998) have investigated the mechanism of transdermal permeation enhancer activity of chitosan and its derivatives and suggested that it could be due to the effects on the secondary structure of keratin and water content in stratum corneum, cell membrane potential, and fluidity. Hydrogels offer attractive drug delivery system structures because of their high water content, providing a comfortable feeling on the patient's skin, leading to better compliance over the duration of the therapy. Glimepride, a third-generation oral antidiabetic sulfonylurea drug that has encountered bioavailability problems due to poor solubility during oral administration, has shown potential for effective delivery by chitosan hydrogel. Transdermal patches of carvedilol containing a soybean extract–chitosan mixture have been developed, which exhibited better performance in controlling hypertension in deoxycorticosterone acetate-induced hypertensive rats

TABLE 11.2
Chitosan-Based Carriers for Ocular Delivery

Carrier System	Drug	Utilization/Application	References
Nanoparticles	Benzalkonium chloride	Prepared and delivered chitosan nanoparticles on ocular surface and evaluate for its toxicity, uptake mechanism, and *in vivo* tolerance.	Salamanca et al., 2006
Chitosan-coated liposomes	Cyclosporin A	Prepared low molecular weight chitosan-coated liposomes for ocular delivery of Cyclosporin A and found that the concentrations of Cyclosporin A in cornea, conjunctiva, and sclera were remarkably increased.	Li et al., 2012
Trimethyl chitosan coated liposomes	Coenzyme Q10	Prepared trimethyl chitosan-coated liposomes, which were loaded with coenzyme Q10 and studies for tolerance, precorneal retention, and anticataract effect.	Zhang et al., 2009
Chitosan nanoparticles	Indomethacin	Indomethacin loaded chitosan nanoparticles developed, which were able to contact intimately with the cornea, providing slow gradual release with long-term drug level, thereby increasing delivery to both external and internal ocular tissues.	Badawi et al., 2008
Alginate-chitosan film	Gatifloxacin sesquihydrate	Films showed a constant drug release, and results demonstrate that the surface treated alginate–chitosan film could be a potential vehicle to enhance ocular gatifloxacin sesquihydrate bioavailability and patient compliance.	Gilhotra et al., 2008
Chitosan nanoparticles	Plasmid pEGFP	Developed novel hyaluronic acid–chitosan nanoparticles and delivered gene successfully through ocular route.	de la Fuente et al., 2008
Mucoadhesive chitosan nanoparticles	Natamycin	Prepared mucoadhesive nanoparticles for prolonged ocular delivery of natamycin and evaluate it for *in vitro* and pharmacokinetic profit.	Bhatta et al., 2012
Lipid nanoparticles with partially deacetylated chitosan	Flurbiprofen	Developed novel surface-modified nanostructured lipid carriers with partially deacetylated water-soluble chitosan demonstrate high potential for ocular drug delivery.	Tian et al., 2012

(*Continued*)

TABLE 11.2 (CONTINUED)
Chitosan-Based Carriers for Ocular Delivery

Carrier System	Drug	Utilization/Application	References
Chitosan nanoparticles	5-fluorouracil	5-fluorouracil-loaded chitosan nanoparticles for ophthalmic delivery showed diffusion controlled release and evaluated for their bioavailability performance.	Nagarwal et al., 2011
Inserts	Pilocarpine	Hybrid polymeric hydrogels were prepared by the reaction of acrylic acid–functionalized chitosan with either N-isopropylacrylamide or 2-hydroxyethyl methacrylate monomers and investigated for controlled release system for ocular drug delivery.	Verestiuc et al., 2006
Chitosan-coated niosomes	Timolol	Timolol-loaded niosomes and coated with chitosan prolonged the drug release and also helped in lowering of intraocular pressure with minimum side effects.	Aggarwal et al., 2005
Solution	Vancomycin	The 0.1% and 0.3% chitosan solutions were used for the ocular drug delivery of vancomycin.	Khangtragool et al., 2009
Microspheres	Rokitamycin	The spray-dried microspheres of new quaternary ammonium chitosan derivatives were prepared and showed better characteristics (solubility, penetration enhancement) compared with chitosan itself. The *in vitro* release behavior and good mucoadhesiveness are making them more suitable for ocular or nasal administration.	Rassu et al., 2009
Nanoparticles	DNA	The chitosan-DNA nanoparticles of NOVAFECT (ultrapure chitosan oligomers) were prepared. *In vitro* transfection studies show the ability of nanoparticles to effectively transfect COS-7 cells. The formulation injected into the stroma showed increased luciferase gene expression.	Eytan et al., 2010
Thermosensitive liposomal hydrogel	Ofloxacin	The *in situ* thermosensitive ofloxacin liposomal hydrogel ensures steady and prolonged transcorneal permeation, which improves the ocular bioavailability and minimizes frequency of administration, and ocular side effect of ofloxacin.	Hosny, 2009

(Sapra et al., 2009). Kahlig et al. (2009) developed an adhesive matrix of chitosan–glycolic acid for a transdermal application of progesterone exhibiting excellent skin adhesiveness and permeation properties. Permeation enhancement along with the bioadhesive nature of chitosan makes it a preferred polymer for the designing of the transdermal delivery systems.

Nasal Delivery

Nasal mucosa is an attractive site for the delivery of protein, peptide, vaccines, and other bioactive molecules because it has a relatively large absorptive surface and low proteolytic activity. However, most proteins are not well absorbed from the nasal cavity when administered as simple solutions. Major factors limiting the absorption of nasally administered proteins are their poor ability to cross nasal membranes and the mucociliary clearance mechanism, which rapidly removes protein solutions from the absorption site (Hejazi, 2003; Mina et al., 2004; Tiyaboonchai et al., 2003). There are many approaches to improve the absorption of peptides and proteins through the nasal mucosa by the use of absorption enhancers, enzyme inhibitors, and solutions of bioadhesive polymers or bioadhesive microspheres. Among the various bioadhesive materials that have been proposed for nasal delivery of proteins, chitosan, a copolymer of glucosamine and N-acetylglucosamine, has received particular interest. Chitosan has been studied as a biomaterial and as a pharmaceutical excipient for drug delivery because of its favorable biological properties (Tiyaboonchai et al., 2003) in addition to its ability to facilitate paracellular transport of peptides and proteins across mucosal barriers. Moreover, chitosan microparticles or nanoparticles loaded with macromolecules are able to enhance the absorption of these molecules at mucosal sites. Alhalaweh et al. (2009) prepared mucoadhesive dry powders of the zolmitriptan (antimigraine drug), in combination with chitosan, for nasal administration using a spray-drying method. Several studies have shown the ability of chitosan microparticles to enhance both systemic and local immune responses against various antigens after oral or nasal administration (Jain et al., 2007, 2008). Wang et al. (2008) prepared estradiol-loaded chitosan nanoparticles, and their *in vivo* studies on male Wistar rats revealed that the drug can be directly transported from the nasal cavity into the cerebrospinal fluid in rats with an improved drug delivery to central nervous system (CNS) using chitosan nanoparticles. Also, insulin-loaded chitosan nanoparticles have shown enhanced nasal absorption of insulin resulting in a reduction of plasma glucose levels (Tozaki et al., 1997). And recently, Vila et al. (2004) reported that low-molecular-weight chitosan nanoparticles containing tetanus toxoid could induce long-lasting immune responses after nasal administration in mice. Modification of chitosan with PEG can resist adsorption of plasma proteins in contact with blood through the steric repulsion mechanism, and PEG-g-chitosan nanoparticles as a delivery vehicle for nasal administration of proteins and peptides give a better result (Zhang et al., 2008).

Jain et al. (2007) prepared multivesicular liposomes coated with chitosan for intranasal delivery of insulin and performed *in vivo* studies on streptozotocin-induced diabetic rats. The chitosan-coated formulation showed a better hypoglycemic profile as compared to plain insulin solution. Intranasal administration is another route for gene therapy. Kumar et al. reported that mice vaccinated with a cocktail of RSV (respiratory syncytial virus) cDNAs complexed to chitosan, in nanoparticulate form, exhibited a significant reduction in RSV titer and antigen load as compared to untreated and naked DNA administered controls after intranasal administration.

The nasal route is a promising immunization site, and chitosan-based nasal delivery systems for various antigens have now been developed and studied by some researchers due to bioadhesion and paracellular transport effects (Bacon et al., 2000; Gill et al., 1998). The influence of N, N, N-trimethylchitosan on the intranasal delivery of whole inactivated influenza virus was studied in mice for nasal residence time and the specific location in the nasal cavity of formulation.

Liver-Targeted Drug Delivery

Liver targeting for treatment of many fatal conditions, including chronic hepatitis, enzyme deficiency, and hepatoma, that occur in hepatocytes is becoming a major challenge in the drug delivery field. In general, liver-targeting systems employ passive trapping of microparticles by reticuloendothelium or active targeting based on recognition between hepatic receptor and ligand bearing particulates (Ogawara et al., 1999). There is potential of lactosaminated N-succinyl-chitosan, synthesized by reductive amination between N-succinyl-chitosan and lactose in the presence of sodium cyanoborohydride, as a liver-specific drug carrier (Kato et al., 2001). Lactosaminated N-succinyl-chitosan found maximum binding to the asialoglycoprotein receptors and presence in liver parenchymal cells. This concept has been utilized in targeting the early metastatic stage of liver cancer (Kato et al., 2002). Liu et al. prepared polyion complex micelles based on methoxy poly (ethylene glycol) (PEG)–graft chitosan and lactose-conjugated PEG-graft–chitosan for liver-targeted delivery of diammonium glycyrrhizinate for the treatment of chronic hepatitis and immune deficiency virus infection (Yang et al., 2009; Lin et al., 2008). Lin et al. (2008) prepared glycyrrhizin conjugated to the surface of chitosan nanoparticles bearing adriamycin for targeting the liver through a specific interaction between glycyrrhizin and hepatocytes.

Gene Delivery

Chitosan is a naturally occurring cationic mucopolysaccharide. It is generally biocompatible, biodegradable, mucoadhesive, nonimmunogenic, and nontoxic. Chitosan is able to condense nucleic acids (NA) (both DNA and RNA) and protect them from nuclease degradation. pDNA encoding therapeutic genes have been extensively studied in NA therapy. Those encoded genes include metabolic suicide genes (e.g., herpes simplex thymidine kinase, varicella zoster thymidine kinase, and Escherichia coli cytosine deaminase) and genes encoding the following proteins: angiogenesis inhibitors, proapoptotic proteins, prodrug activators, or immune response modulators. In addition to pDNA, small RNA like micro-RNA (miRNA), small interfering RNA (siRNA), and antisense RNA have also been widely explored as tools for genetic treatments. Because of its biodegradability, biocompatibility, nonallergenicity, and nucleic acid binding ability, chitosan has been widely studied as a pDNA carrier.

Chitosan-based pDNA transfer depends greatly on both the ionic and nonionic interactions between the carbohydrate backbone of chitosan and surface proteins of transfected cells. These interact electrostatically with negatively charged DNA and form complexes (poly-plexes). Like many other polymeric vectors, chitosan-mediated pDNA delivery may involve a number of cellular barriers, including enzymatic degradation, inefficient cellular uptake, encapsulation in endo-lysosomes, failure of polymer dissociation, and nuclear localization (Lee at al., 2001; Liu et al., 2007; Song et al., 2009; Borchard et al., 2001; Yoo et al., 2005).

On the contrary, chitosan is a cationic polymer with significantly lower toxicity than poly-L-lysine and PEI, and it also enhances the transport of drug across the cell membrane. The transfection efficiency was shown to be lower than that of other cationic polymer vehicles, such as polyethyleimine (MacLaughlin et al., 1998), and it depends on the cell type, serum concentration, pH, and molecular weight of chitosan. The transfection efficiency is found to be higher at pH 6.9 than that at pH 7.6. Transfection efficiency meditated by chitosan of high molecular weight, >100 kDa, is less than that of low molecular weight, 15 and 52 kDa. To increase their transfection efficiency, two approaches have been developed. Park et al. (2000) developed a liver-targeted delivery system by preparing galactosylated-chitosan-graft-dextran DNA complexes as galactose is known as a liver-targeting ligand. Similarly, Mao et al., (2001) have prepared transferrin-chitosan-DNA nanoparticles as a targeted drug delivery. However, when KNOB (C-terminal globular domain of fiber protein) conjugated to the chitosan, the transfection efficiency in *Hela* cells can be improved by 130-fold. All this indicates the use of chitosan as promising nonviral vector for gene delivery, which comes with a bonus pack of reduced toxicity, biodegradability, and nonimmunogenecity.

In fact it has been argued that the most important application of alkylated chitosan is in DNA delivery, such as proven with dodecyl chitosan (Borchard et al., 2001). The high transfection efficiency of alkylated chitosan was attributed to the increasing entry into cells facilitated by hydrophobic interactions and easier unpacking of DNA from alkylated chitosan carriers due to the weakening of electrostatic attractions between DNA and alkylated chitosan. Some works related with intracellular delivery for gene therapy using modified chitosan-based materials were reported (Bielinska et al., 2000). Very recently, novel water-soluble nanoparticles that consist of a PAMAM dendrimer core with grafted carboxymethyl chitosan chains were successfully synthesized (Oliveira et al., 2008). In another work, deoxycholic acid, which is the main component of bile acids, was used to modify chitosan hydrophobically and to obtain self-assembling macromolecules for a nonviral gene delivery system. The self-aggregated DNA complex from deoxycholic acid–modified chitosan was shown to enhance the transfection efficiency over monkey kidney cells. The feasibility of these chitosan self-aggregates for the transfection of genetic material in mammalian cells was investigated. Self-aggregates can form charge complexes when mixed with plasmid DNA. These self-aggregated DNA complexes are considered to be useful for transfer of genes into mammalian cells *in vitro* and served as good delivery systems composed of biodegradable polymeric materials, PEGylation of chitosan in order to increase its solubility, prolong the plasma circulation time and gene transfer. For example, Liu et al. (2007) prepared chitosan–DNA complexes conjugated with alphamethoxy-omega-succinimidyl PEG, and the gene expression was improved in comparison with the chitosan–DNA complex both *in vitro* and *in vivo*. Microspheres physically combining PEG-grafted chitosan (PEG-*g*-CHI) with poly(lactide-co-glycolide) (PLGA) were formulated by Yun et al. (2005). They reported that these microspheres were capable of sustained release of PEG-*g*-CHI/DNA for at least 9 weeks, and the rate of DNA release was not modulated by varying the amount of PEG-*g*-CHI. In another work, folate-PEG-grafted chitosan was synthesized and proposed for targeted plasmid DNA delivery to tumor cells. The authors found that folate conjugation in this system significantly improved gene transfection efficiency due to promoted uptake of folate receptor bearing tumor cells. *In vitro* and *in vivo* studies of gene transfection are being conducted in the laboratory to evaluate its gene transfection efficiency (Gao et al., 2009; Liu et al., 2002; Cheng et al., 2009).

Chitosan Bioconjugates as Drug Delivery

Chitosan has been found to be used as a support material for gene delivery, cell culture, and tissue engineering. However, practical use of chitosan has been mainly confined to the unmodified forms. It has been found that chitosan itself has no recognizable moiety in respect to cellular surface or biological fluid. The introduction of a new moiety or making the conjugate with the chitosan molecule increases the recognization potential of chitosan. Chemical modification of chitosan is useful for the association of bioactive molecules to polymer and controlling the drug release profile. Advance utilization of chitosan, especially in the field of controlled drug delivery, graft copolymerization onto chitosan can function as a key point in the delivery. The bioconjugation approaches and strategies may transform into enhanced specificity, reproducibility, targetabilty, and sustained-release profile and may be used for the treatment of different diseases. This introduces desired properties to the therapeutic molecules and enlarges the field of the potential applications of chitosan by choosing various types of side chains and subsequently is helpful to conjugate many drugs; bioactive macromolecules, such as antibodies, ligonucleotides, interleukins, and interferons, transferrin, folic acid, and so on; enzymes; glycoproteins; and some polymers, such as PEG, poly-l-lysine, and related polymers. Some important examples of such bioconjugates have been presented in Table 11.3 for a brief overview.

FORMULATION ASPECTS OF CHITOSAN

Conventional Drug Delivery Systems

Conventional drug delivery includes those delivery systems that have been utilized for the treatment since the advent of the pharmaceutical sciences or the formulation science where the prime aim is to release the drug after it is administered into the body. These include tablets, capsules, pills, ointments, suspensions, and so on. The chitosan has been deployed in some of these dosage forms with the aim of adding advancement to the existing system. Some of these uses and attributes are discussed below.

TABLE 11.3
Bioconjugates of Chitosan and Their Role in Therapeutics

Conjugate	Delivery System	Purpose/Target Cell	Activity	Reference
Chitosan–kojic acid	Film	Food industry, cosmetics, or pharmacy	Antioxidant	Synytsya et al., 2008
Doxorubicin–chitosan	Thermo-responsive and photo-cross-linkable hydrogels	Sustained-release profiles—lung adenocarcinoma	Anticancer activity	Cho et al., 2009
Doxorubicin-conjugated glycol chitosan	Microsphere	Oral delivery for target colon cancer	Anticancer activity	Son et al., 2003
N,N,N-trimethyl-chitosan/tetragalactose antenna conjugate		Gene delivery—HepG2 human hepatoma cells	Galactosidase activity	Murata et al., 1997
Chitosan-paclitaxel	Microsphere	Oral delivery for colon cancer	Anticancer activity	Lee et al., 2008
Chitosan-amino acid	Chitosan beads	Increase the adsorption capacity	Removal of heavy metals (Cu, Ni, Co, and Mn)	Ishii et al., 1995
Chitosan-conjugated docetaxel	Solution	Evaluate *in vivo* antitumor efficacy and subacute toxicity of docetaxel-human non-small cell lung carcinoma (NCIH358) and glioblastoma (U87MG)	Antitumor effects	Lee et al., 2009

(Continued)

TABLE 11.3 (CONTINUED)
Bioconjugates of Chitosan and Their Role in Therapeutics

Conjugate	Delivery System	Purpose/Target Cell	Activity	Reference
N-succinyl-chitosan-mitomycin	Nanoparticles	Different type of solid tumor targeting	Antitumor effect	Song et al., 1992
Eudragit-coated chitosan–prednisolone conjugate	Microspheres	Gastrointestinal distribution and absorption behavior, reducing toxicity and inflammation	Treatment of inflammatory bowel disease	Oosegi et al., 2008
Chitosan-polyaspartic acid-5-fluorouracil	Nano- and microsphere	Treatment of colon cancer	Antitumor	Zhang et al., 2008
Cholesterol-modified chitosan conjugate	Epirubicin-loaded nanoparticles	Release rate modification	Drug loading and sustained release	Wang et al., 2007
PEG-chitosan	Water-soluble dispersion	Solubility enhancement of chitosan	Suitable carrier for DNA, protein, anionic drug	Hiroshi et al., 1997
Lipase-chitosan conjugate	Particulate system	To improve lipase activity	Increase activity of lipase from simple lipase (40%) to chitosan conjugate (93%)	Kwon et al., 2007
Cholesterol-modified glycol chitosan conjugate	Nanoparticles	Evaluate for drug entrapment and release profile	Anti-inflammatory	Yu et al., 2008
Glycol-chitosan	Micelles	Improve tumor uptake efficacy	Antitumor	Yu et al., 2012

Tablets

Beacause of its biodegradable, nontoxic property and no interaction with other excipients, chitosan may be used as a diluent and coating material with other diluents, such as lactose, microcrystalline cellulose, and potato starch in tablets, capsules, and other pharmaceutical preparations. Amrutkar et al. (2009) prepared chitosan–chondroitin sulfate-based matrix tablets for colon-specific delivery of indomethacin. A researcher prepared chitosan–chodroitin sulfate complex granules loaded with 5-flourouracil anticancer drug for colon cancer–specific targeting. Bigucci et al. (2008) prepared polyelectrolyte complexes between CH and pectin in various pH regions using different molar ratios by simple mixing. These complexes were used for the preparation of tablets containing vancomycin, which exhibited mucoadhesive and pH-dependent swelling properties for colon-specific delivery.

Knapczyk (1992) developed antimycotic buccal and vaginal tablets utilizing chitosan as an auxillary substance for direct tableting. These tablets contained a mixture of deacetylated chitosans as a slow disintegrating agent, which retained their properties during storage while chitosan has also been assessed for its role as a binder (Upadrashta et al., 1992). Nunthanid et al. (2004) utilized chitosan acetate as a binder for the tablets and assessed its properties. They suggested that the simple incorporation of spray-dried chitosan acetate as a tablet binder could exhibit sustained drug release. An oral mucoadhesive tablet containing diltiazem was developed using chitosan and sodium alginate as diluents (Miyazaki et al., 1995).

Novel Delivery Systems

Chitosan has been extensively investigated in the formulation of novel drug delivery systems. These systems are novel in the sense that these are more advanced than the conventional dosage forms with respect to drug delivery. These are controlled drug delivery systems that deliver drug in a controlled way with uniform drug release pattern. Moreover, these can be targeted to a specific site, surpassing the other organs of the body and thus eventually lessen the side effects along with the maintenance of therapeutic concentrations in the body for a longer period of time. These include microspheres, nanoparticles, gastrointestinal patches, niosomes, hydrogel, beads, and so on.

Chitosan hydrogels have been used for the delivery of macromolecular compounds, such as peptides, proteins, antigens, oligonucleotides, and genes. The chitosan-based hydrogels have also been used for cancer therapeutics, subcutaneous release, and oral delivery. Chitosan is one of the water-soluble polymers that possesses cell adhesion and has potential uptake properties due to the positive charge.

Chitosan nanoparticles in this respect are most favorable due to their attraction to negatively charged cell membranes. Due to these properties of the chitosan, it has a valuable role in the treatment of many diseases, such as solid tumors, local GIT deasease, and targeting different body organs. Chitosan nanoparticles are highly preferred because they show promise in drug delivery systems. Such nanoparticles provide controlled or sustained release properties, subcellular size and biocompatibility with tissue and cells (Janes et al., 2001; Panyam et al., 2003; Campos et al., 2001). Apart from this, these nanomedicines are stable in blood; nontoxic, nonthrombogenic, nonimmunogenic, and noninflammatory; do not activate neutrophils; are biodegradable; avoid the reticuloendothelial system; and are applicable to various molecules such as drugs, proteins, peptides, or nucleic acids. Microspheres are matrix-type controlled drug delivery systems, which can be targeted to a specific site as well as formulated in different ways. Recently, microspheres of chitosan have been prepared on a large scale for drug delivery. Microspheres of chitosan can be formulated through various methods depending upon the properties of the therapeutic agent to be encapsulated and other attributes of the system to be designed. Sinha et al. (2004) discussed the potential of chitosan microspheres as a delivery system. It has been shown that chitosan and its derivatives, such as *N*-trimethyl chitosan or *N*-carboxymethyl chitosan, have the special feature of adhering to mucosal surfaces, being useful for mucosal drug delivery. Acrylic acid grafts of chitosan are possible means of creating hydrophilic and mucoadhesive polymers. Chitosan-grafted poly(acrylic acid) particles have been proposed as hydrophilic drug carriers for hydrophilic drugs and sensitive proteins (Dutta et al., 2004; Rassu et al., 2009; Sinha et al., 2004). Some of the delivery systems formulated with chitosan are discussed below and also summarized in Table 11.4.

TABLE 11.4
Chitosan Used in Novel Drug Delivery Systems

Novel Drug Delivery System	Type/Activity/Drug	Utilization/Methodology	Reference
Hydrogel	pH-responsive hydrogel beads	Ionotropic gelation reaction prepared for the controlled release study of protein drugs in the small intestine	El-Sherbiny et al., 2010
	Hydrogel membrane	Evaluate for cell cytotoxicity and proliferation effect on skin	Lu et al., 2010
	Injectable temperature sensitive chitosan hydrogels	*In situ* gel-like implants carrier systems for drug delivery and tissue engineering	Schuetz et al., 2008
	Thiol-containing chitosan beads	Used as a controlled and pH-responsive drug delivery system	No et al., 1989
	Chitosan-based systems bearing β-cyclodextrin cavities	Proposed as a matrix for controlled release	Krauland et al., 2007
	Metal ion-composite chitosan beads	To retain antigenicity and infectivity enterovirus 71 after adsorption on chitosan beads	Lin et al., 2012
Nanoparticles	Cyclosporin A	For the improvement of the delivery of drugs to the ocular surface	Campos et al., 2001
	Tacrine	Chitosan nanoparticles as a new delivery system for the anti-Alzheimer's drug	Wilson et al., 2009

(*Continued*)

TABLE 11.4 (CONTINUED)
Chitosan Used in Novel Drug Delivery Systems

Novel Drug Delivery System	Type/Activity/ Drug	Utilization/Methodology	Reference
	Doxorubicin	Chitosan nanoparticles as delivery systems for target cancer cell	Janes et al., 2001
	Gene delivery	Evaluate *in vitro* uptake and transfection efficiency of chitosan N-betainates/DNA self-assembly nanoparticles for gene delivery	Gao et al., 2009
	Antisense oligonucleotides	Chitosan-coated PLGA transfection effect of nanoparticles for DNA/RNA delivery	Nafee et al., 2007
	Antiangiogenesis peptide	Antiangiogensis loaded chitosan-dextran sulfate nanoparticles for peptide delivery	Chen et al., 2003
Microsphere	Insulin	Cross linked chitosan microspheres for oral delivery of insulin and testing for Taguchi design and *in vivo* performance	Jose et al., 2012
	Carvedilol	Mucoadhesive bilayer buccal tablet of carvedilol-loaded chitosan microspheres and evaluate for *in vitro*, pharmacokinetic, and pharmacodynamic performance	Yedurkar et al., 2012
	Gliclazide	Microparticles for oral sustained drug delivery	Barakat et al., 2011
	Naproxen	Alginate-chitosan microparticles for oral delivery of naproxen, which shows good encapsulation efficiency and release profile	Calija et al., 2011
	Hepatitis B surface antigen	Chitosan microspheres loaded with hepatitis B surface antigen (HBsAg)-for the purpose of oral immunization against hepatitis	Premaletha et al., 2012
	Insulin	Hollow quaternized chitosan microspheres to increase the therapeutic effect of orally administered insulin	Wei et al., 2010
	Protein and peptide	Chondroitin sulphate-chitosan microspheres as carrier for the delivery of proteins	Maculotti et al., 2009
	5-FU	pH-dependent chitosan microsphere for the delivery of 5-FU to the colon cancer	Zhao et al., 2008
	Insulin	Insulin loaded chitosan phthalate microspheres for effective management of blood glucose level after oral delivery	Ubaidulla et al., 2007
	Tetanus toxoid	Oral immunization against tetanus by tetanus toxoid-loaded chitosan microparticles	Ahire et al., 2007
	Plasmid DNA	Chitosan microparticles bearing plasmid DNA for oral immunization and it is found that chitosan is potent material for transfection	Guliyeva et al., 2006
	Antigen	Eudragit-coated chitosan microparticles as an oral immune delivery system	Hori et al., 2005

Hydrogel

Chitosan is one of the most suitable polymers for hydrogel due to its biocompatible, biodegradable, and hydrophilic nature along with functional amino groups and a net cationic charge. Chitosan hydrogels have been used for the delivery of macromolecular compounds, such as peptides, proteins, antigens, oligonucleotides, and genes. The chitosan-based hydrogels have also been used for cancer therapeutics, subcutaneous release, and oral delivery. Chitosan hydrogel has shown strong potential for use as a new tissue adhesive in surgical applications and wound dressing (Lu et al., 2010). The hydrogel membrane maintains a moist environment over the wound bed for enhancing re-epithelialization and also exhibits barrier function as it was impermeable to bacteria but permeable to oxygen. These studies on skin revealed that the hydrogel membrane has neither cytotoxicity nor an effect on cell proliferation (Lu et al., 2010). The pH-responsive hydrogel beads based on chitosan and sodium alginate were prepared using an ionotropic gelation reaction and have been subsequently characterized for the controlled release study of protein drugs in the small intestine (El-Sherbiny et al., 2010). pH change occurs at many specific or pathological body sites, which is one of the important environmental parameters for drug delivery systems. In this system, the swelling depends not only on the chemical composition but also on the pH of the surrounding medium. The pH-sensitive polymers show dramatic changes on the pH and on the composition of the external solutions. The mechanism of drug release from the different types of hydrogel, such as drug-loaded normal hydrogel, pH-sensitive hydrogel, and glucose-sensitive hydrogel, are clearly explained in Figure 11.6. Injectable temperature-sensitive chitosan hydrogels are attractive carrier systems for drug delivery and tissue engineering to form *in situ* gel-like implants (Schuetz et al., 2008). Thiol-containing chitosan beads were synthesized as a controlled and pH-responsive drug delivery system (No et al., 1989). It has been shown that pH-sensitive chitosan beads have a great potential in controlled drug release through oral administration since the release in the highly acidic gastric fluid region of the stomach is avoided (Prabaharan et al., 2005). Chitosan-based systems bearing β-cyclodextrin cavities have been proposed as a matrix for controlled release (Prabaharan et al., 2005; Krauland et al., 2007). Due to the presence of the hydrophobic β-cyclodextrin rings, these systems provide a slower release of the entrapped hydrophobic drug. Finally, stimuli-responsive hydrogels have shown an improved drug-loading capacity and a sustained release behavior. In particular, systems that combine chitosan and PNIPAAm have shown drug release profiles that can be controlled by both pH and temperature, constituting very promising materials (Bhattarai et al., 2005). The chitosan-based hydrogels have been extensively studied by many researchers and established as a potential chemotherapeutic delivery system.

Nanoparticles

There are many biodegradable polymers available that can be utilized to formulate their nanopaticulate formulation for drug delivery, of which some polymers are water-soluble and some are water-insoluble. Chitosan is one of the water-soluble polymers that possess cell adhesion and have potential uptake properties due to their positive

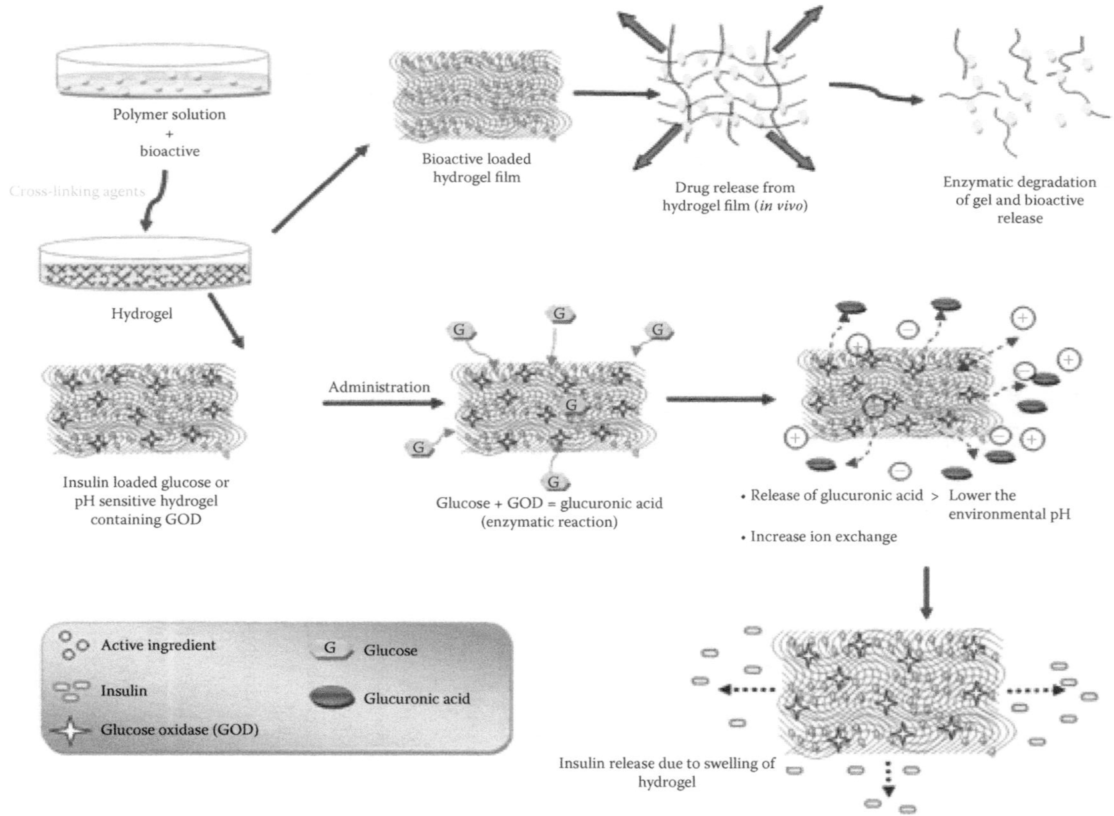

FIGURE 11.6 Chitosan-based pH-sensitive hydrogel-loaded active biomolecules.

charge. Chitosan particles in this respect are most favorable due to their attraction to negatively charged cell membranes. Due to these properties of the chitosan, it has a valuable role in the treatment of solid tumors. Careful design of chitosan-based delivery systems with respect to target and route of administration may solve some of the problems faced by new classes of active molecules. Most of the reported methods are frequently used for the synthesis of biodegradable nanomedicines. Polymeric nanoparticles have been prepared using various methods of solvent evaporation, ionic gelation, *in situ* polymerization, and so on, according to the needs of its application and the type of drugs to be encapsulated. These nanoparticles are extensively used for the nanoencapsulation of various useful bioactive molecules and medicinal drugs to develop nanomedicine. Chitosan nanoparticles are highly preferred because they show promise in drug delivery systems. Such nanoparticles provide controlled or sustained release properties, subcellular size, and biocompatibility with tissue and cells (Panyam et al., 2003) Apart from this, these nanomedicines are stable in blood, nontoxic, nonthrombogenic, nonimmunogenic, noninflammatory; do not activate neutrophils; are biodegradable; avoid the reticuloendothelial system; and are applicable to various molecules, such as drugs, proteins, peptides, or nucleic acids (Rieux et al., 2006). The drug molecules are either bound to the surface as nanospheres or encapsulated inside as nanocapsules. Other examples are related to the production of polymeric vesicles for encapsulation of hydrophobic compounds like bleomycin. The noncytotoxicity and successful internalization of these dendrimer nanoparticles by two different types of cells—that is, cell lines and primary cultures—was demonstrated in this work. The authors also showed that the dexamethasone-loaded nanoparticles induced the osteogenic differentiation of rat bone marrow stem cels *in vitro*. So these novel dendrimer nanoparticles may be used as targeted drug-delivery carriers to cover a wide range of applications that involve the efficient intracellular delivery of biological agents to modulate the behavior of cells.

Microspheres

Microspheres are matrix-type controlled drug delivery systems that can be targeted to a specific site as well as formulated in different ways. Recently, microspheres of chitosan have been prepared on a large scale for drug delivery. Microspheres of chitosan can be formulated through various methods, depending upon the properties of the therapeutic agent to be encapsulated and other attributes of the system to be designed. Sinha et al. (2004) discussed the potential of chitosan microspheres as a delivery system. It has been shown that chitosan and its derivatives, such as *N*-trimethyl chitosan or *N*-carboxymethyl chitosan, have the special feature of adhering to mucosal surfaces, being useful for mucosal drug delivery (Barakat et al., 2011; Yedurkar et al., 2012; Wei et al., 2010). Acrylic acid grafts of chitosan are a possible means of creating hydrophilic and mucoadhesive polymers. Chitosan-grafted poly(acrylic acid) particles have been proposed as hydrophilic drug carriers for hydrophilic drugs and sensitive proteins (Verestiuc et al., 2006). Zhao et al. (2008) and Jain et al. (2007, 2009) prepared pH enzyme–dependent chitosan microspheres coated with enteric polymers, which were to remain intact in the upper part of the GIT and delivered drugs, such as 5-FU, insulin, and other antiinflammatory drugs to the colon (Figure 11.7).

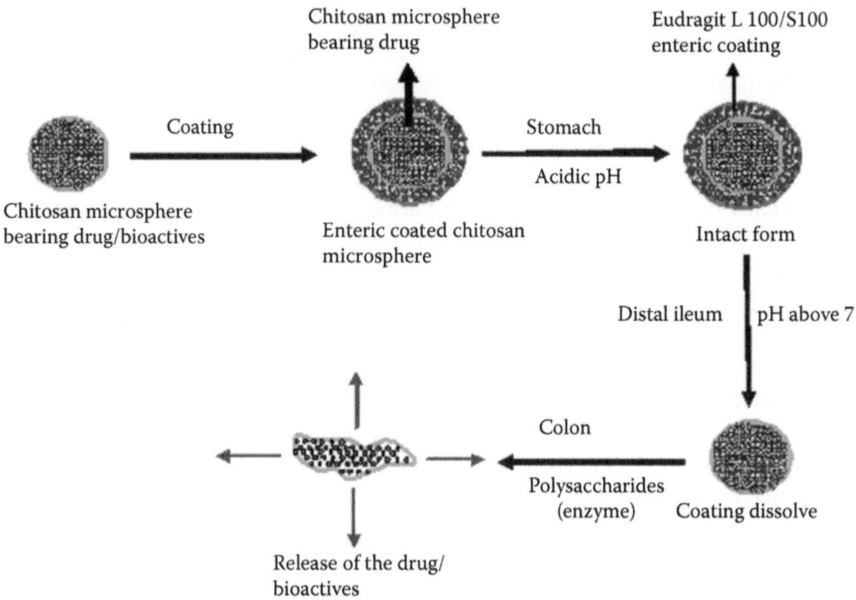

FIGURE 11.7 Schematic representation of polymer-based colon-specific microspheres.

Kumbar et al. (2003) prepared microspheres of polyacrylamide-grafted-chitosan cross-linked with glutaraldehyde to encapsulate indomethacin (IM), a nonsteroidal anti-inflammatory drug used in the treatment of arthritis. Microspheres of grafted chitosan cross-linked with glutaraldehyde were prepared to encapsulate nifidifine (NFD), a calcium channel blocker and an antihypertensive drug. *N*-Lauryl carboxymethyl chitosan with both hydrophobic and hydrophilic groups was studied for the delivery of taxol to cancerous tissues (Miva et al., 1998).

CONCLUSION

This chapter has focused on physicochemical and biological properties of chitosan and uses in the fabrication of drug delivery systems especially for targeted and controlled applications. It is a more defined biodegradable, biocompatible, natural polymer, which contributes to new generations of biomimetic nanostructures and vehicles for carrying biomolecules or therapeutic drugs. Chitosan and its derivatives have antibacterial, fungistatic, hemostatic, anticancer, immunoadjuvant, spermicidal, antioxidant, preservative, metal chelate, wound healing, hypocholeteromic, analgesic, anti-inflammatory, and immunomodulator activity.

The chitosan also plays a very important role in the delivery of proteins/peptidal drugs. Chitosan and its derivatives possess various advantages, such as biocompatibility, biodegradability, mucoadhesivity, and other unique biological properties, which help in the targeted and controlled delivery of proteins or peptides. The properties of chitosan are greatly influenced by its molecular weight and degree of deacetylation. The presence of reactive functional groups in chitosan provides great opportunity for chemical modification, which affords a wide range of derivatives possessing unique properties.

Chitosan and its derivatives are widely used in the fabrication of novel drug delivery systems like nanoparticles, microsphere, dendrimers, micelles, hydrogels, and polymerosomes, which can securely deliver drugs, genes, proteins, vaccines, enzymes, and other biomolecules for the treatment of different diseases. Overall, it is evident that chitosan and its derivatives are useful carriers for a wide category of drugs requiring targeted delivery. Thus, it is stated that chitosan and its derivatives have a remarkable impact on the science of drug delivery and in human health care.

REFERENCES

Aggarwal, D., & Kaur, I. P. 2005. Improve pharmacodnamics of timolol maleate from a mucoadhesive niosomal ophthalmic drug delivery system. *Int. J. Pharm.* 290: 155–159.

Ahire, V. J., Sawant, K. K., Doshi, J. B., & Ravetkar, S. D. 2007. Chitosan microparticles as oral delivery system for tetanus toxoid. *Drug. Dev. Ind. Pharm.* 33(10): 1112–1124.

Alhalaweh, A., Andersson, S., & Velaga, S. P. 2009. Preparation of zolmitriptan-chitosan microparticles by spray drying for nasal delivery. *Eur. J. Pharm. Sci.* 38(3): 206–214.

Amrutkar, J. R., & Gattani, S. G. 2009. Chitosan–chondroitin sulfate based matrix tablets for colon specific delivery of indomethacin. *AAPS PharmSciTech.* 10(2): 670–677.

Andriy, S., Petra, B., Alla, S., Jana, C., Jiri, S., & Michal, U. 2008. Conjugation of kojic acid with chitosan. *Carbohydr. Polym.* 72: 21–31.

Artursson, P., Lindmark, T., Davis, S. S., & Illum, L. 1994. Effect of chitosan on the permeability of monolayers of intestinal epithelial cells (Caco-2). *Pharm. Res.* 11: 1358–1361.

Artursson, P., Lindmark, T., Davis, S. S. et al. 1994. Effect of chitosan on the permeability of monolayers of intestinal epithelial cells (Caco-2). *Pharm. Res.* 11: 1358–1361.

Bacon, A., Makin, J., Sizer, P. J. et al. 2000. Carbohydrate biopolymers enhance antibody responses to mucosally delivered vaccine antigens. *Infect. Immun.* 68: 5764–7570.

Badawi, A. A., El-Laithy, H. M., El Qidra, R. K., El Mofty, H., & El dally, M. 2008. Chitosan based nanocarriers for indomethacin ocular delivery. *Arch. Pharm. Res.* 31(8): 1040–1049.

Barakat, N. S., & Almurshedi, A. S. 2011. Design and development of gliclazide-loaded chitosan microparticles for oral sustained drug delivery: In-vitro/in-vivo evaluation. *J. Pharm. Pharmacol.* 63(2): 169–178.

Bhatta, R. S., Chandasana, H., Chhonker, Y. S., Rathi, C., Kumar, D., Mitra, K., & Shukla, P. K. 2012. Mucoadhesive nanoparticles for prolonged ocular delivery of natamycin: In vitro and pharmacokinetics studies. *Int. J. Pharm.* 432(1–2): 105–112.

Bhattarai, N., Gunn, J., & Zhang, M. 2010. Chitosan-based hydrogels for controlled, localized drug delivery. *Adv. Drug Deliv. Rev.* 62(1): 83–99.

Bhattarai, N., Ramay, H. R., Gunn, J., Matsen, F. A., & Zhang, M. 2005. PEG-grafted chitosan as an injectable thermosensitive hydrogel for sustained protein release. *J. Control. Release* 103(3): 609–624.

Biagini, G., Bertani, A., Muzzarelli, R. et al. 1991. Wound management with N-carboxybutyl chitosan. *Biomaterials* 12(3): 281–286.

Bielinska, A. U., Yen, A., Wu, H. L. et al. 2000. Application of membrane based dendrimer/DNA complexes for solid phase transfection in vitro and in vivo. *Biomaterials* 21: 877–887.

Bigucci, F., Luppi, B., Cerchiara, T., Sorrenti, M., Bettinetti, G., Rodriguez, L., & Zecchi, V. 2008. Chitosan/pectin polyelectrolyte complexes: Selection of suitable preparative conditions for colon-specific delivery of vancomycin. *Eur. J. Pharm. Sci.* 35(5): 435–441.

Borchard, G. 2001. Chitosan for gene delivery. *Adv. Drug Deliv. Rev.* 52: 145–150.

Calija, B., Cekic, N., Savic, S., Krajisnik, D., Daniels, R., & Milic, J. 2011. An investigation of formulation factors affecting feasibility of alginate-chitosan microparticles for oral delivery of naproxen. *Arch. Pharm. Res.* 34(6): 919–929.

Chang, H. Y., Chen, J. J., Fang, F., & Chen, Z. 2004. Enhancement of antibody response by chitosan, a novel adjuvant of inactivated influenza vaccine. *Chin. J. Biol.* 17(6): 21–24.

Chen, Y. M., Chung, Y. C., Wang, L. W., Chen, K. T., & Li, S. Y. 2002. Designing chitosan-dextran sulfate nanoparticles using charge ratios. *J. Environ. Sci. Health A.* 37: 1379–1390.

Chen, Y., Mohanraj, V. J., & Parkin, J. E. 2003. Chitosan-dextran sulfate nanoparticles for delivery of an antiangiogenesis peptide. *Lett. Pept. Sci.* 10: 621–627.

Cheng, X., Zhang, F., Zhou, G. et al. 2009. DNA/chitosan nanocomplex as a novel drug carrier for doxorubicin. *Drug Deliv.* 16: 135–144.

Cho, Y. I., Park, S., Jeong, S. Y., & Yoo, H. S. 2009. In vivo and in vitro anticancer activity of thermo-sensitive and photo-crosslinkable doxorubicin hydrogels composed of chitosan–doxorubicin conjugates. *Eur. J. Pharm. Biopharm.* 73: 59–65.

Chung, Y. C., Fang, C., & Fung, C. 2006. Preparation and characterization of water-soluble chitosan produced by Maillard reaction. *Fisheries Sci.* 72: 1096–1103.

Coma, V., Martial-Gros, A., Garreau, S., Copinet, A., Salin, F., & Deschamps, A. 2002. *J. Food Sci.* 67: 1162–1169.

De Campos, A. M., Sanchez, A., & Alonso, M. J. 2001. Chitosan nanoparticles: A new vehicle for the improvement of the delivery of drugs to the ocular surface: Application to cyclosporin A. *Int. J. Pharm.* 224: 159–168.

de la Fuente, M., Seijo, B., & Alonso, M. J. 2008. Novel hyaluronic acid-chitosan nanoparticles for ocular gene therapy. *Invest. Ophthalmol. Vis. Sci.* 49(5): 2016–2024

de Salamanca, A. E., Diebold, Y., Calonge, M., Garcia-Vazquez, C., Callejo S., Vila, A. & Alonso, M. J. 2006. Chitosan nanoparticles as a potential drug delivery system for the ocular surface: Toxicity, uptake mechanism and in vivo tolerance. *Invest. Ophthalmol. Vis. Sci.* 47(4): 1416–1425.

Deacon, M. P., McGurk, S., Roberts, C. J. et al. 2000. Atomic force microscopy of gastric mucin and chitosan mucoadhesive systems. *Biochem. J.* 348: 557–563.

des Rieux, A., Fievez, V., Garinot, M., Schneider, Y. J., & Preat, V. 2006. Nanoparticles as potential oral delivery systems of proteins and vaccines: A mechanistic approach. *J. Control. Release* 116(1): 1–27.

Dhawan, S., Singla, A. K., & Sinha, V. R. 2004. Evaluation of mucoadhesive properties of chitosan microspheres prepared by different methods. *AAPS PharmSciTech.* 67: 1–7.

Dodane, V., Khan, M. A., & Merwin, J. R. 1999. Effect of chitosan on epithelial permeability and structure. *Int. J. Pharm.* 182: 21–32.

Dutta, P. K., Dutta, J. & Tripathi, V. S. 2004. Chitin and Chitosan: Chemistry, properties and Application. *J. Sci. Ind. Res.* 63: 20–31.

El Ghaouth, A., Arul, J., Grenier, J., & Asselin, A. 1992. Antifungal activity of chitosan on two postharvest pathogens of strawberry fruits. *Phytopathology* 82: 398–402.

El-Sherbiny, I. M., Abdel-Bary, E. M., & Harding, D. R. K. 2010. Preparation and in vitro evaluation of new pH-sensitive hydrogel beads for oral delivery of protein drugs. *J. Appl. Polym. Sci.* 115(5): 2828–2837.

Eytan, A. K., Zhong, Z., Robert, L. C., Richard F. M., & Michael, V. V. 2010. Ultrapure chitosan oligomers as carriers for corneal gene transfer. *Biomaterials* 31: 1814–1820.

Fang, N., Chan, V., Mao, H.-Q. et al. 2001. Interactions of phospholipid bilayer with chitosan: Effect of molecular weight and pH. *Biomacromolecules* 2: 1161–1168.

Gao, Y., Zhang, Z., Chen, L., Gu, W., & Li, Y. 2009. Chitosan N-betainates/DNA self-assembly nanoparticles for gene delivery: In vitro uptake and transfection efficiency. *Int. J. Pharm.* 371: 156–162.

Gil, E. S., & Hudson, S. M. 2004. Selective antimicrobial activity of chitosan on beer spoilage bacteria and brewing yeasts. *Prog. Polym. Sci.* 29: 1173–1222.

Gilhotra, R. M., & Mishra, D. N. 2008. Alginate-chitosan film for ocular drug delivery: Effect of surface cross-linking on film properties and characterization. *Pharmazie.* 63(8): 576–579.

Gu, R., Sun, W., Zhou, H., Wu, Z. et al. 2010. The performance of a fly–larva shell–derived chitosan sponge as an absorbable surgical hemostatic agent. *Biomaterials* 31(6): 1270–1277.

Guliyeva, U., Oner, F., Ozsoy, S., & Haziroglu, R. 2006. Chitosan microparticles containing plasmid DNA as potential oral gene delivery system. *Eur. J. Pharm Biopharm.* 62(1): 17–25.

Hadwiger, L. A., Kendra, D. G., Fristensky, B. W., & Wagoner, W. 1981. Chitosan both activated genes in plants and inhibits RNA synthesis in fungi, In: *Chitin in Nature and Technology*. Muzzarelli, R. A. A., Jeuniaux, C., & Gooday, G. W. (Eds.), Plenum, New York.

He, P., Davis, S. S., & Illum, L. 1998. In vitro evaluation of the mucoadhesive properties of chitosan microspheres. *Int. J. Pharm.* 166: 75–88.

Hejazi, R, & Amiji, M. 2003. Chitosan-based gastrointestinal delivery systems. *J. Control. Release* 89: 151–165.

Helander, I. M., Nurmiaho-Lassila, E. L., Ahvenainen, R., Rhoades, J., & Roller, S. 2001. *Int. J. Food Microbiol.* 30: 235–244.

Henriksen, K. L., Green, J. D., Smart, G., Smistad, J., & Karlsen. 1996. Bioadhesion of hydrated chitosans: An in vitro and in vivo study. *Int. J. Pharm.* 145: 231–240.

Hirano, S. 1996. Chitin biotechnology applications. *Biotechnol. Annu. Rev.* 2: 237–258.

Hirano, S., & Nagao, N. 1989. Effects of chitosan, pectic acid, lysozyme, and chitinase on the growth of several phytopathogens. *Agric. Biol. Chem.* 53(11): 3065–3066.

Hiroshi, I., Maiko, M., Boonma, L. & Tomoyo, I. 1995. Synthesis of chitosan-amino acid conjugates and their use in heavy metal uptake. *Int. J. Biol. Macromol.* 17(1): 21–23.

Hori, M., Onishi, H., & Machida, Y. 2005. Evaluation of Eudragit-coated chitosan microparticles as an oral immune delivery system. *Int. J. Pharm.* 97(1–2): 223–234.

Hosny, K. M. 2009. Preparation and evaluation of thermosensitive liposomal hydrogel for enhanced transcorneal permeation of ofloxacin. *AAPS PharmSciTech.* 1–7.

Hsu, S. C., Don, T. M., & Chiu, W. Y. 2002. Free radical degradation of chitosan with potassium persulfate. *Polym. Degrad. Stab.* 75: 73–83.

Huang, M., Fong, C. W., Khor, E. et al. 2005. Transfection efficiency of chitosan vectors: Effect of polymer molecular weight and degree of deacetylation. *J. Control. Release* 106: 391–406.

Huang, R. H., Mendis, E., Rajapakse, N., & Kim, S. K. 2006. Strong electronic charge as an important factor for anticancer activity of chitooligosaccharides (COS). *Life Science* 78(20): 2399–2408.

Ishihara, M., Nakanishi, K., Ono, K. et al. 2002. Photocrosslinkable chitosan as a dressing for wound occlusion and accelerator in healing process. *Biomaterials* 23: 833–840.

Jabbal-Gill, I, Fisher, A. N., Rappuoli, R., Davis, S. S., & Illum, L. 1998. Stimulation of mucosal and systemic antibody responses against Bordetella pertussis filamentous haemagglutinin and recombinant pertussis toxin after nasal administration with chitosan in mice. *Vaccine* 16: 2039–2046.

Jain, S. K., Jain, A., Gupta, Y. et al. 2007. Design and development of hydrogel beads for targeted drug delivery to the colon. *AAPS PharmSciTech.* 8: E56.

Jain, S. K., Jain, A., Gupta, Y. et al. 2008. Targeted delivery of 5-ASA to colon using chitosan hydrogel microspheres. *J. Drug Deliv. Sci. Tech.* 18(5): 315–321.

Janes, K. A. et al. 2001. Chitosan nanoparticles as delivery systems for doxorubicin. *J. Control. Release* 73(2–3): 255–267.

Janvikul, W., Uppanan, P., Thavornyutikarn, B., Krewraing, J., & Prateepasen, R. 2006. *In vitro* comparative hemostatic studies of chitin, chitosan, and their derivatives. *J. Appl. Polym. Sci.* 102: 445–451.

Jayakumar, R., Nwe, N., Tokura, S., & Tamura, H. 2007. Sulfated chitin and chitosan as novel biomaterials. *Int. J. Biol. Macromol.* 40: 175–181.

Jeon, Y. J., Park, P. J, & Kim, S. K. 2001. Antimicrobial effect of chitooligosaccharides produced by bioreactor. *Carbohydr. Polym.* 44: 71–76.

Jeon, Y. J., Shahidi, F., & Kim, S. K. 2000. Preparation of chitin and chitosan oligomers and their application in physiological functional foods. *Food Rev. Int.* 16: 159–176.

Jose, S., Fangueiro, J. F., Smitha, J., Cinu, T. A., Chacko, A. J., Premaletha, K., & Souto, E. B. 2012. Cross-linked chitosan microspheres for oral delivery of insulin: Taguchi design and in vivo testing. *Colloids Surf. B Biointerfaces* 92: 175–179.

Kahlig, H., Hasanovic, A., Biruss, B., Holler, S., Grim, J., & Valenta, C. 2009. Chitosan-glycolic acid: A possible matrix for progesterone delivery into skin. *Drug Dev. Ind. Pharm.* 14: 1–6.

Kato, Y., Onishi, H., & Machida, Y. 2001. Biological characteristics of lactosaminated N-succinyl-chitosan as a liver-specific drug carrier in mice. *J. Control. Release* 70: 295–307.

Kato, Y., Onishi, H., & Machida, Y. 2002. Efficacy of lactosaminated and intact N-succinylchitosan–mitomycin C conjugates against M5076 liver metastatic cancer. *J. Pharm. Pharmacol.* 54: 529–537.

Kean, T., & Thanou, M. 2009. Chitin and chitosan sources, production and medical applications. In: Williams, P. A., Arshady, R., editors. *Desk Reference of Natural Polymers, their Sources, Chemistry and Applications.* Kentus Books; London: 327–361.

Khangtragool, A., Ausayakhun, S., Leesawat, P., Molloy, R., & Laokul, C. 2009. Evaluation of the use of chitosan in ocular drug delivery of Vancomycin. *CMU J. Natural Sci* 8(1): 1–10.

Kim, S. J., Shin, S. R., Lee, S. M., Kim, I. Y., & Kim, S. I. 2003. Physical properties and degradability of PHB/*chitosan* blend films. *J. Appl. Polym. Sci.* 88(88): 2721–2724.

Knapczyk, J. 1992. Antimycotic buccal and vaginal tablets with chitosan. *Int. J. Pharm.* 88: 9–14.

Knorr, D. 1984. Use of chitinous polymers in food challenge for food research and development. *Food Technol.* 38: 85–97.

Kockisch, S., Rees, G. D., Young, S. A. et al. 2003. Polymeric microspheres for drug delivery to the oral cavity: An in vitro evaluation of mucoadhesive potential. *J. Pharm. Sci.* 92: 1614–1623.

Krauland, A. H., & Alonso, M. J., 2007. Chitosan/Cyclodextrin nanoparticles as macromolecular drug delivery systems. *Int. J. Pharm.* 340: 134–142.

Kumbar, S. G., Soppimath, K. S., & Tejraj, M. A. 2003. Synthesis and characterization of polyacrylamide-grafted chitosan hydrogel microspheres for the controlled release of indomethacin. *J. Appl. Polym. Sci.* 87(9): 1525–1536.

Lee, E., Kima, H., Lee, I.-H., & Jon, S. 2009. In vivo antitumor effects of chitosan-conjugated docetaxel after oral administration. *J. Control. Release* 140: 79–85.

Lee, E., Lee, J., Lee, I. H., Yu, M. H., Kim, S. Y. & Chae, S. J. 2008. Conjugated chitosan as a novel platform for oral delivery of paclitaxel. *J. Med. Chem.* 51: 6442–6449.

Lee, M., Nah, J. W., Kwon, Y., Koh, J. J., Ko, K. S., & Kim, S. W. 2001. Water-soluble and low molecular weight chitosan-based plasmid DNA delivery. *Pharm. Res.* 18: 427–431.

Lehr, C. M., Bouwstra, J. A., Schacht, E. H. et al. 1992. In vitro evaluation of mucoadhesive properties of chitosan and some other natural polymers. *Int. J. Pharm.* 78: 43–48.

Li, N., Zhuang, C. Y., Wang, M., Sui, C. G., & Pan, W. S. 2012. Low molecular weight chitosan-coated liposomes for ocular drug delivery: In vitro and in vivo studies. *Drug Deliv.* 19(1): 28–35.

Lim, C. K., Halim, A. S., Lau, H. Y., Ujang, Z., & Hazri, A. 2007. In vitro cytotoxicology model of oligo-chitosan and n, o-carboxymethyl chitosan using primary normal human epidermal keratinocyte cultures. *J. Appl. Biomater. Biomech.* 5(2): 82–87.
Lin, A., Liu, Y., Huang, Y., Sun, J., Wu, Z., Zhang, X., & Ping, Q. 2008. Glycyrrhizin surface modified chitosan nanoparticles for hepatocyte-targeted delivery. *Int. J. Pharm.* 359: 247–253.
Lin, Y. C., Lin, S. T., Chen, C. Y., & Wu, S. C. 2012. Enterovirus 71 adsorption on metal ion-composite chitosan beads. *Biotechnol. Prog.* 28(1): 206–214.
Liu, W. G. & Yao, K. D. 2002. Chitosan and its derivatives-a promising non-viral vector for gene transfection. *J. Control. Release* 83: 1–11.
Liu, X., Howard, K. A., Dong, M., Andersen, M. O., Rahbek, U. L., Johnsen, M. G. et al. 2007. The influence of polymeric properties on chitosan/siRNA nanoparticle formulation and gene silencing. *Biomaterials* 28: 1280–1288.
Liu, X. F., Guan, Y. L., Yang, D. Z., Li, Z., & Yao, K. D. 2001. Antibacterial action of chitosan and carboxymethylated chitosan. *J. Appl. Polym. Sci.* 79: 1324–1335.
Lorenzo-Lamosa, M. L., Remunan-Lopez, C., Vila-Jato, J. L., & Alonso, M. J. 1998. Design of microencapsulated chitosan microspheres for colonic drug delivery. *J. Control. Release* 52(1–2): 109–118.
Lu, G., Ling, K., & Zhao, P. 2010. A novel in situ-formed hydrogel wound dressing by the photocross-linking of a chitosan derivative. *Wound Repair Regen.* 18(1): 70–79.
MacLaughlin, F. C., Mumper, R. J., Wang, J. et al. 1998. Chitosan and depolymerized chitosan oligomers as condensing carriers for in vivo plasmid delivery. *J. Control. Release* 56: 259–272.
Maculotti, K., Tira, E. M., Sonaggere, M., Perugini, P., Conti, B., Modena, T., & Pavanetto, F. 2009. In vitro evaluation of chondroitin sulphate-chitosan microspheres as carrier for the delivery of proteins. *J. Microencapsul.* 26(6): 535–543.
Maezaki, Y., Tsuji, K., Nakagawa, Y., Kawai, Y., Akimoto, M., Tsugita, T. et al. 1996. *Chitin enzymology*. Italy: Lyon and Ancona: European Chitin Society. 217–232.
Mao, C., Zhao, W. B., Zhu, A. P., Shen, J., & Lin, S. C. 2004. A photochemical method for the surface modification of poly(vinyl chloride) with *O*-butyrylchitosan to improve blood compatibility. *Process Biochem.* 39: 1151–1157.
Mao, H. Q., Roy, K., Troung-Le, V. L. et al. 2001. Chitosan-DNA nanoparticles as gene carrier: Synthesis, characterization and transfection efficiency. *J. Control. Release* 70: 399–421.
Mina, B. M., Leeb, S. W., Limb, J. N. et al. 2004. Chitin and chitosan nanofibers: Electrospinning of chitin and deacetylation of chitin nanofibers. *Polymer* 45: 7137–7142.
Miwa, A., Ishibe, A., Nakano, M., Yamahira T., Itai, S., Jinno, S., & Kawahara, H. 1998. Development of novel chitosan derivatives as micellar carriers of taxol. *Pharm. Res.* 12: 1844–1850.
Miyazaki, S. Nakayama, A. Oda, M, Takada, M. & Atwood, D. 1995. Drug release from oral mucosal adhesive tablets of chitosan and sodium alginate. *Int. J. Pharm.* 118: 257–263.
Mucha, M. 1997. Rheological characteristics of semi-dilute chitosan solutions. *Macromol. Chem. Phys.* 198: 471–484.
Murata, J.-I., Ohya, Y., & Ouchi, T. 1997. Design of quaternary chitosan conjugate having antennary galactose residues as a gene delivery tool. *Carbohydr. Polym.* 32: 105–109.
Muzzarelli, R. A. A., Xia, W., Tomasetti, M., Ilari, P. et al. 1995. Depolymerization of chitosan and substituted chitosans with the aid of a wheat germ lipase preparation. *Enzyme Microb. Technol.* 17(6): 541–545.
Muzzarelli, R., Baldassare, V., Conti, F. et al. 1988. Biological activity of chitosan: Ultrastructure study. *Biomaterials* 9: 247–252.

Nafee, N., Taetz, S., Schneider, M., Schaefer, U. F., & Lehr, C. M. 2007. Chitosan-coated PLGA nanoparticles for DNA/RNA delivery: Effect of the formulation parameters on complexation and transfection of antisense oligonucleotides. *Nanomedicine* 3(3): 173–183.

Nagarwal, R. C., Singh, P. N., Kant, S., Maiti, P., & Pandit, J. K. 2011. Chitosan nanoparticles of 5-fluorouracil for ophthalmic delivery: Characterization, in-vitro and in-vivo study. *Chem. Pharm. Bull.* (Tokyo) 59(2): 272–278.

Ngo, D. N., Kim, M. M., & Kim, S. K. 2008. Chitin oligosaccharides inhibit oxidative stress in live cells. *Carbohydr. Polym.* 74(2): 228–234.

Nishimura, K., Nishimura, S., Nishi, N., Saiki, I., Tokura, S., & Azuma, I. 1984. Immunological activity of chitin and its derivatives. *Vaccine* 2(1): 93–99.

No, H. K., Meyers, J. S. P., & Lee, K. S. 1989. Isolation and characterization of chitin from crawfish shell waste. *J. Agric. Food Chem.* 37 (3): 575–579.

Ogawara, K., Yoshida, M., Higaki, K. et al. 1999. Hepatic uptake of polystyrene microspheres in rats: Effect of particle size on intrahepatic distribution. *J. Control. Release* 59: 15–22.

Okamoto, Y., Yano, R., Miyatake, K., Tomohiro, I., Shigemasa, Y., & Minami, S. 2003. Effects of chitin and chitosan on blood coagulation. *Carbohydr. Polym.* 53: 337–342.

Oliveira, J. M., Kotobuki, N., Marques, A. P. et al. 2008. Surface engineered carboxymethylchitosan/poly(amidoamine) dendrimer nanoparticles for intracellular targeting. *Adv. Funct. Mater.* 18: 1840–1853.

Owens, M., Senrud, A., Teach, J., & Gregory, K. A. 2006. Device for the deployment of internal esophageal chitosan bandage. *Gastrointestinal Endoscopy GIE* 63(5): AB237.

Panyam, J., & Labhasetwar, V. 2003. Biodegradable nanoparticles for drug and gene delivery to cells and tissue, *Adv. Drug Deliv. Rev.* 55(3): 329–347.

Park, I. K., Park, Y. H., Shin, B. A. et al. 2000. Galactosylated chitosan-graft-dextran as hepatocyte-targeting DNA carrier. *J. Control. Release* 69: 97–108.

Prabaharan, M., & Mano, J. F. 2005. Hydroxypropyl chitosan bearing beta-cyclodextrin cavities: Synthesis and slow release of its inclusion complex with a model hydrophobic drug. *Macromol. Biosci.* 5(10): 965–973.

Prabaharan, M., Rodriguez-Perez, M. A., de Saja, J. A., & Mano, J. F. 2007. *J. Biomed. Mater. Res. Part B: Appl. Biomater.* 81B: 427–434.

Prashanth, K. V. H., & Tharanathan, R. N. 2007. Chitin/chitosan: Modifications and their unlimited application potential: An overview. *Trends Food Sci. Technol.* 18: 117–131.

Premaletha, K., Licy, C. D., Jose, S., Saraladevi, A., Shirwaikar, A., & Shirwaikar, A. 2012. Formulation, characterization and optimization of hepatitis B surface antigen (HBsAg)-loadedchitosan microspheres for oral delivery. *Pharm. Dev. Technol.* 17(2): 251–258.

Rassu, G., Gavini, E., Jonassen, H., Zambito, Y., Fogli, S., Breschi, M. C., & Giunchedi, P. 2009. New chitosan derivatives for the preparation of rokitamycin loaded microspheres designed for ocular or nasal administration. *J. Pharm. Sci.* 98(12): 4852–4865.

Razdan, A., & Pettersson, D. 1994. Effect of chitin and chitosan on nutrient digestibility and plasma lipid concentrations in broiler chickens. *Br. J. Nutr.* 7: 277–288.

Razdan, A., & Pettersson, D. 1996. Hypolipidaemic, gastrointestinal and related responses of broiler chickens to chitosans of different viscosity. *Br. J. Nutr.* 76: 387–397.

Ren, D., Yi, H., Wang, W. et al. 2005. The enzymatic degradation and swelling properties of chitosan matrices with different degrees of N-acetylation. *Carbohydr. Res.* 340: 2403–2410.

Rha, C. K., Rodriguez-Sanchez, D., & Kienzle-Sterzer, C. 1984. Novel applications of chitosan. In: Colwell, R. R., Pariser, E. R., Sinskey, A. J., editors. *Biotechnology of Marine Polysaccharides.* Hemisphere; Washington. 284–311.

Sapra, B., Jain, S., & Tiwary, A. K. 2009. Transdermal delivery of carvedilol in rats: Probing the percutaneous permeation enhancement mechanism of soybean extract-chitosan mixture. *Drug Dev. Ind. Pharm.* 35(10): 1230–1241.

Schipper, N. G., Varum, K. M., & Artursson, P. 1996. Chitosans as absorption enhancers for poorly absorbable drugs. 1: Influence of molecular weight and degree of acetylation on drug transport across human intestinal epithelial (Caco-2) cells. *Pharm. Res.* 13: 1686–1692.

Schuetz, Y. B., Gurny, R., & Jordan, O. 2008. A novel thermoresponsive hydrogel based on chitosan. *Eur. J. Pharm. Biopharm.* 68(1): 19–25.

Shahidi, F., Arachchi, J. K. V., & Jeon, Y. J. 1999. Food applications of chitin and chitosans. *Trends Food Sci. Technol.* 10: 37–51.

Sinha, V. R., Singla, A. K., Wadhawan, S., Kaushik, R., Kumria, R., Bansal, K., & Dhawan, S. 2004. Chitosan microspheres as a potential carrier for drugs. *Int. J. Pharm.* 274: 1–33.

Snyman, D., Hamman, J. H., & Kotze, A. F. 2003. Evaluation of the mucoadhesive properties of N-trimethyl chitosan chloride. *Drug. Dev. Ind. Pharm.* 29: 61–69.

Son, Y. J., Jang, J. S., Cho, Y. W. et al. 2003. Biodistribution and antitumor efficacy of doxorubicin loaded glycol chitosan nanoaggregates by EPR effect. *J. Control. Release* 91(1–2): 135–145.

Song, B., Zhang, W., Peng, R., Huang, J., Nie, T., Li, Y. et al. 2009. Synthesis and cell activity of novel galactosylated chitosan as a gene carrier. *Colloids Surf.* 70: 181–186.

Stossel, O., & Leuba, J. L. 1984. Effect of chitosan, chitin and some aminosugars on growth of various soilborne phytopathogenic fungi. *J. Phytopathol.* 111: 82–90.

Sugano, M., Fujikawa, T., Hiratsuji, Y., Nakashima, K., Fukuda, N., & Hasegawa, Y. 1980. A novel use of chitosan as a hypocholesterolemic agent in rats. *Am. J. Clin. Nutr.* 33: 787–793.

Sun, S. K., Sang, H. J., Jeong, K. S., Duck, H. K., Ih, S. C., & Ji, M. K. 2007. Preparation and stabilization of chitosan-lipase composite within mesoporous silica material. *Solid State Phenom.* 124–126: 1717.

Suzuki, K., Mikami, T., Okawa, Y., Tokoro, A., Suzuki, S., & Suzuki, M. 1986. Antitumor effect of hexa-N-acetylchitohexaose and chitohexaose. *Carbohydr. Res.* 151: 403–408.

Takayama, K., Hirata, M., Machida, Y., Masada, T., Sannan, T. & Nagai, T. 1990. Effect of interpolymer complex formation on bioadhesive property and drug release phenomenon of compressed tablet consisting of chitosan and sodium hyaluronate. *Chem. Pharm. Bull.* 38(7): 1993–1997.

Taveira, S. F., Nomizo, A., & Lopez, R. F. V. 2009. Effect of the iontophoresis of a chitosan gel on doxorubicin skin penetration and cytotoxicity. *J. Control. Release* 134: 35–40.

Tian, B., Luo, Q., Song, S. et al. 2012. Novel surface-modified nanostructured lipid carriers with partially deacetylated water-soluble chitosan for efficient ocular delivery. *J. Pharm. Sci.* 101(3): 1040–1049.

Tiyaboonchai W. 2003. Chitosan nanoparticles: A promising system for drug delivery. *Naresuan Univ. J.* 11: 51–66.

Tokoro, A., Tatewaki, N., Suzuki, K., Mikami, T., Suzuki, S., & Suzuki, M. 1988. Growth-inhibitory effect of hexa-N-acetylchitohexaose and chitohexaose against meth-A solid tumor. *Chem. Pharm. Bull.* 36: 784–790.

Tozaki, H., Komoike, J., Tada, C. et al. 1997. Chitosan capsules for colon-specific drug delivery: Improvement of insulin absorption from the rat colon. *J. Pharm. Sci.* 86: 1016–1021.

Tuzlakoglu, K., Alves, C. M., Mano, J. F., & Reis, R. L. 2004. *Macromol. Biosci.* 4: 811–819.

Ubaidulla, U., Khar, R. K., Ahmed, F. J., & Panda, A. K. 2007. Development and in-vivo evaluation of insulin-loaded chitosan phthalate microspheres for oral delivery. *J. Pharm. Pharmacol.* 59(10): 1345–1351.

Upadrashta, S. M., Katikaneni, P. R., & Nuessle, N. O. 1992. Chitosan as a tablet binder. *Drug. Dev. Ind. Pharm.* 18(15): 2701– 2708.

Verestiuc, L., Nastasescu, O., Barbu, E., Sarvaiya, I., Green, K. L., & Tsibouklis, J. 2006. Functionalized chitosan/NIPAM (HEMA) hybrid polymer networks as inserts for ocular drug delivery: Synthesis, *in vitro* assessment, and *in vivo* evaluation. *J. Biomed. Mater. Res.* 77: 726–735.

Vila, A., Sánchez, A., Janes, K., Behrens, I., Kissel, T., Vila Jato, J. L., & Alonso, M. J. 2004. Low molecular weight chitosan nanoparticles as new carriers for nasal vaccine delivery in mice. *Eur. J. Pharm. Biopharm.* 57(1): 123–131.

Wang, X., Yan, Y., & Zhang, R. 2006. A comparison of chitosan and collagen sponges as hemostatic dressings. *J. Bioact. Compat. Polym.* 21: 39–54.

Wang, Y.-S., Liu, L.-R., Jiang, Q., & Zhang, Q.-Q. 2007. Self-aggregated nanoparticles of cholesterol-modified chitosan conjugate as a novel carrier of epirubicin. *Eur. Polym. J.* 43: 43–51.

Wei, W., Ma, G. H., Wang, L. Y., Wu, J., & Su, Z. G. 2010. Hollow quaternized chitosan microspheres increase the therapeutic effect of orally administered insulin. *Acta Biomater.* 6(1): 205–209.

Wei, W., Wang, L. Y., Yuan, L., Yang, X. D., Su, Z. G., & Ma, G. H. 2008. Bioprocess of uniform-sized crosslinked chitosan microspheres in rats following oral administration. *Eur. J. Pharm. Biopharm.* 69(3): 878–886.

Wei, X. L., & Xia, W. S. 2003. Research development of chitooligosaccharides physiological activities. *Chem. Pharm. Bull.* 19(6): 614–617.

Wilson, B., Samanta, M. K., Santhi, K., Kumar, K. P., Ramasamy, M., & Suresh, B. 2010. Chitosan nanoparticles as a new delivery system for the anti-Alzheimer drug tacrine. *Nanomedicine* 6(1): 144–152.

Xia, W. S. 2003. Physiological activities of chitosan and its application in functional foods. *J. Chin. Inst. Food Sci. Technol.* 3(1): 77–81.

Xu, J., McCarthy, S. P., Gross, R. A. et al. 1996. Chitosan film acylation and effects on biodegradability. *Macromolecules* 29: 3436–3440.

Yang, K. W., Li, X. R., Yang, Z. L., Li, P. Z., Wang, F., & Liu, Y. 2009. Novel polyion complex micelles for liver-targeted delivery of diammonium glycyrrhizinate: In vitro and in vivo characterization. *J. Biomed. Mater. Res. A.* 2009: 140–148.

Yang, Y. M., Hu, W., Wang, X. D. et al. 2007. The controlling biodegradation of chitosan fibers by n-acetylation in vitro and in vivo. *J. Mater. Sci. Mater. Med.* 18: 2117–2121.

Yedurkar, P., Dhiman, M. K., Petkar, K., & Sawant, K. 2012. Mucoadhesive bilayer buccal tablet of carvedilol-loaded chitosan microspheres: In vitro, pharmacokinetic and pharmacodynamic investigations. *J. Microencapsul.* 29(2): 126–137.

Yoo, H. S., Lee, J. E., Chung, H., Kwon, I. C., & Jeong, S. Y. 2005. Self-assembled nanoparticles containing hydrophobically modified glycol chitosan for gene delivery. *J. Control. Release* 103: 235–243.

Young, D. H., Kohle, H., & Kauss, H. 1982. Release of calcium from suspension-cultured Glycine max cells by chitosan, other polycations, and polyamines in relation to effects on membrane permeability. *Plant Physiol.* 70: 1449–1454.

Yu, J. M., Li, Y. J., Qiu, L. Y., & Jin, Y. 2008. Self-aggregated nanoparticles of cholesterol-modified glycol chitosan conjugate: Preparation, characterization, and preliminary assessment as a new drug delivery carrier. *Eur. Polym. J.* 44(3): 555–565.

Yu, J., Xie, X., Zheng, M., Yu, L. Zhang L., Zhao, J., Jiang, D., & Che, X. 2012. Fabrication and characterization of nuclear localization signal-conjugated glycol chitosan micelles for improving the nuclear delivery of doxorubicin. *Int. J. Nanomedicine.* 7: 5079–5090.

Zhang, J., & Wang, S. 2009. Topical use of coenzyme Q10-loaded liposomes coated with trimethyl chitosan: Tolerance, precorneal retention and anti-cataract effect. *Int. J. Pharm.* 372(1–2): 66–75.

Zhang, M., Tan, T., Yuan, H. & Rui, C. 2003. Insecticidal and fungicidal activities of chitosan and oligo-chitosan. *J Bioactive Compatible Polym.* 18: 391–400.

Zhang, Y., Wei, W., Lv, P., Wang, L., & Ma, G. 2011. Preparation and evaluation of alginate-chitosan microspheres for oral delivery of insulin. *Eur. J. Pharm. Biopharm.* 77(1): 11–19.

Zhao, X. L., Li, K. X., Zhao, X. F., Pang, D. H., & Chen, D. W. 2008. Study on colon-specific 5-Fu pH-enzyme Di-dependent chitosan microspheres. *Chem. Pharm. Bull. (Tokyo).* 56(7): 963–968.
Zhao, X. R., & Xia, W. S. 2006. Antimicrobial activities of chitosan and application in food preservation. *Chin. Food Res. Dev.* 27(2): 157–160.
Zoldners, J., Kiseleva, T., & Kaiminsh, I. 2005. Influence of ascorbic acid on the stability of chitosan solutions. *Carbohydr. Polym.* 60: 215–218.

12 Gene Delivery by Electroporation

Julie Gehl

CONTENTS

INTRODUCTION

By applying brief electric pulses, it is possible to transfer molecules into cells and tissues. The use of electroporation for delivery of chemotherapy is now quite widely used and in further development. Electrochemotherapy is in routine use for cutaneous tumors [1] in more than 100 cancer centers, and several thousand patients have been treated. Response rates are high and side effects limited [2–8]. An important perspective about the success of electrochemotherapy is that electroporation equipment approved for clinical use is now available in many hospitals, allowing its use for gene therapy.

And what are the possibilities for gene therapy using electroporation? Arguably the most important future use could be gene delivery for vaccination [9]. As more than one DNA sequence may be delivered at the same time, vaccination for several epitopes is a possibility using electroporation. Equipment is being developed that allows small, easily transportable units, and as DNA is heat stable, this means that vaccines can be transported into remote areas without cold chain transportation. There is an increasing understanding that vaccinations may be used both to prevent spread of infectious disease, such as measles and HIV [10], but also to prevent cancer as about one of six cancers worldwide are caused by infectious agents, such as human papilloma virus and hepatitis virus [11].

The most extensively studied area of use for gene therapy is cancer treatment, and although considerable progress has been made over the past decades in surgery, radiotherapy, and drug therapy, it remains the fact that cancer is a leading cause of death and morbidity worldwide. Over 70% of cancer cases are found in low- and middle-income countries [12], underlining the need for less expensive therapies, and here gene therapy might provide a solution. Thus, by transfecting tissues in a patient, the desired therapeutic molecule may be produced in that tissue, and the patient actually may become his own medicine's producer (Figure 12.1). Furthermore, gene delivery allows concomitant attack on several pathways, possibly giving a brighter future for cancer therapy. Gene therapy trials based on electroporation, as the nonviral means of delivery, are now being published [13–15].

Chronic disease, such as hemophilia, may also be amenable to gene therapy, and here electroporation-based delivery may be of interest as this can be done in an immunologically safe way so that antibodies against the transgene product may be avoided. In a number of diseases, such as hemophilia, correcting a fraction of the anomaly caused by the genetic defect may be sufficient to cause a real difference for the patient. For example, having some ability for coagulation may be hugely different than having very little. Gene transfer may be performed in different ways, for example, to the muscle [16], or with different equipment to the lungs [17], thus targeting very different tissues.

When using gene electrotransfer for vaccination purposes, brief expression of a couple of weeks will be perfect to elicit an immune response, and so gene electrotransfer to skin might be an optimal solution because then the expression will fade quickly (Figure 12.2) [9,18]. On the contrary, ameliorating a protein deficiency disorder by electrotransfer to muscle may be optimal as very long-lived expression may be obtained [16].

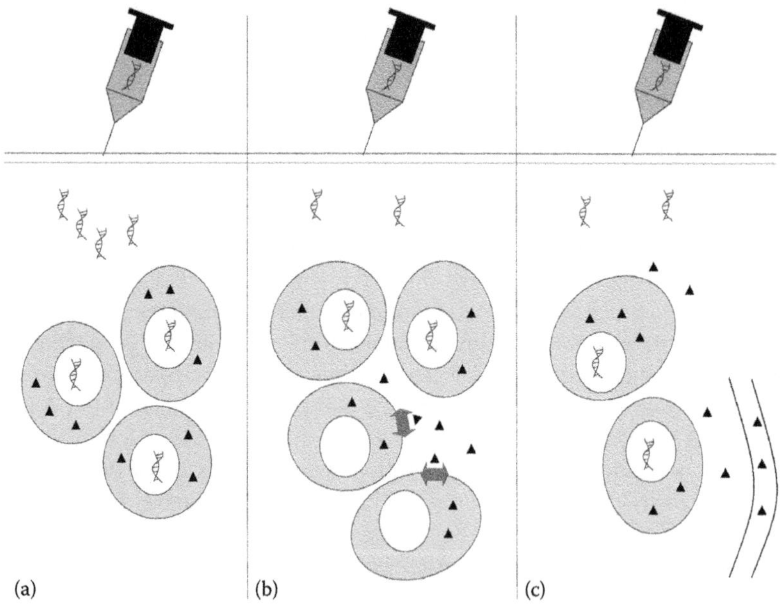

FIGURE 12.1 The three approaches. (a) Single cell approach, in which every single cell in a population has to be transfected with the plasmid in order to benefit from the transgene. An example could be ex vivo transfection of keratinocytes. (b) Paracrine approach, in which few cells in a population are transfected with the plasmid, and the produced protein then acts locally, e.g., by eliciting an immune response. (c) Systemic approach, in which few cells in a population are transfected with the plasmid. The produced protein is then transferred to, e.g., the blood stream, where it can create a systemic response. The distinction of these three approaches is of course theoretical, and the borders between them are arbitrary. (From Gothelf A, Gehl J. *Curr Gene Ther* 2010;10:287–99.)

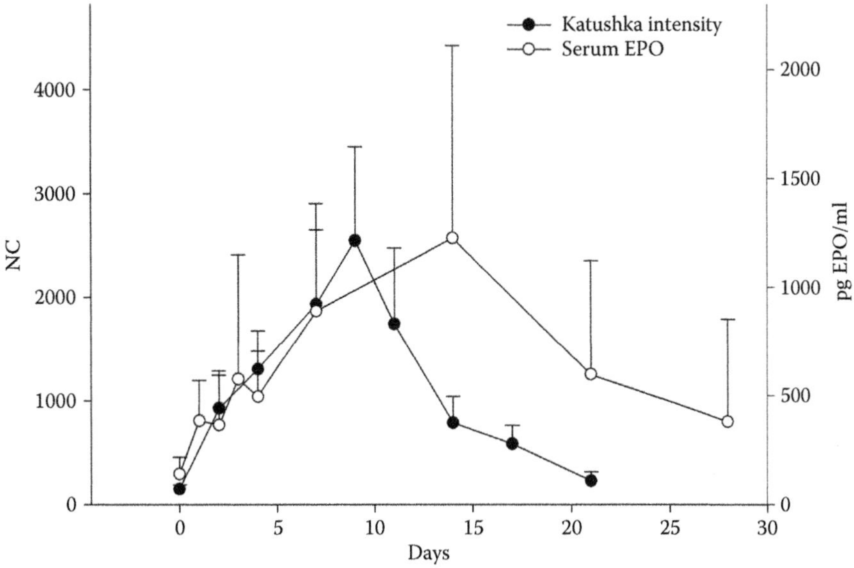

FIGURE 12.2 Comparison of gene electrotransfer to skin with Katushka with EPO in terms of duration and level of expression. With Katushka, a peak in expression (in NC) is reached after 9 days, whereas serum EPO (in pg EPO per ml) seems to peak after 14 days. (From Gothelf A et al. *Gene Ther* 2010;17:839–45.)

GENETIC THERAPY

The term *genetic therapy* has been coined to describe therapy using different nucleotide formulations, and indeed there are a number of possibilities and more on the way in classic gene therapy; utilizing DNA, a transgene is transferred to cells that may then produce a protein with a medicinal effect. DNA is very stable, which facilitates production of DNA drugs, and DNA is easily soluble, allowing injection into tissues.

RNA is a class of nucleotides that may be used in different, even opposite, directions. Thus, RNA may be electrotransferred into dendritic cells, allowing expression of the protein causing an immune response. But using siRNA (silencing RNA), it is possible to quench expression of a particular gene [19].

Oligonucleotides are a broad description for molecules containing nucleotides, but they often have a number of chemical alterations allowing new and different virtues. An example of oligonucleotide therapy would be correction of Duchennes muscular atrophy, where correction of a single mutation may right the wrong. Oligonucleotides are a very heterogeneous group of molecules, and so electroporation parameters optimized for delivery may be quite different [20].

IN VITRO VERSUS IN VIVO

There is a considerable difference between working in vitro and in vivo with gene electrotransfer—or transfer of RNA or oligonucleotides. When working in vitro,

DNA is able to move almost freely in the medium and will adsorb to the cell membrane in the presence of a divalent cation, such as calcium or magnesium. On the other hand, the cells are more vulnerable to electroporation when in solution because the extracellular volume is large compared to the intracellular volume, and therefore, electrolyte exchange over the cell membrane will be much more extensive, posing a challenge to the cell when the transmembrane potential has to be restored [21].

When working in vivo, other challenges appear: DNA diffusion is slow [22], and as the solution is often quite viscous, this is also a contributing factor to slow diffusion. The DNA needs to be present with the electrodes, and so coordination between the two is necessary. When applying an electric field in vivo, mostly needle electrodes are used, and there are inhomogeneities in the field [23], which may lead to a varied uptake but, on the other hand, also sometimes an automatic optimization in that, given a field gradient is present, there will be optimal uptake somewhere in the field [24].

THE ELECTROPORATION PROCEDURE

DNA electrotransfer is a multistep process as reviewed in, for example, Escoffre et al. [25].

The initial step is diffusion toward the cell. As mentioned, diffusion is much simpler in vitro and in vivo, and even between tissues, there are noticeable differences. Thus, in a tumor, cell adherence is often low, and DNA may distribute in the space between cells. Contrarily, DNA diffusion after injection intradermally may be notoriously difficult as there are tight junctions between keratinocytes.

The pulses used for electrotransfer may have an electrophoretic potential, and so the electric pulses may also have an effect on diffusion of the molecule. DNA and RNA have multiple negative charges and therefore move in the electric field.

The next step is an adsorption to the cell membrane [26]. In vitro, often magnesium is added to link the negative exterior of the cells to the negatively charged DNA. When injecting in vivo, it is assumed that divalent cations, such as calcium, may perform this function. It has been shown that, in a field where pulses are reversed, DNA may migrate away from the membrane again, clearly showing the importance of the electric field in the process of approximation and adsorption.

When the electric field is applied, a small water bridge is formed in the cell membrane in a matter of nanoseconds [27,28]. This step facilitates the transfer of DNA through the membrane although it is the electrophoretic push that is the driving force of delivery [16,29].

Trafficking of DNA toward the cell nucleus is now well described in elegant studies, showing that the microtubuli act as highways for DNA transfer [30–32].

CHOICE AND EFFECT OF ELECTRIC PULSES

Using the correct pulse parameters is very important for success in gene electrotransfer. On a positive note, pulse parameters may be chosen in order to target delivery of specific molecules to certain cell types. As discussed below, there are two major ways to go: One is long-duration, low-voltage pulses, and the other is high-voltage pulses. High-voltage pulses do an excellent job permeabilizing the cell membrane. Thus, when the objective is to transfer molecules that enter the cell by diffusion, a series of high-voltage pulses is an excellent choice. It has been shown that there is an almost linear increase in uptake going from a few pulses to approximately 10 pulses, and therefore, a standard for the use of electrochemotherapy (transfer of molecules with cytotoxic potential) is to use eight pulses. DNA or RNA is not transferred into the cell by simple diffusion. Indeed, the molecules are far too large, and the many negative charges stick to the outside of the membrane. It has been shown that DNA transfer is largely dependent on an electrophoretic effect [33], and therefore, administration of the electric pulses needs to relate to this mechanism. An exception to this rule seems to be that certain cells (tumor, liver) may actually take up exogenous DNA using high-voltage pulses [13,34]; however, the exact mechanism behind this is not yet fully elucidated.

When performing gene delivery to bacteria, such as *E. coli*, the object is to obtain one of the few transfected clones, and little attention is paid to the fate of the rest of the batch. Needless to say, when working with humans, this attitude is not applicable. It is very important to look at the side effect profile in normal tissues and adjust pulses to be appropriate for the job but not excessive. When treating tumors, a certain allowance can be made in that there is no concern for the well-being of cancer cells. However, it has been shown that for gene electrotransfer to, for example, muscle it is paramount that cell integrity is preserved [35,36]. Thus, it has been shown that expression is higher with a lower DNA dose and with the lowest pulse parameters that are above the permeabilization threshold. An example of gene eletrotransfer in the clinical setting is shown in Figure 12.3.

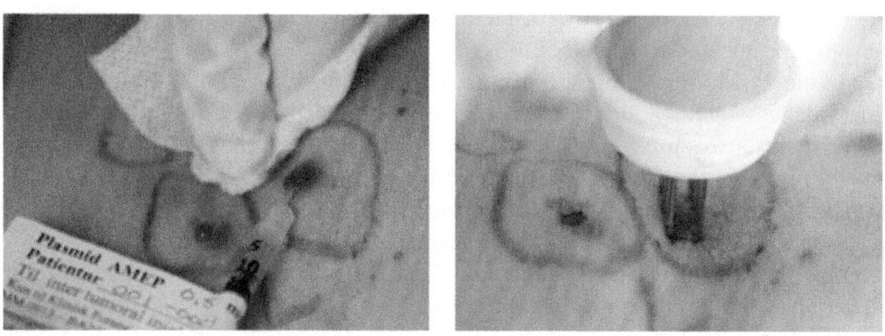

(a) (b)

FIGURE 12.3 Treatment procedure. In each patient, two cutaneous lesions were identified, marked (one treated, one control), and photographed. Treatment was performed at day 1 and day 8 under local anesthesia. The same lesion was treated at the two sessions. The drop of blood seen on the control lesion is because of the fine-needle aspiration taken before injection of plasmid AMEP into the treated lesion. (a) Intratumoral injection of plasmid AMEP. (b) Application of the electric pulses using a linear needle electrode inserted into the cutaneous lesion. AMEP, antiangiogenic metargidin peptide. (From Spanggaard I et al. *Hum Gene Ther Clin Dev* 2013;24:99–107.)

EQUIPMENT

For in vitro or in vivo studies, a number of options exist regarding equipment. For gene delivery, long, low-voltage pulses would be recommended, but a number of different pulse combinations can be used [33,37,38], and some of these conditions may be met by many of the commercially available solutions. For in vivo gene delivery, the situation is different in that the equipment must be approved for clinical use, which dramatically limits the options. Current equipment options include the Cliniporator (Carpi, Italy), which allows a range of options for gene delivery, including the high-voltage, low-voltage pulse combination used preclinically and clinically [14,39], and the Inovio generators for gene delivery to skin and muscle [13,40].

CONCLUSION AND PERSPECTIVES

Electroporation is a delivery technology, which is in expansion for a number of purposes. Within medical indications, the use for vaccines is very promising, and electroporation-based cancer therapy is gaining momentum with regards to both drug and gene delivery. Also, for the treatment of chronic disease, gene delivery by electroporation may become important, in particular because the immune response to the transferred gene is lower when no vira are involved in the process.

REFERENCES

1. National Institute for Health and Care Excellence. Electrochemotherapy for metastases in the skin from tumours of non-skin origin and melanoma. http://publications.nice.org.uk/electrochemotherapy-for-metastases-in-the-skin-from-tumours-of-non-skin-origin-and-melanoma-ipg446. 2013.
2. Quaglino P, Mortera C, Osella-Abate S, Barberis M, Illengo M, Rissone M et al. Electrochemotherapy with intravenous bleomycin in the local treatment of skin melanoma metastases. *Ann Surg Oncol* 2008;15:2215–22.
3. Quaglino P, Matthiessen LW, Curatolo P, Muir T, Bertino G, Kunte C et al. Predicting patients at risk for pain associated with electrochemotherapy. *Acta Oncol* 2015;1–9.
4. Campana LG, Mocellin S, Basso M, Puccetti O, De Salvo GL, Chiarion-Sileni V et al. Bleomycin-based electrochemotherapy: Clinical outcome from a single institution's experience with 52 patients. *Ann Surg Oncol* 2009;16:191–9.
5. Matthiessen LW, Johannesen HH, Hendel HW, Moss T, Kamby C, Gehl J. Electrochemotherapy for large cutaneous recurrence of breast cancer: A phase II clinical trial. *Acta Oncol* 2012;51:713–21.
6. Matthiessen LW, Chalmers RL, Sainsbury DC, Veeramani S, Kessell G, Humphreys AC et al. Management of cutaneous metastases using electrochemotherapy. *Acta Oncol* 2011;50:621–9.
7. Marty M, Sersa G, Garbay JR, Gehl J, Collins CG, Snoj M et al. Electrochemotherapy—An easy, highly effective and safe treatment of cutaneous and subcutaneous metastases: Results of ESOPE (European Standard Operating Procedures of Electrochemotherapy) study. *EJC Suppl* 2006;4:3–13.

8. Mir LM, Gehl J, Sersa G, Collins CG, Garbay JR, Billard V et al. Standard operating procedures of the electrochemotherapy: Instructions for the use of bleomycin or cisplatin administered either systemically or locally and electric pulses delivered by the Cliniporator (TM) by means of invasive or non-invasive electrodes. *EJC Suppl* 2006;4:14–25.
9. Gothelf A, Gehl J. Gene electrotransfer to skin; Review of existing literature and clinical perspectives. *Curr Gene Ther* 2010;10:287–99.
10. Muthumani K, Lambert VM, Kawalekar O, Heller R, Kim JJ, Weiner DB et al. Anti-cancer activity of the HIV accessory molecule viral protein R (Vpr): Delivery as a DNA expression plasmid or biologically active peptides. *Vaccine* 2010;28:2005–10.
11. de Martel C, Ferlay J, Franceschi S, Vignat J, Bray F, Forman D et al. Global burden of cancers attributable to infections in 2008: A review and synthetic analysis. *Lancet Oncol* 2012;13:607–15.
12. Farmer P, Frenk J, Knaul FM, Shulman LN, Alleyne G, Armstrong L et al. Expansion of cancer care and control in countries of low and middle income: A call to action. *Lancet* 2010;376:1186–93.
13. Daud AI, DeConti RC, Andrews S, Urbas P, Riker AI, Sondak VK et al. Phase I trial of interleukin-12 plasmid electroporation in patients with metastatic melanoma. *J Clin Oncol* 2008;26:5896–903.
14. Spanggaard I, Snoj M, Cavalcanti A, Bouquet C, Sersa G, Robert C et al. Gene electrotransfer of plasmid antiangiogenic metargidin peptide (AMEP) in disseminated melanoma: Safety and efficacy results of a phase I first-in-man study. *Hum Gene Ther Clin Dev* 2013;24:99–107.
15. Heller LC, Heller R. Electroporation gene therapy preclinical and clinical trials for melanoma. *Curr Gene Ther* 2010;10:312–7.
16. Mir LM, Bureau MF, Gehl J, Rangara R, Rouy D, Caillaud J-M et al. High efficiency gene transfer into skeletal muscle mediated by electric pulses. *Proc Natl Acad Sci U S A* 1999;96:4262–7.
17. Dean DA, Machado-Aranda D, Blair-Parks K, Yeldandi AV, Young JL. Electroporation as a method for high-level nonviral gene transfer to the lung. *Gene Ther* 2003; 10:1608–15.
18. Gothelf A, Eriksen J, Hojman P, Gehl J. Duration and level of transgene expression after gene electrotransfer to skin in mice. *Gene Ther* 2010;17:839–45.
19. Paganin-Gioanni A, Bellard E, Escoffre JM, Rols MP, Teissie J, Golzio M. Direct visualization at the single-cell level of siRNA electrotransfer into cancer cells. *Proc Natl Acad Sci U S A* 2011;108:10443–7.
20. Joergensen M, Agerholm-Larsen B, Nielsen PE, Gehl J. Efficiency of cellular delivery of antisense Peptide nucleic Acid by electroporation depends on charge and electroporation geometry. *Oligonucleotides* 2011;21:29–37.
21. Gehl J. Electroporation: Theory and methods, perspectives for drug delivery, gene therapy and research. *Acta Physiol Scand* 2003;177:437–47.
22. Zaharoff DA, Barr RC, Li CY, Yuan F. Electromobility of plasmid DNA in tumor tissues during electric field-mediated gene delivery. *Gene Ther* 2002;9:1286–90.
23. Gehl J, Sørensen TH, Nielsen K, Raskmark P, Nielsen SL, Skovsgaard T et al. In vivo electroporation of skeletal muscle: Threshold, efficacy and relation to electric field distribution. *Biochim Biophys Acta* 1999;1428:233–40.
24. Mathiesen I. Electropermeabilization of skeletal muscle enhances gene transfer in vivo. *Gene Ther* 1999;6:508–14.
25. Escoffre JM, Rols MP, Dean DA. Electrotransfer of plasmid DNA. In: Kee S, Gehl J, Lee E, editors. *Clinical aspects of electroporation.* New York: Springer; 2011. pp. 145–57.

26. Faurie C, Rebersek M, Golzio M, Kanduser M, Escoffre JM, Pavlin M et al. Electro-mediated gene transfer and expression are controlled by the life-time of DNA/membrane complex formation. *J Gene Med* 2010;12:117–25.
27. Levine ZA, Vernier PT. Life cycle of an electropore: Field-dependent and field-independent steps in pore creation and annihilation. *J Membr Biol* 2010;236:27–36.
28. Romeo S, Wu YH, Levine ZA, Gundersen MA, Vernier PT. Water influx and cell swelling after nanosecond electropermeabilization. *Biochim Biophys Acta* 2013; 1828:1715–22.
29. Golzio M, Teissie J, Rols MP. Direct visualization at the single-cell level of electrically mediated gene delivery. *Proc Natl Acad Sci U S A* 2002;99:1292–7.
30. Rosazza C, Escoffre JM, Zumbusch A, Rols MP. The actin cytoskeleton has an active role in the electrotransfer of plasmid DNA in mammalian cells. *Mol Ther* 2011;19:913–21.
31. Rosazza C, Buntz A, Riess T, Woll D, Zumbusch A, Rols MP. Intracellular tracking of single-plasmid DNA particles after delivery by electroporation. *Mol Ther* 2013;21:2217–26.
32. Vaughan EE, Dean DA. Intracellular trafficking of plasmids during transfection is mediated by microtubules. *Mol Ther* 2006;13:422–8.
33. Andre FM, Gehl J, Sersa G, Preat V, Hojman P, Eriksen J et al. Efficiency of high- and low-voltage pulse combinations for gene electrotransfer in muscle, liver, tumor, and skin. *Hum Gene Ther* 2008;19:1261–71.
34. Heller R, Jaroszeski M, Atkin A, Moradpour D, Gilbert R, Wands J et al. In vivo gene electroinjection and expression in rat liver. *FEBS Lett* 1996;389:225–8.
35. Hojman P, Gissel H, Andre F, Cournil-Henrionnet C, Eriksen J, Gehl J et al. Physiological effect of high and low voltage pulse combinations for gene electrotransfer in muscle. *Hum Gene Ther* 2008.
36. Gehl J, Skovsgaard T, Mir LM. Vascular reactions to in vivo electroporation: Characterization and consequences for drug and gene delivery. *Biochim Biophys Acta* 2002;1569:51–8.
37. Rols MP. Gene transfer by electrical fields. *Curr Gene Ther* 2010;10:255.
38. Ferraro B, Heller LC, Cruz YL, Guo S, Donate A, Heller R. Evaluation of delivery conditions for cutaneous plasmid electrotransfer using a multielectrode array. *Gene Ther* 2011;18:496–500.
39. Andre F, Gehl J, Sersa G, Preat V, Hojman P, Eriksen J et al. Efficiency of high and low voltage pulse combinations for gene electrotransfer in muscle, liver, tumor and skin. *Hum Gene Ther* 2008.
40. Staal LG, Gilbert R. Generators and applicators: Equipment for electroporation. In: Kee S, Gehl J, Lee E, editors. *Clinical aspects of electroporation*. New York: Springer; 2011. pp. 45–65.

13 Drug Delivery Systems for Infectious Diseases

Maximiliano L. Cacicedo, Germán A. Islan, Pablo Gurman, and Guillermo R. Castro

CONTENTS

INTRODUCTION

During the past century, the discovery of penicillin in the 1940s diminished the number of illnesses and death drastically. However, the World Health Organization estimated that the number of deaths attributable to infectious diseases was 18 million in 2012 (WHO, 2015). Poor disease management, inappropriate diagnosis and medication and enhanced drug resistance, including multidrug-resistant bugs, are some of the reasons that account for this high death numbers. Particularly, the challenge of so-called "superbugs" is the requirement for fast diagnosis and the use of new approaches for the development of effective therapies.

Two confluent strategies are currently being pursued to develop novel antibug medicines: the search for new and more efficient antibiotics and the development of novel drug delivery platforms. For the latter, nanotechnology represents an attractive venue for the development of novel carriers to control the pharmacokinetics and pharmacodynamics of antibiotics, and thus reduce drug toxicity and improve efficacy by avoiding drug degradation, extending the circulation time, delivering the drug in the organ/cell target, keeping the drug levels in the therapeutic windows, and increasing patient compliance. In addition, novel nanodevices can be used to combine therapeutic methodologies with diagnostic techniques (theranostics). The estimation of the nanomedicine market accounted for US$72.8 billion in 2011, and it will reach US$130.9 billion in 2016. Particularly, the drug delivery device market is expected to grow to US$31 billion in 2019 (BBC Research, 2013, 2015).

In the present chapter, new advances in the therapeutic procedures for infectious diseases associated to lungs as the primary organ target are covered, including the use of nanotechnology. Cystic fibrosis (CF), leishmaniasis, and tuberculosis (TB) were selected as representative examples where drug delivery devices are expected to have a major clinical impact.

CYSTIC FIBROSIS DISEASE: A DISSEMINATIVE INFECTION FROM LUNG TO INTESTINE

Cystic fibrosis (CF) is a genetic disorder caused by malfunction of a chloride transporter in the membranes of cells in different tissues, which leads to the accumulation of mucus in different organs and brings serious clinical problems, increasing the chances of recurrent infections by opportunistic pathogens. The mucus can be found spread at different tissues and organs, impeding the natural clearance of fluids, which contributes to the establishment of microorganisms at different tissues. The mucus is notoriously thick and sticky, mainly composed of rests of DNA and the bacterial polymer alginate, which represents a huge barrier for drug administration delivered by inhalation (Suci et al., 1994). The main colonizing bacterium in CF pathology is *Pseudomonas Aeruginosa*, and it is responsible for producing the viscous exopolysaccharide alginate. The mucoid strains can survive aggressive antibiotic therapies and become extremely difficult to eradicate. The bacteria are able to spread out from colonized lung to the intestinal tract. As a consequence, proper digestion is impaired because pancreatic enzymes cannot reach the intestine, and patients suffer malnutrition (Pedersen et al., 1992).

Strategies for the treatment of infections produced by opportunistic pathogens involve the delivery of antibiotics entrapped in particles that improve the diffusion across the mucus barrier (i.e., micro- and nanoparticles) or along with other molecules, such as nonantibiotics (i.e., benserazide [a] and loperamide) (Ejim, 2011) or enzymes with hydrolytic functions, like DNAses or alginate lyases (Mrsny et al., 1994). New modalities to potentially treat CF were recently reported whereby size scale and cargo molecules were taken into account.

MICROPARTICLES

A strategy to overcome the challenge posed by diffusional barriers, such as the high-viscosity mucus, was to develop biopolymeric microspheres composed of alginate (2%) and high methoxylated pectin (1%) containing entrapped ciprofloxacin (Cip) and alginate lyase (AL) as dispositive for oral drug delivery (Islan et al., 2013). Both molecules were entrapped with high efficiency in the coacervate formulation, and the molecular cargos were released properly under simulated intestinal conditions, where biofilm formation was produced by *Pseudomonas Aeruginosa*. The presence of methoxylated regions (hydrophobic zones) on pectin probably retarded the fast enzyme inactivation when exposed to the gastric pH levels, and also were playing a key role in controlling the ciprofloxacin release. The developed system is a promising alternative to treat chronic infections in CF patients because the enzyme is able to reduce the viscoelasticity of the mucus accumulated in the intestine, improving the diffusion of the antibiotic to kill the bacteria (Figure 13.1).

Another modality for delivering active alginate lyase to the intestine, extending the biocatalyst half-life, was the development of cross-linked enzyme aggregates (CLEAs). This technique not only is an immobilization method that allows the improvement of enzyme stability in the digestive tract, avoiding the deleterious effect of lytic enzymes (e.g., proteases, esterases, and lipases), but it also extends the biocatalyst half-life for long periods of time (Islan et al., 2004). The alginate lyase (AL) from *Sphingobacterium multivorum* was selected as the enzyme for oral delivery. The AL was 100% precipitated with 95% ammonium sulfate in the presence of

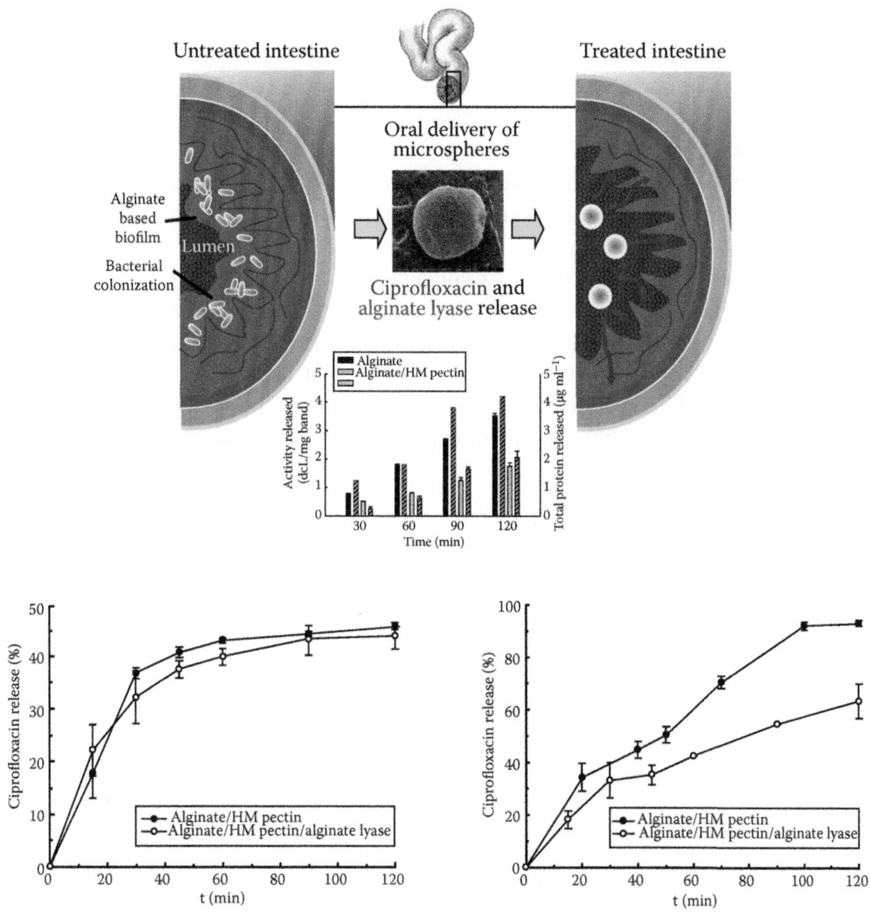

FIGURE 13.1 Top: Scheme of the mechanism of *Pseudomonas aeruginosa* eradication by oral delivery of alginate/pectin microparticles containing ciprofloxacin and alginate lyase in the intestine of CF patients; bottom: release profile of ciprofloxacin at simulated gastric (left) and intestinal (right) environments. (From Islan G. A., Bosio V. E., Castro G. R., *Macromolecular Bioscience* 13, 1238–1248, 2013.)

low methoxylated pectin (LMP), followed by cross-linking with glutaraldehyde. In order to prevent AL inactivation by glutaraldehyde, bovine serum albumin (BSA) was added during AL-CLEA synthesis to obtain an activity yield of 14.7%. SEM images revealed the presence of micro- to nano-aggregates (Figure 13.2a). When AL-CLEA was exposed to acidic gastric conditions (pH 1.2 to 3.0) for 2 hours, more than 70% of enzymatic residual activity was observed, providing a new way to reach the intestine in an active form. Moreover, considering that, after infections, the body temperature increases over 37°C, the AL-CLEA showed increased thermal stability in comparison with the free enzyme. In addition, a 25% viscosity reduction was observed when the AL-CLEA was exposed to an alginate solution at 2.0% (w/v).

In order to provide antibacterial properties to the AL-CLEAs, the biocatalyst was immersed in a levofloxacin solution. The system was able to load 10% of the fluoroquinolone antibiotic by an absorption mechanism and to release it in a period of 24 hours (Figure 13.2b). In this sense, the CLEAs aggregates not only are capable of reducing the alginate covering the tissues, but also delivering a broad spectrum antibiotic that would enhance the eradication of *Pseudomonas aeruginosa* infection in CF patients.

On the other hand, microparticles were developed as inhalable carriers for lung drug delivery in CF patients. In this case, inhalable dry powders showed some advantages in chronic pulmonary infections of patients with CF compared with nebulized solutions of antibiotics. Chronic administration of drugs using nebulized solutions requires specific and uncomfortable equipment, intensive cleaning, and reiterative administration frequency and is, above all, time consuming. On the other side, dry powder formulations have the advantages of improving the intrapulmonary deposition efficiency, significant fast drug delivery, no special equipment is needed (except an aerosolization apparatus), and precise control over the drug dose. Among them, PulmoSphere® technology emerged as an alternative to nebulized solutions for delivery of antipseudomonal antibiotics to lungs. It consists of light

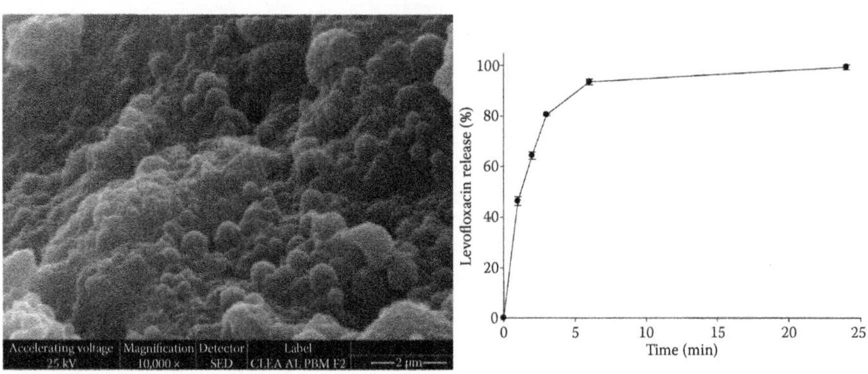

(a) (b)

FIGURE 13.2 (a) SEM image of an alginate lyase CLEAs. (From Islan G. A., Martinez Y. N., Illanes A., Castro G. R., *RSC Advances*, 4, 11758–11765, 2014. Reproduced by permission of The Royal Society of Chemistry.) (b) Levofloxacin release at 37°C and neutral pH from AL aggregates (unpublished results).

porous particles formulated in dry powder–containing tobramycin, which can be dosed with passive dry powder inhalers using desirable flow and dispersion (Geller et al., 2011). They were prepared by an emulsion-based spray-drying process that results in fine dry powders. The tobramycin was dissolved in the continuous phase of the emulsion.

The resulting microparticles showed an average geometric diameter ranging from 1.7 to 2.7 μm (determined by laser diffraction) and a mass average aerodynamic diameter less than 4 μm, which represents an ideal size range for targeting the powder aerosol to the infection site of *Pseudomonas aeruginosa* in the lungs. After administration, the serum pharmacokinetic profiles for tobramycin indicated a rapid dissolution of the amorphous dry powder into the epithelial lining fluid. The system provides a more efficient and convenient treatment option to improve treatment compliance and therapeutic outcomes in CF.

Another lung delivery system recently developed was based on the synthesis of hybrid biopolymer/$CaCO_3$ microparticles containing Levofloxacin, another antibiotic commonly used in CF treatment against *Pseudomonas aeruginosa* (Islan et al., 2015). Hybrid microparticles were developed by colloidal precipitation of $CaCO_3$ in the presence of biopolymers: alginate (Alg) or Alg-high methoxylated pectin (HMP) coacervates. After their synthesis, microparticles were treated with alginate lyase (AL) to increase the surface porosity and obtain new architectures. The changes were confirmed by SEM images, which revealed a "hairy" surface for $CaCO_3$/Alg microparticles and "nanoballons" in the whole surface of the $CaCO_3$/Alg-HMP microparticles (Figure 13.3, left). The increase in surface-to-volume ratio was at least two times higher and was confirmed by BET isotherms. This parameter directly affected the loading capacity of the microparticles, which incorporated higher amounts of Levofloxacin by absorption. Microparticles showed prolonged release profiles of the antibiotic and an enhanced antimicrobial activity against *Pseudomonas Aeruginosa* (Figure 13.3, right). The present work demonstrates significant progress toward the development of new drug delivery systems with potential application for lung infection treatment.

Nanoparticles

An interesting application of nanotechnology in CF treatment consists of biodegradable polymer nanoparticles with the ability for fast penetration across the human mucus barrier composed of sputum expectorated from the lungs of patients with cystic fibrosis. Nanoparticles composed of a diblock copolymer of poly (sebacic acid) and poly (ethylene glycol) (PSA-PEG) were synthetized via melt polycondensation of sebacic acid (SA) and methoxy-PEG prepolymers (Tang et al., 2009). The PSA-PEG nanoparticles can penetrate fresh, undiluted sputum expectorated from CF patients, which usually showed a bulk viscosity around ten- to a hundredfold higher than that of mucus from healthy volunteers. The rapid nanoparticle transport across the mucus can be possible by the efficient partitioning of PEG to the particle surface during formulation. The dense surface coating of low MW PEG allows for the mucus-penetrating capacity of nanoparticles. These properties make the biodegradable polymeric nanoparticles capable of overcoming human mucus barriers and providing sustained drug release at mucosal surfaces.

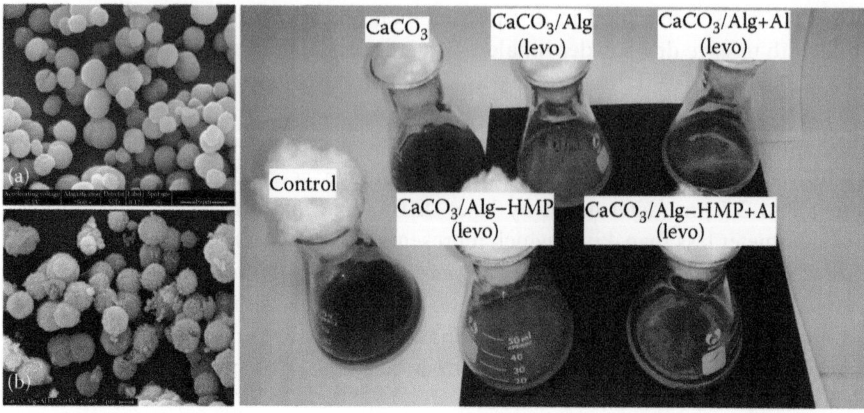

FIGURE 13.3 Left: SEM images of (a) $CaCO_3$/Alg microparticles; (b) $CaCO_3$/Alg microparticles after alginate lyase treatment observed at 5000×; right: antimicrobial assay against *Ps. aeruginosa* after 24 hours exposition to hybrid biopolymer/$CaCO_3$ microparticles loading Levofloxacin. (From Islan G. A., Cacicedo M. L., Bosio V. E., Castro G. R., *Journal of Colloid and Interface Science*, 439, 76–87, 2015.)

In another approach, nanoparticles composed of biodegradable PEGylated PLGA (PLGA-PEG) of 121.5 ± 15 nm in size were developed to provide a controlled and sustained drug delivery in CF disease (Vij et al., 2010) (Figure 13.4). The encapsulated drug was PS-341 (pyrazylcarbonyl-Phe-Leuboronate, a.k.a. Velcade or bortezomib), which is a potent proteosome inhibitor and reduces the inflammatory response of CF cells exposed to an infection. Studies in vitro showed slow release kinetics of the drug from nanoparticles from Day 2–7 with a maximum inhibition at Day 7. In addition, in vivo studies were carried out to determine the biodistribution of fluorescent label tobramycin nanoparticles in C57BL6 mice, demonstrating that PLGA-PEG NPs were efficiently delivered to murine lungs. A murine model of CF ($Cftr^{-/-}$) was used for lung delivery of PS-341–loaded nanoparticles. The decrease (twofold) in proteasomal

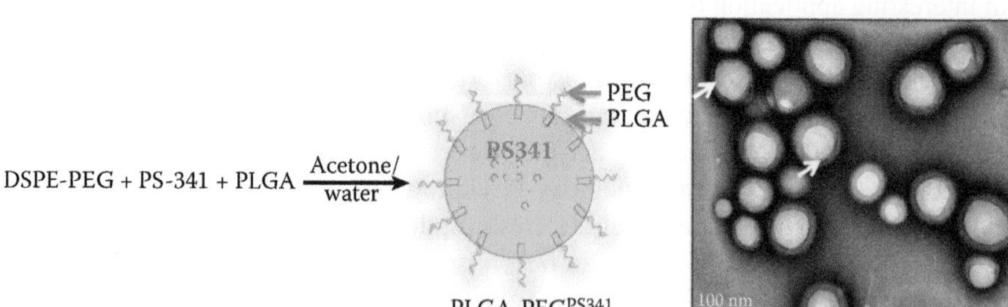

FIGURE 13.4 Scheme of PLGA-PEG nanoparticles containing a fluorescent dye (PS-342) and TEM image of the resulting monodispersed spherical NPs around 200 nm. (From Vij N., Min T., Marasigan R., Belcher C. N., Mazur S., Ding H., Yong K., Roy I., *Journal of Nanobiotechnology*, 8, 22, 2010.)

activity and the reduction of inflammation induced with the *Pseudomonas Aeruginosa* LPS (Pa-LPS) validates the ability of nanoparticles to treat CF lungs.

Other works describe the encapsulation of antibiotics into liposomes as inhalable or nebulizable nanoparticles for infected CF lungs. An investigation in biofilm penetration revealed that a nanoscale liposomal formulation (fluorescently labeled) of amikacin (aminoglycoside antibiotic) is capable of diffusing across sputum or *P. aeruginosa* biofilm (Meers et al., 2009). It was found that inhaled liposomal amikacin was slowly released in normal rat lungs and was more efficacious than inhaled free amikacin in infected lungs, highlighting the important of this therapy for chronic lung infections (Figure 13.5).

A more recent study emphasized the relevance of the synergic effect of simultaneous presence in a formulation of DNase and alginate lyase for enhancing free and liposomal aminoglycoside (e.g., gentamicin, amikacin, and tobramycin) activity against *Pseudomonas aeruginosa* (Alipour et al., 2009). The encapsulation improves the delivery and bioavailability of the antibiotics as was reflected by the similar or lower MIC values of the liposomal aminoglycosides in comparison with free aminoglycosides. Also, the coadministration of DNase and AL is essential for enhanced activity in reducing biofilm growth and sputum bacterial counts.

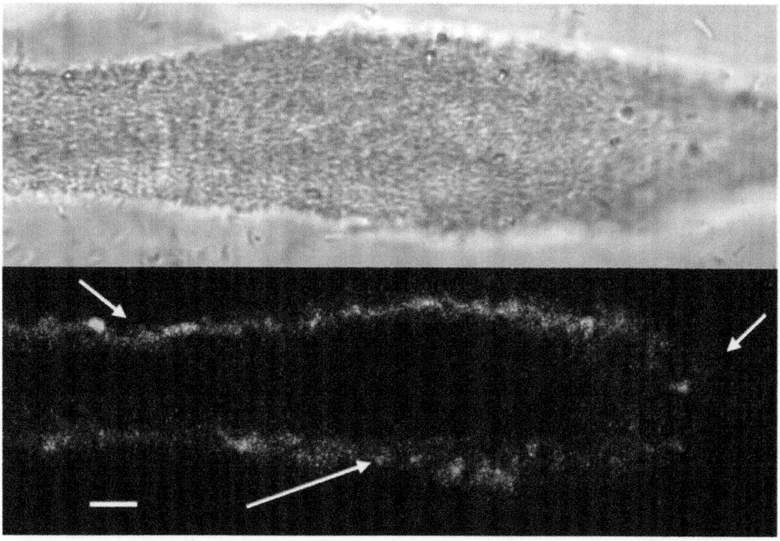

FIGURE 13.5 Penetration of liposomes into Pseudomonas biofilms and cystic fibrosis sputum. The upper photo shows a light microscopic image of a section of biofilm whereas the lower image shows the corresponding confocal fluorescence image taken 50 min after addition of liposomes. Bar represents 10 mm. (From Meers P., Neville M., Malinin V., Scotto A. W., Sardaryan G., Kurumunda R., Mackinson C., James G., Fisher S., Perkins W. R. *Journal of Antimicrobial Chemotherapy*, 61, 859–868, 2008.)

LEISHMANIASIS: CURRENT ADVANCES AND NEW STRATEGIES FOR THE TREATMENT OF AN ENDEMIC DISEASE

Infection Mechanism

Leishmaniasis is considered a neglected tropical disease by the World Health Organization and reported in 98 countries. Among infectious diseases, leishmaniasis is considered the ninth largest disease for humans and one of the most relevant in terms of mortality and high number of people affected (Vélez et al., 2012). It was estimated that about 1.3 million new leishmaniases cases occur per year, resulting in 20,000 to 30,000 deaths (WHO, 2014a). Leishmaniasis is a disease produced by parasites from the genus *Leishmania* containing more than 20 *Leishmania* species that belong to the typanosomatid protozoa. Leishmaniasis is transmitted to humans by the bites of certain infected female types of sand flies (*Lutzomyia*, *Phlebotomus*, *Psychodopygus*). There are three different types of infections, and each one presents distinctive characteristics, which lead to different approaches for infection removal. The infectious forms include the cutaneous (CL), mucocutaneous, and visceral form (VL). VL or kala-azar is the most severe form of Leishmaniasis if left untreated. In VL, the parasite migrates to vital organs, in particular the spleen, but also liver and bone marrow, resulting in hypoalbuminemia and pancytopenia, leading to death if left untreated. However, following strict treatment, the disease can be limited to the skin and manifest as a cutaneous pathology. Cutaneous leishmaniasis infection is the most common form of the disease and can exhibit a wide range of manifestations, such as cutaneous nodules and gross mucosal and tissue destruction. Moreover, it is reported that CL causes high morbidity levels because of the continued presence of skin ulcers and the terrible psychological effects caused by the disfiguring effects of the disease, especially in children (Bern et al., 2008).

The infectious strategies of Leishmania parasites are very complex, and in order to understand effective treatments, herein a brief description is introduced. Leishmania are unicellular eukaryotes belonging to a genus of trypanosomatid protozoa and possessing two different morphological and physiological forms: amastigote and proamastigote, which are present in the infected mammals and in the flies, respectively. Once an infected sand fly bites the skin, the protozoan is transmitted to the mammal. Soon after, macrophages and other cells from the reticuloendothelial system (RES) are invaded via phagocytosis and serve as host to the proliferative form of the parasite, the amastigote form. Therefore, the parasite can easily replicate and survive inside the cell, being also resistant to the macrophage's immune response, especially VL, which is resistant to lysis by lysosomes and resides in macrophages from the liver and spleen. Also, amastigote multiplication disseminates the infection to other organs and tissues, such as the lymph nodes and bone marrow (Harhay et al., 2011; van Griensven and Diro, 2012). A synthesized scheme of the parasite cycle is depicted in Figure 13.6.

Conventional Treatment Strategies

Classical treatment for leishmaniasis still involves traditional chemotherapeutic drugs used for decades, such as pentavalent antimonials (Glucantime and Pentosam),

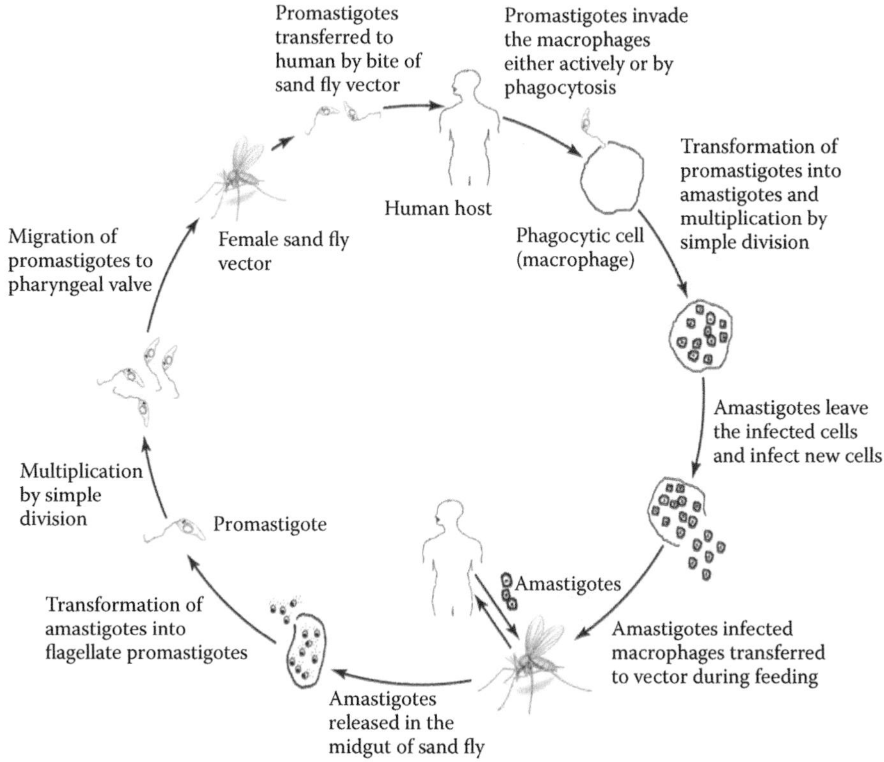

FIGURE 13.6 Diagrammatic depiction of digenetic life cycle of parasite of visceral leishmaniasis. (From Jain K., and Jain N. K., *Drug Discovery Today*, 18, 1272–1281, 2013.)

pentamidine, and Amphotericin B (AmB). Although some of these therapies are usually successful, the treatment takes long time periods with increasing highly toxic effects. In addition, leishmania-resistant strains have become more common (Tiuman et al., 2011).

Nowadays, the most utilized drug is Amphotericin B (AmB). In addition, it is the most studied active principle, and some improvements on drug pharmacokinetics and bioavailability have been achieved with different pharmaceutical formulations (Torrado et al., 2008). It is relevant to understand that AmB is a polyene antibiotic widely used in systemic fungal infections, produced by Streptomyces sp. with low solubility at physiological pH (about 100 μg/mL). Administration of AmB leads to kidney toxicity among other severe adverse reactions. Indeed, the association of AmB with low-density lipoproteins (LDL) and the slow elimination of the drug is well known and associated with nephrotoxicity in patients (Lemke et al., 2005).

Some drug delivery systems (DDSs) have been developed to overcome adverse effects. Most of these systems are lipid-based and have shown improvements in therapeutic efficiency and reduction on drug toxicity. Some examples are AmBisome®, Amphocil®, and Abelcet®. In spite of these achievements, toxic levels are still significant, and the costs of these new treatments are also expensive (Costa Lima et al., 2014).

As a common treatment, systemic administration of the aforementioned drugs is used for different types of leishmaniasis. The strongest therapy protocols are often applied to VL patients. Additionally, some local treatments are being applied to ulcers in CL patients. These dermal wounds can be easily infected by other opportunistic pathogenic microorganisms because of the host's weak immune response. In this case, some topical creams with antibiotics (i.e., Paromomycin), have been used. Paromomycin is an antibacterial aminoglycoside that, for unknown reasons, also has efficacy against leishmania. A combination between this anti-leishmania drug and other wide-spectrum antibacterial compounds exhibited improvements in the treatment of CL (Salah et al., 2013).

The development of biocompatible film matrices containing active drugs can be an alternative for the local treatment of skin wounds. Bacterial cellulose films loaded with an antibiotic (Levofloxacin) were developed in our laboratory (Cacicedo et al., 2015). These films are able to perform sustained release of antibiotics and create a dermal protection for wound healing (Figure 13.7).

Recent Advances in Nanotechnology for the Treatment of Leishmaniasis

Nanotechnology tools have improved pharmacological efficacy for treatment of several diseases. The aim of developing nanoparticle systems has been the protection of the drug against extracellular degradation treatment, reduction time, and decreased dose frequency. Moreover, a great advantage of these nanosystems in leishmaniasis treatment is the inherent phagocytic properties of the macrophages over nano- and microparticulate compounds.

Recently, the use of green synthesis of gold nanoparticles by use of quercetin was reported as an effective treatment for wild and resistant types of visceral leishmaniasis (VL). The strategy was the functionalization of gold nanoparticles with quercetin, a plant flavonoid displaying antioxidant and anti-leishmanial activities (Das et al., 2013).

One of the most widely used drugs for leishmaniasis research is AmB, as described. This drug is the most effective against several Leishmania types in spite of its very high toxicity and the side effects (Tiuman et al., 2011). In this sense, scientists have been investigating new nanoparticle systems that can carry high loads of AmB and release it only inside of infected cells. Liposomes have been the first colloidal systems studied for this use because of their biocompatibility, flexibility for surface modifications, and versatility to carry either hydrophilic or hydrophobic drugs (Date et al., 2007). Liposomes can be formed by one or more phospholipid bilayers, which surround an aqueous area that can be loaded with hydrophilic drugs. Considering the phospholipid bilayer as a dynamic structure that can load hydrophobic drugs, several environmental agents, such as UV light, magnetic fields, hyperthermia, and others can be used to trigger the cargo (Figure 13.8). Lipids with a cylindrical shape, such as phosphatidylcholine, phosphatidylserine, phosphatidylglycerol, and sphingomyelin, that form stable bilayers in aqueous solution are commonly used. Phosphatidylcholine is the most employed lipid in liposomal formulation studies

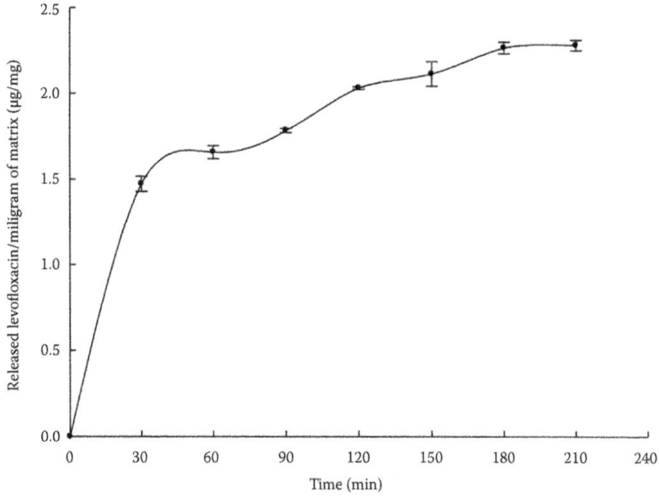

(a)

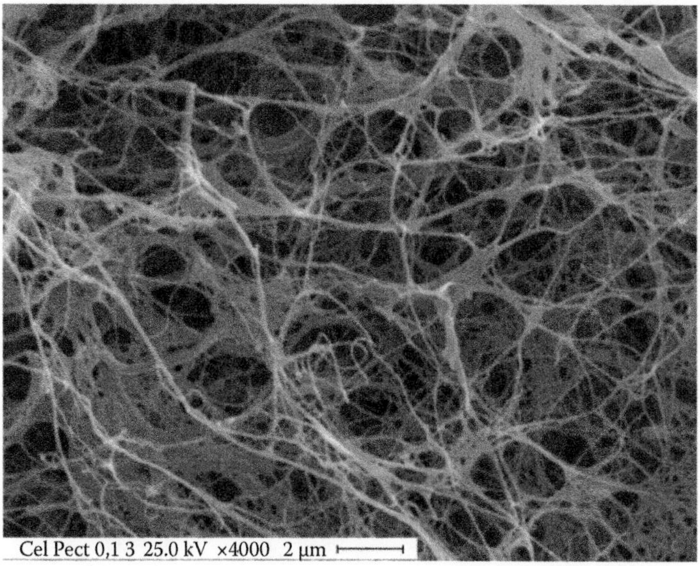

(b)

FIGURE 13.7 Bacterial cellulose membrane loaded with Levofloxacin for topical treatment of dermal wounds. (a) Release profile. (b) SEM image from inside bacterial cellulose matrix where the drug is encapsulated. (From Cacicedo et al., unpublished results.)

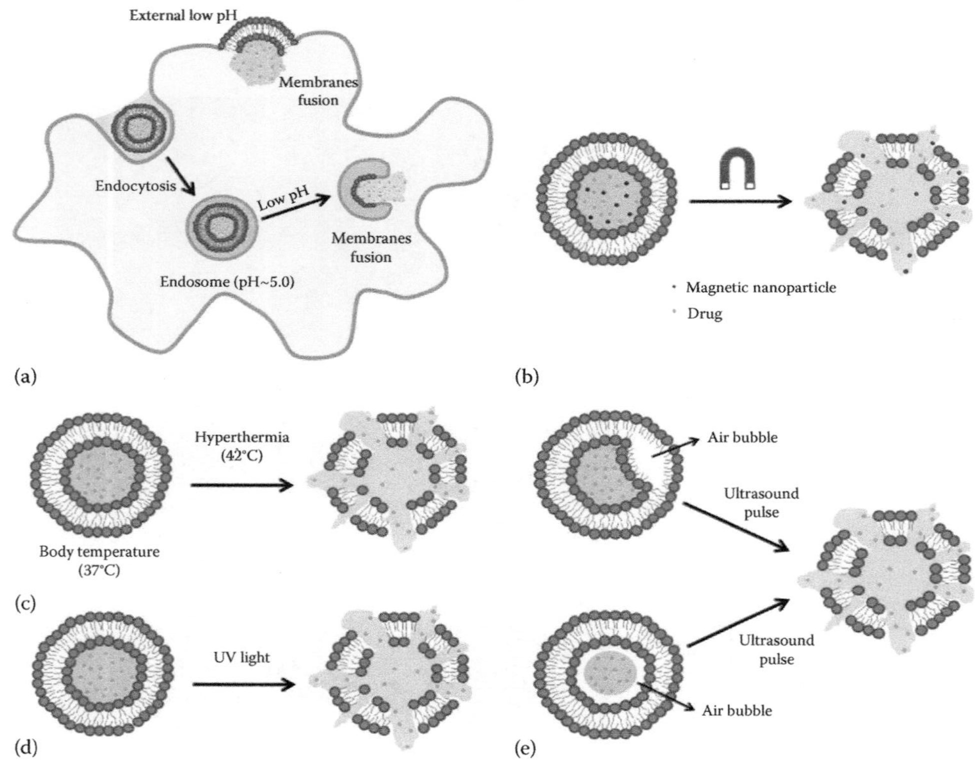

FIGURE 13.8 Liposomal triggered release mechanisms. (a) pH decrease; (b) external alternating magnetic field; (c) hyperthermia; (d) light; (e) ultrasound. (From Eloy J. O., de Souza M. C., Petrilli R., Abriata Barcellos J. P., Leeb R. J., Maldonado Marchetti J., *Colloids and Surfaces B: Biointerfaces*, 123, 345–363, 2014.)

due to its great stability against pH or salt concentration variations in the medium (Vermelho et al., 2014).

As mentioned above, several formulations, such as Ambisome®, Amphocil®, and Abel-cet®, showed superior therapeutic effects over Leishmania, which was attributed to an improved intracellular drug uptake (Moen et al., 2009; Jain and Jain, 2013). Further review information about clinical trials of liposomal systems for leishmaniasis treatment has been recently reported (Sundar and Chakravarty, 2010; Balasegaram et al., 2012).

Alternatively, polymeric nanoparticles have been described as a better option in comparison to liposomes, mainly because of their higher stability under stress conditions of preparation and storage, biocompatibility, and the fact that this type of nanoparticles can be synthesized with a wide range of different polymers in order to specifically target infected cells and release the drug only under certain conditions. Usually, synthetic biodegradable polymers, such as poly (cyanoacrylates), poly (methacrylate), poly (lactic-co-glycolic acid), poly (lactic acid), and poly (caprolactone), are utilized for these nanosystems. Other natural polymers, such as gelatin or albumin, have also been used. The mechanisms of polymeric particles as carriers of antibiotics to overcome tissue barriers are still being discussed and investigated. Figure 13.9 (Xiong et al., 2014) provides a summary of a well-described scheme.

There are several methods for synthesis of polymeric nanoparticles (NPs), and the variations depend especially on the type of drug that is going to be encapsulated. Figure 13.10 schematically exposes the different types of polymeric NPs. PLGA (poly-d, l-lactide-co-glycolide) is one of the most successfully used polymers for the preparation of NPs because of the several advantages that this polymer exhibits, including biodegradability and excellent biocompatibility.

Kumari et al. explained how polymeric NPs can be prepared by several methods. One such example involves PLGA nanoparticles, and one of most common methods for their synthesis involves emulsification–diffusion, solvent emulsion–evaporation, interfacial deposition, and nanoprecipitation (Figure 13.11). Another example of this concept is a study performed by Van de Ven et al. (2011) where they reported an increase in therapeutic efficacy and a reduction in drug toxicity. They synthesized nanoparticles of PLGA by the solvent emulsion–evaporation method for saponin ß-aescin encapsulation. Briefly, the synthesis consisted of making an emulsion between the drug and PLGA in the presence of a surfactant (Polysorbate 80). The mixture was sonicated, and then the solvent was evaporated. PLGA NPs in vitro toxicity was evaluated over macrophages infected with *Leishmania infantum*. Results suggested a good reduction on drug toxicity while therapeutic effects were the same in comparison with free drug exposition.

Moreover, active targeting is another strategy using nanosystems. This strategy basically involves the modification of a particle's surface with the attachment of different molecules that can interact with specific receptors in the macrophage's membrane. Those receptors include scavenger receptors, integrins, and lectins, including mannose and Fc-receptors. Thus, this kind of targeting presents a very promising alternative to attack specifically infected cells and overcome the limitations of common drugs (Jain and Jain, 2013). Furthermore, multiple types of carriers have

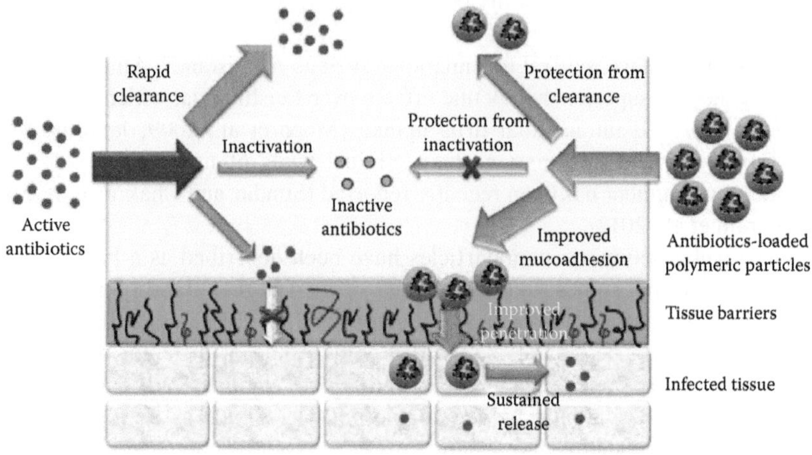

FIGURE 13.9 Mechanisms of polymeric particles as a carrier of antibiotics to overcome tissue barriers. Antibiotic treatment is usually complicated by the rapid clearance of antibiotics from organs, the inactive of the drug, and the barriers of tissues. Polymeric particles are able to protect the drug against degradation and the body's clearing mechanisms as well as facilitate transport across critical and specific barriers, thus drugs are sustained release to maintain a proper drug concentration for a relatively long time. (From Xiong M., Bao Y., Yang X., Zhu Y., Wang J., *Advanced Drug Delivery Reviews*, 78, 63–76, 2014.)

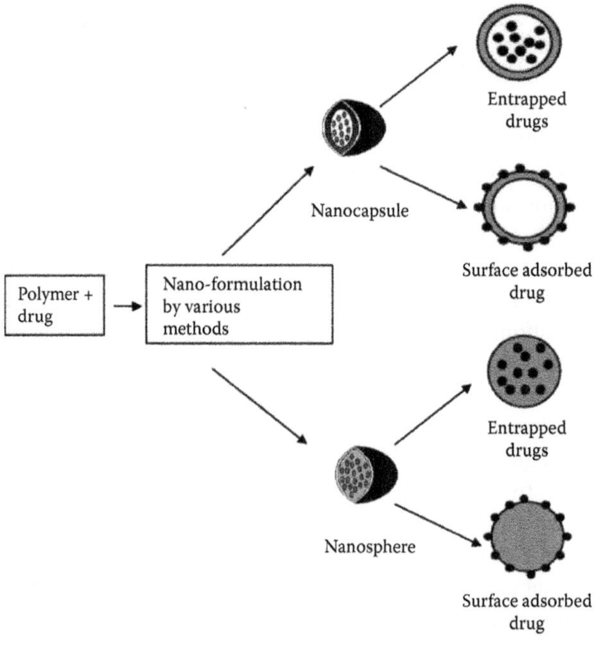

FIGURE 13.10 Types of biodegradable nanoparticles. (From Kumari A., Kumar A., Yadav S., Yadav S. C., *Colloids and Surfaces B: Biointerfaces*, 75, 1–18, 2010.)

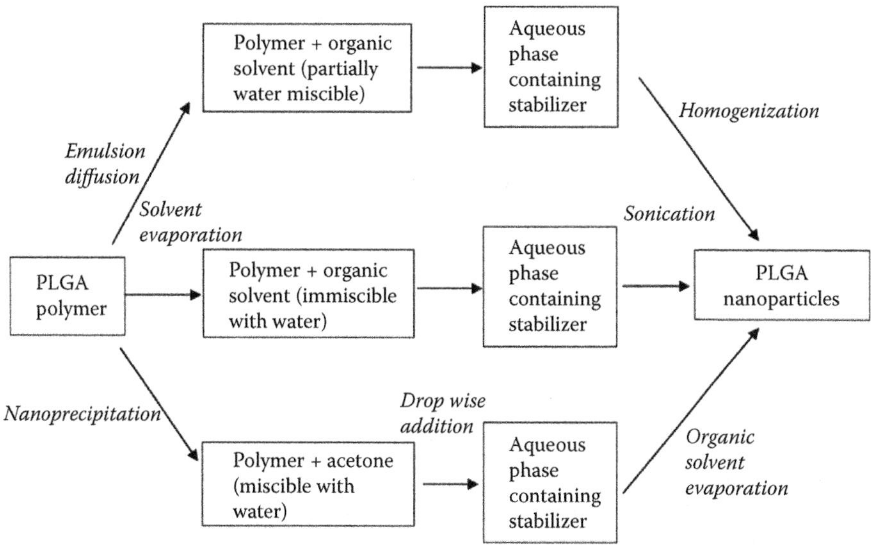

FIGURE 13.11 Different method for the synthesis of PLGA nanoparticles. (From Kumari A., Kumar A., Yadav S., Yadav S. C., *Colloids and Surfaces B: Biointerfaces*, 75, 1–18, 2010.)

been modified for active targeting, including liposomes, niosomes, microspheres, nanoparticles, and carbon nanotubes (Singodia et al., 2012; Alsaadi et al., 2012; Jain, N. K. et al., 2013; Jain K. et al., 2012; Jain and Jain, 2013).

One of the most studied ligands for active targeting is mannose. In this case, Nahar et al. demonstrated a considerable enhancement in anti-leishmanial activity when they surface funtionalized gelatin nanoparticles conjugating mannose, achieving a 5.4-fold reduction on IC50 in comparison with plain AmB (Nahar et al., 2010). Subsequently, Singodia et al. worked with the surface modification of AmB-loaded liposomes. This work involved attaching two different types of ligands to the liposomal surface, mannose (Man-Lip) and 4-sulfated N-acetyl galactosamine (Sulf-Lip). They demonstrated that both systems (Sulf-Lip and Man-Lip) better localized AmB inside macrophages in comparison with unmodified liposomes. Moreover, intracellular localization was much higher for the Sulf-Lip system (Singodia et al., 2012; Khalil et al., 2013).

Finally, another very promising strategy to take into account is the targeting of a carrier to the Leishmania parasite machinery itself—that is, topoisomerases, kinetoplast, trypanothione reductase, cysteine protease, mitochondria, fatty acid, and sterol pathways—without directly targeting the host (Asthana et al., 2013). Additionally, a very recent study suggested that the induction of macrophage immune system activation by certain compounds, such as fucoidan, can develop a positive reaction against both antimony-sensitive and antimony-resistant visceral leishmania (Sharma et al., 2014). This mayor discovery has led to improved treatments. Thus, future therapies will probably rely on the use of nanocarrier systems targeting macrophage cells with the capacity to release some compounds with immune activation properties to kill the leishmania parasite.

TUBERCULOSIS: A RECURRENT AIRBORNE DISEASE

Tuberculosis (TB) is an infectious disease caused by the gram-positive bacteria *Mycobacterium tuberculosis*, which is primarily invading alveolar macrophages of the lungs but also other organs in humans. In 2013, TB caused 9 million infections and 1.5 million deaths, and it is considered by the World Health Organization (WHO) to be one of the most lethal diseases. The re-emergence of TB globally can be ascribed in part to the concomitant HIV pandemic that allowed the reactivation of TB in otherwise asymptomatic patients (Gandhi et al., 2010; Lalloo and Ambaram, 2010).

After World War II, several anti-TB drugs were synthesized and extensively used, but since 1952, however, no new anti-TB was found in the market (Lalloo and Ambaram, 2010; Sosnik et al., 2010) (Figure 13.12). Current anti-TB drugs include Ethionamide, Isoniazid, Pyrazinamide, and Rifampicin (Mehanna et al., 2014; Kaur and Singh, 2014). Two key problems with current anti-TB drugs exist, namely 1) achieving high concentrations of the drug in the macrophages located in the lungs, the major bacilli reservoirs, remains a challenging endeavor and 2) the emergence of multiple drug–resistant (MDR) and drug-resistant (DR) *Mycobacterium tuberculosis* (Mtb), which turned these drugs ineffective (Pandey and Khuller, 2005).

In order to overcome these limitations, several therapeutic modalities were developed. First, based on recent problems with coinfection of TB in HIV-positive patients, new molecule candidates are being developed and are now in different stages of clinical development. Table 13.1 summarizes novel anti-TBC drug candidates' key features.

Second, recent advances in molecular biology and physiology are providing new strategies based on small interfering RNA (siRNA) to treat several lung pathologies, including TB (Merkel et al., 2014). Different strategies to deliver siRNA were reviewed recently (Lam et al., 2012; Merkel et al., 2014). The mechanism of siRNA is based on inhibiting the post-transcriptional gene expression of the target cells using interference RNA (RNAi), which initiates the mRNA degradation process. Briefly, the mechanisms of RNAi can be triggered by delivering the small interfering RNA, which generally is composed of 21 to 26 synthetic nucleotides, inside the Mtb cells or by introducing long double-strand RNA or by the presence of plasmid DNA encoding for short hairpin RNA, which, in both cases, are processed by a Dicer biocatalyst into siRNA. Recent in vitro and in vivo studies of siRNA anti-TB in mice have shown promising results (Dhiman et al., 2008; Rosas-Taraco et al., 2011).

In vitro studies of human monocyte–derived macrophages infected with two strains of Mtb showed promising results using siRNA technology by targeting the expression of specific antiapoptotic bfl-1/A1protein. Inhibition of bfl-1/A1 protein synthesis expressed by Mtb by siRNA induces infected macrophage apoptosis, indicating a potential new target for anti-TB therapy (Dhiman et al., 2008). Also, the siRNA approach was used to improve the immune system of chronic infection of Mtb in mice. The siRNA target was the immunosuppressive cytokine TGFb1 interfering with the synthesis of TGFb1 protein, which enhances the expression of Th1 and macrophage activation, both involved in the mice immune response. Additionally, the reduced expression of TGFb1 protein increased the expression of the antimicrobial mediators (NO and iNOS), and consequently, the bacterial load is reduced in mice (Rosas-Taraco et al., 2011). However, the main challenge for anti-TB

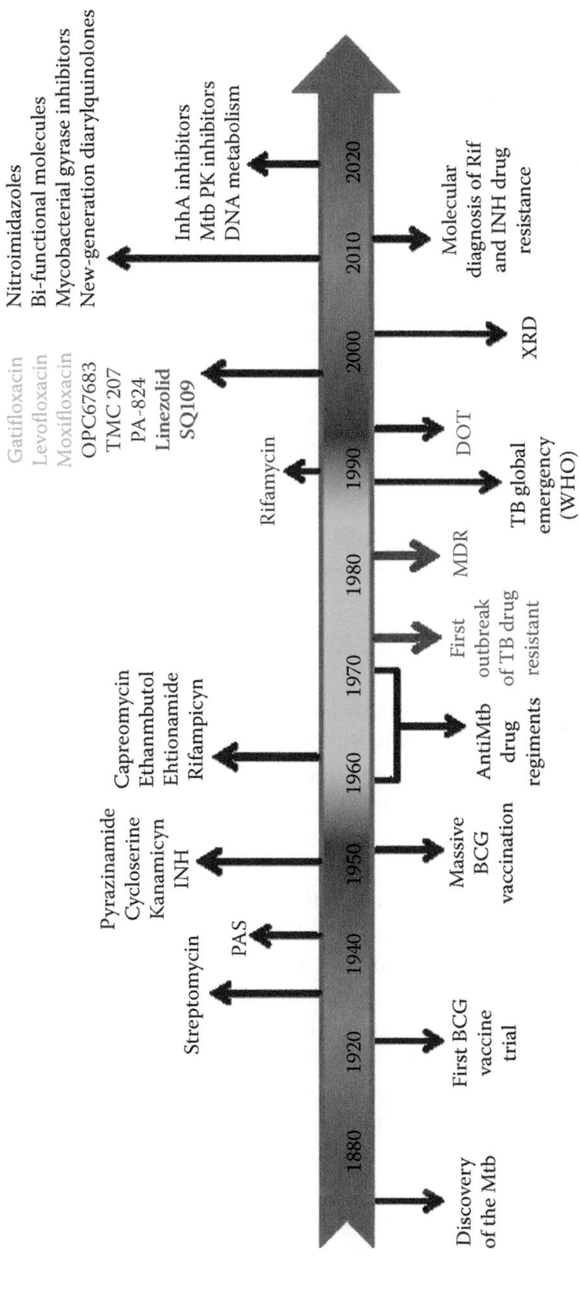

FIGURE 13.12 Chronological diagram of TB and anti-TB therapy facts. (Modified from Lalloo U. G., and Ambaram A., *Current HIV/AIDS Reports* 7, 143–151, 2010.)

TABLE 13.1
Recent Development of New Drugs

Drug			
Class	**Molecule**	**Main Targets**	**Clinical Phase**
Diarylquinoline	Bedaquiline TMC 207	ATP synthase	IIb
Ethylenediamine	SQ109	Cell wall (mycolic acid)	I
Flouroquinolones	Gatifloxacin Levofloxacin Moxifloxacin	DNA gyrase	III
Iminophenazine	Clofazimine	DNA synthesis and enhance phospholipase A2	In the market
Nitroimidazole	Delanamid PA-824 TBA354	Cell wall (blocking synthesis of mycolic acid) and release of nitric oxide intracellular	IIa
Rifamycin	Rifabutin Rifampicin Rifapentine	RNA polymerase	IIb

Source: Lalloo U. G., and Ambaram A., *Current HIV/AIDS Reports* 7, 143–151, 2010.

therapies remains with the choice of the RNAi and the drug delivery system to the targeted cells in vivo.

Third, the anti-TB therapies mentioned above are complex since they must be extended for long peirods of time (4 to 9 months, depending on the severity of the disease). The requirement of high compliance is associated with treatment failure in a significant number of patients. This is particularly true for those patients with rapid improvements in their symptoms who decide to withdraw the treatment before completing the scheduled regimen.

In addition, side effects related to anti-TB drugs constitute another major issue that attempts against a successful treatment. These factors provide an undesirable scenario for the patients, and new approaches are required to improve TB pharmacotherapies. In this sense, new strategies based on passive and active drug delivery systems plus the recent progress in nanotechnologies are bringing alternative avenues for the development of novel anti-TB therapies.

Different approaches for the development of nanodevices have been reported, but most of them can be grouped into the following main strategies or a combination of them:

- Nanoparticles made of polymers, such as PGLA, acrylate derivatives, alginate, chitosan, gelatin and mixtures.
- Nanostructures based on lipids, such as niosomes, solid lipid nanoparticles, liposomes, and micelles, were reported as potential systems. Different types of lipids were used, from natural, such as stearic, oleic, linoleic,

phosphatidylcholine-cholesterol, to synthetic, such as Spams (®), and also mixtures.
- Hybrid systems based in the development of coacervates to mixtures, such as caprolactone-cogliycolide, chitosan-PLA, wheat germ agglutinin, and PGLA.

A detailed review of the nano drug delivery systems, including main advantages, has recently been reported (Kaur and Harinder, 2014; Mehanna et al., 2014). A summary of nanosystems is shown in Figure 13.10.

CONCLUSIONS

The advent of modern pharmacotherapies for infectious diseases following World War II has allowed a dramatic decrease in morbidity and mortality worldwide. In spite of this fact, several limitations, including poor pharmacokinetics (e.g., due to poor bioavailability at the biophase), poor pharmacodynamics (poor drug selectivity toward the target), high drug toxicity, and more recently, the dramatic increase in antibiotic resistance among bacteria, have prompted the search for new therapeutic strategies. With current advances in micro- and nanotechnologies for medical applications, novel delivery systems based on micro- and nanoparticles have been developed to improve drug pharmacokinetics and/or pharmacodynamics.

Cystic fibrosis (CF), leishamaniasis, and tuberculosis represent clinical entities where poor access of the drug to the site of infection, unwanted toxicity, and the emergence of highly resistant bacteria and parasites, have limited the therapeutic success of current best management therapies. Therefore, new therapeutic strategies are urgently needed in order to overcome disease progression and death due to poor response to current treatments.

In CF, a thick layer of mucus produced by defective transport of Cl^- ions across the cell membrane constitute the site where *Pseudomonas aeruginosa* (PA) colonizes tissues. The bacteria become difficult to eradicate due to the impaired transport of drugs across the mucus layer. Several approaches using micro- and nanotechnology are being explored for the treatment of CF patients who are colonized by PA. Microparticles loaded with ciprofloxacin-alginate lyase were developed with promising results. The preparation of enzyme cross-linked aggregates of alginate lyase represents an improvement in the strategy to eradicate *Pseudomonas* spp. from CF patients. This technology provides exciting results as the enzyme stability was increased as well as its biocatalytic lifetime.

The development of microparticle powder systems delivered through inhalers became another novel strategy, overcoming some of the limitations of nebulized solutions. In this case, the delivery of tobramycin entrapped in porous microparticles was successfully demonstrated.

Leishmaniasis, a disease produced by parasites from the genus *Leishmania* is responsible for high morbidity and mortality in the world with current treatment modalities, such as Amphotericin, facing unwanted toxicity. Liposomes containing amphotericin were developed and are currently in the market. These liposomes formulations were developed to overcome kidney toxicity associated with amphotericin treatment. Liposomes, however, suffer from poor stability, and novel formulations containing polymeric nanoparticles were developed. Polymeric nanoparticles represent a versatile technology platform whereby different types of polymers allow tailoring the delivery system with the desired pharmacokinetic and pharmacodynamic profiles. A remarkable example of polymeric materials currently being tested includes PLGA nanoparticles.

In order to improve the pharmacodynamics of nanoparticle delivery systems, active targeting, consisting of surface functionalization of nanoparticles with monoclonal antibodies or other ligands, are being pursued to increase target selectivity, thus allowing an increasing number of drug molecules to reach the interior of macrophages without affecting healthy tissues.

Tuberculosis (TB) is an infectious disease caused by the gram-positive bacteria *Mycobacterium tuberculosis.* Due to the HIV pandemic, tuberculosis has reemerged as a significant public health threat, becoming an important burden worldwide. Tuberculosis pharmacotherapies include the drugs Isoniazid, Riphampicin, Ethambutol, and Pyrazinamide, which were developed during the Second World War and remained as the cornerstone in TB for the last 70 years. Unfortunately, although these drugs have played a major role over the control of the TB epidemic, the requirement of high payload to achieve therapeutic concentrations and the emergence of multidrug-resistant TB became a major problem in the management of TB. New strategies based on novel small molecules, RNAi technology, and drug delivery systems based on nanoparticles are expected to overcome current limitations in anti-TB therapies.

Leishmaniasis, cystic fibrosis, and tuberculosis represent three typical examples of diseases where novel therapeutic strategies are urgently needed. Several issues include drug toxicity and lack of efficacy due to antibiotic resistance, which have become a major problem in public health. Drug delivery systems based on micro- and nanoparticles represent an attractive modality to overcome some of these limitations. Overcoming these challenges will still demand a successful clinical translation and commercialization to fully exploit the potential of these novel technologies.

REFERENCES

Alipour M., Suntres Z. E., Omri A. 2009. Importance of DNase and alginate lyase for enhancing free and liposome encapsulated aminoglycoside activity against *Pseudomonas aeruginosa. Journal of Antimicrobial Chemotherapy* 64: 317–325.

Alsaadi M., Italia J. L., Mullen A. B., Ravi Kumar M. N., Candlish A. A., Williams R. A., Shaw C. D. et al. 2012. The efficacy of aerosol treatment with non-ionic surfactant vesicles containing AmB in rodent models of leishmaniasis and pulmonary aspergillosis infection. *Journal of Controlled Release* 160: 685–691.

Asthana S., Gupta P. K., Chaurasia M., Dube A., Chourasia M. K. 2013. Polymeric colloidal particulate systems: Intelligent tools for intracellular targeting of antileishmanial cargos. *Expert Opinion in Drug Delivery* 10: 1633–1651.

Balasegaram M., Ritmeijer K., Lima M. A., Burza S., Ortiz Genovese G., Milani B., Gaspani S., Potet J., Chappuis F. 2012. Liposomal amphotericin B as a treatment for human leishmaniasis. *Expert Opinion in Emerging Drugs* 17: 493–510.

BCC Research 2013. Nanotechnology in medical applications: The global market (HLC069B), http://www.bccresearch.com/report/nanotechnology-medical-applicationsglobal-market-hlc069b.html, (accessed on January 2015).

BCC Research 2015. Global Markets for Drug-Device Combinations. http://www.bccresearch.com/Report Code: PHM045D (accessed on January 2015).

Berman J., Ransom J., Magill A. J., Grogl M. 2013. Topical paromomycin with or without gentamicin for cutaneous leishmaniasis. *New England Journal of Medicine* 368: 524–532.

Bern C., Maguire J. H., Alvar J. 2008. Complexities of assessing the disease burden attributable to leishmaniasis. *PLoS One Neglected Tropical Diseases* 2(10): e313.

Cacicedo M. L., Cesca K., Bosio V. E., Porto L. M., Castro G. R. 2015. Development of bacterial cellulose films containing carrageenin-$CaCO_3$ microparticles for the sustained delivery of doxorubicin. *Journal of Applied Biomedicine.* Submitted.

Costa Lima S. A., Silvestre R., Barros D., Cunha J., Baltazar M. T., Dinis-Oliveira R. J., Cordeiro-da-Silva A. 2014. Crucial CD8+ T-lymphocyte cytotoxic role in amphotericin B nanospheres efficacy against experimental visceral leishmaniasis. *Nanomedicine: Nanotechnology, Biology, and Medicine* 10: 1021–1030.

Das S., Roy P., Mondal S., Bera T., Mukherjee A. 2013. One pot synthesis of gold nanoparticles and application in chemotherapy of wild and resistant type visceral leishmaniasis. *Colloids Surfaces B: Biointerfaces* 107: 27–34.

Date A. A., Joshi M. D., Patravale V. B. 2007. Parasitic diseases: Liposomes and polymeric nanoparticles versus lipid nanoparticles. *Advances in Drug Delivery Reviews* 59: 505–521.

Dhiman R., Kathania M., Raje M., Majumdar S. 2008. Inhibition of bfl-1/A1 by siRNA inhibits mycobacterial growth in THP-1 cells by enhancing phagosomal acidification. *Biochimica et Biophysical Acta* 1780: 733–742.

Ejim L., Farha M. A., Falconer S. B., Wildenhain J., Coombes B. K., Tyers M., Brown E. D., Wright G. D. 2011. Combinations of antibiotics and non-antibiotic drugs enhance antimicrobial efficacy. *Nature Chemical Biology* 7: 348–335.

Eloy J. O., de Souza M. C., Petrilli R., Abriata Barcellos J. P., Leeb R. J., Maldonado Marchetti J. 2014. Liposomes as carriers of hydrophilic small molecule drugs: Strategies to enhance encapsulation and delivery. *Colloids and Surfaces B: Biointerfaces* 123: 345–363.

Gandhi N. R., Shah N. S., Andrews J. R. et al. 2010. Tugela Ferry Care and Research (TF CARES) Collaboration: HIV co-infection in multidrug- and extensively drug-resistant tuberculosis results in high early mortality. *American Journal of Respiratory Critical Care Medical* 181: 80–86.

Geller D. E., Weers J., Heuerding S. 2011. Development of an inhaled dry-powder formulation of tobramycin using PulmoSphere technology. *Journal of Aerosol Medicine and Pulmonary Drug Delivery* 24: 175–182.

Harhay M. O., Olliaro P. L., Costa D. L., Costa C. H. N. 2011. Urban parasitology: Visceral leishmaniasis in Brazil. *Trends in Parasitology* 27: 403–409.

Islan G. A., Bosio V. E., Castro G. R. 2013. Alginate lyase and ciprofloxacin co-immobilization on biopolymeric microspheres for cystic fibrosis treatment. *Macromolecular Bioscience* 13: 1238–1248.

Islan G. A., Martinez Y. N., Illanes A., Castro G. R. 2014. Development of novel alginate lyase cross-linked aggregates for the oral treatment of cystic fibrosis. *RSC Advances* 4: 11758–11765.

Islan G. A., Cacicedo M. L., Bosio V. E., Castro G. R. 2015. Development and characterization of new enzymatic modified hybrid $CaCO_3$ microparticles to obtain nano-architectured surfaces for enhanced drug loading. *Journal of Colloid and Interface Science* 439: 76–87.

Jain K., Kesharwani P., Gupta U., Jain N. K. 2012. A review of glycosylated carriers for drug delivery. *Biomaterials* 33: 4166–4186.

Jain K. and Jain N. K. 2013. Novel therapeutic strategies for treatment of visceral leishmaniasis. *Drug Discovery Today* 18: 1272–1281.

Jain N. K., Mishra V., Mehra N. K. 2013. Targeted drug delivery to macrophages. *Expert Opinion in Drug Delivery* 10: 353–367.

Kaur I. P. and Singh H. 2014. Nanostructured drug delivery for better management of tuberculosis. *Journal of Controlled Release* 184: 36–50.

Khalil N. M., de Mattos A. C., Moraes Moreira Carraro T. C., Ludwig D. B., Mainardes R. M. 2013. Nanotechnological strategies for the treatment of neglected diseases. *Current Pharmaceutical Design* 19: 7316–7329.

Kumari A., Kumar A., Yadav S., Yadav S. C. 2010. Biodegradable polymeric nanoparticles based drug delivery systems. *Colloids and Surfaces B: Biointerfaces* 75: 1–18.

Lalloo U. G., and Ambaram A. 2010. New antituberculous drugs in development. *Current HIV/AIDS Reports* 7: 143–151.

Lam J. K.-W., Liang W., Hak-Kim Chan H. K. 2012. Pulmonary delivery of therapeutic siRNA. *Advanced Drug Delivery Reviews* 64: 1–15.

Lemke A., Kiderlen A., Kayser O. 2005. Amphotericin B. *Applied Microbiology and Biotechnology* 68: 151–162.

Meers P., Neville M., Malinin V., Scotto A. W., Sardaryan G., Kurumunda R., Mackinson C., James G., Fisher S., Perkins W. R. 2008. Biofilm penetration, triggered release and in vivo activity of inhaled liposomal amikacin in chronic *Pseudomonas aeruginosa* lung infections. *Journal of Antimicrobial Chemotherapy* 61: 859–868.

Mehanna M. M., Mohyeldin S. M., Elgindy N. A. 2014. Respirable nanocarriers as a promising strategy for antitubercular drug delivery. *Journal of Controlled Release* 187: 193–197.

Merkel O. M., Rubinstein I., Kissel T. 2014. siRNA delivery to the lung: What's new? *Advanced Drug Delivery Reviews* 75: 112–128.

Moen M. D., Lyseng-Williamson K. A., Scott L. J. 2009. Liposomal AmB a review of its use as empirical therapy in febrile neutropenia and in the treatment of invasive fungal infections. *Drugs* 69: 361–392.

Mrsny R. J., Lazazzera B. A., Daugherty A. L., Schiller N. L., Patapoff T. W. 1994. Addition of a bacterial alginate lyase to purulent CF sputum in vitro can result in the disruption of alginate and modification of sputum viscoelasticity. *Pulmonary Pharmacology* 7, 357–366.

Nahar M., Dubey V., Mishra D., Mishra P. K., Dube A., Jain N. K. 2010. In-vitro evaluation of surface functionalized gelatin nanoparticles for macrophage targeting in the therapy of visceral leishmaniasis. *Journal of Drug Targeting* 18: 93–105.

Pandey R. and Khuller G. K. 2005. Antitubercular inhaled therapy: Opportunities, progress and challenges. *Journal of Antimicrobial and Chemotheraphy* 55: 430–435.

Pedersen S. S., Høiby N., Espersen F., Koch C. 1992. Role of alginate in infection with mucoid *Pseudomonas aeruginosa* in cystic fibrosis. *Thorax* 47: 6–13.

Rosas-Taraco A. G., Higgins D. M., Sánchez-Campillo J., Lee E. J., Orme I. M., González-Juarrero M. 2011. Local pulmonary immunotherapy with siRNA targeting TGFb1 enhances antimicrobial capacity in *Mycobacterium tuberculosis* infected mice. *Tuberculosis* 91: 98–106.

Salah A. B., Messaoud N. B., Guedri E., Zaatour A., Alaya N. B., Bettaieb J., Gharbi A. et al. 2012. Investigations into an alternate approach to target mannose receptors on macrophages using 4-sulfated N-acetyl galactosamine more efficiently in comparison with mannose-decorated liposomes: An application in drug delivery. *Nanomedicine* 8: 468–477.

Sharma G., Kar S., Ball W. B., Ghosh K., Das P. K. 2014. The curative effect of fucoidan on visceral leishmaniasis is mediated by activation of MAP kinases through specific protein kinase C isoforms. *Cellular and Molecular Immunology* 11: 263–274.

Sosnik A., Carcaboso A. M., Glisoni R. J., Moretton M. A., Chiappetta D. A. 2010. New old challenges in tuberculosis: Potentially effective nanotechnologies in drug delivery. *Advanced Drug Delivery Reviews* 62: 547–559.

Suci P. A., Mittelman M. W., Yu F. P., Geesey G. G. 1994. Investigation of ciprofloxacin penetration into *Pseudomonas aeruginosa* biofilms. *Antimicrobial Agents and Chemotherapy* 38: 2125–2133.

Sundar S., Chakravarty J. 2010. Liposomal Amphotericin B and Leishmaniasis: Dose and Response. *Journal of Global Infectious Diseases* 2: 159–166.

Tang B. C., Dawson M., Lai S. K., Wang Y., Soo Suk J., Yang M., Zeitlin P., Boyle M. P., Fu J., and Hanes J. 2009. Biodegradable polymer nanoparticles that rapidly penetrate the human mucus barrier. *PNAS (USA)* 106: 19268–19273.

Tiuman T. S., Santos A. O., Ueda-Nakamura T., Dias Filho B. P., Nakamura C. V. 2011. Recent advances in leishmaniasis treatment. *International Journal of Infectious Diseases* 15: 525–532.

Torrado J., Espada R., Ballesteros M., Torrado-Santiago S. 2008. Amphotericin B formulations and drug targeting. *Journal of Pharmaceutical Sciences* 7: 2405–2425.

Van de Ven H., Vermeersch M., Matheeussen A., Vandervoort J., Weyenberg W., Apers S., Cos P., Maes L., Ludwig A. 2011. PLGA nanoparticles loaded with the antileishmanial saponin ß-aescin: Factor influence study and *in vitro* efficacy evaluation. *International Journal of Pharmacy* 420: 122–132.

Van Griensven J. and Diro E. 2012. Visceral leishmaniasis. *Infectious Disease Clinics of North America* 26: 309–322.

Vélez J., Bern I. D., Herrero C. M. Desjeux P. et al. 2012. Leishmaniasis worldwide and global estimates of its incidence. *PLoS One* 7(5): e35671. doi: 10.1371/journal.pone.0035671.

Vermelho A. B., Supuran C. T., Cardoso V., Menezes D., Rocha de Andrade Silva J., Pinto Ferreira J. L., Fernandes Amaral A. C., Rodrigues I. A. 2014. Leishmaniasis: Possible New Strategies for Treatment (Charper 15). In: *Leishmaniasis—Trends in Epidemiology, Diagnosis and Treatment.* Intech Open. ISBN 978-953-51-1232-7.

Vij N., Min T., Marasigan R., Belcher C. N., Mazur S., Ding H., Yong K., Roy I. 2010. Development of PEGylated PLGA nanoparticle for controlled and sustained drug delivery in cystic fibrosis. *Journal of Nanobiotechnology* 8: 22.

WHO. 2014a. Leishmaniasis. WHO Fact sheet N° 375. Web site: http://www.who.int/mediacentre/factsheets/fs375/en/ (accessed on January 17, 2015).

WHO. 2014b. WHO Global tuberculosis report 2014. 171 pages. Web site: http://www.who.int/tb/publications/global_report/en/ (accessed on January 17, 2015).

Xiong M., Bao Y., Yang X., Zhu Y., Wang J. 2014. Delivery of antibiotics with polymeric particles. *Advanced Drug Delivery Reviews* 78: 63–76.

14 Nanotechnology in Drug Delivery to Chronic Inflammatory Diseases

Mazen M. El-Hammadi and José L. Arias

CONTENTS

INTRODUCTION

Inflammation is a protective response of living tissues to injury or illness through which the body defends itself against foreign bodies and repairs tissue damage.

The inflammation response can be caused by a number of stimulants, resulting in acute or chronic inflammation. Acute inflammation is typically triggered by external stimuli and lasts for a relatively short period of time (hours to days). It is characterized by pain, redness, warmth, and swelling (tumor), and complete recovery can be achieved by the help of anti-inflammatory drugs and other remedies used to eliminate the cause (such as antibiotics for bacterial infection). Chronic inflammation, however, requires no external stimulus and is often a sign of a more serious condition, which requires a longer period of treatment. While conventional treatment with nonsteroidal anti-inflammatory drugs (NSAIDs) and corticosteroids may improve symptoms, these drugs lack the ability to selectively target their sites of action, which necessitates the use of elevated doses in order to achieve the desired therapeutic response [1,2]. Consequently, extensive amounts of the drug are biodistributed into healthy tissues, causing unwanted side effects, and therefore, proper medical supervision is important when these medicines are to be used for prolonged periods as in chronic inflammatory conditions. The long-term use of these drugs has been associated with a high incidence of serious adverse reactions, including cardiovascular effects (myocardial infarction, stroke, and hypertension), renal effects (decreased renal blood flow and glomerular filtration rate), hepatic effects, bleeding, ulcers, skin bruising, weight gain, cataract, abdominal pain, bone thinning, bone marrow depression, diabetes, pain, and possibility of infections at the injection site.

The entrapment of active molecules into nanocarriers for the treatment of chronic inflammation has been suggested as an effective approach for increasing specificity of drugs and thus minimizing administrated dose and associated toxicity. In addition, nanocarriers can also be employed to protect the entrapped drug against environmental degradation, modify its absorption and transport at the biological barriers, and thus alter its pharmacokinetics characteristics.

The current chapter is dedicated to providing an overview of current approaches of formulating nanocarrier-based drug delivery systems for the management of four common groups of chronic inflammatory diseases (CIDs), namely arthritis, inflammatory bowel disease (IBD), chronic airway inflammation, and uveitis. Characteristics and design requisites of nanocarriers for CIDs, in vivo challenges against their delivery, and passive and active targeting strategies are also discussed.

CHARACTERISTICS AND DESIGN REQUISITES OF NANOCARRIERS FOR CHRONIC INFLAMMATORY DISEASES

Engineering flexibility is a major advantage for drug nanocarriers. Particles of various shape, size, and surface characteristics using numerous materials can be engineered rather easily. It is these characteristics that will determine the fate and biodistribution of the encapsulated drug with no or minimal effect from the drug's physicochemical properties. An ideal nanocarrier should retain the drug and prevent its leakage and quick degradation in vitro and in vivo, exert an improved pharmacokinetic profile of the drug (uniform oral absorption, long biological half-life, etc.), exhibit controllable drug release exclusively into the site of action, minimize the frequency and severity of adverse drug reactions, and show minimal immunogenicity and toxicity.

Particle Characteristics

In general, a nanoparticle (NP) with a spherical shape, a small particle size of under 200 nm, a relatively good hydrophilic character (or negligible hydrophobic nature), and almost null surface electrical charge is highly desirable. These optimal characteristics ensure that the drug–nanocarrier system is physically and chemically stable in biological media, can go unrecognized by the reticuloendothelial system (RES) and the immune system in the body, and as a consequence, exhibit long-circulating times and improved immunogenicity and toxicity profiles.

Materials Used to Formulate Nanoparticles

Besides producing stable NPs with a capacity to load adequate amounts of the therapeutic agent, the NP-forming material is selected based on several criteria. It is essential for the material to be biodegradable and biocompatible with rapid elimination in order to prevent accumulation in the body. In addition, the material and its degradation products must exhibit no toxicity and no immunogenicity. According to the formulating material, NPs for CIDs can be primarily classified in two categories: polymeric and lipid-based NPs.

Polymers

Polymers are considered the most promising materials to be used in the formulation of drug nanocarriers. They are very versatile and can be easily engineered to assure the maximum drug-loading capacity along with an ideal sustained drug release. Despite recent advances in polymer science, only a limited number of biodegradable polymers are safe enough to be used in formulating NPs for biomedical applications; among these, chitosan, poly(D,L-lactide-*co*-glycolide) (PLGA), and poly(ε-caprolactone) (PCL) are the most widely investigated in the treatment of CIDs (Table 14.1).

Lipid-Based Materials

Lipid-based nanocarriers have emerged as an efficient platform for drug delivery; however, due to stability and potential toxicity issues, their use has been less favorable than biodegradable polymers. Lipid-based nanovehicles developed for CID therapy include principally liposomes, niosomes, and solid lipid nanoparticles (SLNs).

In Vivo Challenges against Nanocarrier Delivery in Chronic Inflammatory Diseases

The entire journey of a drug molecule from the site of administration to its site of action can be divided into a series of distinctive steps, at each of which the delivery system is challenged by several obstacles. A successful delivery requires the NPs to be equipped with suitable tools to surmount most, if not all, of these challenges. Regardless of the route of administration, the nanoparticulate system will come into contact with biological media of various composition and pH, such as blood and stomach fluids, in which the delivery system must preserve the drug; maintain physical and chemical stability of both drug and carrier; and avoid aggregations resulting from steric, electrostatic, or hydrophobic interactions with components from these fluids. Systemic delivery, in particular, is problematic, and particle characteristics, including large size, high net surface charge, and hydrophobic surface, may lead to its recognition and subsequent elimination by the RES. Therefore, local administration may be desirable, although sometimes less appealing, when possible as in

TABLE 14.1
Most Studied Materials for Formulating Nanocarriers for CIDs Therapy

Material	Type (Description)	General Method of NP Preparation	Specific Properties and Applications
		Polymeric NPs	
Chitosan	Natural polysaccharide	Coacervation	Mucoadhesive. Colon-specific drug delivery system
Poly(ε-caprolactone)	Synthetic homopolymer	Interfacial polymer disposition and dialysis	Long-term degradation resulting in slow drug release
Poly(D,L-lactide-*co*-glycolide)	Synthetic copolymer	Emulsion or double-emulsion technique followed by solvent evaporation or spray drying, using poly(vinyl alcohol) as a stabilizer	Sustained drug release
		Lipid-Based NPs	
Liposomes	Vesicular systems made of phospholipid bilayer(s)	Lipids are dissolved in an organic solvent, and then a dry lipid film is obtained by solvent evaporation, which is next dispersed into an aqueous phase. Liposomes are often obtained by sonication, extrusion, or thin lipid film hydration.	Lipophilic drugs can be incorporated into the lipid bilayer(s). Hydrophilic drugs can be loaded into the aqueous compartments
Niosomes	Vesicular systems made of nonionic amphiphilic bilayer(s)	Self-assembly of lipids in aqueous media	Similar to liposomes, but exhibit larger stability, lower cost, and relative higher storage stability
Solid lipid nanoparticles	Solid matrices of biodegradable lipids	Lipids are melted and dispersed into nanometer-sized lipid droplets using mostly solvent emulsification–evaporation or diffusion, high-using pressure homogenization, or microemulsification.	Physical stability. Remain in solid form at physiological temperature. Easy to scale up.

intra-articular injection in arthritis, oral and colonic administration in IBD, topical application in uveitis, and pulmonary delivery in lung inflammatory conditions. However, disease-specific pathophysiologic barriers may present a significant challenge for local delivery and, thus, NPs must be specifically designed to bypass them. For example, respiratory secretions, such as respiratory mucus and alveolar fluids, in lung inflammatory diseases present an obstructive barrier to the delivery of the inhaled drug-loaded NPs. NPs captured by the mucus are lost as they will be eliminated via coughing.

Cellular uptake and internalization of NPs are usually mediated by endocytosis although other mechanisms, such as macropinocytosis, may be involved [3]. Efficient uptake necessitates interaction of the particulate system with the cell membrane, which can be facilitated by the electrostatic interaction between cationic NPs and the negatively charged cell membrane and via binding to specific cell-surface receptors.

After internalization by endocytosis, NPs may be transferred into lysosomes where they and their loaded therapeutic cargo may face destruction under the effect of the local acidic pH and lysosomal enzymes. Therefore, endosomal escape is of particular importance, especially with extra-delicate therapeutic molecules, such as deoxyribonucleic acid (DNA).

Extracellular and intracellular challenges against NP delivery to inflammatory diseases are addressed using various strategies of drug targeting.

DRUG TARGETING STRATEGIES TO CHRONIC INFLAMMATORY DISEASES

Passive Targeting

The major advantage of using nanocarrier-based drug delivery systems in comparison with conventional systems is the possibility to improve drug selectivity by increasing its localization at the site of pathology. Drug targeting can be achieved by designing nanocarriers of various shape, size, composition, and physical characteristics that are able to identify sites of action and deliver active molecules to these sites. Systemically administered nanoparticulate drug delivery systems with a hydrophobic surface are recognized by the RES, including Kupffer cells and related organs (spleen, liver, lungs, and bone marrow), and taken up by macrophages, leading to their rapid clearance from the blood circulation (plasma half-life ≈3 minutes). Since macrophages play a key role in the immune response in inflammatory diseases, this can be advantageously exploited as a therapeutic strategy for passive targeting of drug-loaded NPs into these cells [2,4–6].

Although this strategy is efficient in selective targeting of macrophage-producing organs, in particular the spleen and liver, a successful anti-inflammatory therapy may require the targeting of other tissues, such as the synovial in arthritis.

Another passive targeting approach is to take advantage of the locally enhanced capillary permeability of inflamed tissues [7,8]. This effect can be improved by surface engineering of drug-loaded nanocarriers to increase their systemic circulation time. This is usually achieved by the physical or chemical attachment of hydrophilic polymers, such as poly(ethylene glycol) (PEG), poloxamers, poloxamines, or polysaccharides, onto the surface of the NP to produce a hydrophilic neutral shell of polymeric chains able to repel plasma proteins and prevent opsonization, thus, resulting in longer biological half-life [1,9–12].

One study investigated mechanisms underlying the anti-inflammatory effect of PEGylated NPs using NPs made by a blend of poly(D,L-lactide) (PLA) and PEG-PLA block copolymer, which were loaded with betamethasone disodium 21-phosphate (BP). Based on in vitro and in vivo observations, it was suggested that initial accumulation of NPs in the inflammatory lesion was because of the enhanced permeation

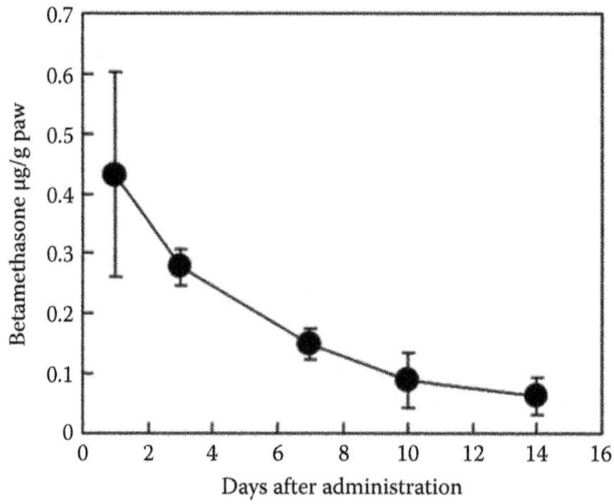

FIGURE 14.1 Accumulation (μg/g tissue) of betamethasone disodium 21-phosphate-loaded nanoparticles (synthesized by using a blend of PLA and PEG-PLA copolymer) in the inflammatory lesion (left hind paw, adjuvant arthritis rat model, $n = 3$). Each data point represents the mean value ± standard deviation. (Reprinted with permission from Ishihara, T., Takahashi, M., Higaki, M., Mizushima, Y., and Mizushima, T., *Int. J. Pharm.* 385, 170–175. Copyright Elsevier 2010.)

and retention (EPR) effect, followed by internalization in inflammatory macrophages as the NPs lose their PEG segment, and consequently, BP was released in macrophages during the hydrolysis of the polymer [13]. In fact, the amount of BP at Day 1 after the administration of the NPs in the lesion was considerably high (Figure 14.1). Conversely, after the administration of free BP, the amount of drug was below the detection limit (0.04 μg/g tissue). It was hypothesized that the EPR effect was responsible for the prolonged residence of the drug-loaded nanocarriers in blood, thus leading to higher accumulation in the inflamed paw.

Nanoparticulate oral and colonic deliveries have also been reported to target inflamed intestine and to be taken up by presenting macrophages. Small particle size and negative surface charge were found to enhance drug targeting of inflamed regions of the intestine [14–16].

Active Targeting

Despite advantages brought in by passive targeting, the engineering of actively targeted drug nanocarriers can ensure more specific accumulation of the drug at the site of pathology and much less nonspecific distribution to undiseased tissues. Active targeting after systemic administration can be achieved by modification of the particles' surface with a ligand (targeting entity) for specific recognition of a receptor and/or by the manipulation of stimuli-sensitive "smart" drug nanoplatforms.

Drug Targeting through a Specific Recognition Mechanism

Surface-functionalized NPs with ligand moieties are able to bind to unique targeted molecules in the inflamed lesions. This conceptualization is the basis of the so-called ligand- or receptor-mediated drug targeting. Several biomolecules have the potential to target inflamed regions and can be recruited as targeting ligands [1,2], such as cell-adhesion molecules (P-selectin, E-selectin, and L-selectin), RGD (arginine–glycine–aspartic acid) peptides and integrins, folate moieties, and monoclonal antibodies (MAbs).

Zhou et al. prepared targeted perfluorooctylbromide (PFOB) NPs loaded with a lipase-labile prodrug of fumagillin, a mycotoxin produced by *Aspergillus fumagatus* with anti-angiogenic activity. PFOB was microfluidized under high pressure, and the highly hydrophobic fumagillin prodrug was incorporated as a component of the outer monolayer membrane composed of a mixture of phospholipid surfactants. The $\alpha_v\beta_3$-integrin antagonist conjugated to PEG2000-phosphatidylethanolamine was then added to the lipid surfactant mixture. The resulting NPs had diameters within 230–260 nm and zeta potential values of ≈25 mV. Following intravenous injection into the KRN serum-mediated inflammatory arthritis mouse model, $\alpha_v\beta_3$-targeted NPs accumulated mainly in the small blood vessel wall at the arthritic paw whereas no similar accumulation was observed with the nontargeted NPs. Furthermore, nanotherapy slowed the progression of synovial inflammation, as evidenced by ≈50% decrease in ankle thickness and arthritic score, a noticeable decrease in the number of inflammatory cells recruited into the subsynovial space, and preservation of bone and cartilage integrity [17]. Another report for receptor-targeting joint inflammation utilized folate surface–modified NPs to target the folate receptor found in synovial mononuclear cells and $CD14^+$ cells in patients with rheumatoid arthritis (RA). Chitosan NPs surface-decorated with folate moieties and loaded with IL-1Ra gene remarkably reverted alterations in bone turnover in arthritic rats by modulating the osteocalcin level as well as the activities of alkaline phosphatase and tartrate-resistant acid phosphatise, compared to nontargeted NPs. These protective effects were evidenced by the decrease in the expression levels of interleukine-1β and prostaglandin E_2. Furthermore, surface-functionalized NPs had a better cytotoxicity profile and promoted IL-1Ra protein synthesis compared to control formulations [18].

Galactosylated trimethylchitosan (GTC)-cysteine NPs were used for active delivery of a small interfering ribonucleic acid (*si*RNA) to suppress tumor necrosis factor-alpha (TNF-α) production in macrophages at the inflamed intestine. The galactosylated NPs demonstrated enhanced uptake by activated macrophages due to galactose receptor-mediated endocytosis and led to efficient localization of the orally delivered DNA in the colon [19]. Similarly, CyD1–*si*RNA loaded liposomes surface functionalized with a MAb against β_7 integrins were successfully delivered to the inflamed intestines after intravenous injection [20].

Selective targeting of the inflamed eyes in mice was achieved after intravenous injection of dexamethasone (DEX)-loaded sialyl-Lewis X (SLX)-conjugated liposomes, which were able to target both E-selectin and P-selectin on the activated endothelial cells [21].

Mannose- and specific peptide-grafted NPs have also been investigated for targeting the inflamed colon in IBD [22]. Orally administered multifunctional mannose-modified trimethylchitosan (MTC)-cysteine conjugate NPs loaded with *si*RNA against TNF-α successfully suppressed TNF-α production in macrophages of mice with acute hepatic injury [3].

Drug Delivery by Stimuli-Sensitive Nanoparticles

Stimuli-sensitive NPs can be formulated using nanoparticulate materials with the capacity to change their physical properties (e.g., disruption/aggregation, swelling/deswelling) in response to a specific external stimulus. This property can be advantageous in active drug targeting and can be exploited to trigger drug release exclusively into the targeted site (light-, enzyme-, acid-, or thermosensitive-triggered drug release) or, instead, to localize the therapeutic agent into the targeted site of action before allowing its release (e.g., magnetically responsive nanoparticulate materials) [1].

Light-Triggered Drug Release

In particular, liposomes have shown potential for drug targeting through light-triggered drug release. Photooxidation or photofragmentation of the liposome components using different exciting light waves can trigger the release of encapsulated drugs [1]. Similarly, multifunctional ultra-small (13.33 nm–sized) nanoassemblies were formulated by conjugating magnetite NPs to the glucocorticoid DEX through a photosensitive linker. Exposure to near-infrared (NIR) radiation was found to trigger DEX release as a result of the photocleavage of the linker [23].

Enzyme-Triggered Drug Release

Enzyme-triggered drug release can be achieved by formulating nanovehicles that are cleaved by enzymes specifically overexpressed at the targeted site. These carriers retain the drug as they circulate in the body while at the site of action they are disrupted by the enzyme, thus releasing the entrapped drug. It is common to formulate long-circulating liposomes that are susceptible to enzyme-triggered drug release [1], such as secretory phospholipase A2, elastase, sphingomyelinase, phospholipase C, alkaline phosphatase, or transglutaminase.

Conjugates of the drug can be synthesized with linkers that are specifically cleaved by a particular enzyme. For example, a polyamidoamine dendrimer conjugated with a linear methoxiPEG-ibuprofen was found to release the NSAID molecules in diluted plasma in response to esterase activity [24].

pH-Triggered Drug Release

pH-responsive nanocarriers are formulated to maintain their stability at physiological pH value while they degrade under acidic pH and drug release occurs [1]. An example of this group is the NP formulated using poly(vinylpyrrolidone-*co*-dimethylmaleic anhydride) (PVD).

Conjugates of dextran with ibuprofen and naproxen with the ability to self-assemble into NPs were shown to have a pH-dependent drug release, which was influenced by the degree of substitution [25]. Poly(β-benzyl-L-aspartate)-*b*-poly(vinylpyrrolidone) diblock copolymeric NPs loaded with prednisone acetate were also found to have a very slow drug release at pH 7.4 compared to that at pH 2.1 [26].

In colon-specific delivery, however, where a drug must be retained in the nanocarrier in the acidic stomach pH and released in the colonic neutral pH, other pH-responsive materials have been proposed for drug delivery to the inflamed colon, for example, Eudragit® S100, which dissolves when the pH is above 7 [22]. Mesoporous silica nanoparticles (MSNs) were also studied as a nanocarrier for pH-dependent controllable release of anionic drugs. For instance, sulfasalazine-loaded MSNs were able to retain the drug in the acidic environment (pH 2–5), while drug release occurred at pH 7.4 due to deprotonation of silanol groups and the consequent electrostatic repulsion with the loaded drug molecules [27].

Thermoresponse-Triggered Drug Release

Although this mechanism has not been described for nanocarriers used in CLDs, it may be proposed as an efficient approach for controlled drug release. It is based on the physical behavior of temperature-sensitive polymers, which show a remarkable change in the hydration degree below and above their lower critical solution temperature (LCST) [1].

Combining receptor-mediated targeting with a stimuli-sensitive drug release strategy in one multifunctional nanoparticulate system can be highly attractive for efficient therapy.

Methotrexate (MTX)-loaded PEGylated gold half-shell PLGA NPs were developed, and the RGD peptide, a targeting moiety for inflammation, was conjugated to the surface of the gold half-shell. After intravenous injection into collagen-induced arthritic (CIA) mice, the targeting peptides resulted in enhanced accumulation of NPs in the inflamed joints while the gold half-shell allowed photothermally controlled drug release from the NPs upon exposure to NIR irradiation. The multifunctional NPs exhibited a superior therapeutic efficacy with a much smaller dosage of MTX in CIA mice in comparison with conventional treatment [28].

Magnetic Drug Targeting

NPs containing a magnetic core (i.e., an iron oxide: magnetite or maghemite) can be employed to drive drug-loaded nanocarriers to the desired site of action by applying a magnetic gradient. As a consequence, the nanocarrier will accumulate in the targeted site and remain there until the drug is entirely released.

Along this line, Arias et al. developed magnetic nanocomposites consisting of a magnetic core (iron) and an ethylcellulose shell in which diclofenac sodium was effectively incorporated. It is expected that this nanosystem could very efficiently deliver diclofenac sodium to an arthritic site with the help of a magnetic gradient and may also lead to a remarkable decrease in drug dose required to achieve an adequate therapeutic response [29].

ADVANCES IN NANOCARRIERS FOR COMMON CHRONIC INFLAMMATORY DISEASES

ARTHRITIS

Arthritis is a serious health problem, which has been described to provoke in the United States alone that more than 20 million new patients develop work disability every day. Chronic arthritis encompasses a plethora of inflammatory disorders characterized by a progressive joint degeneration and severe pain. The most common forms of chronic arthritis are RA, an autoimmune inflammatory disorder, and osteoarthritis (OA), the most frequent cause of pain, loss of function, and disability in adults.

Although the pathophysiologic cause remains uncertain, chronic inflammation and immune response appear to play a role in the destruction of the joint in arthritis. Additionally, trauma, infection, and age are the major key factors involved in the origin and development of this degenerative joint disease.

Despite recent advances in pharmacotherapy, curing of arthritis still represents an unmet medical need because of safety and efficacy concerns with currently marketed drugs. Current medicinal approaches aim at reducing pain and local inflammation, helping patients to feel better. As a result, these treatments can only slow the progressive joint damage but not completely prevent it. In addition to NSAIDs and corticosteroids, disease-modifying antirheumatic drugs (DMARDs) are also used in the management of arthritis, including MTX, actarit, and anti-TNF-α MAbs, such as infliximab and adalimumab.

The incorporation of antiarthritis molecules into nanocarriers represents an attractive and effective approach for the treatment of arthritis due to the expected improvement in drug efficacy and the reduction of the associated adverse reactions [1,2,29,30].

In this context, NPs loaded with NSAIDs have gained particular interest. Diclofenac sodium-loaded PCL NPs prepared by interfacial polymer disposition (average size $\approx$200 nm; drug entrapment efficiency $\approx$45%; drug loading $\approx$20%) showed a desired sustained drug release profile in which a burst effect was observed in the first 2 hours ($\approx$40% drug release), followed by a slow liberation over the next 94 hours [31]. Türker et al. demonstrated that the incorporation of diclofenac sodium into a liposomal formulation enhanced the therapeutic effect of the drug against RA after a single dose intra-articular administration in comparison with the topically applied commercial product [32]. Histopathological examination revealed that joints treated with the lipid-based nanomedicine had significantly ($p < 0.05$) less synovial inflammatory-related changes than observed in control joints.

Similarly, celecoxib-loaded SLNs were explored for their ability to improve the drug retention in the joint and produce prolonged drug release [33]. Drug-release studies performed in vitro demonstrated that the celecoxib-loaded NPs resulted in sustained release of the drug and the release pattern followed quasi-Fickian diffusion. Histopathology studies of the rat joints after intra-articular injection in normal rats proved that NSAID-loaded SLN were biocompatible and suitable for intra-articular use. The biodistribution studies showed that the NPs had greater retention in the inflamed articular joints and lower distribution to the RES organs compared to free drug. In another study, celecoxib-loaded niosomes were prepared as a gel formulation with the aim to enhance local accumulation, prolong drug release, and improve site specificity of this NSAID [34]. The niosomal gel provided 6.5-fold greater drug deposition in deep skin layer and muscle compared to carbopol gel (195.2 ± 8.7 and 30.0 ± 1.5 μg, respectively). In addition, while the muscle-to-plasma concentration ratio for niosomal gel formulation was six (2.16 ± 0.12 μg/g vs. 0.34 ± 0.01 μg/mL), it was only one for carbopol gel (0.36 ± 0.01 μg/g vs. 0.43 ± 0.02 μg/mL). As a result, remarkable diminution of rat paw edema compared to that after application of the conventional gel was obtained.

NPs loaded with corticosteroids, such as BP and DEX, have been formulated and studied for their antiarthritic effects. A study by Higaki et al. reported the formulation of PLGA NPs loaded with BP (average size ≈100–200 nm) by an oil-in-water emulsion solvent diffusion method [8]. The PLGA–nanosteroid was assessed after intravenous administration to rats with adjuvant arthritis and to mice with anti-type II collagen antibody–induced arthritis. After 1 day of a single injection of the NPs into rats, a 30% reduction in paw inflammation was observed and maintained for 1 week. In addition, diminished soft tissue swelling was obtained 7 days after the treatment. Similar findings were also achieved in the mouse model. The observed antiarthritic effect of the nanosteroid was hypothesized to be the result of a selective targeting of the inflamed joint and the prolonged in situ drug release.

Gene therapy with nonviral vectors offers great promise as a therapeutic strategy to overcome inflammatory conditions in arthritis. In particular, chitosan-based NPs have been suggested as an appropriate carrier for DNA delivery. Chitosan NPs loaded with interleukin-1 receptor antagonist (IL-1Ra) gene were utilized against OA [35]. After direct injection of IL-1Ra–loaded chitosan NPs into the knee joint cavities of OA rabbits, apparent expression of IL-1Ra was measured in the knee joint synovial fluid (unlike control groups). In addition, chitosan-DNA injection produced a significant reduction in the severity of histological cartilage lesions. Similar findings were obtained when chitosan NPs were used to incorporate anti-TNF-α Dicer-substrate small interfering ribonucleic acid (D*si*RNA) [5]. When given intraperitoneally to CIA mice, *si*RNA-chitosan NPs were able to knockdown the TNF-α expression in macrophages and, as a consequence, they effectively downregulated TNF-α-induced inflammatory responses and prevented joint swelling. Histological examination of joints showed minimal cartilage destruction and inflammatory cell infiltration in treated mice. It was hypothesized that a prophylactic use of this nanosystem could delay the onset of arthritis.

DMARDs, such as MTX and actarit, have also been incorporated into nanocarriers to improve their therapeutic efficiency against arthritis. Actarit-loaded SLN were produced using a solvent diffusion–evaporation method, and the resulting NPs showed a mean size of 241 ± 23 nm, a zeta potential value of −17.1 ± 1.6 mV, and an average drug entrapment efficiency and loading of ≈50% and 8%, respectively [4]. Pharmacokinetic studies showed that actarit-loaded SLNs had a longer mean retention time (MRT ≈14 hours) than the corresponding actarit propylene glycol (PG) solution (MRT ≈1 hour) after intravenous injection to New Zealand rabbits. Moreover, the area under the curve of plasma concentration–time (AUC) of the nanomedicine was 1.88 times greater than that of the free drug solution. Additionally, the biodistribution study in intravenously injected mice revealed that the encapsulation of actarit increased its accumulation in the spleen from ≈6% to ≈16% and reduced its renal distribution (and consequently, its nephrotoxicity) compared to the actarit PG solution. These findings suggest that actarit-loaded SLNs could be used for passive targeting of the spleen in RA. Likewise, MTX was incorporated into stealth liposomes made using a PEGylated phospholipid and into conventional liposomes coated with chitosan. In vitro studies revealed that both formulations produced a prolonged drug release profile in comparison with the uncoated conventional liposomes. In vivo studies in rats with induced RA showed that MTX-loaded liposomes significantly reduced edema volume after intravenous injection while PEGylated lipid vesicles produced the highest antirheumatoid efficacy. These intravenous lipid nanovesicles of MTX may be an interesting alternative for intra-articular and oral delivery of MTX.

A recent study reported on the oral delivery of *Tripterygium wilfordii Hook* f. (TWHF), a traditional Chinese herb with anti-inflammatory and immunosuppressive effects, loaded into SLNs (mean particle size ≈116 nm and zeta potential ≈−45 mV) [36]. The SLNs showed enhanced anti-inflammatory activity and reduced hepatotoxicity compared to free TWHF after oral administration to rats with adjuvant-induced arthritis.

Although extensive research has been done to develop nanoparticulate systems for selective therapy of arthritis, no registered products for human administration are available yet, which may be owing to stability issues and lack of definite evidence of clinical efficacy.

Inflammatory Bowel Disease

The IBD is a relapsing and remitting chronic disease with incidences ranging from 0.1% to 0.15% in the population of Western countries. IBD encompasses a number of chronic inflammatory conditions, among which Crohn's disease (CD) and ulcerative colitis (UC) are the most common. Both diseases share many similar symptoms, such as diarrhea, bloody stools, weight loss, abdominal pain, fever, and fatigue. However, they differ from each other in terms of the pathogenesis and the typical clinical manifestations. In CD, the inflammation is transmural, extending through the bowel wall to the serosal layer, and can affect the small and the large intestines whereas in the case of UC the inflammation affects only the colon and rectum, and the innermost mucosa is completely inflamed. It is noteworthy that the strategies involving the development of an appropriate drug delivery system in CD and UC are challenging and quite different, depending on the inflamed region in the intestines. Drug administration via the rectal route is preferred in UC while it is indicated to administer drugs orally in CD, which frequently impacts the ileum.

The conventional pharmacotherapy of IBD involves the administration of 5-aminosalicylic acid (5-ASA) and corticosteroids. When these drugs are given orally, they are absorbed during their transit in the gastrointestinal tract, and only a proportion can reach the inflamed sites of the intestinal mucosa. In addition, increased permeability in the intact noninflamed tissues of the upper intestinal tract has been reported in patients with IBD [37,38]. Therefore, high doses of the therapeutic agents are normally required to achieve and maintain remission in IBD, which may result in serious side effects. To address these problems, the use of nano-based drug carriers has been suggested.

The rationale behind using nanocarriers in the treatment of IBD is based on the ability of NPs to selectively adhere to the inflamed tissues of the intestines, owing to pathophysiological changes in these tissues [14]. The disruption of the intestinal barrier, the increased levels of mucus production, and the uptake by immune-related cells, including macrophages and dendritic cells, presented in high numbers at the inflamed regions in IBD can lead to selective accumulation of the orally administrated drug-loaded NPs. Additionally, the microvascular permeability and endothelial fenestration can result in the accumulation of nanocarriers in the ulcerated tissues after parenteral systemic administration. Moreover, unlike conventional dosage forms, such as tablets, NPs are not affected by diarrhea, a major symptom in IBD.

Many experimental animal models have been used to study human IBD. One well-characterized animal model for the study of human UC is dextran sodium sulfate (DSS)–induced acute and chronic colitis with ulceration in mice, which is characterized by a marked loss in body weight, rectal bleeding, reduction in colon length, and destruction of the intestinal epithelium.

First works by Lamprecht et al. investigated the effect of particle size on potential targeting of IBD. Fluorescent polystyrene particles with a size of 0.1, 1, or 10 μm were administered orally over a period of 3 days to rats with induced UC. The absorption was found to be size-dependent; while 16% of the 100-nm-sized particles were absorbed over a 10-day period, only ≈2% of the 1-μm-sized particles were absorbed under the same conditions [14].

These encouraging results in animals were not in line with clinical findings in humans. A similar study in human patients with IBD showed obvious deposition of microparticles (average size: 3.0 μm) in ulcerous lesions while NPs (250 nm) were detectable only in traces in the inflamed mucosa after rectal administration [39]. The study also found that microparticles adhered to the ulcerated tissue were not absorbed across the epithelial barrier. On the contrary, NPs were translocated to the serosal compartment in IBD, probably resulting in undesired systemic absorption. This may explain the increased accumulation in inflamed mucosa with larger particle size.

The incorporation of drug-loaded nanocarriers into a second carrier that can adhere to the inflamed lesions and provide a controlled liberation of the NPs may be suggested to improve their therapeutic efficiency. A polysaccharide hydrogel system composed of alginate and chitosan (1:1, molar ratio), which was shown to collapse in colonic pH between pH 5 and 6, has been proposed as a carrier for drug-loaded PLA NPs [40,41]. The alginate–chitosan solution containing NPs was orally gavaged to animals first, followed by a chelation solution containing calcium chloride and sodium sulfate. A hydrogel solution encapsulated with NPs was formed in situ by the mixture of these two solutions in the mouse stomach. Two drugs were investigated using this technique: lysine–proline–valine (KPV) [40], a tripeptide with anti-inflammatory properties, and prohibitin 1 (PHB1) [41], a multifunctional protein implicated in cellular processes whose expression from intestinal epithelial was found to be inhibited by proinflammatory cytokines. In the first study [40], the KPV-containing formulation appeared to protect DSS-induced colitis mice against inflammatory and histologic parameters. The effective dose of KPV in free solution (200 μg/day) was ≈12,000 times higher compared with encapsulated KPV-loaded NPs (25.2 ng/day). In the second study [41], recombinant human PHB1 (negatively charged) was complexed to polyethyleneimine (PEI) (positively charged) by electrostatic interaction, followed by the addition of bovine serum albumin (BSA) to neutralize the extra charge of PEI. This complex was loaded into PLA NPs before the resulting NPs were encapsulated into the polysaccharide solution. Oral administration of the PHB1-loaded nanoparticulate hydrogel system was found to increase the levels of PHB1 in the surface epithelial cells of the colon, thus leading to reduced severity of the inflammation in mice with DSS-induced colitis. These findings were comparable to the effects produced by enema administration of a recombinant adenovirus comprising a plasmid encoded for the PHB1 gene.

Effects of particle surface charge, the other influential factor in NP efficiency, in IBD treatment has also been explored. Jubeh et al. studied the adhesion properties of charged liposomes to the intestinal tissues of healthy and colitis-induced rats after rectal administration [15]. Anionic liposomes adhered two times more to the inflamed colonic mucosa than neutral or cationic liposomes. On the contrary, the adherence of cationic liposomes to the healthy colonic mucosa was three times that of either neutral or anionic liposomes. The study also found that adherence was directly correlated with charge density. Promoted adherence of negatively charged particles to ulcerated tissues is explained by the overexpression of transferrin, a positively charged protein, in these tissues. While in this study the stability of liposomes was maximized by direct administration to the inflamed regions, the development of an oral formulation would require additional arrangements to address stability issues in the stomach and duodenum. Nonetheless, positively charged Eudragit® RL NPs (hydrodynamic diameter: 119 ± 13 nm; zeta potential: 47 ± 2 mV) loaded with clodronate, an antiosteoporotic drug with macrophage suppressive and potent anti-inflammatory effects, were found to improve the therapeutic efficiency of the negatively charged hydrophilic drug after rectal application in 2,4,6-trinitrobenzenesulfonic acid (TNBS) and oxazolone (OXA) mice models of colitis [16]. This enhanced effect seems to stem from improved uptake by macrophages with local administration into the inflamed intestine. However, an oral administration may not be expected to exert such efficient effect as interactions with mucous may impede the transport of cationic NPs through the intestinal tube to the site of action.

Interestingly, therapeutic variances have also been observed among different animal species. PLGA NPs loaded with tacrolimus, an immune-suppressant with nephrotoxic effects, did not seem to improve the therapeutic efficiency of the drug when given orally to colitis-induced rats although rectal administration of NPs resulted in an enhanced and selective drug deposition into the inflamed tissues [42]. On the contrary, orally administered PLGA and Eudragit® P-4135F NPs of tacrolimus were more efficient in mitigating experimental colitis in mice compared to a drug solution although less efficient if the drug solution is administered as a subcutaneous injection [43]. Furthermore, tacrolimus-loaded NPs of both types showed reduced nephrotoxicity in comparison with free drug solutions (oral and subcutaneous). With longer and slower passage of the drug carriers throughout the intestinal tract in rats compared to mice, it is probable that the efficiency of these carriers may be reduced due to several factors, such as degradation by digestive enzymes and efficient uptake by Peyer's patches. Another effect that has to be taken into account is the mean particle size of NPs administered to rats and mice, in these two reports, which was 107 ± 8 nm and ≈450 nm, respectively.

NPs formulated using drug–polymer conjugates have also been suggested to improve their therapeutic efficiency and selectivity. 5-ASA was covalently coupled to either PCL [44] or silica, and NPs of the two conjugates were produced [45]. Both nanoparticulate formulations were observed to accumulate selectively in the inflamed regions, enabling a considerable reduction in the necessary drug dose compared with free 5-ASA solution. In vitro drug release demonstrated a slow leakage of the drug from both NPs, which is desirable to ensure no drug release before reaching the inflamed regions in the colon.

A number of studies assessed the potential of nanocarriers for gene therapy using a *si*RNA strategy. Laroui et al. prepared a TNF-α *si*RNA/PEI nanocomplex, which was then loaded into PLA NPs [46]. The resulting NPs had a diameter of ≈380 nm and zeta potential of −8 mV at pH 7.2 and were noncytotoxic. Furthermore, complexation of TNF-α *si*RNA with PEI protected it from ribonuclease. In vitro studies revealed that TNF-α *si*RNA/PEI-loaded PLA NPs were taken up by macrophages and inhibited the lipopolysaccharide-induced TNF-α secretion in these cells. To deliver the NPs to mice colonic lumen, they were encapsulated into a hydrogel comprised of alginate and chitosan (described above). Following oral administration, TNF-α *si*RNA/PEI-loaded PLA NPs encapsulated in this hydrogel system were efficiently taken up by inflamed macrophages leading to a specific inhibition of TNF-α expression/secretion in the colonic tissue in lipopolysaccharide-treated mice.

More recently, similar oral delivery of *si*RNA was reported using GTC NPs [19]. A *si*RNA of mitogen-activated protein kinase kinase kinase kinase 4 (Map4k4), a key upstream mediator of TNF-α action, was employed as a means to suppress TNF-α production in macrophages. *si*RNA-loaded GTC NPs were made using ionic gelation of GTC with tripolyphosphate (TPP) or hyaluronic acid (HA) as an anionic cross-linker. GTC/TPP NPs resulted in enhanced in vitro uptake by activated macrophages due to galactose receptor–mediated endocytosis. In vivo studies showed that Map4k4 *si*RNA-loaded GTC/TPP NPs efficiently localized orally delivered *si*RNA to the colon, inhibited TNF-α production, and improved pathological symptoms.

Interestingly, liposomes comprising a MAb against β_7 integrins, which are highly expressed in gut mononuclear leukocytes, were loaded with protamine-condensed CyD1-*si*RNA for active targeted delivery to the inflamed intestines by intravenous injection [20]. Cyclin D1 is a pivotal cell cycle–regulatory molecule, which is strongly upregulated at sites of inflammation in IBD. The administration of *si*RNA-loaded liposomes remarkably decreased CyD1 messenger ribonucleic acid (*m*RNA) to a level similar to that of the uninflamed gut, leading to a drastic reduction in intestinal tissue damage, a potent suppression of leukocyte infiltration into the colon, and a reversal in body weight loss and hematocrit reduction.

Other targeting approaches have also been under investigation. MSNs with a positive surface charge were proposed as a nanocarrier for pH-dependent loading and controllable release of anionic drug molecules [27]. MSNs loaded with sulfasalazine (an anionic anti-inflammatory prodrug used for IBD) were found to retain the drug in an acidic environment (pH 2–5) while the incubation in physiological buffer solution (pH 7.4) generated a partial negative charge to the surface of NPs, owing to the deprotonation of silanol groups, triggering a sustained release of the loaded molecules due to an electrostatic repulsion. As a result, it can be speculated that loaded drugs would remain trapped in the nanovehicle when passing through the stomach's acidic environment and be released in the intestine where the environmental pH is close to neutral. A recent report by Coco et al. compared several colon-specific delivery strategies using polymeric NPs loaded with ovalbumin (OVA) as a model drug [22]. NPs were formulated using Eudragit® S100 for pH-responsiveness, which dissolves when the pH is above 7; trimethylchitosan (TMC) for mucoadhesion; or a mix of PLGA, PEG-PLGA, and PEG-PCL for sustained drug delivery. In addition, active targeting of NPs was done using the latter mix of polymers after grafting mannose (for targeting immune cells) or specific peptides (for targeting the inflamed colon) on the PEG chain of PCL. In vitro studies using Caco-2 cells showed that TMC NPs produced the highest permeability for OVA in the untreated model while all formulations had similar efficiency in the inflamed model. Furthermore, in vivo studies revealed that mannose-grafted NPs assured the highest accumulation of the drug (quantified by liquid scintillation counting) in the inflamed colon ($p < 0.05$) (Figure 14.2). Based on

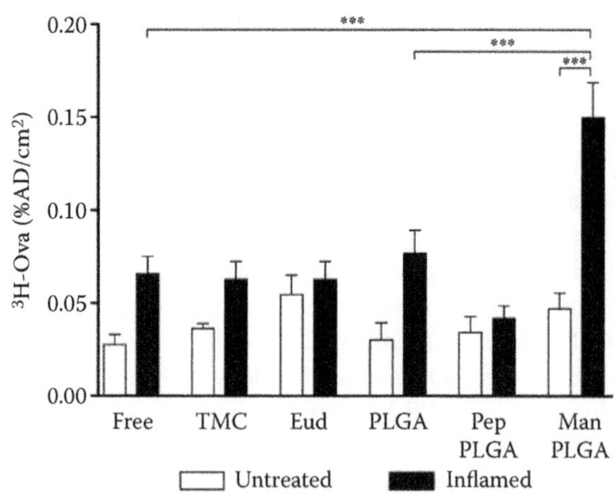

FIGURE 14.2 Uptake (percentage of administered dose per cm^2, %AD/cm^2) of ^{3}H-OVA in untreated colonic samples (white bars) and inflamed colonic samples (black bars) ($n = 7$). Data are mean ± standard error of the mean. OVA formulations (drug dose: 10 μg): free (ovalbumin solution); PLGA; Pep-PLGA (mix of the polymers PLGA, PLGA-PEG, and PEG-PCL, the later grafted with the peptidic ligand Gly-Ser-Gln-Ser-His-Pro-Arg-His); Man-PLGA (mix of the polymers PLGA, PLGA-PEG, and PEG-PCL, the later grafted with a mannose derivative, i.e., 2-aminoethyl-α-D-mannopyroside); TMC (*N,N,N*-trimethylchitosan chloride); and, Eud (Eudragit® S100). (Reprinted with permission from Coco, R., Plapied, L., Pourcelle, V., Jérôme, C., Brayden, D. J., Schneider, Y. J., and Préat, V., *Int. J. Pharm.*, 440, 3–12. Copyright Elsevier 2013.)

these results, active targeting of macrophages and dendritic cells may be a promising approach for targeting the colon in IBD.

Despite the promise demonstrated by in vivo studies of drug-loaded nanovehicles in animals with IBD, clinical findings in humans have not been equally successful [39]. Nonetheless, in vitro treatment of patients' peripheral blood mononuclear cell (PBMC) culture supernatants with butyrate- and DEX-loaded SLNs has led to significant reduction in cytokine production, compared to free drug [47]. Therefore, optimization of the particulate system properties seems to be crucial in order to circumvent in vivo obstacles in humans and species differences in the intestinal surface area, lumen conditions, and mucosal physiology.

Chronic Lung Inflammatory Diseases

Chronic lung inflammatory diseases (CLIDs) are characterized by chronic airway inflammation and mucous hypersecretion and considered major global health problems. The most common CLIDs are asthma and chronic obstructive pulmonary disease (COPD). In asthma, the inflammatory response seems to be mediated by allergen-specific T-helper type-2 (Th2) cells, resulting in eosinophilia, whereas in COPD, the inflammation is neutrophilic driven [48]. In addition, in asthma all airways, apart from the lung parenchyma, are involved in the inflammatory response while in COPD the inflammation affects the peripheral airways (bronchioles) as well as lung parenchyma [48]. Excessive inflammation contributes to mucous hypersecretion and the widespread damage affecting the bronchial epithelium in the chronic stage of these diseases. Moreover, inflammation and the associated immune response and mucous hypersecretion are the major obstacles in the delivery and efficacy of therapeutic molecules. Therefore, the management of inflammation is an important strategy in the treatment of these lung inflammatory conditions.

There is no curative treatment for these conditions. Pharmacotherapy involves the use of bronchodilators, anti-inflammatory agents, and glucocorticoids. Nanonization of drugs has been suggested to improve steric stability and facilitate rapid dissolution of drugs administrated by inhalation, such as budesonide [49]. Interestingly, inhaled silver NPs (mean particle size ≈6 nm) appeared to attenuate airway inflammation and hyper-responsiveness in OVA-induced murine model of asthma although the mechanism remains unknown [50]. Furthermore, drug formulation as nano-based systems may be an efficient approach to override delivery challenges and provide sustained drug delivery in CLIDs. A variety of NPs forming polymers has been assessed via different routes of administration including oral, pulmonary, and nasal routes.

Among these polymers, chitosan has a great potential for topical delivery across mucosal surfaces because of its mucoadhesiveness and ability to facilitate drug absorption through the opening of tight junctions between epithelial cells [51]. Several reports investigated small drug molecules, macromolecules, and DNA delivery using chitosan-based NPs via the nasal route.

In one study, the ability of thiolated chitosan NPs to enhance the capacity of theophylline, a bronchodilator that possesses anti-inflammatory properties, to alleviate allergic asthma was investigated in a mouse model of allergic asthma [52]. Thiol groups were coupled to the polymer to enhance its mucoadhesiveness and permeation properties without compromising biodegradability. The conjugated NPs were produced by ionic cross-linking with sodium TPP followed by sonication (diameter: 220 ± 23 nm; zeta potential: 15 ± 2 mV), and theophylline was allowed to adsorb to the resulting NPs. The anti-inflammatory effects of intranasally administrated theophylline were remarkably augmented when the drug was formulated as chitosan-based NPs. This was evident by reduction in eosinophils in bronchoalveolar lavage fluid (BALF), inhibition of mucus hypersecretion, decreased bronchial damage, and increased apoptosis of lung cells.

The macromolecular drug heparin, an anticoagulant that possesses potent anti-allergic and anti-inflammatory properties, was also loaded to chitosan-based NPs for enhanced asthma treatment efficiency. Unfractionated or low-molecular-weight heparin-loaded chitosan/HA NPs [53] and chitosan/carboxymethyl-β-cyclodextrin NPs [54] were obtained by ionotropic gelation between the positively charged amino groups of chitosan and the negatively charged HA/carboxymethyl-β-cyclodextrin, heparin as well as pentasodium TPP. The resulting NPs had a diameter between 162 and 729 nm, a positive zeta potential ranging from +28.1 to +40.7 mV, and, in general, a high drug association efficiency up to more than 70%. Ex vivo studies with rat mast cells were performed to determine the capacity of NPs to prevent histamine release in comparison with heparin solution. While chitosan/HA NPs had a similar effect to that obtained with free heparin solution, heparin-loaded chitosan/carboxymethyl-β-cyclodextrin NPs significantly improved heparin efficacy in preventing degranulation of mast cells but only at the highest heparin dose used in this study. Taking into account that the conditions of these ex vivo experiments are different from those present in vivo, the chitosan-based NPs may have potential for pulmonary delivery of heparin because of their mucoadhesive properties and ability to protect the loaded drug from enzymatic degradation.

Gene therapy was explored using chitosan-based NPs of plasmid encoded for interferon-γ, a pleiotropic cytokine that promotes T-helper type-1 (Th1) responses that downregulate Th2-associated airway inflammation and hyper-responsiveness, and were reported to effectively reduce OVA-induced airway inflammation in mice after intranasal administration [55]. Another gene delivery experiment involved the loading of chitosan NPs with a plasmid encoded for vessel dilator, an *N*-terminal natriuretic peptide of proatrial natriuretic factor. The intranasal administration of DNA-chitosan NPs appeared to inactivate extracellular-signal regulated receptor kinase (ERK1/2) and downregulate atrial natriuretic peptide receptor (NPRA) expression, thus leading to protection of mice from airway inflammation [56].

For systemic delivery of anti-inflammatory agents to the lungs, PLGA-based NPs have been suggested. Pyridine 6, a pan-Janus kinase (JAK) inhibitor that may potentially inhibit allergic asthma, was loaded into PLGA NPs using an emulsion–solvent evaporation technique. The method allowed the encapsulation of a 10 times higher dose than the maximum dose that could be injected of free pyridine 6. These NPs were administrated intraperitoneally to mice sensitized and challenged by OVA [57]. These nanovehicles were found to improve pyridine 6 therapeutic potency in inhibiting Th2 inflammation, thus resulting in suppressed asthmatic responses. Similarly, PLGA was suggested as a nanocarrier for the macromolecule α1-antitrypsin, a 54 kDa glycoprotein inhibiter of different proteases, which can protect the lung from cellular inflammatory enzymes, as a means of improving stability and efficacy of the protein and providing a sustained release of it [58].

Despite the fact that inhaled steroids are the first choice treatment to control asthma, systemic administration of steroids is necessary for treatment of intractable asthma and of asthmatic exacerbation. In this context, stealth NPs prepared using a blend of PLA homopolymers and PEG-PLA block copolymers were proposed to improve accumulation of BP at the site of airway inflammation (Figure 14.3) [10]. After intravenous administration to mice with OVA-induced asthma, the nanomedicines were found to exert significant anti-inflammatory effects (and reduce the drug adverse effects) as evidenced by a decrease in BALF eosinophil number and attenuated airway responsiveness.

Recently, SLNs (based on the combination of stearic acid and lecithin) were used to incorporate curcumin, a natural polyphenol compound with anti-inflammatory properties, and tested in an OVA-induced allergic rat model of asthma [59]. NPs made using a solvent injection method had an average size of 190 nm with a mean zeta potential value of −20.7 mV and 75% drug entrapment efficiency. The biodistribution study (in mice) revealed that SLNs could augment the tissue distribution of curcumin, especially in the liver and lung. In fact, curcumin-loaded SLNs

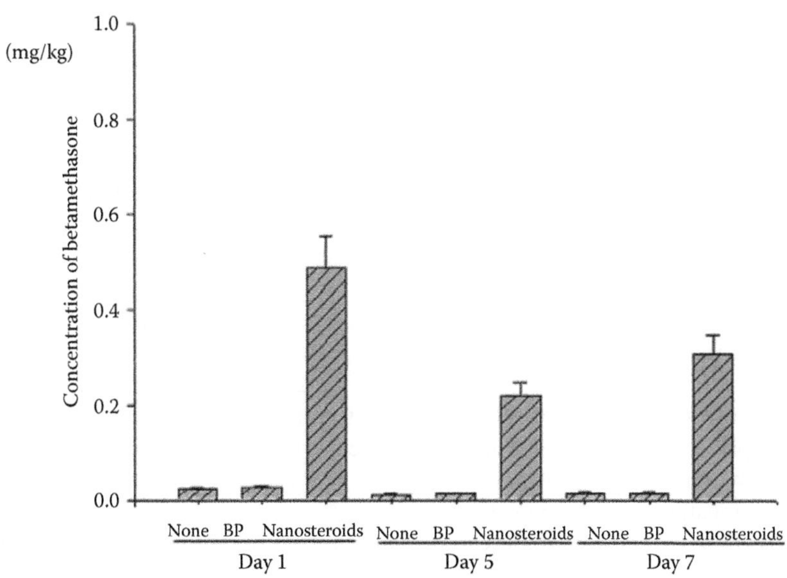

FIGURE 14.3 Enhanced accumulation (mg/Kg) of betamethasone disodium 21-phosphate (BP) in the lung when administered as a nanosteroid form ($p < 0.01$). Mice were divided into three groups ($n = 6$): nanosteroids administered through the tail vein (drug dose: 40 μg), (free) BP administered intraperitoneally (drug dose: 40 μg), and saline administered intravenously ("none"). Mean ± standard error of the mean are shown from Days 1, 5, and 7. Reprinted with permission from Matsuo, Y., Ishihara, T., Ishizaki, J., Miyamoto, K., Higaki, M., and Yamashita, N., *Cell Immunol.*, 260, 33–38. Copyright Elsevier 2009.)

administrated by intraperitoneal injection increased drug concentration in the lung and significantly inhibited airway inflammation as observed by suppressed inflammatory cell infiltration and inhibited expression of Th2 cytokines.

It is important to note that NPs made for pulmonary delivery should be carefully formulated to avoid any undesired adverse reaction. Reports have shown that inhalation of NPs can lead to serious health consequences, such as oxidative inflammatory reactions and pulmonary diseases. Furthermore, inhaled NPs may be absorbed to the systemic circulation and consequently target the central nervous system and immune system, presumably leading to systemic side effects [60]. Nonetheless, NPs still have great potential for CLIDs treatment via both local and systemic administration.

Uveitis

Uveitis is the inflammation of the tissues forming the uvea, which consists of the iris, ciliary body, choroids, and contiguous structures. It is considered to be one of the leading causes of blindness.

Because of the complex structure of the eye, it shows a high resistance to foreign substances, including drugs, and topical administration comprises a number of limitations. The defensive mechanisms of the eye, including tearing and blinking, lead to a quick elimination of the topically administrated drug into the nose through the nasolacrimal drainage. In addition, drugs must diffuse a great distance penetrating the corneal tight junctions to reach the intraocular tissues. Consequently, only a very small proportion of the drug dose, down to 5% or less, reaches its intraocular targets. This requires the use of higher drug concentrations, which, in turn, may result in an increased likelihood of systemic side effects caused by drug absorption from the nose. Additionally, intraocular injection is associated with certain complications, such as accelerated cataract formation, hemorrhage, retinal detachment, endophthalmitis, and increased intraocular pressure [61]. Furthermore, conventional systemic therapy does not provide effective intraocular concentrations because of the ocular–blood barrier.

It has been reported that the administration of nanosized therapeutic agents enhances the ophthalmic drug absorption and therapeutic efficiency [62]. The use of nanocarriers in uveitis is desirable because it can improve absorption by topical administration, particularly for poorly soluble drugs; improve localization by systemic administration; reduce frequency of dosing by intraocular injection; protect the encapsulated drug; and prolong the drug action by sustained release. Because of their very small particle size and composition, NPs ensure low irritation, low toxicity, biocompatibility, and mucoadhesiveness.

Most in vivo delivery studies have been performed in experimental animals with endotoxin (i.e., lipopolysaccharide)-induced uveitis (EIU). In these studies, the anti-inflammatory properties of the delivery systems were assessed using clinical examinations (Hogan's classification method is normally employed) and measuring the intensity of local inflammation by quantifying leukocyte infiltration and other inflammatory mediators in the aqueous humor.

Eudragit® RS100–based NPs were among the first to be used for the ophthalmic delivery of anti-inflammatory agents. Eudragit® RS100 is a copolymer of poly(ethyl-acrylate, methyl-methacrylate, and chlorotrimethyl-ammonioethyl methacrylate) in which the amount of quaternary ammonium groups ranges from 4.5% to 6.8%. Because of these positively charged groups, the copolymer can interact with negatively charged drugs or cellular membranes leading to drug complexation and improved cellular uptake, respectively. Adibkia et al. formulated piroxicam-loaded Eudragit® RS100-based NPs (particle size ≈240 nm and zeta potential ≈35 mV) using a solvent evaporation/extraction technique [63]. The anti-inflammatory properties of the piroxicam-loaded NPs were compared with a microsuspension of piroxicam alone (particle size ≈1.7 μm and zeta potential ≈0.4 mV) in rabbits with EIU. It was demonstrated that piroxicam-loaded NPs were significantly more effective in inhibiting inflammation than the pure drug microsuspension.

In the same way, triamcinolone acetonide (TA)-loaded PLGA NPs prepared using an emulsification/solvent diffusion method were evaluated for their efficacy in an EIU rabbit model (Figure 14.4) [64]. Inflammation was indirectly assessed by determination of cells and proteins infiltrated into the anterior chamber and by measurement of inflammatory mediators (e.g., prostaglandin E2 and nitric oxide) in the aqueous humor. The nanomedicine proved to be superior in treating inflammation over a TA microsuspension and a prednisolone acetate microsuspension and showed comparable effects to a TA subconjunctive injection.

The use of nanovehicles has also been suggested for intraocular injection with the aim to reduce dosing frequency in the treatment of uveitis. Lajavardi et al. encapsulated the vasoactive intestinal peptide (VIP), an immunosuppressive factor, in PEGylated liposomes to increase its stability in biological media and to control its release [65]. A single intravitreal injection of these VIP-containing sterically stabilized liposomes was effective at minimizing clinical and pathological ocular inflammation signs in rats when injected simultaneously with induction of EIU [65] or experimental autoimmune uveoretinitis (EAU) [66]. Further incorporation of the VIP-loaded liposomes within a HA gel was found to improve the anti-inflammatory effect of VIP and prolong its activity by slowing the release from liposomes, when the gel was intravitreally injected 7 days before EIU induction [65].

Besides administration by local routes, systemic delivery has also been explored by injecting PEG- and ligand surface–engineered NPs. It was shown that the incorporation of BP into stealth (PEGylated) PLA NPs improved drug accumulation in inflamed eyes and enhanced the efficiency of treatment after a single intravenous injection in rats with EAU [11]. Confocal microscope images showed the improved NP localization in the inflamed retina of EAU rats until 7 days after injection. However, further studies are needed to define whether repeated injections of BP-loaded stealth NPs improve the anti-inflammatory effect. Similarly, DEX was loaded into SLX conjugated liposomes and injected intravenously into mice with EAU [21]. SLX liposomes were found to selectively target inflamed eyes in EAU mice where the concentration of DEX was two times higher than that measured after the injection with a free drug solution. A binding inhibition assay revealed that SLX liposomes were able to target both E-selectin and P-selectin on the activated endothelial cells.

The studies described above have paved the way for new possibilities for the treatment of intraocular inflammation. However, the implementation of nanoparticulate therapy in humans would first require more functional studies to exclude any possibility of immune response development or loss of vision.

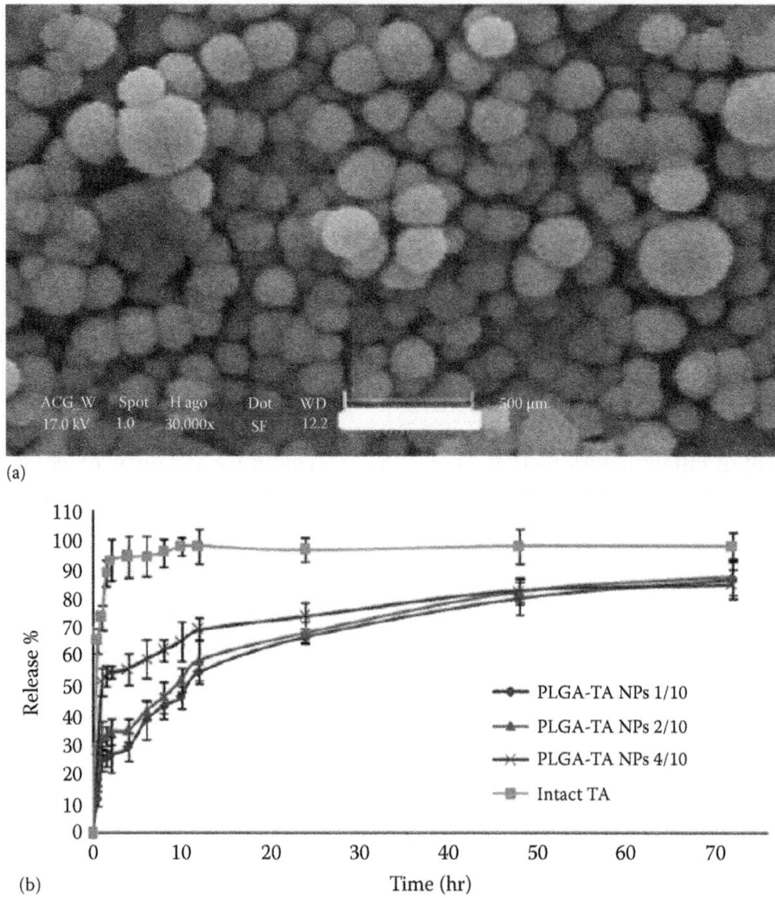

FIGURE 14.4 (a) Scanning electron microphotography of spherical PLGA-TA NPs (bar length: 500 nm) and (b) TA release profiles (%) from PLGA-TA NPs formulated by using different ratios of PLGA and TA (w/w, total mass: 110 mg) as a function of the incubation time (hours). Data represents the mean value of three replications ± standard deviation. (Adapted with permission from Sabzevari, A., Adibkia, K., Hashemi, H., Hedayatfar, A., Mohsenzadeh, N., Atyabi, F., Ghahremani, M. H., and Dinarvand, R., *Eur. J. Pharm. Biopharm.*, 84, 63–71. Copyright Elsevier 2013.)

CONCLUSIONS

Nano-based drug delivery systems have demonstrated great potential in the treatment of CIDs by allowing accumulation of therapeutic molecules at the site of inflammation and enhancing uptake by inflammation cells. Consequently, drug-loaded nanocarriers have improved drug pharmacokinetics and reduced incidence of adverse effects. Intensive work has been done with the aim of optimizing nanocarrier geometry and surface characteristics, leading to the development of multifunctional nanoparticulate drug delivery vehicles, which combine several strategies for drug targeting and release. Unfortunately, it is not currently possible to develop a universal nanocarrier for all CIDs, and the specificity of each disease must be considered when formulating the appropriate nanomedicine device. Generation of adequate in vivo toxicity data is crucial before these systems can find their way to the clinic. Industrial scale-up of nanovehicles will also be another challenging step owing to the inherent complexity of these systems and the associated costs of development, which are generally considered economically unprofitable in the health care system.

LIST OF ABBREVIATIONS

5-ASA	5-aminosalicylic acid
AUC	Area under the curve of plasma concentration–time
BALF	Bronchoalveolar lavage fluid
BP	Betamethasone disodium 21-phosphate
BSA	Bovine serum albumin
CD	Crohn's disease
CIA	Collagen-induced arthritic
CID	Chronic inflammatory disease
CLID	Chronic lung inflammatory disease
COPD	Chronic obstructive pulmonary disease
DEX	Dexamethasone
DMARD	Disease-modifying antirheumatic drug
DNA	Deoxyribonucleic acid
DSS	Dextran sodium sulfate
EAU	Experimental autoimmune uveoretinitis
EIU	Endotoxin-induced uveitis
EPR	Enhanced permeation and retention
ERK1/2	Extracellular signal regulated receptor kinase
GTC	Galactosylated trimethylchitosan
HA	Hyaluronic acid
IBD	Inflammatory bowel disease
IL-1Ra	Interleukin-1 receptor antagonist
JAK	Janus kinase
KPV	Lysine–proline–valine
LCST	Lower critical solution temperature
MAb	Monoclonal antibody
Map4k4	Mitogen-activated protein kinase kinase kinase kinase 4
***m*RNA**	Messenger ribonucleic acid
MRT	Mean retention time
MSN	Mesoporous silica nanoparticle
MTC	Mannose-modified trimethylchitosan
MTX	Methotrexate
NIR	Near-infrared
NP	Nanoparticle
NPRA	Natriuretic peptide receptor
NSAID	Nonsteroidal anti-inflammatory drug

OA	Osteoarthritis
OVA	Ovalbumin
OXA	Oxazolone
PBMC	Peripheral blood mononuclear cell
PCL	Poly(ε-caprolactone)
PEG	Poly(ethylene glycol)
PEI	Polyethyleneimine
PFOB	Perfluorooctylbromide
PG	Propylene glycol
PHB1	Prohibitin 1
PLA	Poly(D,L-lactide)
PLGA	Poly(D,L-lactide-*co*-glycolide)
PVD	Poly(vinylpyrrolidone-*co*-dimethylmaleic anhydride)
RA	Rheumatoid arthritis
RES	Reticuloendothelial system
RGD	Arginine–glycine–aspartic acid
***si*RNA**	Small interfering ribonucleic acid
D*si*RNA	Dicer-substrate small interfering ribonucleic acid
SLN	Solid lipid nanoparticle
SLX	Sialyl-Lewis X
TA	Triamcinolone acetonide
Th1	T-helper type-1
Th2	T-helper type-2
TMC	Trimethylchitosan
TNBS	2,4,6-trinitrobenzenesulfonic acid
TNF-α	Tumor necrosis factor-alpha
TPP	Tripolyphosphate
TWHF	*Tripterygium wilfordii Hook* f.
UC	Ulcerative colitis
VIP	Vasoactive intestinal peptide.

REFERENCES

1. Arias, J. L. 2009. Micro- and nano-particulate drug delivery systems for cancer treatment. In *Anticancer Drugs: Design, Delivery and Pharmacology*, P. Spencer, and W. Holt, ed., pp. 1–85. New York: Nova Science Publishers Inc.
2. Ulbrich, W., and Lamprecht, A. 2010. Targeted drug-delivery approaches by nanoparticulate carriers in the therapy of inflammatory diseases. *J. R. Soc. Interface* 7: S55–66.
3. He, C., Yin, L., Tang, C., and Yin, C. 2013. Multifunctional polymeric nanoparticles for oral delivery of TNF-alpha siRNA to macrophages. *Biomaterials* 34: 2843–2854.
4. Ye, J., Wang, Q., Zhou, X., and Zhang, N. 2008. Injectable actarit-loaded solid lipid nanoparticles as passive targeting therapeutic agents for rheumatoid arthritis. *Int. J. Pharm.* 352: 273–279.
5. Howard, K. A., Paludan, S. R., Behlke, M. A., Besenbacher, F., Deleuran, B., and Kjems, J. 2009. Chitosan/siRNA nanoparticle-mediated TNF-alpha knockdown in peritoneal macrophages for anti-inflammatory treatment in a murine arthritis model. *Mol. Ther.* 17: 162–168.

6. Lo, C. T., Van Tassel, P. R., and Saltzman, W. M. 2010. Poly(lactide-co-glycolide) nanoparticle assembly for highly efficient delivery of potent therapeutic agents from medical devices. *Biomaterials* 31: 3631–3642.
7. Paleolog, E. M., and Fava, R. A. 1998. Angiogenesis in rheumatoid arthritis: Implications for future therapeutic strategies. *Springer Semin. Immunopathol.* 20: 73–94.
8. Higaki, M., Ishihara, T., Izumo, N., Takatsu, M., and Mizushima, Y. 2005. Treatment of experimental arthritis with poly(D,L-lactic/glycolic acid) nanoparticles encapsulating betamethasone sodium phosphate. *Ann. Rheum. Dis.* 64: 1132–1136.
9. Schroeder, A., Sigal, A., Turjeman, K., and Barenholz, Y. 2008. Using PEGylated nano-liposomes to target tissue invaded by a foreign body. *J. Drug Target.* 16: 591–595.
10. Matsuo, Y., Ishihara, T., Ishizaki, J., Miyamoto, K., Higaki, M., and Yamashita, N. 2009. Effect of betamethasone phosphate loaded polymeric nanoparticles on a murine asthma model. *Cell Immunol.* 260: 33–38.
11. Sakai, T., Ishihara, T., Higaki, M., Akiyama, G., and Tsuneoka, H. 2011. Therapeutic effect of stealth-type polymeric nanoparticles with encapsulated betamethasone phosphate on experimental autoimmune uveoretinitis. *Invest. Ophthalmol. Vis. Sci.* 52: 1516–1521.
12. Prabhu, P., Shetty, R., Koland, M., Vijayanarayana, K., Vijayalakshmi, K. K., Nairy, M. H., and Nisha, G. S. 2012. Investigation of nano lipid vesicles of methotrexate for anti-rheumatoid activity. *Int. J. Nanomedicine* 7: 177–186.
13. Ishihara, T., Takahashi, M., Higaki, M., Mizushima, Y., and Mizushima, T. 2010. Preparation and characterization of a nanoparticulate formulation composed of PEG-PLA and PLA as anti-inflammatory agents. *Int. J. Pharm.* 385: 170–175.
14. Lamprecht, A., Schäfer, U., and Lehr, C. M. 2001. Size-dependent bioadhesion of micro- and nanoparticulate carriers to the inflamed colonic mucosa. *Pharm. Res.* 18: 788–793.
15. Jubeh, T. T., Barenholz, Y., and Rubinstein, A. 2004. Differential adhesion of normal and inflamed rat colonic mucosa by charged liposomes. *Pharm. Res.* 21: 447–453.
16. Niebel, W., Walkenbach, K., Béduneau, A., Pellequer, Y., and Lamprecht, A. 2012. Nanoparticle-based clodronate delivery mitigates murine experimental colitis. *J. Control. Release* 160: 659–665.
17. Zhou, H. F., Yan, H., Senpan, A., Wickline, S. A., Pan, D., Lanza, G. M., and Pham, C. T. 2012. Suppression of inflammation in a mouse model of rheumatoid arthritis using targeted lipase-labile fumagillin prodrug nanoparticles. *Biomaterials* 33: 8632–8640.
18. Fernandes, J. C., Wang, H., Jreyssaty, C., Benderdour, M., Lavigne, P., Qiu, X., Winnik, F. M., Zhang, X., Dai, K., and Shi, Q. 2008. Bone-protective effects of nonviral gene therapy with folate-chitosan DNA nanoparticle containing interleukin-1 receptor antagonist gene in rats with adjuvant-induced arthritis. *Mol. Ther.* 16: 1243–1251.
19. Zhang, J., Tang, C., and Yin, C. 2013. Galactosylated trimethyl chitosan-cysteine nanoparticles loaded with Map4k4 siRNA for targeting activated macrophages. *Biomaterials* 34: 3667–3677.
20. Peer, D., Park, E. J., Morishita, Y., Carman, C. V., and Shimaoka, M. 2008. Systemic leukocyte-directed siRNA delivery revealing cyclin D1 as an anti-inflammatory target. *Science* 319: 627–630.
21. Hashida, N., Ohguro, N., Yamazaki, N., Arakawa, Y., Oiki, E., Mashimo, H., Kurokawa, N., and Tano, Y. 2008. High-efficacy site-directed drug delivery system using sialyl-Lewis X conjugated liposome. *Exp. Eye Res.* 86: 138–149.
22. Coco, R., Plapied, L., Pourcelle, V., Jérôme, C., Brayden, D. J., Schneider, Y. J., and Préat, V. 2013. Drug delivery to inflamed colon by nanoparticles: Comparison of different strategies. *Int. J. Pharm.* 440: 3–12.

23. Banerjee, S. S., and Chen, D. H. 2009. A multifunctional magnetic nanocarrier bearing fluorescent dye for targeted drug delivery by enhanced two-photon triggered release. *Nanotechnology* 20: 185103.
24. Kurtoglu, Y. E., Mishra, M. K., Kannan, S., and Kannan, R. M. 2010. Drug release characteristics of PAMAM dendrimer-drug conjugates with different linkers. *Int. J. Pharm.* 384: 189–194.
25. Hornig, S., Bunjes, H., and Heinze, T. 2009. Preparation and characterization of nanoparticles based on dextran-drug conjugates. *J. Colloid Interface Sci.* 338: 56–62.
26. Wang, L., Zeng, R., Li, C., and Qiao, R. 2009. Self-assembled polypeptide-block-poly(vinylpyrrolidone) as prospective drug-delivery systems. *Colloids Surf. B Biointerfaces* 74: 284–292.
27. Lee, C. H., Lo, L. W., Mou, C. Y., and Yang, C. S. 2008. Synthesis and characterization of positive-charge functionalized mesoporous silica nanoparticles for oral drug delivery of an anti-inflammatory drug. *Adv. Funct. Mater.* 18: 3283–3292.
28. Lee, S. M., Kim, H. J., Ha, Y. J., Park, Y. N., Lee, S. K., Park, Y. B., and Yoo, K. H. 2013. Targeted chemo-photothermal treatments of rheumatoid arthritis using gold half-shell multifunctional nanoparticles. *ACS Nano* 7: 50–57.
29. Arias, J. L., López-Viota, M., López-Viota, J., and Delgado, A. V. 2009. Development of iron/ethylcellulose (core/shell) nanoparticles loaded with diclofenac sodium for arthritis treatment. *Int. J. Pharm.* 382: 270–276.
30. Arias, J. L. 2010. *Drug Targeting by Magnetically Responsive Colloids.* New York: Nova Science Publishers Inc.
31. Arias, J. L., López-Viota, M., Sáez-Fernández, E., and Ruiz, M. A. 2010. Formulation and physicochemical characterization of poly(epsilon-caprolactone) nanoparticles loaded with ftorafur and diclofenac sodium. *Colloids Surf. B Biointerfaces* 75: 204–208.
32. Türker, S., Erdoğan, S., Ozer, Y. A., Bilgili, H., and Deveci, S. 2008. Enhanced efficacy of diclofenac sodium-loaded lipogelosome formulation in intra-articular treatment of rheumatoid arthritis. *J. Drug Target.* 16: 51–57.
33. Thakkar, H., Kumar Sharma, R., and Murthy, R. S. 2007. Enhanced retention of celecoxib-loaded solid lipid nanoparticles after intra-articular administration. *Drugs R. D.* 8: 275–285.
34. Kaur, K., Jain, S., Sapra, B., and Tiwary, A. K. 2007. Niosomal gel for site-specific sustained delivery of anti-arthritic drug: In vitro–in vivo evaluation. *Curr. Drug Deliv.* 4: 276–282.
35. Zhang, X., Yu, C., Xushi, Zhang, C., Tang, T., and Dai, K. 2006. Direct chitosan-mediated gene delivery to the rabbit knee joints in vitro and in vivo. *Biochem. Biophys. Res. Commun.* 341: 202–208.
36. Xue, M., Jiang, Z. Z., Wu, T., Li, J., Zhang, L., Zhao, Y., Li, X. J., Zhang, L. Y., and Yang, S. Y. 2012. Anti-inflammatory effects and hepatotoxicity of Tripterygium-loaded solid lipid nanoparticles on adjuvant-induced arthritis in rats. *Phytomedicine* 19: 998–1006.
37. Teahon, K., Somasundaram, S., Smith, T., Menzies, I., and Bjarnason, I. 1996. Assessing the site of increased intestinal permeability in coeliac and inflammatory bowel disease. *Gut* 38: 864–869.
38. Bruewer, M., Luegering, A., Kucharzik, T., Parkos, C. A., Madara, J. L., Hopkins, A. M., and Nusrat, A. 2003. Proinflammatory cytokines disrupt epithelial barrier function by apoptosis-independent mechanisms. *J. Immunol.* 171: 6164–6172.
39. Schmidt, C., Lautenschlaeger, C., Collnot, E. M., Schumann, M., Bojarski, C., Schulzke, J. D., Lehr, C. M., and Stallmach, A. 2013. Nano- and microscaled particles for drug targeting to inflamed intestinal mucosa: A first in vivo study in human patients. *J. Control. Release* 165: 139–145.

40. Laroui, H., Dalmasso, G., Nguyen, H. T., Yan, Y., Sitaraman, S. V., and Merlin, D. 2010. Drug-loaded nanoparticles targeted to the colon with polysaccharide hydrogel reduce colitis in a mouse model. *Gastroenterology* 138: 843–853.el–2.
41. Theiss, A. L., Laroui, H., Obertone, T. S., Chowdhury, I., Thompson, W. E., Merlin, D., and Sitaraman, S. V. 2011. Nanoparticle-based therapeutic delivery of prohibitin to the colonic epithelial cells ameliorates acute murine colitis. *Inflamm. Bowel Dis.* 17: 1163–1176.
42. Lamprecht, A., Yamamoto, H., Takeuchi, H., and Kawashima, Y. 2005. Nanoparticles enhance therapeutic efficiency by selectively increased local drug dose in experimental colitis in rats. *J. Pharmacol. Exp. Ther.* 315: 196–202.
43. Meissner, Y., Pellequer, Y., and Lamprecht, A. 2006. Nanoparticles in inflammatory bowel disease: Particle targeting versus pH-sensitive delivery. *Int. J. Pharm.* 316: 138–143.
44. Pertuit, D., Moulari, B., Betz, T., Nadaradjane, A., Neumann, D., Ismaïli, L., Refouvelet, B., Pellequer, Y., and Lamprecht, A. 2007. 5-amino salicylic acid bound nanoparticles for the therapy of inflammatory bowel disease. *J. Control. Release* 123: 211–218.
45. Moulari, B., Pertuit, D., Pellequer, Y., and Lamprecht, A. 2008. The targeting of surface modified silica nanoparticles to inflamed tissue in experimental colitis. *Biomaterials* 29: 4554–4560.
46. Laroui, H., Theiss, A. L., Yan, Y., Dalmasso, G., Nguyen, H. T., Sitaraman, S. V., and Merlin, D. 2011. Functional TNFalpha gene silencing mediated by polyethyleneimine/TNFalpha siRNA nanocomplexes in inflamed colon. *Biomaterials* 32: 1218–1228.
47. Serpe, L., Canaparo, R., Daperno, M., Sostegni, R., Martinasso, G., Muntoni, E., Ippolito, L. et al. 2010. Solid lipid nanoparticles as anti-inflammatory drug delivery system in a human inflammatory bowel disease whole-blood model. *Eur. J. Pharm. Sci.* 39: 428–436.
48. Barnes, P. J., Shapiro, S. D., and Pauwels, R. A. 2003. Chronic obstructive pulmonary disease: Molecular and cellular mechanisms. *Eur. Respir. J.* 22: 672–688.
49. El-Gendy, N., Gorman, E. M., Munson, E. J., and Berkland, C. 2009. Budesonide nanoparticle agglomerates as dry powder aerosols with rapid dissolution. *J. Pharm. Sci.* 98: 2731–2746.
50. Park, H. S., Kim, K. H., Jang, S., Park, J. W., Cha, H. R., Lee, J. E., Kim, J. O. et. al. 2010. Attenuation of allergic airway inflammation and hyperresponsiveness in a murine model of asthma by silver nanoparticles. *Int. J. Nanomedicine* 5: 505–515.
51. Fernández-Urrusuno, R., Romani, D., Calvo, P., Vila-Jato, J. L., and Alonso, M. J. 1999. Development of a freeze-dried formulation of insulin-loaded chitosan nanoparticles intended for nasal administration. *S.T.P. Pharma Sciences* 9: 429–436.
52. Lee, D. W., Shirley, S. A., Lockey, R. F., and Mohapatra, S. S. 2006. Thiolated chitosan nanoparticles enhance anti-inflammatory effects of intranasally delivered theophylline. *Respir. Res.* 7: 112.
53. Oyarzun-Ampuero, F. A., Brea, J., Loza, M. I., Torres, D., and Alonso, M. J. 2009. Chitosan-hyaluronic acid nanoparticles loaded with heparin for the treatment of asthma. *Int. J. Pharm.* 381: 122–129.
54. Oyarzun-Ampuero, F. A., Brea, J., Loza, M. I., Alonso, M. J., and Torres, D. 2012. A potential nanomedicine consisting of heparin-loaded polysaccharide nanocarriers for the treatment of asthma. *Macromol. Biosci.* 12: 176–183.
55. Kumar, M., Kong, X., Behera, A. K., Hellermann, G. R., Lockey, R. F., and Mohapatra, S. S. 2003. Chitosan IFN-gamma-pDNA nanoparticle (CIN) therapy for allergic asthma. *Genet. Vaccines Ther.* 1: 3.
56. Wang, X., Xu, W., Kong, X., Chen, D., Hellermann, G., Ahlert, T. A., Giaimo, J. D. et al. 2009. Modulation of lung inflammation by vessel dilator in a mouse model of allergic asthma. *Respir. Res.* 10: 66.

57. Matsunaga, Y., Inoue, H., Fukuyama, S., Yoshida, H., Moriwaki, A., Matsumoto, T., Matsumoto, K. et al. 2011. Effects of a Janus kinase inhibitor, pyridone 6, on airway responses in a murine model of asthma. *Biochem. Biophys. Res. Commun.* 404: 261–267.
58. Pirooznia, N., Hasannia, S., Lotfi, A. S., and Ghanei, M. 2012. Encapsulation of alpha-1 antitrypsin in PLGA nanoparticles: In vitro characterization as an effective aerosol formulation in pulmonary diseases. *J. Nanobiotechnology* 10: 20.
59. Wang, W., Zhu, R., Xie, Q., Li, A., Xiao, Y., Li, K., Liu, H., Cui, D., Chen, Y., and Wang, S. 2012. Enhanced bioavailability and efficiency of curcumin for the treatment of asthma by its formulation in solid lipid nanoparticles. *Int. J. Nanomedicine* 7: 3667–3677.
60. Madl, A. K., and Pinkerton, K. E. 2009. Health effects of inhaled engineered and incidental nanoparticles. *Crit. Rev. Toxicol.* 39: 629–658.
61. Parke, D. W. 2003. Intravitreal triamcinolone and endophthalmitis. *Am. J. Ophthalmol.* 136: 918–919.
62. Kassem, M. A., Abdel Rahman, A. A., Ghorab, M. M., Ahmed, M. B., and Khalil, R. M. 2007. Nanosuspension as an ophthalmic delivery system for certain glucocorticoid drugs. *Int. J. Pharm.* 340: 126–133.
63. Adibkia, K., Siahi Shadbad, M. R, Nokhodchi, A., Javadzedeh, A., Barzegar-Jalali, M., Barar, J., Mohammadi, G., and Omidi, Y. 2007. Piroxicam nanoparticles for ocular delivery: Physicochemical characterization and implementation in endotoxin-induced uveitis. *J. Drug Target.* 15: 407–416.
64. Sabzevari, A., Adibkia, K., Hashemi, H., Hedayatfar, A., Mohsenzadeh, N., Atyabi, F., Ghahremani, M. H., and Dinarvand, R. 2013. Polymeric triamcinolone acetonide nanoparticles as a new alternative in the treatment of uveitis: In vitro and in vivo studies. *Eur. J. Pharm. Biopharm.* 84: 63–71.
65. Lajavardi, L., Bochot, A., Camelo, S., Goldenberg, B., Naud, M. C., Behar-Cohen, F., Fattal, E., and de Kozak, Y. 2007. Downregulation of endotoxin-induced uveitis by intravitreal injection of vasoactive intestinal Peptide encapsulated in liposomes. *Invest. Ophthalmol. Vis. Sci.* 48: 3230–3238.
66. Camelo, S., Lajavardi, L., Bochot, A., Goldenberg, B., Naud, M. C., Brunel, N., Lescure, B. et al. 2009. Protective effect of intravitreal injection of vasoactive intestinal peptide-loaded liposomes on experimental autoimmune uveoretinitis. *J. Ocul. Pharmacol. Ther.* 25: 9–21.

15 Intrathecal Drug Delivery

SriKrishna Chandran

CONTENTS

INTRODUCTION

Intrathecal drug delivery systems are a means to provide direct administration of medications into the cerebrospinal fluid (CSF). Bypassing the blood–brain barrier allows a significantly lower dose of medication to be administered to attain analgesia when compared to oral, intravenous, transdermal, or epidural routes. Within the dorsal horn of the spinal cord reside various receptors targeted in intrathecal drug delivery, including opioid receptors, alpha 2 adrenergic receptors, NMDA receptors, sodium and calcium channels, and GABA receptors.

The administration of medications directly into the intrathecal space to achieve analgesia has many benefits. The direct administration of medications allows a more rapid response at a fraction of the oral dose. The use of lower medication doses may reduce the systemic side effects. Intrathecal drug delivery systems have become a useful and effective option in the management of recalcitrant cancer and noncancer pain.

In 1898, August Bier documented the first spinal analgesia by injecting cocaine into the intrathecal space of six patients undergoing lower extremity surgery (Bier 1899). The discovery of opiate receptors in the spinal cord in 1973 provided scientific rationale for intrathecal analgesia (Pert and Snyder 1973). In 1979, Wang et al. first reported the successful use of intrathecal morphine in the treatment of intractable cancer pain (Wang, Nauss, and Thomas 1979). In 1981, the first use of an implantable intrathecal drug delivery system was reported for the management of cancer pain (Wang, Nauss, and Thomas 1979). In the 1980s, intrathecal drug delivery systems allowed a fixed continuous infusion rate of drug delivery. In 1991, externally programmable, battery-powered intrathecal drug delivery system pumps were introduced, allowing for noninvasive dose changes using an external programmer (Wallace and Yaksh 2000).

There are two general classes of patients for which intrathecal drug delivery systems are utilized in pain management: those with cancer and noncancer pain. In 1994, the

Mayo Clinic symposium on pain management extended the World Health Organization's three-step "ladder" approach to cancer pain by introducing a fourth step that included interventional pain therapies, such as spinal analgesia, nerve stimulation, and neurolytic blocks (Lamer 1994). In 2000, the Polyanalgesic Consensus Conference panel first convened to address the use of intrathecal infusion of analgesic medications to patients with chronic refractory pain. While there are no universally accepted guidelines for patient selection, those suffering from intolerable side effects of oral, intravenous, or transdermal therapies as well as those unable to obtain adequate analgesia despite high opioid doses should also be considered for intrathecal drug delivery systems.

CSF FLOW DYNAMICS

Cerebrospinal fluid exists within the intracerebral ventricles and subarachnoid spaces as well as the central canal of the spinal cord. CSF is formed at a rate of 0.3–0.4 mL/min (approximately 500 mL/day). The total volume of CSF is 90–150 mL in adults. CSF is formed in the choroid plexus, parenchyma of the brain and spinal cord, and ependymal lining of the ventricles (Segal and Pollay 1977).

The absorption of CSF occurs primarily through the arachnoid villi and lymphatic vessels. The arachnoid villi drains cerebrospinal fluid into the great dural sinuses while the true lymphatic vessels drain CSF by means of an indirect perineural (ophthalmic, optic, and vagal nerves) course and the CNS capillary bed (Battal et al. 2011).

The classical view of cerebrospinal spinal fluid movement is termed bulk flow. CSF is created in the choroid plexus and spreads in a cranio-caudal direction propelled by hydrostatic pressure. More recent studies have shown that CSF movement is more of a pulsatile flow (Henry-Feugeas et al. 2000). Arterial pulsations and intrathoracic respiratory pressures predominantly govern pulsatile flow. At cranial and cranio-thoracic levels, arterial pulsations during diastole create a cranial flow of cerebrospinal fluid while systole creates a caudal flow (Henry-Feugeas et al. 2000). At more caudal levels, respiratory flow governs flow, causing cranial flow during deep inspiration and caudal flow during deep exhalation (Yamada et al. 2013). Cerebrospinal fluid flow is more pronounced in the cervical when compared to the lumbar region (Enzmann and Pelc 1991). CSF flow is therefore a heterogeneous, oscillatory, bidirectional, cranio-caudal movement. This movement is further influenced by the presence of venous plexuses, nerve rootlets, and epidural fat, each of which creates a barrier to flow, creating focal mixing (Stockman 2006).

TYPES OF PUMPS: EXTERNALIZED VERSUS IMPLANTED AND RATES/MODES

Externalized and internalized pumps are two general classes of intrathecal drug delivery systems. Externalized pumps can be further classified as those with a percutaneous catheter (tunneled or not tunneled) and those with a fully implanted catheter with a subcutaneous injection port. A percutaneous catheter involves a procedure where the catheter used to infuse the intrathecal medication is introduced into the body via a needle. The catheter tip is positioned in the appropriate position using fluoroscopy. The catheter is then attached to an externalized pump, which delivers the medication. Its limitations are the risks of infection and catheter migration. Therefore, it is usually considered a temporary solution. Externalized pumps are less invasive to place and can be useful in patients with a limited life expectancy (Bhatia et al. 2013; Cohen and Dragovich 2007).

Internalized pumps can be subdivided into those with fixed rate delivery systems and those that are programmable. Fully implanted, fixed rate intrathecal drug delivery systems deliver a constant rate of medication. They usually possess a larger reservoir, allowing for lengthier time intervals between refills. They do not require a battery to operate and are less expensive than variable rate delivery systems. Variable rate delivery systems are fully implantable devices that can either deliver an intermittent or continuous amount of intrathecal medication. Variable rate delivery systems can be programmed to administer medications at a simple continuous or variable rate. In addition, they provide the option for patient-controlled analgesia via a wireless radiofrequency transmitter. Programmable devices are battery operated and have a lifespan usually between 5 and 7 years, after which surgical revision is required to implant a new pump (Bhatia et al. 2013).

The decision to use an externalized or implanted pump is based on several factors, including life expectancy, cost, patient wishes, professional expertise, and medication requirements.

MECHANISMS OF IMPLANTED PUMPS

There are several components to an intrathecal drug delivery system. The medication reservoir contains the solution to be infused. The Medtronic synchromed II model 8637 reservoir is constructed using a bellows design. The reservoir expands and contracts based on the drug volume. Pressurized gas surrounding the reservoir exerts a constant pressure at normal body temperatures, propelling medication into the pump tubing. The motor and battery-powered electronics cause the roller arm in the peristaltic pump to rotate. This mechanism allows the administration of a precise, programmed amount of medication through the catheter port and into the catheter. A valve within the system prevents reservoir overfilling or overpressurization. A catheter access port located on the device allows direct access to the catheter and cerebrospinal fluid. A separate reservoir fill port allows access to the pump reservoir for medication refills. Figure 15.1 shows a labeled image of the SynchroMed II pump (Medtronic Inc. 2010).

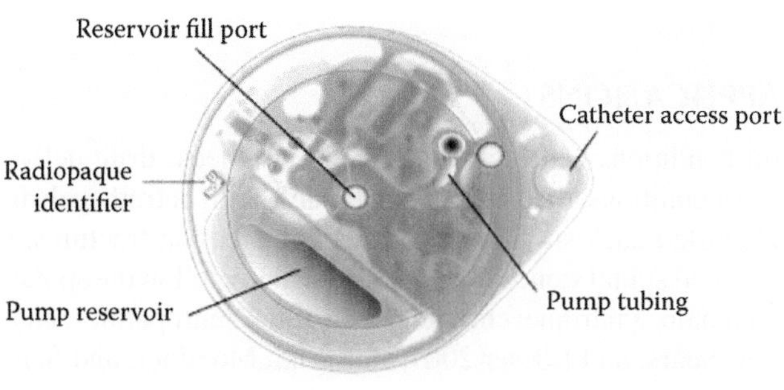

FIGURE 15.1 SynchroMed II pump. (Image courtesy of Medtronic, Inc.)

CHALLENGES IN INTRATHECAL DRUG DELIVERY

Once a decision to employ intrathecal therapy has been made, there are several variables that must be considered. Currently, only three medications are approved by the Federal Drug Administration for intrathecal use: morphine, ziconitide, and baclofen. Of these, morphine and ziconitide are approved for use in chronic pain. Other intrathecal medications for which extensive clinical experience and published clinical and preclinical data exist include hydromorphone, fentanyl, bupivacaine, clonidine, and sufentanyl. Medication can be dosed in a continuous or intermittent fashion using a programmable pump. Patient-controlled analgesia can be employed using a personal therapy manager in cases where patients are able to identify activities or times when their pain is exacerbated.

There are no studies defining the best rate to deliver intrathecal medications. It has been theorized that the use of lower flow rates may result in higher medication concentrations at the catheter tip, increasing the risk of granuloma formation. However, this is yet to be proven.

The physiologic properties of medications administered influence their distribution within the cerebrospinal fluid and spinal cord. Opioid medications primarily exert their effect in the gray matter of the dorsal horn (primarily lamina II or the substantia gelatinosa). The lipid solubility of an agent determines its ability to diffuse to its site of action. Lipid solubility can be expressed in terms of an agent's octanol/water partition coefficient. In order for intrathecal medications to reach their receptors, they must pass through the pia mater and white matter (containing myelinated axons) to reach their site of action within the gray matter. The myelinated fibers within the white matter make it more hydrophobic while the gray matter is more hydrophilic. As a result, hydrophilic opioids have a greater spinal bioavailability and spread more widely in the cerebrospinal fluid (Ummenhofer et al. 2000). Lipophilic agents have a more focal area of action in part due to their more rapid diffusion out of the cerebrospinal fluid (Bernards 2004).

Local anesthetic solutions can be classified as being either hypobaric, isobaric, or hyperbaric based on the solution density when compared to the density of the cerebrospinal fluid. The baricity predicts the direction of local anesthetic spread after administration into the cerebrospinal fluid based on the effects of gravity in relation to the location of medication administration, spinal curvature, and patient position. Isobaric solutions undergo limited spread in the subarachnoid space.

CLINICAL APPLICATIONS

Several painful conditions can be treated using intrathecal drug delivery systems. Noncancer pain conditions that have been treated with intrathecal drug delivery systems include failed back surgery syndrome, compression fractures, spondylosis, spondyloisthesis, and spinal stenosis as well as spasticity following spinal cord injury, complex regional pain syndrome, chronic pancreatitis, neuropathies, and rheumatoid arthritis (Turner, Sears, and Loeser 2007; Belverud, Mogilner, and Schulder 2008). A retrospective study performed in 2010 by Atli et al. examined 55 patients with noncancer pain over a 3-year period and showed a statistically significant decrease in visual analog pain scores between the first refill and all subsequent time periods (1, 2, and 3 years postimplant) (Atli et al. 2010). Twenty-eight patients in this study had a diagnosis of failed back surgery syndrome, 16 had neuropathic pain, five had visceral pain, and six had miscellaneous pain (lipomeningomyelocele, necrotizing fasciitis, idiopathic scoliosis, axial back pain of uncertain etiology, and osteomyelitis).

Comorbid conditions, such as depression, anxiety, and addiction, may exist in patients with chronic noncancer-related pain. Evaluation and management of these conditions should occur prior to consideration of an intrathecal drug delivery system. Personality disorders, for example, have been shown to portend poor response to long-term intrathecal therapy (Brown et al. 1999).

Intrathecal drug delivery systems can be especially useful in the management of patients with cancer-related pain. Pain is often the first sign of malignancy (Cohen and Dragovich 2007). In many cases, pain may be the most feared symptom among individuals with cancer, and it can occur at any point during the disease course. Various treatment options have been utilized in the management of cancer-related pain and include nonsteroidal anti-inflammatories, acetaminophen, opioids, neuropathic pain medications, peripheral nerve blocks, sympathetic blocks, and continuous epidural analgesia as well as intrathecal drug delivery systems. The advantage of intrathecal drug delivery is that it may reduce the systemic side effects. Furthermore, direct medication delivery to the site of action allows for more rapid and effective analgesia. Intrathecal drug delivery systems can be useful in alleviating pain in 60%–80% of patients experiencing chronic cancer-related pain (Deer et al. 2012).

In addition to pain, intrathecal drug delivery systems can be used to manage spastic hypertonia though the administration of baclofen. It has been effective in treating spastic hypertonia in spinal cord injury (Ordia et al. 1996; Coffey et al. 1993; Meythaler et al. 1992; Penn et al. 1989), cerebral palsy (Albright et al. 2003; Meythaler et al. 2001), brain injuries (Meythaler, McCary, and Hadley 1997; Becker, Alberti, and Bauer 1997), multiple sclerosis (Rizzo et al. 2004), and stroke (Ivanhoe et al. 2006). Recent studies have shown that the use of intrathecal baclofen can result in reduced impairment, improved, gait, upper extremity function, and pain relief (Francisco et al. 2009; Sadiq and Wang 2006; Francisco and Boake 2003).

Intrathecal drug delivery systems may not be appropriate in all patients with clinical indications. It is contraindicated in patients with significant psychiatric comorbidities, significant emaciation preventing implantation, active infection over the catheter or pump implantation site, sepsis, cerebrospinal fluid outflow obstruction, intracranial hypertension, hemodynamic instability, and significant coagulopathy or who require continuous therapeutic anticoagulation preventing temporary discontinuation (Bottros and Christo 2014; Smith and Coyne 2003).

COMPLICATIONS

Complications of intrathecal drug delivery systems can be classified as mechanical, pharmacologic, surgical, patient specific, and refill related. This chapter focuses on the mechanical complications. These can further be subclassified as catheter-related or pump-related complications.

Catheter-related complications have an incidence of 15%–25% (Follett et al. 2003; Follett and Naumann 2000). They can result from catheter migration, dislodgement, occlusion, kinking, leaking, puncture, or shearing. Proper catheter placement and surgical technique may decrease the incidence of shearing. For example, a paramedian approach to intrathecal catheter insertion may decrease the incidence of catheter shearing (Kamran and Wright 2001). Furthermore, several new catheters have been developed to reduce such complications (Follett and Naumann 2000). Evaluation of catheter placement and integrity can be performed by a fluoroscopic catheter dye study and should include the entire extent of the tubing, connectors, and catheter tip. Subsequently, a catheter access port aspiration may be performed to ensure free flowing CSF. Spiral computed tomography (CT) following isotonic myelogram contrast injection into the catheter access port injection can also be employed to evaluate catheter patency. Following contrast administration, the patient is immediately scanned from two vertebral segments above the catheter tip down through the pump site (Francisco et al. 2009).

Catheter tip granulomas are a rare but potentially devastating complication. A granuloma is a noninfectious collection of inflammatory cells located at the catheter tip. Over time, it can increase in size and cause spinal compression, leading to devastating neurologic complications. It has an incidence of 0.04% at 1 year and 1.16% after 6 years. The cause of these granulomas is unclear. They may arise as a result of a reaction to the infused medication, a low-grade infection, or a catheter tip reaction. Granulomas have been associated with opioids in the intrathecal space; however, they have not been reported with lipophilic opioids, such as fentanyl or sufentanil (Bottros and Christo 2014).

An intrathecal pump malfunction may result in either pump failure, underdosing, or overdosing. In addition to symptoms of medication withdrawal or overdose, an audible alarm or significant variation between the expected and actual reservoir volume may signal pump malfunction or a catheter-related problem. The most common cause of pump malfunction is the rotor (Francisco et al. 2009). Rotor failure will cause a loss of drug delivery. It can be diagnosed with a rotor test. This test involves obtaining a radiograph of the rotor, programming a specific bolus, and using repeated imaging to visualize the expected rotor rotation. The Synchromed II has a three-arm rotor, for example, and is programmed to rotate 120°. A rotor stall requires pump replacement. In some cases, a rotor stall can be seen with severely kinked catheters (Francisco et al. 2009).

FUTURE DIRECTIONS

Future directions of intrathecal drug delivery systems include advancements in technology and medication delivery. Monitoring systems to directly measure the reservoir volume and catheter pressure can improve safety by assisting in troubleshooting and catheter occlusion detection. Material advancements may improve durability and patient outcomes.

The benefits of intrathecal drug delivery are well established; however, decreasing efficacy with prolonged treatment may limit analgesia in long-term therapy. Intrathecal microdosing has been proposed as a means to prevent opioid-induced hyperalgesia and prolong treatment efficacy. Intrathecal microdosing involves utilizing doses as low as 25 to 50 mcg/day to produce long sustained analgesia (Deer et al. 2012). In 2012, Hamza et al. published a 3-year prospective study showing the efficacy of low-dose intrathecal opioid management in the management of chronic noncancer pain. Microdosing may be a promising alternative to traditional dosing promoting long-term efficacy and analgesia.

REFERENCES

Albright, A. L., R. Gilmartin, D. Swift, L. E. Krach, C. B. Ivanhoe, and J. F. McLaughlin. 2003. "Long-term intrathecal baclofen therapy for severe spasticity of cerebral origin." *J Neurosurg* 98 (2): 291–5. doi: 10.3171/jns.2003.98.2.0291.

Atli, A., B. R. Theodore, D. C. Turk, and J. D. Loeser. 2010. "Intrathecal opioid therapy for chronic nonmalignant pain: A retrospective cohort study with 3-year follow-up." *Pain Med* 11 (7): 1010–6. doi: 10.1111/j.1526-4637.2010.00876.x.

Battal, B., M. Kocaoglu, N. Bulakbasi, G. Husmen, H. Tuba Sanal, and C. Tayfun. 2011. "Cerebrospinal fluid flow imaging by using phase-contrast MR technique." *Br J Radiol* 84 (1004): 758–65. doi: 10.1259/bjr/66206791.

Becker, R., O. Alberti, and B. L. Bauer. 1997. "Continuous intrathecal baclofen infusion in severe spasticity after traumatic or hypoxic brain injury." *J Neurol* 244 (3): 160–6.

Belverud, S., A. Mogilner, and M. Schulder. 2008. "Intrathecal pumps." *Neurotherapeutics* 5 (1): 114–22. doi: 10.1016/j.nurt.2007.10.070.

Bernards, C. M. 2004. "Recent insights into the pharmacokinetics of spinal opioids and the relevance to opioid selection." *Curr Opin Anaesthesiol* 17 (5): 441–7.

Bhatia, G., M. E. Lau, K. M. Koury, and P. Gulur. 2013. "Intrathecal Drug Delivery (ITDD) systems for cancer pain." *F1000Res* 2: 96. doi: 10.12688/f1000research.2-96.v4.

Bier, A. 1899. "[Attempts over Cocainisirung of the Ruckenmarkers]." *Langenbecks Arch Klin Chir Ver Dtsch Z Chir* 51: 361–9.

Bottros, M. M., and P. J. Christo. 2014. "Current perspectives on intrathecal drug delivery." *J Pain Res* 7: 615–26. doi: 10.2147/JPR.S37591.

Brown, J., J. Klapow, D. Doleys, D. Lowery, and U. Tutak. 1999. "Disease-specific and generic health outcomes: A model for the evaluation of long-term intrathecal opioid therapy in noncancer low back pain patients." *Clin J Pain* 15 (2): 122–31.

Coffey, J. R., D. Cahill, W. Steers, T. S. Park, J. Ordia, J. Meythaler, R. Herman, A. G. Shetter, R. Levy, B. Gill et al. 1993. "Intrathecal baclofen for intractable spasticity of spinal origin: Results of a long-term multicenter study." *J Neurosurg* 78 (2): 226–32. doi: 10.3171/jns.1993.78.2.0226.

Cohen, S. P., and A. Dragovich. 2007. "Intrathecal analgesia." *Anesthesiol Clin* 25 (4): 863–82, viii. doi: 10.1016/j.anclin.2007.07.001.

Deer, T. R., J. Prager, R. Levy, J. Rathmell, E. Buchser, A. Burton, D. Caraway et al. 2012. "Polyanalgesic Consensus Conference 2012: Recommendations for the management of pain by intrathecal (intraspinal) drug delivery: Report of an interdisciplinary expert panel." *Neuromodulation* 15 (5): 436–64; discussion 464–6. doi: 10.1111/j.1525-1403.2012.00476.x.

Enzmann, D. R., and N. J. Pelc. 1991. "Normal flow patterns of intracranial and spinal cerebrospinal fluid defined with phase-contrast cine MR imaging." *Radiology* 178 (2): 467–74. doi: 10.1148/radiology.178.2.1987610.

Follett, K. A., K. Burchiel, T. Deer, S. Dupen, J. Prager, M. S. Turner, and R. J. Coffey. 2003. "Prevention of intrathecal drug delivery catheter-related complications." *Neuromodulation* 6 (1): 32–41. doi: 10.1046/j.1525-1403.2003.03005.x.

Follett, K. A., and C. P. Naumann. 2000. "A prospective study of catheter-related complications of intrathecal drug delivery systems." *J Pain Symptom Manage* 19 (3): 209–15.

Francisco, G. E., and C. Boake. 2003. "Improvement in walking speed in poststroke spastic hemiplegia after intrathecal baclofen therapy: A preliminary study." *Arch Phys Med Rehabil* 84 (8): 1194–9.

Francisco, G. E., M. F. Saulino, S. A. Yablon, and M. Turner. 2009. "Intrathecal baclofen therapy: An update." *PM R* 1 (9): 852–8. doi: 10.1016/j.pmrj.2009.07.015.

Henry-Feugeas, M. C., I. Idy-Peretti, O. Baledent, A. Poncelet-Didon, G. Zannoli, J. Bittoun, and E. Schouman-Claeys. 2000. "Origin of subarachnoid cerebrospinal fluid pulsations: A phase-contrast MR analysis." *Magn Reson Imaging* 18 (4): 387–95.

Ivanhoe, C. B., G. E. Francisco, J. R. McGuire, T. Subramanian and S. P. Grissom. 2006. "Intrathecal baclofen management of poststroke spastic hypertonia: Implications for function and quality of life." *Arch Phys Med Rehabil* 87 (11): 1509–15. doi: 10.1016/j.apmr.2006.08.323.

Kamran, S., and B. D. Wright. 2001. "Complications of intrathecal drug delivery systems." *Neuromodulation* 4 (3): 111–5. doi: 10.1046/j.1525-1403.2001.00111.x.

Lamer, T. J. 1994. "Treatment of cancer-related pain: When orally administered medications fail." *Mayo Clin Proc* 69 (5): 473–80.

Medtronic Inc. 2010. SynchroMed Programmable Infusion Systems Clinical Reference Guide System Components.

Meythaler, J. M., S. Guin-Renfroe, C. Law, P. Grabb, and M. N. Hadley. 2001. "Continuously infused intrathecal baclofen over 12 months for spastic hypertonia in adolescents and adults with cerebral palsy." *Arch Phys Med Rehabil* 82 (2): 155–61. doi: 10.1053/apmr.2001.19246.

Meythaler, J. M., A. McCary, and M. N. Hadley. 1997. "Prospective assessment of continuous intrathecal infusion of baclofen for spasticity caused by acquired brain injury: A preliminary report." *J Neurosurg* 87 (3): 415–9. doi: 10.3171/jns.1997.87.3.0415.

Meythaler, J. M., W. D. Steers, S. M. Tuel, L. L. Cross, and C. S. Haworth. 1992. "Continuous intrathecal baclofen in spinal cord spasticity. A prospective study." *Am J Phys Med Rehabil* 71 (6): 321–7.

Ordia, J. I., E. Fischer, E. Adamski, and E. L. Spatz. 1996. "Chronic intrathecal delivery of baclofen by a programmable pump for the treatment of severe spasticity." *J Neurosurg* 85 (3): 452–7. doi: 10.3171/jns.1996.85.3.0452.

Penn, R. D., S. M. Savoy, D. Corcos, M. Latash, G. Gottlieb, B. Parke, and J. S. Kroin. 1989. "Intrathecal baclofen for severe spinal spasticity." *N Engl J Med* 320 (23): 1517–21. doi: 10.1056/NEJM198906083202303.

Pert, C. B., and S. H. Snyder. 1973. "Opiate receptor: Demonstration in nervous tissue." *Science* 179 (4077): 1011–4.

Rizzo, M. A., O. C. Hadjimichael, J. Preiningerova, and T. L. Vollmer. 2004. "Prevalence and treatment of spasticity reported by multiple sclerosis patients." *Mult Scler* 10 (5): 589–95.

Sadiq, S. A., and G. C. Wang. 2006. "Long-term intrathecal baclofen therapy in ambulatory patients with spasticity." *J Neurol* 253 (5): 563–9. doi: 10.1007/s00415-005-0060-4.

Segal, M. B., and M. Pollay. 1977. "The secretion of cerebrospinal fluid." *Exp Eye Res* 25 Suppl: 127–48.

Smith, T. J., and P. J. Coyne. 2003. "How to use implantable intrathecal drug delivery systems for refractory cancer pain." *J Support Oncol* 1 (1): 73–6.

Stockman, H. W. 2006. "Effect of anatomical fine structure on the flow of cerebrospinal fluid in the spinal subarachnoid space." *J Biomech Eng* 128 (1): 106–14.

Turner, J. A., J. M. Sears, and J. D. Loeser. 2007. "Programmable intrathecal opioid delivery systems for chronic noncancer pain: A systematic review of effectiveness and complications." *Clin J Pain* 23 (2): 180–95. doi: 10.1097/01.ajp.0000210955.93878.44.

Ummenhofer, W. C., R. H. Arends, D. D. Shen, and C. M. Bernards. 2000. "Comparative spinal distribution and clearance kinetics of intrathecally administered morphine, fentanyl, alfentanil, and sufentanil." *Anesthesiology* 92 (3): 739–53.

Wallace, M., and T. L. Yaksh. 2000. "Long-term spinal analgesic delivery: A review of the preclinical and clinical literature." *Reg Anesth Pain Med* 25 (2): 117–57. doi: 10.1053/rapm.2000.0250117.

Wang, J. K., L. A. Nauss, and J. E. Thomas. 1979. "Pain relief by intrathecally applied morphine in man." *Anesthesiology* 50 (2): 149–51.

Yamada, S., M. Miyazaki, Y. Yamashita, C. Ouyang, M. Yui, M. Nakahashi, S. Shimizu, I. Aoki, Y. Morohoshi, and J. G. McComb. 2013. "Influence of respiration on cerebrospinal fluid movement using magnetic resonance spin labeling." *Fluids Barriers CNS* 10 (1): 36. doi: 10.1186/2045-8118-10-36.

16 Cancer Stem Cell Drug Delivery

Masturah Bte Mohd Abdul Rashid, Lissa Nurrul Abdullah, Tan Boon Toh, and Edward Kai-Hua Chow

CONTENTS

INTRODUCTION

Cancer stem cells (CSCs) are a small, biologically unique subset of cancer cells with the ability to self-renew and generate the diverse repertoire of cells that make up the bulk tumor.[1] These cells are termed cancer stem cells due to their "stem-like" properties shared commonly with normal tissue stem cells. These properties include the ability to self-renew extensively (both symmetrically and asymmetrically) and their capacity to differentiate into different lineages (multipotency). The latter, however, is not a mandatory feature of CSCs. Nevertheless, the concept of CSCs lying at the apex of the hierarchy is of considerable importance as it highlights the need to eradicate the CSC populations to achieve an effective cure.

The first evidence for the existence of CSCs came from the study on human acute myeloid leukemia (AML).[2] Bonnet and Dick showed that using $CD34^+CD38^-$ cell surface markers that normally marks for human primitive hematopoietic progenitors, they could induce AML in irradiated transplanted nonobese diabetic (NOD)/severe combined immunodeficient (SCID) mice. Importantly, this study highlights the importance of in vivo serial transplantation assays for repopulation capacity and the identification of CSCs. Subsequently, using similar experimental approaches, CSCs have been prospectively isolated in a variety of solid tumors, including breast, colon, brain, prostate, liver, and skin.[3–8] Al-Hajj et al. showed that $CD44^+CD24^{-/low}Lineage^-$ breast cancer cells enriched for a tumor-initiating population. When implanted into the mammary fat pad of NOD/SCID mice, these cells generated tumors with as few as 1×10^3 cells whereas injection of as many as 1×10^5 unsorted breast tumor cells failed to initiate tumor growth. Subsequently, Singh et al. demonstrated that CD133/Prominin-1 marks for brain tumor–initiating cells in the pediatric and adult brain tumors with increased capacity for self-renewal and proliferation in vitro. They demonstrated that as few as 100 $CD133^+$ cells were sufficient and necessary to initiate and recapitulate the tumor upon transplantation into immunodeficient mice.

Tumors formed from these xenograft experiments showed that these isolated CSCs recapitulate the heterogeneity of the original tumor. Since then, the gold standard to identify CSC functionally is the ability of these cells to reform a phenotypic copy of the original tumor in an orthotopic transplantation model, more often than not performed as a limiting dilution assay. Non-CSCs, by definition, lack this ability and fail in the transplantation model. Recently, the rarity of these CSCs was challenged by Quintana et al., who demonstrated that the frequency of CSCs could be altered based on several experimental parameters. These include the addition of extracellular matrix in the form of matrigel, using a more severe immune-compromised strain of mouse, and prolonging the duration of the experimental end point. This demonstrates that the tumor-initiating capacity, at least in melanoma and some AML and acute lymphocytic leukemia (ALL) cases, is an artifactual consequence of the conditions employed in the xenograft models.[9–11] Nevertheless, other cancers continue to show rare tumorigenic cells in the repopulation of bulk tumor, and syngeneic transplantation of mouse cancer cells have all been consistent with the cancer stem cell model.

Key signaling pathways that are crucial in the normal development of stem cells, for example, Notch, Wnt, and Hedgehog, have been a focus of increasing interest in cancer therapy as these pathways are commonly found to be altered in CSCs. Although the roles of these pathways have been studied extensively, the effectiveness of targeting these pathways, specifically the CSCs, the long-term self-renewing population, is of immense interest in designing a therapy with an effective cure, abrogating the sustenance of the tumors. In this chapter, we discuss the roles of several important mediators of resistance in tumors, including the ABC family of transporters, CSC-related stem-like markers, self-renewal pathways, and DNA damage repair proteins. We also present current ways of enhanced drug delivery in tumors as a potential treatment strategy in the future medicine.

DRUG RESISTANCE IN CANCER STEM CELLS (CSCs)

Multidrug resistance is the key stammer in eliminating cancer via chemotherapy. Ninety percent of chemotherapy failures in metastatic cancers result from chemoresistance.[12] Recurring tumors and cancer relapse are problematic as both acquire resistance to chemotherapy and radiation. This is worrying as, apart from local surgical resection, both conventional therapies remain as the mainstay in the treatment of cancers. Cancer patients can acquire chemoresistance through desensitization of tumor cells after periodic exposure to chemotherapeutics or preexisting intrinsic factors that contribute toward drug resistance prior to treatment. Intrinsic chemoresistance is of immense interest as it highlights the importance and complexity of tumor heterogeneity and the hierarchical concepts of cancer stem cells. These factors are likely to contribute to intrinsic resistance to therapies.

Compelling evidence in different solid tumors and hematological cancers has emphasized the presence of a fraction of stem cell–like cells that is highly tumorigenic and capable of self-renewal and multidirectional differentiation and possibly recapitulating the whole heterogeneity of human cancer in xenograft mouse models. This invigorating discovery and subsequent understanding eventually gave rise to the cancer stem cell (CSC) hypothesis. Of note, these putative CSCs demonstrated in different malignant solid tumors are chemo- and radio-resistant. By targeting these putative CSCs demonstrated in reported malignant solid tumors, regression of the tumor bulk and the chances of reducing risk of metastasis are optimistic. It is now clear that chemoresistance is one of the major modalities in functional characterization of CSCs. Therefore, overcoming chemoresistance mediated by CSCs has tremendous implications in eradicating cancer.

CSCs and ABC Transporters

Drug transporters are crucial in defining the pharmacokinetic profile of chemotherapeutics across target tissues systemically. They are also one of the major factors to consider during drug discovery and development. Impaired drug transporters can lead to insufficient drug influx or excessive drug efflux. These transporters are the main cause of multidrug resistance and pose a great challenge to clinicians in treating various diseases. ATP binding cassette (ABC) transporters are ATP-power driven pumps that have been well studied for more than 35 years and function mainly as exporters in eukaryotes. ATP transporters may differ in tissue distribution, but they all function to protect host cells against a diverse array of substrates, including endogenous metabolites, toxins, antibiotics, and drugs. Deficits in these ABC transporters are deleterious, and their presence is critical in maintaining homeostasis in cell biology.[13] In cancer, three ABC superfamily multidrug efflux transporters are well documented in driving chemoresistance. These include ABCB1 (P-glycoprotein or multidrug resistance protein 1), ABCC1 (multidrug resistance-associated protein 1), and ABCG2 (Breast Cancer Resistance Protein).

In general, ABC transporters evolved from a single ancestral gene, thereby sharing highly conserved domains with overlapping similarities. They typically consist of four domains: two transmembrane domains (TMD) and two nucleotide-binding domains (NBD). TMDs bear the substrate binding sites whereas NBDs mediate the catalytic activity of ATP within the cytoplasm. ABCB1 transporters are one of the widely studied ABC transporters since 1976.[14] This protein is strategically located at the epithelial lining of major organs and blood vessels: brain, inner ear, testes, small intestines, colon, and pancreatic and bile ducts. It is normally lowly expressed and is responsible to ward off potential xenobiotics from entering sensitive organs. ABCB1 has a wide array of drug substrates, including the anticancer drugs Doxorubicin, Paclitaxel, and Vincristine.[15] ABCG2 transporters, similar to their ABCB1 counterpart, are localized in the apical surface of polarized membranes, including the milk ducts of the mammary glands and the endothelium of blood capillaries and veins. ABCC1 transporters, on the other hand, are associated with glutathione homeostasis and keep bilirubin levels in check. Due to its structural conformation, ABCG2 interacts poorly with most ABCB1 substrates and effluxes anionic drugs, such as tyrosine kinase inhibitors Imatinib and Geftinib. ABCG2 have been implicated as a potential cancer prognostic marker and possess clinical relevance for drug resistance. Diestra et al. supported this idea through developing a monoclonal antibody BXP21 that targets ABCG2 in a large panel of human solid tumors: endometrium, stomach, lung, liver, gastrointestinal tract, and skin.[16] Therefore, identifying ABC transporter overexpression in different cancers provides a means to identify CSCs.

One such method is the enhanced efflux activity of a fluorescence substrate Hoechst 33342 by ABC drug transporters. The Hoechst 33342 dye exclusion assay was originally discovered by Margaret Goodell when isolating hematopoietic stem cells from mouse bone marrow.[17] Cells capable of excluding the Hoechst 33342 dye were defined as side population (SP). SP cells display high expression of both ABCB1 and ABCG2 transporters. They are capable to initiate and sustain tumor growth when implanted into immune-compromised mice. Zhou and colleagues first demonstrated that ABCG2 mediate chemoresistance in the hematopoietic stem cells (HSCs) as defined by the SP phenotype.[18] Using the ABCG2 knockout mouse model, they showed that ABCG2 expression is required for preserving the SP properties, and the absence of ABCG2 expression confers increased sensitivity toward Mitoxantrone in HSCs. Similarly, when ABCG2 expression was reduced using short interfering RNA in thyroid cancer cells, marked increased TUNEL stainings were observed after exposure to Doxorubicin.[19] Hence, identifying ABCG2 via the SP approach seems to be a robust marker to identify CSCs. However, recent studies have shown that other ABC efflux pumps are also involved in chemotherapeutic resistance. For instance, both MDR1 and ABCG2 render chemoresistance to Doxorubicin whereas only MDR1 effluxes Paclitaxel. Identification of CSCs via SP phenotype were also reported in a number of solid tumors and hematological cancers, including C6 glioma and gastric cell lines as well as in primary human cancer tumor samples. Studies from our lab have demonstrated that hepatic tumors are driven by Myc as indicated by a significant number of SP cells enriched with chemoresistant CSCs.[20] On the same note, SP phenotype in cancer is also determined by the predominating specific oncogenic activation, and exploiting SP analysis enriches CSCs.

It is now clear that ABC transporters are the main causes of chemoresistance. However, most ABC protein inhibitors/modulators, such as Verapamil displayed a high toxicity profile in early clinical trials.[21] In addition, other phenotypes contributing to resistance in cancer are also discouraging. The use of an enhanced drug delivery platform, for example, nanodiamonds, showed promising efficacy against tumors via drug transporter inhibition. Our recent data have shown that using Mitoxantrone physically adsorbed onto nanodiamonds (ND-MTX) with the drug-resistant triple-negative breast cancer cell line MDA-MB-231 showed increased sensitivity and increased drug retention in the cells.[22] Hence, our work suggests that using nanodiamonds to deliver mitoxantrone may have potential clinical benefits, particularly in patients with drug-resistant cancers or recurrences.

ALDH AND CHEMORESISTANCE

Recent investigations have corroborated the role of cytosolic enzyme aldehyde dehydrogenase (ALDH) in CSC-mediated chemoresistance. Of note, ALDH also serves as a pivotal CSC marker in several types of cancer. To date, there are 19 isoforms of ALDH in humans, distributed within the membrane, cytosol, and nucleous.[23] ALDH are critical in detoxification through catalyzing oxidation of aldehydes to carboxylic acids. Importantly, this metabolic marker concentrates in the liver and kidneys and forms part of the Phase I non P450 cytochrome aldehyde reduction enzymes that are heavily involved in biotransformation of xenobiotics and drugs.[24] Aldehydes are produced by a number of metabolic processes, such as lipid peroxidation, and if not cleared efficiently, these accumulated aldehydes become cytotoxic to the cells. The biotransforming capability also potentiates ALDH to function as an antioxidant by scavenging hydroxyl radicals, absorbing UV rays, and NADPH production. This may, in part, explain how CSCs contribute to radio-resistance.

Retinoic acid (RA) signaling is also an important metabolic pathway that modulates cell proliferation and differentiation, promoting cell cycle arrest and apoptosis. Out of the 19 isoforms, ALDH1 catalyzes the conversion of retinol to retinoic acids in an irreversible manner.[25] Through RA signaling, ALDH is also involved in early embryonic development and differentiation of progenitor/multipotent stem cells.[26,27] Hence, ALDH activity is being extensively studied as it suggests a potential metabolic marker for CSCs. Indeed, elevated ALDH activities are commonly shown in cancer through the ALDEFLUOR assay. Using a fluorescent substrate-based assay that allows quantification of ALDH activity in live cells, the "ALDEFLUOR" assay was first shown in the isolation of hematopoietic stem cells from human umbilical cord blood and is now widely used to identify and isolate CSCs.[26] Using the ALDEFLUOR assay, Ginestier et al. demonstrated high ALDH activity in both normal human breast and breast carcinomas.[28] The observation that normal and malignant stem/progenitor cells are marked by the same marker further supports the cancer stem cell hypothesis. Of note, the authors showed that as few as 500 $ALDH^+$ cells from human breast tumors were capable of inducing tumor growth in a xenograft model whereas as many as 50000 $ALDH^-$ cells did not, highlighting that ALDH marks a population of highly tumorigenic cells in breast cancer.

Since ALDH has been shown to be a potential marker to identify CSCs, it is crucial to find out if these $ALDH^+$ cells also mark for a population of chemoresistant clones. In 1984, the anticancer drug cyclophosphoamide was first studied in a population of chemoresistant L1210 leukemic cells where ALDH was implicated to confer drug resistance.[29] ALDH-mediated cyclophosphamide resistance was also demonstrated in medulloblastoma.[30] The role of ALDH1, a specific isoform of ALDH, is of particular interest when it comes to targeting cancer cells. ALDH1 overexpression has been well documented in a variety of drug-resistant cancer cell lines, including the lung, breast, and colon cancers. Moreb et al. demonstrated that pretreatment of drug-resistant lung adenocarcinoma cell line A549 with all-trans retinoic acid (ATRA) resulted in increased sensitivity of the cancer cells to 4-hydroperoxycyclophosphamide (4-HC) in vitro, through the downregulation of ALDH1A1 and ALDH3A1 enzymatic activities but not their mRNAs levels.[31] This highlights that both ALDH1A1 and ALDH3A1 are both potential molecular targets and that ATRA regulates ALDH activity at the protein level. In breast cancer, Alysha et al. showed that ALDH1$^+$ cells were more resistant to conventional chemotherapeutics, for example, epirubicin and paclitaxel.[32] However, when these ALDH1$^+$ breast cancer cells were pretreated with ATRA, the sensitivity of the cells to these chemotherapeutics increased significantly, but not the ALDH1$^-$ cells, therefore, suggesting that ALDH1 can serve as a potential molecular target for combating drug resistance in cancers. The use of ATRA has been widely used in the differentiation of normal stem cells.[26,33] Since CSCs have been identified as the culprit of drug resistance, the use of ATRA or another differentiation agent can drive these stem-like cancer cells to a more differentiated state, rendering them more sensitive to chemotherapy. One good example for the use of ATRA in the clinics is the treatment of acute promyelocytic leukemia (APL).[34] Treatment of APL cells with ATRA increases the RA levels in the cells, which results in the decrease of ALDH1A1 and ALDH3A1 levels. This drives the APL cells to a more mature neutrophil state, enhancing the use of chemotherapeutics. Therefore, ALDH activity and its possible role in driving drug resistance in CSCs deserves more in depth study and focus.

Antiapoptotic BCL-2 Protein Family Members in CSCs

Evasion of apoptosis is one of the hallmarks in cancer.[35] An attractive mechanism by which CSC drives chemoresistance is through the upregulation of prosurvival proteins, such as B-cell lymphoma-2 (BCL-2) protein, B-cell lymphoma extra-large (BCL-XL), BCL-2-like-2 (BCL-W), BCL-2-related protein A1A (BCL-A1A), and myeloid cell leukemia sequence-1 (MCL1).[36] These prosurvival proteins share similar Bcl-2 homology domains. The overexpression of these prosurvival proteins is able to protect cells from apoptotic stimuli. BCL-2 promotes prosurvival signals via binding to the proapoptotic proteins Bax and Bak, perturbing their ability to release apoptotic proteins, such as cytochrome c, through mitochondrial outer membrane permeabilization (MOMP) or by modulation of Ca^{2+} signaling by inhibiting inositol 1,4,5-trisphosphate receptors (IP3Rs) in the endoplasmic reticulum.[36,37]

The highlight of Bcl-2 in cancer was first demonstrated in 14:18 chromosomal translocation leukemic cell lines transfected with Bcl-2 to induce overexpression. This resulted in resistance to killing by cytotoxic drugs.[38] Bcl-2 and related proteins are crucial in normal development, such as tissue homeostasis, the regulation of apoptosis, and protection against pathogens and the survival of many progenitor cells, including the hematopoietic stem cells, sperm cells, neuronal cells, fetal erythroid progenitors, renal epithelial progenitors, and melanocyte progenitors.[39–42] In tumors, Bcl-2 was shown to be activated by many oncogenic signaling pathways, such as PI3K–AKT, RAS–RAF–MEK–ERK, SRC, and signal transducer and activator of transcription 3 (STAT3) and Janus kinase (JAK)–signal transducer pathways. Activation of these oncogenic pathways promotes cell survival, proliferation, invasion, and metastasis. Additionally, it was shown in an acute lymphoblastic leukemia patient that one of the joining segments on the 14q chromosome arm is rearranged with a segment on chromosome 8, where the c-myc oncogene resides.[43] The cooperation of myc and Bcl2 in driving tumorigenesis in lymphomas is further supported by other convincing evidence in a double knock-in mice model where mice overexpressing both Bcl2 and myc showed hyperproliferation of pre-B and B-cells and are terminally ill from leukemia much faster as compared to transgenic mice that overexpress myc only.[44]

There is increasing evidence that CSCs-mediated chemoresistance is fueled in part by the regulation of Bcl-2 in resisting apoptosis. Madjd et al. demonstrated that the breast cancer stem cell marker CD44 correlated with Bcl-2 expression in a panel of 146 breast cancer tumor patients.[45] This suggests that Bcl-2 may play a role in conferring chemoresistance in a subset of CSCs by evading apoptosis. In AML, chemoresistance has been attributed to the presence of quiescent $CD34^+$ AML cells. These quiescent $CD34^+$ AML cells expressed high levels of antiapoptotic genes BCL-2 and BCL-XL, suggesting a role for these antiapoptotic genes in chemoresistance. Treating these chemoresistant quiescent $CD34^+$ AML cells with ATRA significantly reduced the prosurvival signals and rendered them sensitive to the drug Arabinoside, a common chemotherapeutic agent for treating AML and non-Hodgkins lymphomas. However, it is still unclear as to how Bcl-2 drives chemoresistance, but its correlation with common CSC markers and their associated oncogenic pathways suggests its importance in the contribution of CSC-mediated resistance. For instance, $CD133^+$ colon CSCs displayed significant sensitivity to Oxaliplatin, 5-fluorouracil (5-FU), and death ligand TRAIL treatments after combined treatment with interleukin-4 (IL-4) neutralizing antibodies and IL-4 antagonist.[46] This suggests a role of IL-4 in conferring chemoresistance through the autocrine survival signals most likely by key anti-apoptotic pathways that includes downregulation of Bcl-xl. In addition, using an Akt1 inhibitor specific to the Akt pathway significantly reduced the expression of prosurvival proteins, such as Bcl2 in $CD133^+$ HCC CSCs.[47] It was also demonstrated that through Akt inhibition, these $CD133^+$ HCC CSCs were more sensitive to conventional chemotherapeutics, such as Doxorubicin and 5-fluorouracil. Cammareri et al. showed that Aurora-A, a serine threonine kinase involved in mitosis regulation, is highly expressed in the CSC fraction of colorectal cancer cells.[48] Interestingly, knockdown of Aurora A resulted in significant growth inhibition and enhanced sensitivity to chemotherapeutic treatments with 5-FU and oxaliplatin of these colorectal CSCs. Importantly, Aurora A knockdown resulted in downregulation of several prosurvival Bcl-2 members. Taken together, these results demonstrated a crucial role for Bcl-2 survival response in conferring chemoresistance in CSCs and a potential therapeutic target to overcome chemoresistance.

DNA Damage Response and Radio-Resistance in CSCs

Enhanced DNA repair mechanisms and DNA damage responses are frequently observed in CSCs. Understanding the molecular mechanisms underlying altered DNA damage response and repair pathways are crucial as they correlate significantly with chemoresistance in CSCs. Ataxia Telangiectasia Mutated (ATM) and ATM and Rad-3-related (ATR) are two key DNA damage response signaling proteins in the cells.[49] Upon activation, Chk1 and Chk2 are phosphorylated, and together with other DNA damage response proteins, such as p53, lead to the downregulation of cyclin-dependent kinases (CDKs) activities.[50] This will result in cell cycle arrest at G1/S, S, and G2/M phases. Cell cycle arrest provides a time lapse to enable cells to repair their corresponding damaged DNA or drive cells with irreversible DNA damage to apoptosis. DNA damage can be induced in tumor cells by chemotherapy or ionizing radiation. By hijacking the DNA damage response as described earlier, CSCs can evade apoptosis by prolonging cell cycle arrest for the recruitment of DNA repair effectors. This is evident in recurrent tumors as subsequent use of radiation in these tumors is not effective due to the acquired mutations conferring resistance to DNA damage response.

Work by Bao et al. demonstrated that the CSC population within the highly malignant glioma glioblastoma multiforme (GBM) contributes to enhance radio-resistance.[51] They showed that $CD133^+$ CSCs contribute to glioma radio-resistance through the preferential activation of DNA damage checkpoint response and an increased capacity for DNA repair compared to the non-CSC fraction marked by $CD133^-$. Importantly, by using a specific inhibitor of Chk1 and Chk2 checkpoint kinases, the radio-resistance of these $CD133^+$ glioma CSCs could be reversed. This suggests that inhibition of Chk1 and Chk2 kinases may be of therapeutic value in the treatment of radio-resistant GBMs. A follow-up study by the same group showed that LICAM, a neural cell adhesion molecule, marks $CD133^+$ glioma CSCs and is responsible for mediating the DNA damage checkpoint response via the NBS1-ATM axis.[52] The authors showed that lentiviral-mediated shRNA knockdown of NBS1 attenuated checkpoint activation in glioma CSCs in response to IR-induced DNA damage and that by ectopic expression of NBS1, they were able to rescue the effects of reduced checkpoint activation and restore the preferential survival of glioma CSCs after radiation. Collectively, they identified the L1CAM-mediated checkpoint activation via the NBS1-ATM axis as one of the critical regulatory mechanisms underlying the preferential DNA damage checkpoint response and radio-resistance of glioma CSCs. Resistance to the chemotherapeutic agent, Temozolomide (TMZ) is frequently observed in a subset of GBM patients. TMZ resistance has been attributed to the enhanced expression of O6-methylguanine-DNA-methyltransferase (MGMT), an enzyme that catalyzes the repair of DNA double-strand breaks (DSBs). Liu et al. demonstrated that glioma CSCs display enhanced resistance to several chemotherapeutic agents and express elevated *MGMT* expression as compared to non-CSC counterparts.[53]

Radiotherapy is an indispensable tool to regress local tumors by the use of precisely targeted X-rays. Ionizing radiation (IR) and radiomimetic drugs are aimed at killing cancer cells through the induction of DSBs in DNA. A host of factors have been identified to cause radio-resistance in cancers, including DNA repair ability, cell cycle status, and prosurvival pathways that protect the cells from extracellular stress. As the bulk tumor is usually heterogeneous, radiation may selectively kill the cancer cells that are radiosensitive while leaving behind a CSC population that are radio-resistant, and these surviving CSCs may repopulate and contribute to radio-resistance. Indeed, both reports by Bao et al. and Tamura et al. showed enrichment of the $CD133^+$ glioma CSC fraction after IR, contributing to recurrence in glioma patients.[51,54] In breast cancers, Philips and colleagues demonstrated that the levels of γ-H2AX foci (a marker of DSBs in DNA) in $CD24^{-/low}/CD44^+$ breast CSCs decreased after irradiation.[55] The enhanced radioresistance in $CD24^{-/low}/CD44^+$ breast CSCs is in part attributed to the decrease in reactive oxygen species (ROS) production and high intracellular levels of radical scavengers, contributing to a decrease in DSB formation. On the same note, Diehn et al. reported marked differences in ROS levels of both the normal breast stem cells and breast CSCs.[56] They showed that breast CSCs accumulate fewer DNA DSBs after IR, and that correlates with the increased persistence of CSCs in vitro. More importantly, these radio-resistant breast CSCs expressed enhanced levels of genes, such as glutamate cysteine ligase, glutathione synthetase, and FoxO1, all of which are involved in the production of an important ROS scavenger, glutathione (GSH).

In addition, Woodward et al. demonstrated that radiotherapy results in enrichment for the stem and progenitor cell–containing population in a murine mammary epithelial cell culture, and particularly augments the stem-cell antigen (Sca)–positive compartment of the side population cells.[57] Consistent with this, CSCs from a p53-null mouse mammary tumor had upregulation of active β-catenin and were able to undergo DNA damage repair more efficiently compared to the non-CSCs after exposure to IR.[58]

Another mechanism that contributes to the development of radio-resistance in cancer cells is the activation of autophagic pathways. Autophagy is a cellular conservatory catabolic process that involves intracellular double membrane sequestration of damaged organelles or misfolded proteins for degradation and turnover.[59] Autophagy is paradoxical as it can lead to cell death in a nonapoptotic manner in some circumstances or serve as a survival mechanism providing metabolic support in times of cellular stress such as exposure to radiation. Autophagy is frequently activated in cancer following radiation and/or chemotherapy. Lomonaco et al. demonstrated that autophagy was preferentially activated in $CD133^+$ glioma CSCs after gamma radiation.[60] It was also observed that various autophagy-related proteins including ATG5, ATG12, and LC3 were expressed at higher levels as compared to the $CD133^-$ non-CSCs. Furthermore, using the autophagy inhibitor bafilomycin A1 and the silencing of ATG5 and beclin1 sensitized the $CD133^+$ glioma CSCs to gamma radiation and significantly decreased the viability of the irradiated cells and their ability to form tumor spheres. In breast cancer, Han et al. evaluated the role of autophagy and transforming growth factor–activated kinase 1 (TAK1) in radio-resistance. The authors showed that inhibition of autophagy-enhanced radio sensitivity through suppression of radiation-induced TAK1 activation, suggesting that the modulation of TAK1-induced autophagy may be a good therapeutic strategy to treat radio-resistant breast cancer.

The role of the tumor microenvironment has been of great interest as a potential avenue for therapeutic targeting. It has been proposed that CSCs reside in a specific tumor microenvironment or vascular niches that tightly regulate oxygen and nutrition to maintain these CSCs, facilitating their invasiveness and tumor-propagating properties. A disorganized neovasculature is frequently observed in many cancers and has a protective role in shielding CSCs from therapeutic insults. Calabrese et al. identified a fraction of $CD133^+/Nestin^+$ glioma CSCs enriched in areas of high microvessel density, suggesting that tumor vasculature generates a specialized niche microenvironment in which the formation and maintenance of CSCs proceeds.[61] In addition, coimplantation of tumor cells with endothelial cells led to rapid tumor formation, implicating the influence of the vascular niche on tumor initiation. Glioma CSCs are enriched in functional aberrant niches, predominantly the perivascular niche, which provides microenvironmental cues for the maintenance of CSCs. Abrogation of this niche via antiangiogenic drugs, for example, Bevacizumab, resulted in abrogation of CSC self-renewal and depletion of tumor growth, further validating the importance of the perivascular niche in the regulation of tumorigenesis.

CURRENT STRATEGIES TO TARGET CSCs

Traditional chemotherapy targets cancer cells that are highly proliferative, which shrinks the bulk of the tumor but leaves behind a small proportion of CSCs that are spared from the treatment due to their quiescent nature. In this section, we lay out several current therapeutic approaches that are used to treat these resistant cancer stem cells. These approaches serve to complement chemo- and radiotherapy so as to prevent tumor relapse and to nip the tumor at its bud.

Targeting Cancer Stem Cell–Specific Pathway

Signaling pathways are vital for self-renewal, proliferation, and differentiation of normal stem cells. Cancer stem cells and normal stem cells share many similarities in terms of self-renewal, differentiation processes, expression of specific surface markers and oncogenes, utilization of common signaling pathways, and regulation of stem cell niche.[62] In this section, we highlight the aberration of these signaling pathways, which include Notch, Hedgehog, Wnt/β-catenin, STAT3, PI3K/AKT, Bmi-1, and c-Met in cancer stem cells.[62]

The Notch Signaling Pathway

The Notch pathway determines cell fate decisions and is involved in cell–cell communication in normal stem cells.[63,64] Notch signaling is activated when one of the five Notch ligands (Delta-like 1, 3, 4 and Jagged1, 2) binds to one of the four transmembrane receptors (Notch 1–Notch 4) on an adjacent cell. This will result in the γ-secretase-mediated proteolytic cleavage and the subsequent release of Notch intracellular domain (NICD), which translocates into the nucleus and regulates transcription of target genes.[63] Studies have shown a context-dependent aberrant notch signaling pathway in several cancers.[65] Notch signaling has been implicated in a variety of cancers, both as an oncogene and as a tumor suppressor, depending on the relevant context. The function of Notch signaling as an oncogene is first demonstrated in T-lineage acute lymphoblastic leukemia (T-ALL), a neoplastic disorder accounting for approximately 15% of all acute lymphoblastic leukemias. It has been shown that overexpression or activating mutations of the NOTCH1 gene are the main oncogenic drivers in majority of T-ALL patients.[66,67] The role of Notch signaling in tumor suppression is observed in skin, pancreatic epithelium, and hepatocytes.[68] In the keratinocytes of the skin, Notch activation induces differentiation and cell cycle arrest by inducing p21WAF1/Cip1 expression. More importantly, they showed that keratinocyte-specific deletion of the Notch1 gene evoked marked epidermal hyperplasia and aberrant expression of multiple differentiation markers.

In the context of cancer stem cells, Notch signaling is involved in self-renewal, differentiation, and apoptosis. It has been demonstrated by Purow et al. that targeting overexpressed components of the Notch signaling pathway, such as Notch-1, Delta-like-1, or Jagged-1 by RNA interference induced apoptosis and inhibited the proliferation of several glioma cell lines.[69] More importantly, pretreatment of glioma cells with short interfering RNAs targeting Notch components significantly prolongs the survival of mice in an orthotopic xenograft model. Collectively, these results highlight the therapeutic significance of targeting the Notch signaling pathway in glioma.

Inhibiting the proteolytic process, which is crucial for the formation of NICD, is one of the most efficient ways to inhibit the Notch signaling pathway. Fan et al. showed that γ-secretase inhibitors (GSIs) blocked the Notch pathway in glioblastoma by decreasing the proliferation of $CD133^+$ stem-like cells derived from glioma patients with the mRNA levels of the stem cell markers *NESTIN*, *BMI1*, and *OLIG2* decreasing in a dose-dependent manner.[70] In addition, GSI also inhibited the growth of tumor neurospheres in vitro and tumor propagation in vivo. The activity of GSI against CSCs has also been demonstrated in breast cancer, whereby using a GSI MRK-003 also reduced the frequency of tumor-initiating cells in primary mammary epithelial cell and tumor cell populations as assessed by cell transplantation into syngeneic mice.[71] However, the main drawback for GSIs is that they are nonselective drugs as they block the cleavage of all four Notch ligands and various γ-secretase substrates. A promising drug that is currently in clinical trials targeting the Notch pathway is an antibody that targets Delta-like 4 ligand (DLL4).[72] Upon treatment with anti-DLL4, there was a decline in the population of colon CSCs expressing cell markers $ESA^+/CD44^+/CD166^+$. Furthermore, administering anti-DLL4 together with irinotecan further decreased the percentage of this population of colon CSCs. This therapeutic efficacy was also seen in breast, lung, and prostate cancer.

Hedgehog Signaling Pathway

There are three members in the Hedgehog family; Sonic (SHH), Indian (IHH), and desert hedgehog (DHH), which are essential for development and patterning during mammalian embryogenesis.[73] It is triggered when the secreted peptide binds to the 12-span transmembrane receptor, patching and inactivating it. This results in the phosphorylation and stabilization of smoothened (SMO), which in turn activates downstream target genes via the glioma-associated oncogene homolog (Gli) family of zinc-finger transcription factors. *SHH* and *IHH* RNA expression have been shown to be elevated in CSCs of multiple primary pancreatic tumor explant models.[74] Pancreatic tumor spheres, which are enriched in CSCs, have increased levels of hedgehog pathway components.[75] Inhibiting the key signaling molecule, SMO, is effective in arresting the Hedgehog pathway. Some examples of compounds that bind and inactivate SMO include cyclopamine and the recently FDA-approved drug, GDC-0449 (Vismodegib).[76,77] Vismodegib is used to treat patients with recurrent, locally advanced or metastatic basal cell carcinoma.[77] However, these drugs would not be as effective on tumors that have dysregulation of components downstream of SMO in the signaling pathway.

It has been shown that the Hedgehog signaling pathway is crucial for the maintenance of self-renewal and tumorigenesis of CSCs in brain tumors.[78] Differentiation of tumor neurospheres derived from GBM patients reduced both stemness and Hedgehog signaling pathways. Importantly, not all glioma patients have an activated Hedgehog signaling pathway as determined by Gli expression, highlighting the importance of molecular subgroups of brain tumors, whereby targeting this pathway would be ineffective.[79] Nevertheless, it was demonstrated that by treating glioma CSCs with cyclopamine or using RNA interference against *GLI*, a reduction in the self-renewal capability and proliferation while enhanced apoptosis was observed in these cells in vitro while inhibition of tumor propagation was observed in vivo.[78]

Tang et al. showed that an active compound in green tea, (-)-epigallocatechin-3-gallate (EGCG), inhibited the expression of SMO, Patched 1 and 2 as well as the transcription factors, Gli1 and Gli2.[80] EGCG also suppressed the transcriptional activity of Gli1 and Gli2 in a dose-dependent fashion as demonstrated via luciferase assay. This highlights the advantage that ECGC has over the aforementioned compounds as it targets the downstream Hedgehog pathway as well. In addition, EGCG inhibited the early metastasis of pancreatic cancer stem cells and their spheroid and colony formation. The addition of Quercetin to ECGC, a flavonoid with multiple effects, synergistically enhanced the mentioned inhibitory effects.

Wnt/β-Catenin Signaling Pathway

The Wnt signaling pathway is another developmental pathway involved in multiple biological processes, such as embryogenesis, cell proliferation, survival, and differentiation.[81] The canonical Wnt/β-catenin pathway involves secreted Wnt ligands that bind to the Frizzled family and either low-density lipoprotein receptor-related protein 5 or 6 (LRP 5/6). This prevents the GSK3-dependent phosphorylation of β-catenin, thus stabilizing its levels. β-catenin will then accumulate in the cytosol, translocate to the nucleus, and interact with the members of the T-cell factor (TCF)/lymphoid enhancer factor (LEF) family of DNA binding proteins, resulting in the release of transcriptional repressors like Groucho proteins from target genes. Recruitment of coactivators, like cAMP response element-binding protein (CREB)-binding protein (CBP), will initiate the expression of downstream target genes.[81] In cancer, the Wnt pathway is important for the self-renewal and maintenance of CSCs.[82] Oncogenic mutations of β-catenin or inactivating mutations of tumor suppressors, such as adenomatous polyposis coli (APC) or Axin, may result in the dysregulation of the Wnt/β-catenin pathway in CSCs, which induces neoplastic proliferation.

The Wnt pathway can be targeted at different steps of the transduction pathway; antagonists of the Wnt ligand that prevents ligand–receptor interactions, transcriptional coactivator antagonists, or targeting the PDZ domain of Dishevelled (Dvl). Small molecule inhibitors include nonsteroidal anti-inflammatory drugs (NSAIDs) and the CBP/β-catenin antagonist, ICG-001. NSAIDs, like aspirin and celecoxib, inhibit the activity of cyclooxygenase (COX) or promote degradation of TCF. The lead compound, ICG-001, selectively inhibits CBP, thus preventing its interaction with β-catenin. As such, β-catenin will bind to another coactivator, p300, instead of which it initiates differentiation with minimum proliferative ability. ICG-001 was shown to eliminate imatinib-resistant leukemic stem cells both in vitro and in vivo.[83,84] This antagonist of the coactivator would be more effective for tumors that are activated by mutations in adenomatous polyposis coli (APC) or β-catenin as compared to antagonists of the Wnt ligands, which act upstream of the mutations.

An example of a biologic interfering in the Wnt pathway is through RNA interference (RNAi). Teng et al.[85] showed that this resulted in a decrease in CSC properties; decreased expression of the Wnt target gene cyclin D1, proliferation, clone formation, and migration of Cisplatin-resistant lung cancer A549 cells. These studies showed the importance of the Wnt signaling pathway in CSCs, evident in the decreased properties of the CSCs upon inhibition. The caveat of this therapeutic target is that normal stem cells may also be affected as they are also critical in maintaining normal somatic stem cell homeostasis. As such, these inhibitors have to be used in tandem with other CSC-targeting therapies to exclusively target the CSCs more effectively and specifically.

Differentiation of CSCs

Besides the inhibitory approaches against self-renewal pathways listed earlier, another promising way to control tumor progression is to induce terminal differentiation in CSCs. This arrests their self-renewal property and limits their tumor-initiating ability.[86] There are mainly two kinds of drugs that can induce differentiation: retinoic acid and drugs targeting epigenetic changes. It has been shown that the population of $CD133^+$ stem-like glioma cells diminished upon treatment with all-trans retinoic acid (ATRA)-containing medium with reduced migratory, angiogenic, and tumorigenic abilities as well. Differentiation also enhanced cell death in response to irradiation and chemotherapeutic treatment, suggesting that this approach can be employed synergistically with existing treatments.[87] Another differentiation factor, bone morphogenetic protein (BMP) 4, has been shown to increase the neural differentiation potential in human glioblastoma cells with a concomitant decrease in proliferation via the Smad pathway upon activating the BMP receptors.[88] A similar response was also exhibited in colonic stem cells upon BMP4 induction.[89] Inducing terminal differentiation also enhanced the sensitivity of colorectal CSCs to chemotherapeutic agents, fluorouracil, and oxaliplatin.

An example of an epigenetic approach to induce differentiation would be the use of histone deacetylase (HDAC) inhibitor, suberoylanilide hydroxamic acid (SAHA). Butler et al. has demonstrated that SAHA inhibited both androgen-sensitive and -insensitive prostate cancer cells in vitro and arrested prostate tumor growth in vivo via hyperacetylation of histones to induce differentiation.[90] These examples show promising potential to induce differentiation before the administration of chemotherapeutic agents to eliminate cancer stem cells.

Immunotherapy against CSCs

Cancer stem cells have been shown to be selectively targeted by dendritic cell-based vaccines. Teitz-Tennenbaum et al. has demonstrated that pulsing mice with a CSC-rich tumor population confers anti-tumor resistance.[91] Syngeneic, immunocompetent mice were inoculated subcutaneously with D5 melanoma or SCC7 squamous cell carcinoma cells, and the CSCs from the heterogeneous tumors were identified based on elevated ALDH activity. Tumor cells with high ALDH activity have self-renewal properties, form transplantable tumors, and phenotypically resemble the parenteral tumor cells. As reported, these cells were labeled as $ALDH^{bright}$ while tumor populations with low ALDH activity were known as $ALDH^{dim}$. These tumor cells were then used to pulse dendritic cell lysate. Dendritic cells pulsed with $ALDH^{bright}$ potently inhibited tumor growth as compared to those pulsed with $ALDH^{dim}$. This study showed that the immune system could be primed to eradicate cancer stem cells with enhanced ALDH activity.

T-cells and natural killer (NK) cells are also known to play roles as a defense mechanism against tumors. NK cells are regulated by inhibitory and triggering surface receptors. Since some of these surface receptors are not found or lost in tumor cells, including melanomas (for example, the MHC class I molecules), NK cells are able to discriminate between normal and tumor cells.[92–94] In the absence of inhibitory signals, activated NK receptors can interact with specific ligands to mediate cell lysis. Pietra et al. showed that in vitro nonadherent spheroid tumor cells in melanoma melanospheres (enriched in CD133 and NESTIN stem cell–associated CSC markers) were targeted and killed by interleukin-2 (IL-2)-cultured polyclonal NK cell populations.[95] The above results suggest that NK-based adoptive immunotherapy could represent a novel therapeutic approach to eradicate or deplete the CSCs in metastatic melanoma.

ENHANCED DRUG DELIVERY AGAINST CSCs

History of the First Nanoparticle Drug Delivery Particle

The advent of nanoparticle drug delivery was to overcome the limitations of administering a drug on its own. With an enhanced delivery system, drugs can be stabilized by protecting them from degradation in blood circulation before reaching the intended target, resulting in higher therapeutic efficacy and decreased toxicity of the drugs.[96] In cancer, nanoparticles preferentially target the tumor cells via the enhanced and permeability retention (EPR) effect. This increases the sensitivity of the drug by specifically targeting the tumor cells.[97] They can be adapted to include biomolecules and other molecular-scale components. For instance, drugs are attached to the nanoparticle either by being encapsulated, dispersed, adsorbed, or conjugated to the nanoparticle.[96]

Liposomes were the first nanoparticle platform applied in medicine since Bangham described them in 1961.[98,99] Thereafter, other research groups followed suit but with a focus on other nanoparticles, such as polyacrylic beads for oral administration.[100,101] Couvreur et al. demonstrated the advantage of using nanoparticles for treating cancer.[102] In 1995, Doxil (pegylated liposome-encapsulated doxorubicin) became the first liposome drug delivery system approved for human use by the U.S. Food and Drug Administration (FDA).[103]

Doxil/Liposomal Drug Delivery

Liposomes are self-assembled vesicles, consisting of phospholipid molecules that form a spherical bilayer structure with an aqueous core, thus enabling them to contain the drugs required. In attaining effective drug delivery, drugs should reach targeted sites with minimal loss in the blood circulation without affecting nondesired sites. Liposomal drug delivery is able to achieve that via passive or active targeting. Passive targeting takes advantage of the characteristics of the blood vessel: enlarged gap junctions between endothelial cells and compromised lymphatic drainage.[96] This allows migration of nanoparticles of up to 400 nm. Doxil is a perfect example of passive targeting.

Doxorubicin is an anthracycline chemotherapeutic drug that is highly toxic, having effects on both the heart and kidney. However, using the liposomal platform to deliver doxorubicin has protected the patients from cardiotoxicity.[104] Doxil is currently used for ovarian cancer and Kaposi's sarcoma.[105,106] Doxil has been shown to improve Doxorubucin levels in Kaposi Sarcoma's tissues by 22-fold as compared to healthy normal skin tissues.[107] The development of Doxil has definitely improved the delivery of Doxorubucin in chemotherapeutics. Besides Doxil, other cancer-therapeutic drugs have been conjugated onto liposomes as well. Some examples include DaunoXome and Marqibo, where Daunorubucin and Vincristine have been conjugated to liposomes, respectively.[107] Not exclusively to cancer, there are liposomal drug delivery systems that have been marketed for antifungal purpose, Amphotec, and for macular degeneration, Visudyne.

Liposomes have also demonstrated selective drug delivery through passive targeting by adding target components.[108] In the targeting of CSCs, CD44 has been chosen as a target of interest as it has been shown to be highly expressed by CSCs from colon and breast cancers.[3,109] Eliaz et al. demonstrated that modifying the surface of liposomes through the addition of the CD44 ligand, hyaluronic acid (HA), increases the delivery and efficacy of Doxorubucin to CD44-overexpressing tumor cells.[110] This seems to be promising for liposomal drug delivery as it excludes unwanted targeting from occurring.

Despite the advances in liposomal drug delivery, liposomes present some shortcomings, such as the burst release of drugs and low encapsulation efficiency. Cells are impermeable to liposomes, and as such, drugs are released into the extracellular space. This raises the efforts to improve their stability and sustaining drug action by increasing their circulation half-life.[96] An illustrative example is provided in Doxil™ where the polymer PEG (poly-ethylene-glycol) was added to protect the liposomes from macrophages so as to increase their lifespan in blood circulation.

Targeted Drug Delivery against CSC Markers

Current therapeutic strategies against cancers are not satisfactory, and treatment efficacy is often hindered by chemoresistance. Overwhelming evidence of the role of CSC in the initiation of cancer and progression over the past century have positioned CSCs at the forefront of cancer research. Therefore, eradicating CSCs through targeted drug delivery is essential. Hitherto, an extensive list of CSC markers in solid tumors is now available.[111] Despite the debates of the reliability of CSC molecular markers in human tumors over cancer cell lines and mice models, many have demonstrated clinical relevance. As such, more can be done to overcome these limitations, such as selecting combinative CSC markers based on functional traits and signaling pathway activities.

The present challenges faced by conventional chemotherapeutic delivery are collectively listed as follows: drug pharmacokinetics and biodistribution, multidrug resistance, clearance by the reticuloendothelial system, and the hydrophobicity of anticancer drugs. To address these obstacles, nanoparticle-based drug delivery systems are highly promising. Nanoparticle-based delivery platforms encompass both passive and active targeting. Passive targeting of drug delivery systems involves manipulating the enhance permeation and retention effect (EPR). The EPR effect was first described in cancer by Matsumura and Maeda in the development of SMANCs, a tumoritropic copolymer of sterene and maleic acid to an antitumor protein, Neocarcinostatin (NCS).[97] The EPR effect increases the pore size of solid tumors from approximately 6 nm to a range of 100 nm to 780 nm in vasculature, resulting in leakier vessels that supply the tumor microenvironment.[112,113] It is this feature through blood circulation and extravasation that enables passive drug delivery to the tumor site. Passive targeting may not be ideal in some cancers as a majority of delivered drug–drug conjugates home to organs such as liver, spleen, and lungs. On the other hand, active targeting through nanoparticles (NPs) requires specific interaction between the drug–drug carrier and target cell via complementary ligand–receptor binding. Nevertheless, this mode of interaction still occurs intravenously, and its uptake largely depends on EPR.

Nanoparticle-based delivery systems largely depend on the rational design, which includes the ability to control drug release or increase retention time in the blood circulation. Nanoparticles act mainly as nanocarriers when conjugated to drugs with considerations of some general properties, including size and stability. NPs come in different forms, such as lipid-based vehicles, polymer carriers, metallic nanoparticles, carbon structures, and inorganic particles. Small size NPs are shown to retain a longer time in the blood circulation while larger NPs are cleared rapidly by the kidneys.[114] Stability of NPs determines the capacity of NPs to accumulate at tumor sites. Polymer micelles were shown to dissociate within minutes to an hour when released into the systemic circulation, rendering its design ineffective to sustain drug release.[115,116]

One of the early developments of NP-platforms consisted of targeting the notorious CSC marker $CD133^+$ that is highly expressed in a subset of glioblastoma patients. The synthetic analogue of Curcumin and its NP-based encapsulated counterpart possess high chemosensitizing properties when used singly or in combination with other chemotherapeutics.[117] Subsequently, a NP-based Curcumin-loaded Nano-Curc™ was shown to reduce CD133⁺ cells in both medulloblastoma and glioblastoma in a dose-dependent fashion as well as perturbing neurosphere formation.[118] In addition, the authors also observed that curcumin specifically blocked the Hedgehog but not Notch signaling pathway. Hyaluronic acid (HA) is a major extracellular matrix component that is bound by $CD44^+$ to facilitate the growth of CSCs during cancer progression or metastasis. Consequently, HA was exploited as a drug carrier for various NP or NP-drug conjugates to target CSCs. In ovarian cancer lines IGROV-1 and OVCAR-3, NP-HA-Paclitaxel bioconjugates were used to target cancer cells via $CD44^+$-mediated endocytosis.[119] Similarly, NP-HA was also used to target CD44 in squamous cell carcinoma SCC7 tumors in the same fashion. Both NP-HA conjugates resulted in tumor growth inhibition.

Lipoprotein-like nanocapsules (LPN) are also useful in generating vectorized nanocarriers. The LPN surface enables the coupling of a monoclonal antibody to CSC marker of interest. Bourseau-Guilmain et al. have successfully demonstrated narrow-size biodistribution of LPNs conjugated to thiolated anti-CD133 monoclonal antibodies (mAbs) in CACO-2 cells. CACO-2 cells have naturally high levels of CD133, and when stimulated by LPN-mAb, there is an increase in CD133 marker detachment.[120]

siRNA Therapy against Cancer

RNA interference (RNAi) is a naturally occurring mechanism in eukaryotic cells. It involves the use of double-stranded ribonucleic acids to silence gene expression. The applications of RNAi in medicine involve the delivery of double-stranded siRNA to the cancer cells. One important advantage of using siRNA technology is the target specificity and the ability to target or inhibit the gene expression of a mutant oncogene without affecting the wild type. This can be achieved through careful design of siRNA target sequences. Henceforth, RNAi has quickly emerged as one of the most promising anticancer strategies since its discovery in 1998 by Andrew Fire and Crag Mello.

siRNAs are short double-stranded nucleotides of approximately 18–23 nucleotides. They induce the cleavage of a specific gene in the cells through their complementary base pairing with the mRNA, leading to degradation of the mRNA. siRNAs are formed from cleavage of long double-stranded (ds) RNAs by the RNase-III-type enzyme named Dicer.[121] Subsequently, siRNAs are recruited to the protein complexes by the dsRNA-binding protein, R2D2, forming RNA-induced silencing complex (RISC).[122] The RISC-siRNA complex will then bind to the complementary sequences on the mRNA and result in its degradation.

One of the major obstacles of siRNA delivery in vivo is their short half-life and poor stability. Due to their low molecular weight, siRNAs are rapidly degraded by endo- and exonucleases before clearance via the kidneys.[123,124] Besides the instability and rapid clearance of siRNAs, it is known that unmodified siRNAs are recognized by Toll-like receptors (TLRs), which subsequently stimulate the immune system that causes an interferon response and cytokine induction as well as complement activation.[125] In addition, since siRNA is capable of multiple transcript regulation, off-target effects are unavoidable. This involves careful use of dosage and backbone design of these siRNAs. Therefore, there is urgent need to develop a delivery system that can present the initiation of such immune-responsive elements within the body while being capable of delivering these siRNAs at the desired site of action.

An attractive strategy for systemic delivery of siRNAs is the use of nanoparticles. These nanoparticles are engineered and designed based on several factors, which include a well-characterized and biocompatible material, extended circulating half-life, ability to evade the immune and the reticuloendothelial systems (RES), long shelf life, and the ability to accumulate in the target cells over normal cells. siRNAs are mainly delivered systemically via two ways: passive and active (targeted) delivery. Passive delivery utilizes the inherited properties of nanoparticles to accumulate in the cancer tissues due to the EPR effect or in organs of the RES. Whereas in active or targeted delivery, specific antibodies or ligands are attached to the nanoparticles to direct them to their specific sites of action for maximal therapeutic efficacy and avoiding nonspecific silencing of nonmalignant cells.

Liposomes were used as a delivery vector for DNA-based drugs due to their protective functions, including reduced nuclease degradation and renal clearance while enhancing cellular uptake. Since then, a number of lipid nanoparticles (LNPs) have been developed using different lipids and lipid-like structures. LNP-mediated siRNA delivery has since entered several clinical trials, including the treatment of hypercholesterolemia and cancer.[126,127] Alnylam pharmaceuticals initiated a trial of ALN-VSP, a LNP-siRNAs formulation to target VEGF and kinesin spindle protein (KSP) in solid tumors.[128] This is the first dual-targeted RNAi drug that inhibits two pathways simultaneously using two different siRNAs. They demonstrated that the use of ALN-VSP in patients was safe and well-tolerated with RNAi activity in both the liver and extrahepatic metastases. This study provides a proof-of-concept for RNAi therapeutics in humans and forms the basis of LNP-siRNAs treatment. Another first-in-human phase I clinical trial reported by Schultheis et al. demonstrated the efficacy of Atu027 (a LNP-siRNA targeting protein kinase N3 in the vascular endothelium) in patients with advanced solid tumors.[129] Specifically, Atu027 was well tolerated in patients with stabilization of the disease achieved in 41% of the patients with some experiencing complete or partial regression of metastases. Together, delivering siRNAs via LNPs seems to be a potential RNAi therapeutics in the future.

Another example of nanoparticle application in RNAi is the use of cyclodextrin-based polymer. The first-in-human phase I clinical trial (NCT00689065) using a targeted, nanoparticle delivery system of siRNA was reported in melanoma patients.[130,131] The nanoparticles consist of a linear, cyclodextrin-based polymer (CDP), a human transferrin protein (TF) ligand to engage the overexpressed TF receptors on the cancer cells, polyethylene glycol (PEG) to promote stability of the nanoparticle, and a siRNA-targeting ribonucleoside-diphosphate reductase subunit M2 (RRM2), which is an established anticancer target. The use of these nanoparticles (CALAA-01) has been demonstrated to be well tolerated in primates, and more importantly, they showed dose-dependent accumulation of targeted nanoparticles in tumors and the consequent reduction of the anticancer target, RRM2.

Another study by Jensen et al. showed that the spherical nucleic acid (SNA) nanoparticle can be effectively delivered across the blood–brain barrier (BBB) into xenogenic glioma explants and reduce the endogenous oncoprotein BclLike12.[132] These SNAs consist of densely packed, highly oriented siRNAs encapsulating an inorganic gold nanoparticle core. In addition, SNAs showed remarkable stability in physiological conditions, exhibited no toxicity, and demonstrated substantial accumulation in the brain tumor tissues with persistent gene knockdown without triggering significant immune response and off-target effects. Taken together, SNAs hold great promise in biotherapeutic gene silencing since they can overcome some of the major challenges, such as BBB in CNS-directed drug therapy. Taken together, it is encouraging to note that several RNAi therapeutics using nanoparticles are undergoing clinical trials with results that will eventually guide rational design and development in the future.

Nanocarbon-Based Drug Delivery

Nanocarbons, including nanotubes, graphene, fullerenes, and nanodiamonds, are an important class of nanomaterials with versatile physical and chemical properties that have attracted particular interest in many fields, including medicine. In medicine, nanocarbon technology has become a potential application for the development of drug delivery systems. Conventional chemotherapeutics, such as doxorubicin, camptothecin, nucleotide, and nucleoside analogs have been a mainstay in chemotherapy. However, these drugs are nondiscriminatory between normal and cancer cells, resulting in unwanted side effects, such as cardiotoxicity and nephrotoxicity. Recent application of nanocarbons in chemotherapeutic delivery offers potential solutions to the above problems.

In the past years, carbon nanotubes, a one-dimensional sp^2 carbon nanomaterial, have been heavily studied in animals. Drug delivery via covalent conjugation or noncovalent adsorption onto carbon nanotubes into cells has been demonstrated. In 2008, Liu et al. first reported the in vivo delivery of single-walled carbon nanotubes (SWNT) conjugated with paclitaxel in a 4T1 murine breast cancer model.[133] Importantly, the authors demonstrated that using SWNT-paclitaxel, they could achieve higher efficacy in suppressing tumor growth than clinical paclitaxel alone, possibly through prolonged blood circulation and higher uptake of the drug via the EPR effect. Subsequently, Wu et al. developed a multiwalled carbon nanotube (MWNT)-based drug delivery system by conjugating carbon nanotubes with the antitumor agent 10-hydroxycamptothecin (HCPT) using hydrophilic diaminotriethylene glycol as the spacer between nanotube and drug moieties.[134] They showed that MWNT-HCPT conjugates were more superior in terms of antitumor efficacy than the clinical HCPT in a hepatic tumor mouse model. Despite the promising potential of drug delivery using carbon nanotubes, more work has to be done in the future to overcome the issue of in vivo toxicity.

Another nanocarbon that has shown promise in the biomedical application is graphene. Graphene is composed of a single layer of sp^2 carbon atoms organized in a honeycomb two-dimensional (2D) crystal lattice. Due to its unique structure and geometry, graphene exhibits remarkable physical and chemical properties, including biocompatibility, large surface area, high fracture strength and high electrical and thermal conductance. The use of graphene for in vivo treatment of cancer in an animal model has been demonstrated. Specifically, graphene sheets were used as drug carriers by functionalization of graphene oxide (GO) with amine-terminated branched PEG, yielding PEGylated nano-graphene oxide (NGO). These NGOs have high stability in physiological solutions and can be effectively loaded with aromatic anticancer drugs, such as doxorubicin via π-π stacking. In a study by Zhang et al., GO conjugated with PEI was used for Bcl-2 siRNA loading.[135] Sequential delivery of Bcl-2 siRNA and doxorubicin into cancer cells by GO-PEI caused a significant decrease in cell viability. The first use of graphene for in vivo cancer therapy was demonstrated by Yang et al. by labeling PEGylated NGO with a near infrared (NIR) fluorescent dye capable of in vivo bioimaging.[136] The authors could observe high uptake of NIR-labeled PEGylated NGO in several xenograft tumor models that is further demonstrated to be effective for in vivo photothermal ablation of tumors. However, there is noticeable in vivo toxicity of using graphene, and its toxicology is dependent on its surface coating chemistry. Hence, more work has to be done to better design graphene as a safe and effective delivery vector in the clinics.

Nanodiamonds (NDs), a carbon-based material of approximately 2–8 nm, has been extensively studied recently due to their unique properties that are suitable for diagnostic and other clinical applications. The most notable application of NDs is their use in drug delivery for cancer therapy. Chemoresistance, either intrinsic or acquired, contributes to treatment failure in more than 90% of metastatic cancers.[12] ABC drug transporters are the main cause of multidrug resistance and present a major hurdle in cancer therapy.[137] The recent focus of overcoming ABC transporter–mediated drug resistance has been made on the reversal of multidrug resistance phenotype by inhibition of ABC transporters. However, many of these ABC transporter inhibitors have failed to produce clinically significant data due to issues with pharmacokinetic or pharmacodynamic interactions and toxicities.[21,138] This caveat can soon be overcome by the use of NDs in drug delivery. The potent drug delivery capability of NDs has been demonstrated in mouse models of anthracycline-resistant liver and mammary cancers.[139] The use of doxorubicin adsorbed onto NDs (NDX) showed increased tumor regression with lower systemic toxicity as compared to the clinical form of free doxorubicin. Furthermore, delivery of anthracyclines by NDs was capable of overcoming ABC transporter-mediated chemoresistance in hepatic CSCs, proving to be an effective modification for killing CSCs and more chemosensitive non-CSCs equally.[140] An even more impressive therapeutic gain in the treatment of cancers would be the use of a specific target component to deliver drugs at their desired site of action. This has been shown by Moore et al. where ND complexes containing chemotherapeutic agent, epirubicin, and a target component, EGFR antibody were delivered into mice bearing breast cancer xenografts. Mice with EGFR-targeted ND complexes survived the treatment with significant tumor regression and drug tolerance as compared to the administration of the clinical standard epirubicin. The safety and efficacy of ND-drug complexes highlight the use of ND-based platforms to support a wide spectrum of treatment modalities.

CONCLUSIONS

In summary, cancer stem cells present an attractive target for therapeutic intervention because this unique subset of cells has been shown to be critical for the initiation, progression, and sustenance of many tumors. The ablation of CSCs offers the promise of durable disease remission and long-term survival of cancer patients. The identification of CSCs based solely on surface markers are proven insufficient, and there is a need to refine and characterize CSCs based on their functional status. Several methods discussed above have showed promising targeting of CSCs, including the inhibition of critical CSC self-renewal pathways, targeting drug delivery using specific CSC surface markers, inducing differentiation in CSCs, and the use of immunotherapy against CSCs. With the current surge in interest in nanomedicine, more work has been done in terms of rational design and development to improve the use of nanoparticles in a biological setting. The use of nanoparticles in the targeting of cancers or CSCs is especially challenging since it requires optimization of these nanomaterials in clinical settings, such as dosing and efficacy, to achieve an effective therapeutic cure.

REFERENCES

1. Reya, T., Morrison, S. J., Clarke, M. F. & Weissman, I. L. Stem cells, cancer, and cancer stem cells. *Nature* 414, 105–111, doi: 10.1038/35102167 (2001).
2. Bonnet, D. & Dick, J. E. Human acute myeloid leukemia is organized as a hierarchy that originates from a primitive hematopoietic cell. *Nature medicine* 3, 730–737 (1997).
3. Al-Hajj, M., Wicha, M. S., Benito-Hernandez, A., Morrison, S. J. & Clarke, M. F. Prospective identification of tumorigenic breast cancer cells. *Proceedings of the National Academy of Sciences of the United States of America* 100, 3983–3988, doi: 10.1073/pnas.0530291100 (2003).
4. O'Brien, C. A., Pollett, A., Gallinger, S. & Dick, J. E. A human colon cancer cell capable of initiating tumour growth in immunodeficient mice. *Nature* 445, 106–110, doi: 10.1038/nature05372 (2007).
5. Singh, S. K. et al. Identification of a cancer stem cell in human brain tumors. *Cancer research* 63, 5821–5828 (2003).
6. Fang, D. et al. A tumorigenic subpopulation with stem cell properties in melanomas. *Cancer research* 65, 9328–9337, doi: 10.1158/0008-5472.CAN-05-1343 (2005).
7. Collins, A. T., Berry, P. A., Hyde, C., Stower, M. J. & Maitland, N. J. Prospective identification of tumorigenic prostate cancer stem cells. *Cancer research* 65, 10946–10951, doi: 10.1158/0008-5472.CAN-05-2018 (2005).
8. Yang, Z. F. et al. Significance of CD90+ cancer stem cells in human liver cancer. *Cancer cell* 13, 153–166, doi: 10.1016/j.ccr.2008.01.013 (2008).
9. Quintana, E. et al. Efficient tumour formation by single human melanoma cells. *Nature* 456, 593–598, doi: 10.1038/nature07567 (2008).
10. Kelly, P. N., Dakic, A., Adams, J. M., Nutt, S. L. & Strasser, A. Tumor growth need not be driven by rare cancer stem cells. *Science* 317, 337, doi: 10.1126/science.1142596 (2007).
11. Rehe, K. et al. Acute B lymphoblastic leukaemia-propagating cells are present at high frequency in diverse lymphoblast populations. *EMBO molecular medicine* 5, 38–51, doi: 10.1002/emmm.201201703 (2013).

12. Longley, D. B. & Johnston, P. G. Molecular mechanisms of drug resistance. *The Journal of pathology* 205, 275–292, doi: 10.1002/path.1706 (2005).
13. Leslie, E. M., Deeley, R. G. & Cole, S. P. Multidrug resistance proteins: Role of P-glycoprotein, MRP1, MRP2, and BCRP (ABCG2) in tissue defense. *Toxicology and applied pharmacology* 204, 216–237, doi: 10.1016/j.taap.2004.10.012 (2005).
14. Juliano, R. L. & Ling, V. A surface glycoprotein modulating drug permeability in Chinese hamster ovary cell mutants. *Biochimica et biophysica acta* 455, 152–162 (1976).
15. Sharom, F. J. ABC multidrug transporters: structure, function and role in chemoresistance. *Pharmacogenomics* 9, 105–127, doi: 10.2217/14622416.9.1.105 (2008).
16. Diestra, J. E. et al. Frequent expression of the multi-drug resistance-associated protein BCRP/MXR/ABCP/ABCG2 in human tumours detected by the BXP-21 monoclonal antibody in paraffin-embedded material. *The Journal of pathology* 198, 213–219, doi: 10.1002/path.1203 (2002).
17. Goodell, M. A., Brose, K., Paradis, G., Conner, A. S. & Mulligan, R. C. Isolation and functional properties of murine hematopoietic stem cells that are replicating in vivo. *The Journal of experimental medicine* 183, 1797–1806 (1996).
18. Zhou, S. et al. Bcrp1 gene expression is required for normal numbers of side population stem cells in mice, and confers relative protection to mitoxantrone in hematopoietic cells in vivo. *Proceedings of the National Academy of Sciences of the United States of America* 99, 12339–12344, doi: 10.1073/pnas.192276999 (2002).
19. Lopez, J. P. et al. Gefitinib inhibition of drug resistance to doxorubicin by inactivating ABCG2 in thyroid cancer cell lines. *Archives of otolaryngology—head & neck surgery* 133, 1022–1027, doi: 10.1001/archotol.133.10.1022 (2007).
20. Chow, E. K., Fan, L. L., Chen, X. & Bishop, J. M. Oncogene-specific formation of chemoresistant murine hepatic cancer stem cells. *Hepatology* 56, 1331–1341, doi: 10.1002/hep.25776 (2012).
21. Dalton, W. S. et al. A phase III randomized study of oral verapamil as a chemosensitizer to reverse drug resistance in patients with refractory myeloma. A Southwest Oncology Group study. *Cancer* 75, 815–820 (1995).
22. Toh, T. B. et al. Nanodiamond-Mitoxantrone Complexes Enhance Drug Retention in Chemoresistant Breast Cancer Cells. *Molecular pharmaceutics*, doi: 10.1021/mp5001108 (2014).
23. Vasiliou, V. & Nebert, D. W. Analysis and update of the human aldehyde dehydrogenase (ALDH) gene family. *Human genomics* 2, 138–143 (2005).
24. Sladek, N. E. Human aldehyde dehydrogenases: potential pathological, pharmacological, and toxicological impact. *Journal of biochemical and molecular toxicology* 17, 7–23, doi: 10.1002/jbt.10057 (2003).
25. Hsu, L. C., Chang, W. C., Hoffmann, I. & Duester, G. Molecular analysis of two closely related mouse aldehyde dehydrogenase genes: Identification of a role for Aldh1, but not Aldh-pb, in the biosynthesis of retinoic acid. *The Biochemical journal* 339 (Pt 2), 387–395 (1999).
26. Storms, R. W. et al. Isolation of primitive human hematopoietic progenitors on the basis of aldehyde dehydrogenase activity. *Proceedings of the National Academy of Sciences of the United States of America* 96, 9118–9123 (1999).
27. Corti, S. et al. Identification of a primitive brain-derived neural stem cell population based on aldehyde dehydrogenase activity. *Stem cells* 24, 975–985, doi: 10.1634/stemcells.2005-0217 (2006).
28. Ginestier, C. et al. ALDH1 is a marker of normal and malignant human mammary stem cells and a predictor of poor clinical outcome. *Cell stem cell* 1, 555–567, doi: 10.1016/j.stem.2007.08.014 (2007).
29. Hilton, J. Role of aldehyde dehydrogenase in cyclophosphamide-resistant L1210 leukemia. *Cancer research* 44, 5156–5160 (1984).

30. Friedman, H. S. et al. Cyclophosphamide resistance in medulloblastoma. *Cancer research* 52, 5373–5378 (1992).
31. Moreb, J. S. et al. Retinoic acid down-regulates aldehyde dehydrogenase and increases cytotoxicity of 4-hydroperoxycyclophosphamide and acetaldehyde. *The Journal of pharmacology and experimental therapeutics* 312, 339–345, doi: 10.1124/jpet.104.072496 (2005).
32. Croker, A. K. & Allan, A. L. Inhibition of aldehyde dehydrogenase (ALDH) activity reduces chemotherapy and radiation resistance of stem-like ALDHhiCD44(+) human breast cancer cells. *Breast cancer research and treatment* 133, 75–87, doi: 10.1007/s10549-011-1692-y (2012).
33. Tonge, P. D. & Andrews, P. W. Retinoic acid directs neuronal differentiation of human pluripotent stem cell lines in a non-cell-autonomous manner. *Differentiation; research in biological diversity* 80, 20–30, doi: 10.1016/j.diff.2010.04.001 (2010).
34. Petrie, K., Zelent, A. & Waxman, S. Differentiation therapy of acute myeloid leukemia: Past, present and future. *Current opinion in hematology* 16, 84–91, doi: 10.1097/MOH.0b013e3283257aee (2009).
35. Hanahan, D. & Weinberg, R. A. Hallmarks of cancer: The next generation. *Cell* 144, 646–674, doi: 10.1016/j.cell.2011.02.013 (2011).
36. Kelly, P. N. & Strasser, A. The role of Bcl-2 and its pro-survival relatives in tumourigenesis and cancer therapy. *Cell death and differentiation* 18, 1414–1424, doi: 10.1038/cdd.2011.17 (2011).
37. Akl, H. et al. A dual role for the anti-apoptotic Bcl-2 protein in cancer: Mitochondria versus endoplasmic reticulum. *Biochimica et biophysica acta* 1843, 2240–2252, doi: 10.1016/j.bbamcr.2014.04.017 (2014).
38. Tsujimoto, Y., Finger, L. R., Yunis, J., Nowell, P. C. & Croce, C. M. Cloning of the chromosome breakpoint of neoplastic B cells with the t(14;18) chromosome translocation. *Science* 226, 1097–1099 (1984).
39. Adams, J. M. & Cory, S. The Bcl-2 protein family: Arbiters of cell survival. *Science* 281, 1322–1326 (1998).
40. Motoyama, N. et al. Massive cell death of immature hematopoietic cells and neurons in Bcl-x-deficient mice. *Science* 267, 1506–1510 (1995).
41. Print, C. G. et al. Apoptosis regulator bcl-w is essential for spermatogenesis but appears otherwise redundant. *Proceedings of the National Academy of Sciences of the United States of America* 95, 12424–12431 (1998).
42. Rinkenberger, J. L., Horning, S., Klocke, B., Roth, K. & Korsmeyer, S. J. Mcl-1 deficiency results in peri-implantation embryonic lethality. *Genes & development* 14, 23–27 (2000).
43. Pegoraro, L. et al. A 14;18 and an 8;14 chromosome translocation in a cell line derived from an acute B-cell leukemia. *Proceedings of the National Academy of Sciences of the United States of America* 81, 7166–7170 (1984).
44. Strasser, A., Harris, A. W., Bath, M. L. & Cory, S. Novel primitive lymphoid tumours induced in transgenic mice by cooperation between myc and bcl-2. *Nature* 348, 331–333, doi: 10.1038/348331a0 (1990).
45. Madjd, Z. et al. CD44+ cancer cells express higher levels of the anti-apoptotic protein Bcl-2 in breast tumours. *Cancer immunity* 9, 4 (2009).
46. Todaro, M., Perez Alea, M., Scopelliti, A., Medema, J. P. & Stassi, G. IL-4-mediated drug resistance in colon cancer stem cells. *Cell cycle* 7, 309–313 (2008).
47. Ma, S., Lee, T. K., Zheng, B. J., Chan, K. W. & Guan, X. Y. CD133+ HCC cancer stem cells confer chemoresistance by preferential expression of the Akt/PKB survival pathway. *Oncogene* 27, 1749–1758, doi: 10.1038/sj.onc.1210811 (2008).
48. Cammareri, P. et al. Aurora-a is essential for the tumorigenic capacity and chemoresistance of colorectal cancer stem cells. *Cancer research* 70, 4655–4665, doi: 10.1158/0008-5472.CAN-09-3953 (2010).

49. Riley, T., Sontag, E., Chen, P. & Levine, A. Transcriptional control of human p53-regulated genes. *Nature reviews. Molecular cell biology* 9, 402–412, doi: 10.1038/nrm2395 (2008).
50. Sanchez, Y. et al. Control of the DNA damage checkpoint by chk1 and rad53 protein kinases through distinct mechanisms. *Science* 286, 1166–1171 (1999).
51. Bao, S. et al. Glioma stem cells promote radioresistance by preferential activation of the DNA damage response. *Nature* 444, 756–760, doi: 10.1038/nature05236 (2006).
52. Cheng, L. et al. L1CAM regulates DNA damage checkpoint response of glioblastoma stem cells through NBS1. *The EMBO journal* 30, 800–813, doi: 10.1038/emboj.2011.10 (2011).
53. Liu, G. et al. Analysis of gene expression and chemoresistance of CD133+ cancer stem cells in glioblastoma. *Molecular cancer* 5, 67, doi: 10.1186/1476-4598-5-67 (2006).
54. Tamura, K. et al. Accumulation of CD133-positive glioma cells after high-dose irradiation by Gamma Knife surgery plus external beam radiation. *Journal of neurosurgery* 113, 310–318, doi: 10.3171/2010.2.JNS091607 (2010).
55. Phillips, T. M., McBride, W. H. & Pajonk, F. The response of CD24(-/low)/CD44+ breast cancer-initiating cells to radiation. *Journal of the National Cancer Institute* 98, 1777–1785, doi: 10.1093/jnci/djj495 (2006).
56. Diehn, M. et al. Association of reactive oxygen species levels and radioresistance in cancer stem cells. *Nature* 458, 780–783, doi: 10.1038/nature07733 (2009).
57. Woodward, W. A. et al. WNT/beta-catenin mediates radiation resistance of mouse mammary progenitor cells. *Proceedings of the National Academy of Sciences of the United States of America* 104, 618–623, doi: 10.1073/pnas.0606599104 (2007).
58. Zhang, M., Atkinson, R. L. & Rosen, J. M. Selective targeting of radiation-resistant tumor-initiating cells. *Proceedings of the National Academy of Sciences of the United States of America* 107, 3522–3527, doi: 10.1073/pnas.0910179107 (2010).
59. Klionsky, D. J. & Emr, S. D. Autophagy as a regulated pathway of cellular degradation. *Science* 290, 1717–1721 (2000).
60. Lomonaco, S. L. et al. The induction of autophagy by gamma-radiation contributes to the radioresistance of glioma stem cells. *International journal of cancer. Journal international du cancer* 125, 717–722, doi: 10.1002/ijc.24402 (2009).
61. Calabrese, C. et al. A perivascular niche for brain tumor stem cells. *Cancer cell* 11, 69–82, doi: 10.1016/j.ccr.2006.11.020 (2007).
62. Han, L., Shi, S., Gong, T., Zhang, Z. & Sun, X. Cancer stem cells: Therapeutic implications and perspectives in cancer therapy. *Acta pharmaceutica sinica B* 3, 65–75 (2013).
63. Wang, Z., Li, Y., Banerjee, S. & Sarkar, F. H. Exploitation of the Notch signaling pathway as a novel target for cancer therapy. *Anticancer research* 28, 3621–3630 (2008).
64. Good, K. et al. The T-box transcription factors TBX-37 and TBX-38 link GLP-1/Notch signaling to mesoderm induction in C. elegans embryos. *Development* 131, 1967–1978 (2004).
65. Radtke, F. & Raj, K. The role of Notch in tumorigenesis: Oncogene or tumour suppressor? *Nature reviews cancer* 3, 756–767 (2003).
66. Ellisen, L. W. et al. TAN-1, the human homolog of the Drosophila notch gene, is broken by chromosomal translocations in T lymphoblastic neoplasms. *Cell* 66, 649–661 (1991).
67. Weng, A. P. et al. Activating mutations of NOTCH1 in human T cell acute lymphoblastic leukemia. *Science* 306, 269–271, doi: 10.1126/science.1102160 (2004).
68. Rangarajan, A. et al. Notch signaling is a direct determinant of keratinocyte growth arrest and entry into differentiation. *The EMBO journal* 20, 3427–3436, doi: 10.1093/emboj/20.13.3427 (2001).
69. Purow, B. W. et al. Expression of Notch-1 and its ligands, Delta-like-1 and Jagged-1, is critical for glioma cell survival and proliferation. *Cancer research* 65, 2353–2363, doi: 10.1158/0008-5472.CAN-04-1890 (2005).

70. Fan, X. et al. NOTCH pathway blockade depletes CD133-positive glioblastoma cells and inhibits growth of tumor neurospheres and xenografts. *Stem cells* 28, 5–16, doi: 10.1002/stem.254 (2010).
71. Kondratyev, M. et al. Gamma-secretase inhibitors target tumor-initiating cells in a mouse model of ERBB2 breast cancer. *Oncogene* 31, 93–103 (2011).
72. Hoey, T. et al. DLL4 blockade inhibits tumor growth and reduces tumor-initiating cell frequency. *Cell stem cell* 5, 168–177 (2009).
73. i Altaba, A. R., Sánchez, P. & Dahmane, N. Gli and hedgehog in cancer: Tumours, embryos and stem cells. *Nature reviews cancer* 2, 361–372 (2002).
74. Li, C. et al. Identification of pancreatic cancer stem cells. *Cancer research* 67, 1030–1037 (2007).
75. Huang, F.-T. et al. Inhibition of hedgehog signaling depresses self-renewal of pancreatic cancer stem cells and reverses chemoresistance. *International journal of oncology* 41, 1707–1714 (2012).
76. Chen, J. K., Taipale, J., Cooper, M. K. & Beachy, P. A. Inhibition of Hedgehog signaling by direct binding of cyclopamine to Smoothened. *Genes & development* 16, 2743–2748, doi: 10.1101/gad.1025302 (2002).
77. Axelson, M. et al. U.S. Food and Drug Administration approval: Vismodegib for recurrent, locally advanced, or metastatic basal cell carcinoma. *Clinical cancer research: An official journal of the American Association for Cancer Research* 19, 2289–2293, doi: 10.1158/1078-0432.ccr-12-1956 (2013).
78. Clement, V., Sanchez, P., de Tribolet, N., Radovanovic, I. & Ruiz i Altaba, A. HEDGEHOG-GLI1 signaling regulates human glioma growth, cancer stem cell self-renewal, and tumorigenicity. *Current biology: CB* 17, 165–172, doi: 10.1016/j.cub.2006.11.033 (2007).
79. Bar, E. E. et al. Cyclopamine-mediated hedgehog pathway inhibition depletes stem-like cancer cells in glioblastoma. *Stem cells* 25, 2524–2533, doi: 10.1634/stemcells.2007-0166 (2007).
80. Tang, S. N. et al. Inhibition of sonic hedgehog pathway and pluripotency maintaining factors regulate human pancreatic cancer stem cell characteristics. *International journal of cancer. Journal international du cancer* 131, 30–40, doi: 10.1002/ijc.26323 (2012).
81. Klaus, A. & Birchmeier, W. Wnt signalling and its impact on development and cancer. *Nature reviews. Cancer* 8, 387–398, doi: 10.1038/nrc2389 (2008).
82. Wend, P., Holland, J. D., Ziebold, U. & Birchmeier, W. Wnt signaling in stem and cancer stem cells. *Seminars in cell & developmental biology* 21, 855–863, doi: 10.1016/j.semcdb.2010.09.004 (2010).
83. Takahashi-Yanaga, F. & Kahn, M. Targeting Wnt signaling: Can we safely eradicate cancer stem cells? *Clinical cancer research: An official journal of the American Association for Cancer Research* 16, 3153–3162, doi: 10.1158/1078-0432.ccr-09-2943 (2010).
84. Emami, K. H. et al. A small molecule inhibitor of beta-catenin/CREB-binding protein transcription [corrected]. *Proceedings of the National Academy of Sciences of the United States of America* 101, 12682–12687, doi: 10.1073/pnas.0404875101 (2004).
85. Teng, Y., Wang, X., Wang, Y. & Ma, D. Wnt/beta-catenin signaling regulates cancer stem cells in lung cancer A549 cells. *Biochemical and biophysical research communications* 392, 373–379, doi: 10.1016/j.bbrc.2010.01.028 (2010).
86. Soltanian, S. & Matin, M. M. Cancer stem cells and cancer therapy. *Tumour biology: The journal of the International Society for Oncodevelopmental Biology and Medicine* 32, 425–440, doi: 10.1007/s13277-011-0155-8 (2011).
87. Campos, B. et al. Differentiation therapy exerts antitumor effects on stem-like glioma cells. *Clinical cancer research: An official journal of the American Association for Cancer Research* 16, 2715–2728, doi: 10.1158/1078-0432.ccr-09-1800 (2010).

88. Piccirillo, S. G. et al. Bone morphogenetic proteins inhibit the tumorigenic potential of human brain tumour-initiating cells. *Nature* 444, 761–765, doi: 10.1038/nature05349 (2006).
89. Lombardo, Y. et al. Bone morphogenetic protein 4 induces differentiation of colorectal cancer stem cells and increases their response to chemotherapy in mice. *Gastroenterology* 140, 297–309, doi: 10.1053/j.gastro.2010.10.005 (2011).
90. Butler, L. M. et al. Suberoylanilide hydroxamic acid, an inhibitor of histone deacetylase, suppresses the growth of prostate cancer cells in vitro and in vivo. *Cancer research* 60, 5165–5170 (2000).
91. Teitz-Tennenbaum, S., Wicha, M. S., Chang, A. E. & Li, Q. Targeting cancer stem cells via dendritic-cell vaccination. *OncoImmunology* 1, 1401 (2012).
92. Moretta, A. et al. Receptors for HLA class-I molecules in human natural killer cells. *Annual review of immunology* 14, 619–648, doi: 10.1146/annurev.immunol.14.1.619 (1996).
93. Moretta, A. et al. Activating receptors and coreceptors involved in human natural killer cell-mediated cytolysis. *Annual review of immunology* 19, 197–223, doi: 10.1146/annurev.immunol.19.1.197 (2001).
94. Moretta, L. & Moretta, A. Unravelling natural killer cell function: Triggering and inhibitory human NK receptors. *The EMBO journal* 23, 255–259, doi: 10.1038/sj.emboj.7600019 (2004).
95. Pietra, G. et al. Natural killer cells kill human melanoma cells with characteristics of cancer stem cells. *International immunology* 21, 793–801, doi: 10.1093/intimm/dxp047 (2009).
96. Bamrungsap, S. et al. Nanotechnology in therapeutics: A focus on nanoparticles as a drug delivery system. *Nanomedicine (London, England)* 7, 1253–1271, doi: 10.2217/nnm.12.87 (2012).
97. Matsumura, Y. & Maeda, H. A new concept for macromolecular therapeutics in cancer chemotherapy: Mechanism of tumoritropic accumulation of proteins and the antitumor agent smancs. *Cancer research* 46, 6387–6392 (1986).
98. Bangham, A. D. & Horne, R. W. Negative staining of phospholipids and their structural modification by surface-active agents as observed in the electron microscope. *Journal of molecular biology* 8, 660–668 (1964).
99. Bangham, A. D., Standish, M. M. & Watkins, J. C. Diffusion of univalent ions across the lamellae of swollen phospholipids. *Journal of molecular biology* 13, 238–252 (1965).
100. Khanna, S. C., Jecklin, T. & Speiser, P. Bead polymerization technique for sustained-release dosage form. *Journal of pharmaceutical sciences* 59, 614–618 (1970).
101. Khanna, S. C. & Speiser, P. Epoxy resin beads as a pharmaceutical dosage form. I. Method of preparation. *Journal of pharmaceutical sciences* 58, 1114–1117 (1969).
102. Couvreur, P. et al. Biodegradable polymeric nanoparticles as drug carrier for antitumor agents. *Polymeric Nanoparticles and Microspheres, CRC Press, Boca Raton, FL,* 27–93 (1986).
103. James, J. S. DOXIL approved for KS. *AIDS treatment news*, 6 (1995).
104. Safra, T. et al. Pegylated liposomal doxorubicin (doxil): Reduced clinical cardiotoxicity in patients reaching or exceeding cumulative doses of 500 mg/m2. *Annals of oncology: Official journal of the European Society for Medical Oncology/ESMO* 11, 1029–1033 (2000).
105. Ludwig, H., Strasser-Weippl, K., Schreder, M. & Zojer, N. Advances in the treatment of hematological malignancies: Current treatment approaches in multiple myeloma. *Annals of oncology: Official journal of the European Society for Medical Oncology/ESMO* 18 Suppl 9, ix64–70, doi: 10.1093/annonc/mdm296 (2007).
106. Perez-Lopez, M. E., Curiel, T., Gomez, J. G. & Jorge, M. Role of pegylated liposomal doxorubicin (Caelyx) in the treatment of relapsing ovarian cancer. *Anti-cancer drugs* 18, 611–617, doi: 10.1097/CAD.0b013e32802623fc (2007).

107. Kraft, J. C., Freeling, J. P., Wang, Z. & Ho, R. J. Emerging research and clinical development trends of liposome and lipid nanoparticle drug delivery systems. *Journal of pharmaceutical sciences* 103, 29–52, doi: 10.1002/jps.23773 (2014).
108. Dubey, P. K., Mishra, V., Jain, S., Mahor, S. & Vyas, S. P. Liposomes modified with cyclic RGD peptide for tumor targeting. *Journal of drug targeting* 12, 257–264, doi: 10.1080/10611860410001728040 (2004).
109. Dalerba, P. et al. Phenotypic characterization of human colorectal cancer stem cells. *Proceedings of the National Academy of Sciences of the United States of America* 104, 10158–10163, doi: 10.1073/pnas.0703478104 (2007).
110. Eliaz, R. E. & Szoka, F. C., Jr. Liposome-encapsulated doxorubicin targeted to CD44: A strategy to kill CD44-overexpressing tumor cells. *Cancer research* 61, 2592–2601 (2001).
111. Medema, J. P. Cancer stem cells: The challenges ahead. *Nature cell biology* 15, 338–344, doi: 10.1038/ncb2717 (2013).
112. Yuan, F. et al. Vascular permeability in a human tumor xenograft: Molecular size dependence and cutoff size. *Cancer research* 55, 3752–3756 (1995).
113. Drummond, D. C., Meyer, O., Hong, K., Kirpotin, D. B. & Papahadjopoulos, D. Optimizing liposomes for delivery of chemotherapeutic agents to solid tumors. *Pharmacological reviews* 51, 691–743 (1999).
114. Moghimi, S. M., Hunter, A. C. & Murray, J. C. Long-circulating and target-specific nanoparticles: Theory to practice. *Pharmacological reviews* 53, 283–318 (2001).
115. Savic, R., Azzam, T., Eisenberg, A. & Maysinger, D. Assessment of the integrity of poly(caprolactone)-b-poly(ethylene oxide) micelles under biological conditions: A fluorogenic-based approach. *Langmuir: The ACS journal of surfaces and colloids* 22, 3570–3578, doi: 10.1021/la0531998 (2006).
116. Chen, H. et al. Fast release of lipophilic agents from circulating PEG-PDLLA micelles revealed by in vivo forster resonance energy transfer imaging. *Langmuir: The ACS journal of surfaces and colloids* 24, 5213–5217, doi: 10.1021/la703570m (2008).
117. Mimeault, M. & Batra, S. K. Potential applications of curcumin and its novel synthetic analogs and nanotechnology-based formulations in cancer prevention and therapy. *Chinese medicine* 6, 31, doi: 10.1186/1749-8546-6-31 (2011).
118. Lim, K. J., Bisht, S., Bar, E. E., Maitra, A. & Eberhart, C. G. A polymeric nanoparticle formulation of curcumin inhibits growth, clonogenicity and stem-like fraction in malignant brain tumors. *Cancer biology & therapy* 11, 464–473 (2011).
119. Banzato, A. et al. A paclitaxel-hyaluronan bioconjugate targeting ovarian cancer affords a potent in vivo therapeutic activity. *Clinical cancer research: An official journal of the American Association for Cancer Research* 14, 3598–3606, doi: 10.1158/1078-0432.CCR-07-2019 (2008).
120. Bourseau-Guilmain, E. et al. Development and characterization of immuno-nanocarriers targeting the cancer stem cell marker AC133. *International journal of pharmaceutics* 423, 93–101, doi: 10.1016/j.ijpharm.2011.06.001 (2012).
121. Bernstein, E., Caudy, A. A., Hammond, S. M. & Hannon, G. J. Role for a bidentate ribonuclease in the initiation step of RNA interference. *Nature* 409, 363–366, doi: 10.1038/35053110 (2001).
122. Hammond, S. M., Bernstein, E., Beach, D. & Hannon, G. J. An RNA-directed nuclease mediates post-transcriptional gene silencing in Drosophila cells. *Nature* 404, 293–296, doi: 10.1038/35005107 (2000).
123. Akhtar, S. & Benter, I. F. Nonviral delivery of synthetic siRNAs in vivo. *The Journal of clinical investigation* 117, 3623–3632, doi: 10.1172/JCI33494 (2007).
124. Weinstein, S. & Peer, D. RNAi nanomedicines: Challenges and opportunities within the immune system. *Nanotechnology* 21, 232001, doi: 10.1088/0957-4484/21/23/232001 (2010).

125. de Fougerolles, A., Vornlocher, H. P., Maraganore, J. & Lieberman, J. Interfering with disease: A progress report on siRNA-based therapeutics. *Nature reviews. Drug discovery* 6, 443–453, doi: 10.1038/nrd2310 (2007).
126. Alabi, C., Vegas, A. & Anderson, D. Attacking the genome: Emerging siRNA nanocarriers from concept to clinic. *Current opinion in pharmacology* 12, 427–433, doi: 10.1016/j.coph.2012.05.004 (2012).
127. Burnett, J. C., Rossi, J. J. & Tiemann, K. Current progress of siRNA/shRNA therapeutics in clinical trials. *Biotechnology journal* 6, 1130–1146, doi: 10.1002/biot.201100054 (2011).
128. Tabernero, J. et al. First-in-humans trial of an RNA interference therapeutic targeting VEGF and KSP in cancer patients with liver involvement. *Cancer discovery* 3, 406–417, doi: 10.1158/2159-8290.CD-12-0429 (2013).
129. Schultheis, B. et al. First-in-Human Phase I Study of the Liposomal RNA Interference Therapeutic Atu027 in Patients With Advanced Solid Tumors. *Journal of clinical oncology: Official journal of the American Society of Clinical Oncology*, doi: 10.1200/JCO.2013.55.0376 (2014).
130. Davis, M. E. et al. Evidence of RNAi in humans from systemically administered siRNA via targeted nanoparticles. *Nature* 464, 1067–1070, doi: 10.1038/nature08956 (2010).
131. Davis, M. E. The first targeted delivery of siRNA in humans via a self-assembling, cyclodextrin polymer-based nanoparticle: From concept to clinic. *Molecular pharmaceutics* 6, 659–668, doi: 10.1021/mp900015y (2009).
132. Jensen, S. A. et al. Spherical nucleic acid nanoparticle conjugates as an RNAi-based therapy for glioblastoma. *Science translational medicine* 5, 209ra152, doi: 10.1126/scitranslmed.3006839 (2013).
133. Liu, Z. et al. Drug delivery with carbon nanotubes for in vivo cancer treatment. *Cancer research* 68, 6652–6660, doi: 10.1158/0008-5472.CAN-08-1468 (2008).
134. Wu, W. et al. Covalently combining carbon nanotubes with anticancer agent: Preparation and antitumor activity. *ACS nano* 3, 2740–2750, doi: 10.1021/nn9005686 (2009).
135. Zhang, L. et al. Enhanced chemotherapy efficacy by sequential delivery of siRNA and anticancer drugs using PEI-grafted graphene oxide. *Small* 7, 460–464, doi: 10.1002/smll.201001522 (2011).
136. Yang, K. et al. Graphene in mice: Ultrahigh in vivo tumor uptake and efficient photothermal therapy. *Nano letters* 10, 3318–3323, doi: 10.1021/nl100996u (2010).
137. Abdullah, L. N. & Chow, E. K. Mechanisms of chemoresistance in cancer stem cells. *Clinical and translational medicine* 2, 3, doi: 10.1186/2001-1326-2-3 (2013).
138. Motzer, R. J. et al. Phase I/II trial of dexverapamil plus vinblastine for patients with advanced renal cell carcinoma. *Journal of clinical oncology: Official journal of the American Society of Clinical Oncology* 13, 1958–1965 (1995).
139. Chow, E. K. et al. Nanodiamond therapeutic delivery agents mediate enhanced chemoresistant tumor treatment. *Science translational medicine* 3, 73ra21, doi: 10.1126/scitranslmed.3001713 (2011).
140. Wang, X. et al. Epirubicin-Adsorbed Nanodiamonds Kill Chemoresistant Hepatic Cancer Stem Cells. *ACS nano*, doi: 10.1021/nn503491e (2014).

17 Cardiac Drug Delivery*

Paula Díaz-Herráez, Simón Pascual-Gil de Gómez, Elisa Garbayo, Teresa Simón-Yarza, Felipe Prósper, and María J. Blanco-Prieto

CONTENTS

* Paula Díaz-Herráez and Simón Pascual-Gil de Gómez contributed equally to this manuscript.

INTRODUCTION

Cardiovascular disease (CVD) is the leading cause of death worldwide. In fact, 17.3 million people died from CVDs in 2008, representing 30% of all global deaths. Although the death rate due to CVD is high, a similar number of people survive. Nevertheless, those patients who survive may still face a difficult recovery process. The ongoing complications that result from CVD greatly contribute to the economic burden on the health care system and on society as a whole. For example, the direct cost of CVD in the United States was $312.6 billion in 2009 (Go et al., 2013), and in 2010, the cost in health care expenditures and loss of productivity amounted to nearly $444 billion (available at CDCs The Million Hearts Initiative, 2012).

CVD is caused by disorders of the heart and blood vessels. CVD includes coronary artery disease (heart attacks), heart failure, cerebrovascular disease (stroke), raised blood pressure (hypertension), peripheral artery disease, rheumatic heart disease, and congenital heart disease. Of all of these, coronary artery disease is the most important disorder, being responsible for 7.3 million deaths each year (available at http://www.who.int/mediacentre/factsheets/fs317/en/index.html). A heart attack, also called myocardial infarction (MI), is usually caused by coronary artery occlusion that produces loss of blood flow in a specific heart region. Artery blockage is mainly due to the combination of a blood clot and an atheroma, formed by a thrombotic and an atherosclerotic process, respectively (Figure 17.1). The final consequence is hypoxia of the surrounding area. The lack of oxygen causes the death of the heart cells, called myocytes, which become apoptotic and/or necrotic over MI progression,

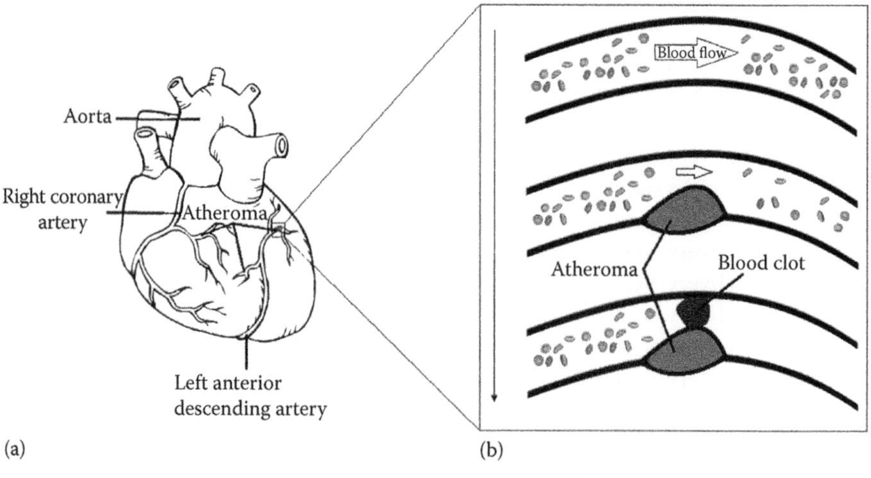

FIGURE 17.1 Myocardial infarction scheme. (a) Heart with several branch arteries blocked. (b) Section of a coronary artery that show the steps during an obstruction process.

generating the infarcted area (Kurrelmeyer et al., 1998). The extent of the damage depends on the blockage location and on the time (Figure 17.1). Interestingly, there is a transitional step in which heart cells lie between the normal, well-vascularized and the necrotic/ischemic myocardium. During that period of time, myocytes are still alive and allow several treatments to avoid irreversible heart tissue loss. If blood flow is restored early enough, much of the heart muscle that could have been damaged might ultimately survive. This is why MI is a medical emergency, and treatment should be given urgently. The quicker the blood flow is restored, the better the outcome.

Current Therapies and Their Limitations

Nowadays there are several options available for those patients suffering from MI. The conventional therapies include the following:

Pharmacological Treatments

Drug therapy is an important component of long-term care following MI. Common medication used for MI treatment includes the use of angiotensin-converting enzyme inhibitors, beta-blockers, diuretics, and vasodilators. These drugs reduce left ventricular filling pressure and volume, allowing cardiac remodeling process control. Other pharmacological treatments are based on antiplatelet agents, such as aspirin or clopidogrel, used to prevent clotting in patients who have had a heart attack. Moreover, antiplatelet drugs can also improve the short- and long-term outcomes of patients treated with coronary stents (Scott et al., 2008).

Balloon Angioplasty

This is a percutaneous intervention where blocked coronary arteries are reopened by inflating a tiny balloon inside the blockage, compressing the fatty plaque against the artery walls and widening the vessel.

Stent

In this strategy, a tiny metal mesh tube or stent, often inserted during angioplasty, is used as a scaffold to help the artery to keep open. The assembly is pushed into the narrowed artery, where the balloon is inflated, expanding the stent. The balloon is then deflated and withdrawn. After several weeks, the artery heals around the stent.

Coronary Bypass

In this type of surgery, one or more blocked coronary arteries are bypassed by blood vessels grafted from patient's chest, legs, or arms with the aim of restoring normal blood flow.

Heart Transplant

This procedure is only performed after all other options have been exhausted.

These classical approaches are useful in mitigating the symptoms and have reduced the MI mortality rate. However, cardiac dysfunction remains an issue due to inadequate heart healing after ischemia (Sy and Davis, 2010). Several factors, including contractile cell loss, inflammatory response, cardiac hypertrophy, and lack of suitable cues for progenitor cells, cause fibrosis in the heart and cardiac function loss. To date, medical and interventional treatments for MI are not able to regenerate the tissue or restore heart function. Moreover, current treatments are either highly invasive or rely on continuous administration of several drugs. Their beneficial effects are only observed when large doses are administered, which is frequently accompanied by side effects. Regarding angioplasty, acute occlusion in the treated vessel as well as restenosis occur in 30%–40% of lesions. The use of bare metal stents reduced restenosis incidence to 25%–30%, and the percentage was further reduced by drug-eluting stents (DES), falling to less than 10% in initial clinical trials (CTs). These results led to the use of DES in more than 85% of all coronary interventions. However, in-stent thrombosis or blood clot formation occurs more frequently in DES as compared to bare metal stents. The most definite solution is perhaps a fully biodegradable scaffolding device that does not leave any struts after drug elution has occurred (Onuba et al., 2011).

Finally, for some patients, the only option is organ transplantation (Formiga et al., 2012) although it has numerous drawbacks, such as the donor waiting list or the immunosuppressive regimen to prevent rejection.

In conclusion, although therapeutic advances have led to significant improvements in the outcomes of MI patients, multiple aspects for treating this pathology remain challenging. Therefore, additional strategies to rescue and regenerate the myocardium are needed.

NEW THERAPEUTIC STRATEGIES FOR CARDIOVASCULAR DISEASES

Clinical and translational research has advanced the available therapeutic options for MI management, and patients have their best survival rates ever. However, the current limitations of conventional therapies have led to an increase in the efforts to develop new strategies. The advent of new molecular and cellular targets, together with advances in genomic and proteomic technologies, have accelerated the discovery of novel pharmaceutical compounds able to regenerate the heart. This emerging class of substances has high specificity and potency and includes proteins, gene therapies, siRNAs, cell-based therapies, or small molecules, among others (Meng and Hoang, 2012).

In this section, we review the therapies based on proteins and cells because these strategies are the ones that have shown the most encouraging results so far.

PROTEIN-BASED THERAPIES

At present, there are numerous protein candidates for MI treatment. The most promising ones are vascular endothelial growth factor (VEGF), fibroblast growth factor (FGF), placental growth factor (PIGF), granulocyte colony stimulating factor (G-CSF), hepatocyte growth factor (HGF), neuregulin (NRG), insulin-like growth factor-1 (IGF), transforming growth factor-β (TGF-β), erythropoietin (EPO), platelet-derived growth factor (PDGF), and stromal cell-derived factor 1-α (SDF) (Segers and Lee, 2010). These growth factors (GFs) have generated interest due to their specific biological functions and roles in MI heart regeneration (Figure 17.2). They have the

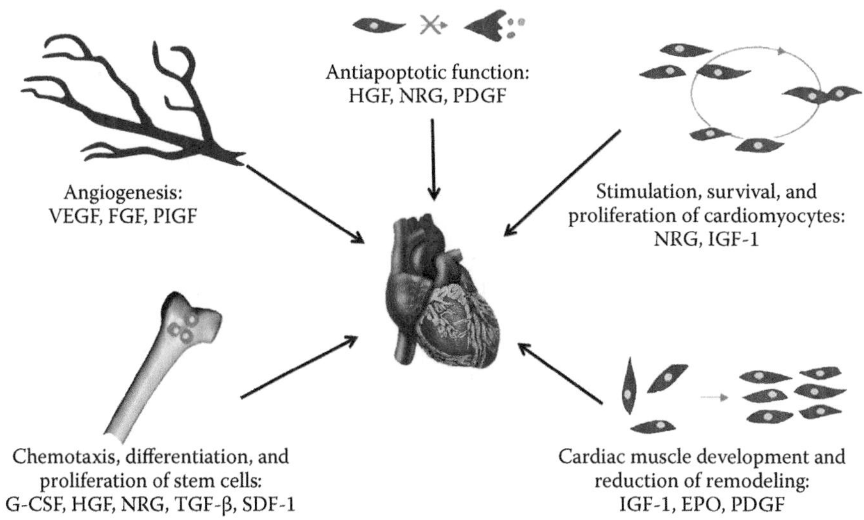

FIGURE 17.2 Scheme of protein candidates for myocardial infarction treatment indicating their specific biological function and roles in heart regeneration.

potential to induce (1) angiogenesis; (2) chemotaxis, differentiation, and proliferation of stem cells; (3) reduction of apoptosis; (4) stimulation, survival, and proliferation of cardiomyocytes; (5) cardiac muscle development; and (6) reduction of remodeling. The current applications of these GFs in CT are detailed next.

Clinical Trials with Proteins

The first CT using therapeutic proteins for cardiac repair involved human FGF-1 (Table 17.1). In this first study, 40 coronary heart disease patients were included. All of them were treated with bypass surgery, and 20 of them also received FGF-1 intramyocardial (IM) injection. A dense capillary network next to the FGF-1 injection area as well as a local blood supply increase were observed after 12 weeks (Schumacher et al., 1998). At the moment, the ongoing ACORD CT Phase II (Clinicaltrials.gov identifier NCT00117936), with an estimated enrollment of 120 patients, is being performed in order to test vessel growth stimulation around the blocked coronary arteries after IM injection of FGF-1 at different dose rates (0, 2, 20, and 40 μg/kg).

Several CTs have been performed to date with FGF-2 (Laham et al., 1999 and 2000; Unger et al., 2000; Udelson et al., 2000). The results of Phase I FGF-2 trials confirmed treatment safety and feasibility and suggested a benefit when applied to ischemic cardiac patients. Based on these results, the FIRST study was then conducted. This Phase II CT included 337 patients with coronary artery disease. They administered intracoronary (IC) FGF-2 in a single bolus at different doses (0, 3, or 30 μg/kg). No improvement was detected until day 90, and only a trend toward symptomatic improvement was observed. However, this benefit disappeared at day 180 due to the continued improvement observed in the placebo group (Simons et al., 2002).

TABLE 17.1
Clinical Trials Using Growth Factors for the Treatment of Myocardial Infarction

Year	GF	Adm. Route	N	Ref.
1998	FGF-1	IM	20	Schummacher et al., 1998
–			estimated 120	ClinicalTrials.gov identifier NCT00117936
1999	VEGF	IV	28	Gibson et al., 1999
2000		IC	14	Hendel et al., 2000
2001			15	Henry et al., 2001
2003		IC/IV	178	Henry et al., 2003
1999	FGF-2	IM	24	Laham et al., 1999
2000		IC	25	Unger et al., 2000
			52	Laham et al., 2000
		IC/IV	59	Udelson et al., 2000
2002		IC	337	Simons et al., 2002
2001	G-CSF	IC/SC	21	Seiler et al., 2001
2005		SC	20	Valgimigli et al., 2005
			50	Ince et al., 2005
			14	Zbinden et al., 2005
2006			114	Zohlnhofer et al., 2006
			78	Ripa et al., 2006
2009			52	Meier et al., 2009
2010			60	Achilli et al., 2010
			44	Engelmann et al., 2010
	G-CSF + sitagliptin	SC	100	Theiss et al., 2010
2009	EPO	IV	44	Tang et al., 2009
2010			529	Voors et al., 2010
2006	long-acting EPO	IV	22	Lipsic et al., 2006
2009	pHGF	IV	49	Wang et al., 2009
2010	NRG	IV	15	Jabbour et al., 2011
			44	Gao et al., 2010
–			331	
		SC	estimated 120	
			120	ClinicalTrials.gov identifier NCT01251406
		IV	estimated 50	ClinicalTrials.gov identifier NCT01258387
			146	ClinicalTrials.gov identifier NCT01439789
			14	ClinicalTrials.gov identifier NCT01439893
			estimated 1,600	ClinicalTrials.gov identifier NCT01541202

VEGF was considered a very promising GF to achieve neovascularization due to the results obtained in preclinical studies. In a Phase I trial with 28 patients, intravenous (IV) VEGF administration showed improvement in myocardial perfusion and in collateral density (Gibson et al., 1999). Two Phase I trials have been performed using IC VEGF administration, concluding the safety and tolerability of the treatment and a dose-dependent effect (Hendel et al., 2000; Henry et al., 2001). The first large CT with VEGF was the VIVA trial, which enrolled 178 patients who received different doses of VEGF administered IV or IC. Despite previously demonstrated beneficial effects, this CT did not show any significant improvement beyond placebo by days 60 and 120. The only significant difference was found by day 120 in the high-dose group, which showed a reduced number of angina events, indicating an improvement in patients' quality of life (Henry et al., 2003).

Several CTs with G-CSF have been conducted in the last decade (Zbinden et al., 2005; Valgimigli et al., 2005). FIRSTLINE-AMI was a trial in which 25 out of 50 patients were randomly assigned to receive a 10 μg/kg daily subcutaneous (SC) dose for 6 days. This treatment promoted mononuclear CD^{34+} cell mobilization, which correlated with better ventricular function preservation and less remodeling (Ince et al., 2005). In the context of the first results obtained in small CTs, the REVIVAL-2 study was conducted. One hundred fourteen patients were included, and half of them received an SC daily dose of 10 μg/kg of G-CSF for 5 days while the rest received placebo. Although stem cell mobilization was significant, it did not have any impact on infarct size, left ventricular function, or coronary restenosis (Zohlnhöfer et al., 2006). The same results were observed in the STEMMI trial performed in 78 patients (Ripa et al., 2006). In spite of these negative results, more CTs with G-CSF have been conducted since then (Meier et al., 2009; Achilli et al., 2010; Theiss et al., 2010; Engelmann et al., 2010).

In a CT with EPO, no improvement in left ventricular ejection fraction (LVEF) was observed 4 months after the long-acting glycoprotein IV administration (Lipsic et al., 2006). Next, in a different trial with acute MI patients, angiogenesis signaling protein expression in peripheral blood mononuclear cells was increased (Tang et al., 2009). Finally, a large Phase II CT, with 529 patients, failed to improve LVEF after 6 weeks (Voors et al., 2010).

In the last years, NRG, a therapeutic protein that has shown great promise in preclinical animal models, has been tested in numerous undergoing CTs. When it was first administered to patients, it appeared to favor hemodynamic effects (Jabbour et al., 2011). In a Phase II trial, it was also demonstrated to improve cardiac function and reduce ventricular remodeling (Gao et al., 2010). Now, larger CTs have been launched to confirm treatment efficacy (ClinicalTrials.gov identifiers NCT01131637, NCT01214096, NCT01251406, NCT01258387, and NCT01541202).

Lessons from Clinical Trials with Proteins

Taking an overview of CT data, some interesting conclusions can be outlined. One of the main limitations is protein half-life. This is because GFs are labile molecules that are degraded in a very short period of time, ranging from some minutes to a few hours, when directly administered into the organism. Therefore, to obtain a more sustained effect over time, many administrations or the use of systems that protect GFs from degradation would be required. This fact justifies the efforts to incorporate therapeutic cytokines into delivery systems that protect them from degradation and that allow their sustained release. This point is extensively discussed in the next sections.

Another drawback concerns the CT design. Studies involving small populations tend to release positive data, but when they are scaled up, no therapeutic benefit can be demonstrated. A better small trial design will help to determine the optimal treatment conditions for larger studies before these are performed. Also, in most of the studies, short-term results do not seem to correlate with long-term effects. For these reasons, patients should be followed up for longer periods of time to obtain more valuable information about the treatment.

Thus, after more than 10 years of CTs with therapeutic proteins, information about several GFs has been accumulated. This will help us to choose the adequate protein or combination of proteins to treat the patients in the future. For instance, VEGF promotes neovascularization but its effect is not powerful enough to affect cardiac function. Thus, in the future, it could be combined with other factors that promote cell recruitment, such as EPO.

Another aspect to take into account is that each patient is different and thus has different requirements. Bearing in mind that most of the GFs are implicated in the acute process, they are always administered to patients at this stage. Nevertheless, NRG is a better candidate to treat not only acute patients, but also chronic patients, based on its ability to promote cardiomyocyte proliferation. Another issue is the preferable route of administration, which also depends on the GF in question. EPO, for instance, has almost always been SC administered in a single dose, being sufficient to promote cell mobilization. Conversely, VEGF and FGF-2 have been IV, IC, and IM administered. In general, IM administration avoids adverse effects associated with systemic administration and allows a better dose control. To reduce the invasiveness of IM administration, novel, commercially available technologies are now being applied, such as the transendocardial injection with the MyoStar™ injection system guided by NOGA®. This method allows direct IM injection with a tissue penetration up to 10 mm and low risk of myocardial perforation or rupture (Kharlamov et al., 2012).

Finally, it can also be concluded that the suitable manner for making these proteins available at the target site with a desired dosage and for a determined period of time remains unclear. Proteins, due to their limited bioactivity, short half-life, pharmacokinetic properties, and instability, require specialized delivery modalities. However, reports of heart-specific drug delivery vehicles are scarce. Thus, there is an unmet need for cardiac drug delivery technologies able to administer biopharmaceuticals. Drug delivery systems (DDS) could also play an important role in multiple GF therapy since they can be made of different materials and can incorporate two or more therapeutic proteins with different release profiles. Currently, these systems are at the preclinical stage of safety and efficacy evaluation (see section "Current status on cardiac drug delivery systems and future trends").

Cell Therapy

On the basis of preclinical data, different cell types have been explored to regenerate infarcted heart (Figure 17.3) (reviewed in Pelacho et al., 2013). Myoblasts were one of the first cells found to differentiate toward cardiomyocytes. However, it has been demonstrated that myoblasts act in a paracrine manner and that they are not able to generate new cardiac cells. Bone marrow–derived stem cells (BMSCs) have been the most widely used adult stem cells used for cardiac repair. BMSCs include hematopoietic stem cells, mesenchymal stem cells (MSCs), and endothelial progenitor stem cell subpopulations. Adipose-derived stem cells (ADSCs), which are easily isolated by liposuction, and umbilical cord blood–derived mesenchymal stem cells are also showing great promise for use in cardiac repair. Contrary to classical conceptions, a population of cardiac progenitor stem cells (CSCs) has been found in the heart, indicating an intrinsic regenerative potential of this organ. These cells appear in clusters that can be isolated and differentiated in vitro toward cardiomyocytes and vascular cells. Fetal cardiomyocytes and embryonic stem cells (ESCs) are also an attractive cell source due to their totipotency. However, they present important concerns that limit their use, such as availability, immunogenicity, teratogenic potential, and ethical issues due to their origin. An alternative to ESCs is induced pluripotent stem cells (iPSs). iPSs are pluripotent cells obtained from adult cell reprogramming. iPSs derived from rodent cells were obtained for the first time in 2006 (Takahashi and Yamanaka, 2006). Next, in 2007, human iPSs were derived from human fibroblasts by the transduction of several transcription factors (Oct3/4, SOX2, Nanog, Lin28) (Takahashi et al., 2007). Improvements in iPS obtention protocol have been performed in recent years in order to avoid integrating virus use. However, the technology to create iPSs is relatively new, and it is still not clear whether these cells are safe for transplantation.

Clinical Trials with Cells

Although many preclinical studies using different cell sources have been performed, only two cell types, BMSCs and myoblasts, have been tested in CTs.

The first CT employing cell therapy for MI regeneration was the Strauer et al. trial in 2002. It enrolled 20 patients that received conventional therapy after MI, 10 of whom also received autologous BMSCs. Three months later, patients in the BMSC group showed significant infarct region reduction along with improvement of the infarction wall movement velocity, stroke volume index, left ventricular end-systolic volume and contractility, and myocardial perfusion of the infarcted region (Strauer et al., 2002). Trials performed later on showed different results. Some of them, such as TOPCARE-AMI, BOOST, REPAIR-AMI, and FINCELL were successful in improving disease progression. On the other hand, LEUVEN-AMI, ASTAMI, and HEBE trials did not confirm the previous positive results. In order to conclude about the effect of BMSC transplantation in acute MI, a meta-analysis was performed by Martin-Rendon et al. in 2008, concluding that BMSC transplantation was not only safe, but also effective in improving the LVEF and reducing the scar size (Martin-Rendon et al., 2008).

On the other hand, the first studies using myoblasts were published 10 years ago (Table 17.2). In 2005, a Phase I CT demonstrated their safety and feasibility for

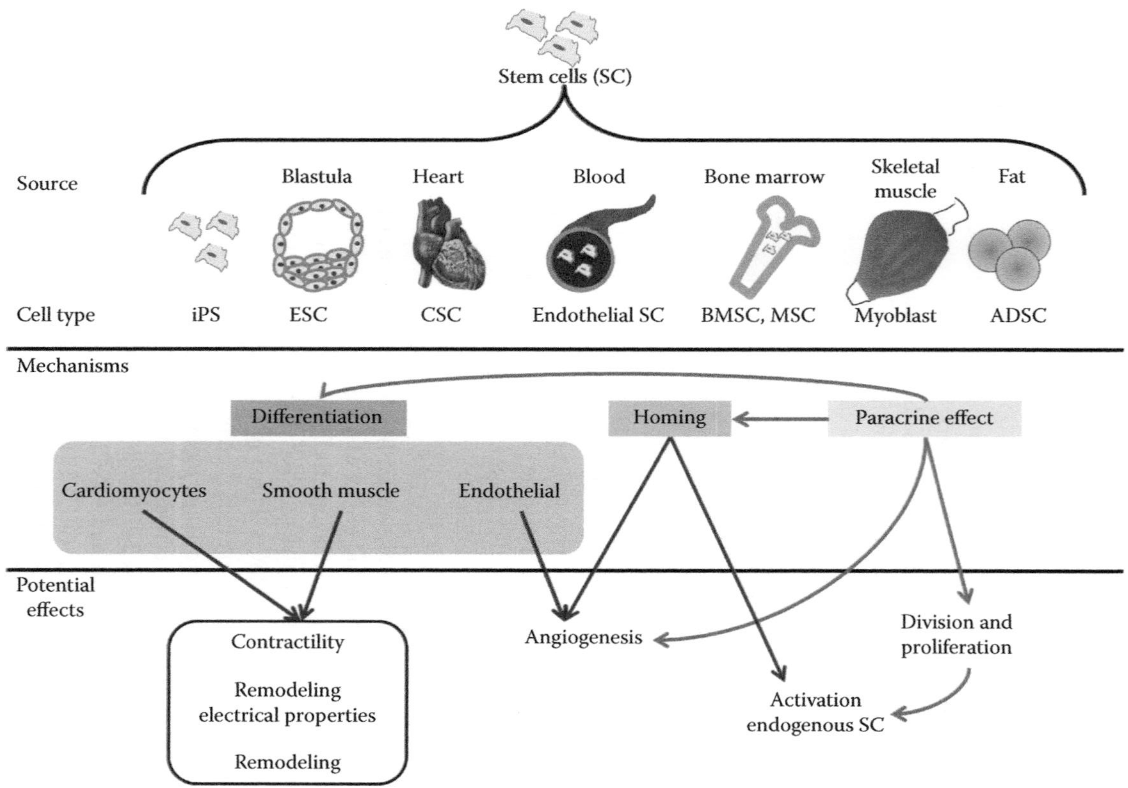

FIGURE 17.3 Schematic representation of the main stem cell sources used for myocardial infarction treatment showing the mechanisms and the potential effects in heart regeneration.

TABLE 17.2
Clinical Trials Using Cell Therapy for the Treatment of Myocardial Infarction

Year	Trial	Cells	Adm. Route	N	Ref.
2003	–	SkM	CABG	10	Menasche et al., 2003
			Tec	5	Smits et al., 2003
2004				12	Ince et al., 2004
			Tep	10	Siminiak et al., 2004
				20	Chachques et al., 2004
2005				30	Dib et al., 2005
	POZNAN		TC	9	Siminiak et al., 2005
2006	–		Tep	26	Gavira et al., 2006
			TEc	10	Biagini et al., 2006
2008	MAGIC		Tep	97	Menasche et al., 2008
2009	CAuSMIC		TEc	23	Dib et al., 2009b
2011	SEISMIC			40	Duckers et al., 2011
2002	–	BMC	IC	20	Strauer et al., 2002
2003	TOPCARE-AMI	BMC/CPC	IC	30	Britten et al., 2003
2006	–	BMC/CPC	IC	75	Assmus et al., 2006
2004	–	BMC	IC	33	Fernandez-Avilés et al., 2004
			Tec	20	Perin et al., 2004
2005			IC	26	Erbs et al., 2005
			dMI	20	Patel et al., 2005
2004	BOOST		IC	60	Wollert et al., 2004
2006	LEUVEN-AMI			66	Janssens et al., 2006
	–		dMI	20	Hendrikx et al., 2006
			IC	60	Meyer et al., 2006
			dMI	36	Mocini et al., 2006
			TEc	27	Fuchs et al., 2006
			IC	10	Briguori et al., 2006
	ASTAMI			97	Lunde et al., 2006 and Beitnes et al., 2009
2007	REPAIR-AMI			204	Schachinger et al., 2006
2006	–			66	Meluzin et al., 2006
2007				10	de la Fuente et al., 2007
	PROTECT-CAD		TEc	28	Tse et al., 2007
	–		dMI	40	Stamm et al., 2007
2008				36	Zhao et al., 2008
			Tep	63	Ang et al., 2008
	FINCELL		IC	77	Huikuri et al., 2008

(Continued)

TABLE 17.2 (CONTINUED)
Clinical Trials Using Cell Therapy for the Treatment of Myocardial Infarction

Year	Trial	Cells	Adm. Route	N	Ref.
2009	–		dMI	50	Akar et al., 2009
			IC	50	van Ramshorts et al., 2009
				67	Herbots et al., 2009
				60	Plewka et al., 2009
	REGENT			120	Tendera et al., 2009
	MYSTAR		IM/IC	60	Gyongyosi et al., 2009
2010	STAR-Heart		IC	391	Strauer et al., 2010
	–			40	Traverse et al., 2011
	HEBE			200	Hirsch et al., 2011
2004	–	MSC	IC	69	Chen et al., 2004
2009			IV	53	Hare et al., 2009
2009			EV	20	Dib et al., 2009b
2010			dMI	30	Viswanathan et al., 2010
–		ADSC	IM/IV	estimated 10	ClinicalTrials.gov identifier NCT01502514 (recruiting)
	APOLLO		IC	estimated 48	ClinicalTrials.gov identifier NCT00442806 (ongoing)
	ADVANCE			estimated 216	ClinicalTrials.gov identifier NCT01216995 (recruiting)
	ATHENA			estimated 45	ClinicalTrials.gov identifier NCT01556022 (recruiting)
	PRECISE		IM	estimated 36	ClinicalTrials.gov identifier NCT00426868 (ongoing)
	–		IC	estimated 6	ClinicalTrials.gov identifier NCT01709279 (recruiting)
2004	MAGIC-cell	G-CSF + PBSC	IC	27	ClinicalTrials.gov identifier Kang et al., 2004
2013	ALCADIA	CPC + bFGF	IM	estimated 6	ClinicalTrials.gov identifier NCT00981006 (ongoing)

cardiac regeneration. Moreover, potential functional benefits were described with an improvement in the ejection fraction even 2 years after implantation. However, the first randomized placebo-controlled trial (MAGIC study) did not show any functional improvement or benefit in the electrocardiography. In fact, patients receiving cell treatment showed a higher number of arrhythmic events (Menasche et al., 2008). The CAuSMIC study included 23 patients with MI and heart failure (Dib et al., 2009a).

Unlike the results of the previous study, these patients did not suffer arrhythmias and showed improvement on the New York Heart Association and Minnesota Living Heart Failure Questionnaires, which are recognized to be representative of the heart failure impact on patients' quality of life.

The Phase IIa study SEISMIC, which also employed myoblasts, concluded that this therapy was safe. However, no improvement in the heart's functional activity was observed (Duckers et al., 2011). In the same way, patients included in the MARVEL-1 study underwent sustained ventricular tachycardia without significant improvement in functional capacity or on the Minnesota Living Heart Failure Questionnaire (Povsic et al., 2011).

Therefore, myoblast therapy is feasible and safe but its beneficial effects are still not clear. Larger studies with long-term follow-up are therefore needed.

Lessons from Clinical Trials with Cells

When cell therapy was suggested as a possible strategy for treating ischemic heart disease, it was hypothesized that cells would be able to engraft and differentiate, contributing to the cellular repopulation of the infarcted area. However, it was soon observed that the benefits were principally due to the paracrine effect of the injected cells (Gnecchi et al., 2008; Reinecke et al., 2008). Cell survival rates in the tissue were very low, partly due to cell escape through capillaries and the stressful environment that the infarcted tissue entails for the cells. Therefore, one of the main lessons from cell CTs is the need to increase cell survival rates. Other lessons concluded from these studies were the need to establish which type of cell is more appropriate for a given application and the best trial end point determination. Other procedural aspects that must be reviewed are related to cell processing for obtaining higher quality cell populations as well as cell dosing, timing, and delivery route optimization. All these issues have recently been reviewed elsewhere (Menasche et al., 2011).

In summary, additional strategies are needed to achieve cardiac regeneration. Improvement of the existing approaches will depend on drug discovery and on the development of new technologies to effectively deliver these compounds.

DRUG DELIVERY SYSTEMS TO ADDRESS UNMET MEDICAL NEEDS IN CARDIOVASCULAR DISEASES

As noted above, the development of new technologies that enable effective drug delivery to the heart would optimize cardiovascular treatment and would address some of the limitations of current therapies. DDS were developed to improve drug therapeutic properties and to render them more safe, effective, and reliable. In general terms, incorporating a medicine into a DDS can significantly improve its performance. The major advantages of these systems could be summarized as drug protection, control over drug release kinetics, minimization of possible side effects, better efficacy, and enhanced patient compliance (Verma and Garg, 2001). Further goals in drug delivery are to target the drug to particular organs or cells in the body or to overcome certain tissue or cellular barriers (Langer and Peppas, 2003). Drug delivery systems can be designed with different mechanical and physical properties, and they can be biodegradable or nonbiodegradable, depending upon the nature of the polymer or the material used for their preparation.

DDS can be used either for local or for systemic delivery. Most strategies for local cardiac therapy have used direct myocardial injection, intrapericardial delivery, or coronary injection, using epicardial surgery or a catheter-based endocardial approach (Reviewed in Rolfes et al., 2012). However, which is the safest and most effective of these delivery strategies is currently unknown.

In the context of heart diseases, DDS could improve the therapeutic properties of standard pharmacological treatments and reduce unwanted side effects. Drug delivery for interventional treatments after MI is one area of great importance under investigation. Drug-eluting metallic stents are an example of DDS developed for localized drug delivery to a specific location and to minimize restenosis associated with bare metal stents (Langer and Peppas, 2003). Various approaches using metal stents delivering paclitaxel (Heldman et al., 2001), sirolimus (Oberhoff et al., 2002), and other drugs have been well developed and tested, showing remarkable results in keeping blood vessels open (Morice et al., 2002). But safety concerns have led to improvements in conventional DES with the use of more biocompatible and biodegradable polymers (Onuba et al., 2011). Regarding their clinical use, only the Absorb™ (Abbot Laboratories) biodegradable DES has been approved for its use in peripheral disease in Europe. However, this device does not have FDA approval yet. Nowadays several CTs using this DES, manufactured with the biodegradable polymer poly-L-lactid acid (PLLA), are ongoing (Table 17.3). Lately, cytokine-eluting stents have been proposed to stimulate arteriogenesis in the peripheral circulation of the rabbit (Grundmann et al., 2007). This intra-arterial delivery platform combines the advantages of therapeutic proteins and DES. With continuing advances in chemical engineering and material sciences, greater progress in this DES application is expected in the future.

The most important potential applications of DDS in the cardiovascular field are without any doubt the development of novel protein and cell delivery systems for cardiac repair. From a therapeutic perspective, proteins offer the advantage of specific mechanisms of action and high potency. However, as pointed out in the preceding sections, one important limitation is the difficulty of administering them efficiently to treat cardiac tissue diseases. The major obstacles, as previously mentioned, are their short half-lives, their low stability, and their immunogenicity. The use of DDS might overcome the limitations associated with protein administration and would improve its potential and efficacy. Notably, such strategies have the potential to become viable therapeutic protein products (Pisal et al., 2010). On the other hand, regarding cell

TABLE 17.3
Clinical Trials Using Bioresorbable Drug-Eluting Stents for the Treatment of Myocardial Infarction

ClinicalTrials.gov Identifier	Trial Name	Drug	Estimated *N*	Situation
NCT01711931	EVERBIOII	EVEROLIMUS	240	Recruiting
NCT01583608	ABSORB		180	Ongoing
NCT01023789	ABSORB EXTEND		1,000	Recruiting
NCT01425281	ABSORBII		501	Recruiting
NCT01308346	ABSORB PHYSIOLOGY		36	Recruiting
NCT01751906	ABSORB RCT		2,000	Recruiting
NCT00856856	ABSORB B		101	Ongoing

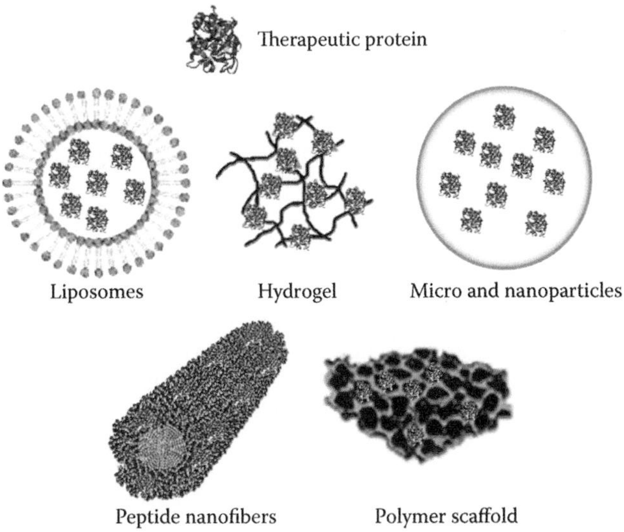

FIGURE 17.4 Schematic representation of the most common vehicles explored for cardiac drug delivery of proteins and cells with therapeutic potential.

therapy, DDS could provide a supportive scaffold for cells to enhance their engraftment and survival in the heart. DDS can be designed to direct cell organization, growth, and differentiation in the process of forming functional tissue by providing physical, mechanical, and chemical cues (Pelacho et al., 2013). They can also reduce acute cell loss after cell transplantation due to the washout from the infarcted myocardium (Dai et al., 2009; Segers and Lee, 2011). Natural polymers like collagen, gelatin, and alginate have inherent peptide sequences that can be easily recognized by the cell-surface receptors and are therefore suitable biomaterials for cell adhesion.

The following are some of the most common vehicles explored so far for cardiac protein and cell delivery (Figure 17.4) (revised in Formiga et al., 2012).

Liposomes

Liposomes are sphere-shaped vesicles that consist of one or more phospholipid bilayers (Akbarzadeh et al., 2013). Due to their size and hydrophobic and hydrophilic characteristics, they are extensively used as carriers for numerous molecules (Figure 17.4).

Hydrogels

Hydrogels are three-dimensional polymer networks swollen by aqueous solvent, which is the major component of the gel system (Silva et al., 2009) (Figure 17.4). They can carry diverse molecules and are very versatile systems. For instance, they can swell in aqueous medium, they can be pH and temperature sensitive, and/or be sensitive toward other stimuli.

Micro- and Nanoparticles

Solid particles in the nanometer (nanoparticles [NP]) or micrometer (microparticles [MP]) size range (Ravi Kumar et al., 2000) (Figure 17.4) can be prepared with many different materials and polymers, and they have been extensively used for protein delivery (Tan et al., 2010; Mundargi et al., 2008; Almeida and Souto, 2007).

Self-Assembling Peptide Nanofibers (NF)

These well-defined scaffolds are made of up to 99% water and amenable to incorporate a variety of bioactive cues. They are peptide repeats that have both hydrophilic and hydrophobic components and alternating charges, allowing them to undergo self-assembly in physiological solutions (Sy et al., 2010), obtaining systems that slowly degrade with low immunogenicity and which are able to release in a sustained pattern (Figure 17.4).

Polymer Scaffolds

Polymer scaffolds are three-dimensional matrices with network architecture that can be manufactured in different forms. They are useful to incorporate and release therapeutic proteins (Chung and Park, 2007) (Figure 17.4).

Examples of DDS used for therapeutic protein and cell delivery in a cardiac context are discussed in deeper detail in the next section.

Finally, a major focus of interest is targeted DDS development (Scott et al., 2008). Targeted therapeutics can be delivered systemically at lower doses and could be used to increase drug concentration to the myocardium. Drug targeting would be possible for all the abovementioned DDS by coupling site-specific ligands like antibodies or receptors. The search for appropriate biomarkers significantly and differentially upregulated in diseased cardiac tissue is another unmet demand necessary to develop targeted drug delivery technologies with fewer toxic effects (Scott et al., 2008).

CURRENT STATUS ON CARDIAC DRUG DELIVERY SYSTEMS AND FUTURE TRENDS

As mentioned in the previous sections, over recent years, research to combine protein and cell therapies with DDS has increased in order to minimize or eliminate possible drawbacks. Here, studies from the last 10 years have been reviewed to show how these delivery systems have the ability to improve MI Clinical outcomes.

Drug Delivery Systems for Growth Factor Delivery

Currently, there are three main ways to incorporate GFs into DDS: immobilization, encapsulation, or embedding. All these strategies have been applied to design an effective therapy for cardiac repair.

Drug Delivery Systems with VEGF

Zhang et al. used a system based on a collagen-binding domain able to bind VEGF. The collagen-binding domain VEGF formed was incorporated into a collagen membrane, which, in an acute MI rat model, produced scar size reduction and cardiac function improvement. The beneficial effect observed is possibly due to high local VEGF concentration and prolongation of the protein's biological effect (Zhang et al., 2009). Similarly, Miyagi et al. covalently immobilized VEGF at two different concentrations in collagen patches and tested them in a rat MI model. Although the VEGF immobilization rate within the cardiac patch was low, positive results were obtained. VEGF-patched hearts were significantly thicker than control ones, which correlated with an increase in neovascularization, which was more significant in the high-dose patch treated group (Miyagi et al., 2011).

Immunoliposomes have also been found to deliver VEGF as the attachment of specific immunogens can facilitate liposome targeting at the infarcted heart. In the study of Scott et al., liposomes were conjugated to anti-P-selectin, one of the major molecules responsible for leukocyte enrollment in inflammation. Immunoliposomes were administered via the rat tail vein and were able to reach the heart infarction area. The immunoliposome-treated group showed a significant improvement in cardiac function compared to controls, showing a moderate left ventricle wall loss and vasculature improvement 4 weeks after DDS administration (Scott et al., 2009).

Synthetic polymers have been studied for VEGF encapsulation. Among them, poly lactic co-glycolic acid (PLGA), a biocompatible and biodegradable polymer approved for human use by the Food and Drug Administration, is a widely used biodegradable polymer for delivery of protein drugs. Our group prepared PLGA MP encapsulating VEGF and examined its potential in a rat MI model. One month after implantation, VEGF MP produced a significant increase in angiogenesis and arteriogenesis, correlating with a positive remodeling of the heart. A significantly greater left ventricle wall thickness was observed when compared to the free-VEGF group (Formiga et al., 2010). Similar results were obtained in the study by Simón-Yarza et al. employing VEGF-PEG-PLGA MP (Simón-Yarza et al., 2013).

Another attractive approach for delivering VEGF to the heart is to embed the protein into hydrogels. Wu et al. prepared an aliphatic polyester hydrogel that allows localized, sustained VEGF release. Their in vivo study, performed in a rat MI model, showed that this hydrogel attenuated the adverse cardiac remodeling and caused ventricular function improvement by increasing blood vessel formation and by preserving the scar thickness (Wu et al., 2011).

Self-assembling peptide NFs are a different strategy to embed VEGF. Guo et al. and Lin et al. tested them in rat and pig MI models, respectively. Fiber administration not only showed an improvement in angiogenesis, arteriogenesis, and cardiac performance, but also transformed the injection site microenvironment into one capable of recruiting endogenous myofibroblasts, which helped in achieving an effective revascularization (Guo et al., 2012; Lin et al., 2012).

Drug Delivery Systems with FGF-2

Fujita et al. studied the efficacy of a chitosan hydrogel encapsulating FGF-2 in a rabbit chronic MI model. The hydrogel was able to retain biologically active FGF-2 and to sustainably release it until the in vivo complete biodegradation of the system 4 weeks after injection. A substantial angiogenesis induction and collateral circulation in the ischemic myocardium was reported (Fujita et al., 2005). Similar results were obtained by Wang et al. who directly injected FGF-2 chitosan hydrogel into the infarcted myocardium border, producing infarction size reduction, cardiac function improvement, collagen deposition reduction, and an increase in arteriole density 4 weeks after administration (Wang et al., 2010).

Sakakibara et al. used FGF-2 incorporated in gelatin microspheres to evaluate their distribution in the rat heart, using different administration methods. They also investigated their efficacy in pigs after MI. In the efficacy study, the mean infarct size was not significantly different between groups. However, the group treated with FGF-2-microspheres showed cardiac function improvement associated with higher angiogenic rates (Sakakibara et al., 2003). In a different approach, Shao et al. studied the effects of the IM injection of FGF-2 incorporated in gelatin hydrogels on neoangiogenesis in a rat MI model. FGF-2-hydrogel produced neoangiogenesis stimulation and also decreased cardiomyocyte apoptosis in the infarct border zone, infarction wall thinning reduction, left ventricular remodeling attenuation, and consequently, cardiac function improvement (Shao et al., 2006).

More recently, FGF-2 was delivered using a pH- and temperature-responsive acrylic polymer hydrogel. This system allowed local FGF-2 retention in the heart apex with minimal diffusion. Not only was the system's beneficial effect demonstrated, which increased microvessel density and regional blood flow and improved cardiovascular function, but it was also shown that the hydrogel produced some benefit on its own. The acrylic polymer hydrogel was able to increase left ventricular thickness and improve cardiac function in the absence of exogenous GF delivery although at a lower rate with respect to the one that contained FGF-2 (Garbern et al., 2011).

Drug Delivery Systems with Other Growth Factors

In the study by Davis et al., IGF was entrapped in peptide NFs resulting in systolic function improvement and ventricular dilation reduction in a rat MI model (Davis et al., 2006). Another study entrapping IGF in peptide NFs revealed that IGF-NF treatment reduced the infarct size, improved the ventricular function, and favored cardiomyocyte regeneration and coronary vessel formation, showing better outcomes than free IGF in a rat MI model (Padin-Iruegas et al., 2009).

The studies by Hsieh et al. also employed peptide NFs for PDGF administration. The NFs were injected in a rat MI model, and it was observed that the system remained at the targeted site 14 days postinjection. Animals treated with PDGF-NFs significantly improved fractional shortening compared with controls. Of particular importance was the point that the improvement of fractional shortening was maintained only in those animals treated with the highest GF dose, implying dose-dependent cardioprotection. Interestingly, these researchers found that cardiac function improvement after PDGF-NF injection may not result from improvement of blood supply directly but from cardiomyocyte apoptosis prevention and myocardial function preservation. The system also improved hemodynamic parameters and cardiac performance 4 months after PDGF-NF injection (Hsieh et al., 2006a,b).

PIGF was encapsulated into chitosan-alginate NP and administered in a rat MI model. LVEF measurement showed that the PIGF-NP beneficial effect had a delay in time but was more sustained than after free PIGF administration. This suggests that chitosan-alginate NP provide a protective sustained-release mechanism to PIGF. These researchers also analyzed scar area, angiogenesis, and arteriogenesis, detecting statistical differences from the control groups (Binsalamah et al., 2011).

More recently, Purcell et al. applied a hyaluronic acid hydrogel containing SDF to a MI mice model. The system was not designed to favor regeneration of the infarcted heart on its own but indirectly due to the capacity to chemoattract BMSCs. SDF-hydrogel increased the circulating BMSC number, but further studies are needed to elucidate post MI remodeling using this system (Purcell et al., 2012).

Drug Delivery Systems for Multiple Growth Factor Delivery

Although DDSs with single GF therapy have shown promising results, restoration of the normal vasculature was not completely achieved. For instance, it has been demonstrated that VEGF delivery may lead to immature and leaky vasculature with poor function (Yancopoulos et al., 2000). This could be due to the requirement of more than one GF as in physiological neovascularization mechanisms in which several GFs are implicated. Thus, the combination of more than one therapeutic protein has produced great interest.

An example of DDS for multiple GF delivery is the work of Hao et al. They evaluated the angiogenic effect of sequential VEGF and PDGF release from an alginate hydrogel in MI rats. The hydrogel was almost degraded in vivo after 4 weeks. At this time point, an increase in capillary density was observed both in the VEGF and VEGF-PDGF hydrogels while PDGF hydrogel did not modify it. However, the capillary density was higher in the group treated with VEGF-PDGF hydrogel than VEGF hydrogel. The authors suggested that PDGF could potentiate VEGF action (Hao et al., 2007). In a similar way, the alginate hydrogel prepared by Ruvinov et al. sequentially delivered IGF and HGF in a rat MI model, based on the different binding affinity of both GFs to alginate. A pronounced beneficial effect in the infarcted area was observed in the cytokine-treated group compared with the control. The system preserved from fibrosis, scar thickness, attenuated infarct expansion, and also increased angiogenesis and mature blood vessel formation 4 weeks after its administration (Ruvinov et al., 2011).

More recently, a PEG based protease-degradable hydrogel combining VEGF with HGF demonstrated that dual factor release from a bioactive hydrogel was feasible and had the capacity to significantly improve the cardiac function in a ischemia/reperfusion rat model (Salimath et al., 2012).

Gelatin microspheres have also been used for multiple GF delivery. For instance, this system was employed for VEGF and IGF administration in a rat MI model by Cittadini et al. IGF antiapoptotic and antiremodeling actions were boosted by the

VEGF neoangiogenic effect. Animals treated with microspheres containing both GFs showed remarkably better effects on infarct size and left ventricular volume reductions, heart function improvement, vascularization enhancement, and apoptosis and inflammation reduction when compared with single GF microsphere administration (Cittadini et al., 2011).

Kim et al. incorporated PDGF and FGF into self-assembling peptide NFs. The system mimicked extracellular matrix porosity and gross structure, which allows cells to reside, migrate, and/or differentiate within the fibers. In the rat MI model, animals treated with the system containing both GFs almost recovered cardiac function. This effect correlated with a decrease in cardiomyocyte apoptosis, capillary, and arterial density recovery with stable vessel formation, higher reduction in the infarction size and improvement in wall thickness. Both GFs were detected 1 month after administration, a much longer period of time than after free GF administration (Kim et al., 2011).

Recently, our group examined whether the administration of MP containing NRG1 and FGF1 in a rat MI model promoted cardiac regeneration (Formiga et al., 2013). Three months after treatment, cardiac function improvement was observed in rats treated with FGF1-MP, NRG1-MP, or FGF1/NRG1-MP in comparison with the control group. Positive cardiac remodeling with smaller infarct size, a lower degree of fibrosis, and induction of tissue revascularization was also noticed. Cardiomyocyte proliferation and progenitor cell recruitment were also detected. Based on NRG1 and FGF1 putative activities, we hypothesized that a combination therapy involving administration of both cytokines would be more beneficial than each individually; however, we did not observe a consistent synergistic effect in vitro or in vivo. This important observation should be considered when designing new studies involving combination therapies.

Drug Delivery Systems for Cell Therapy

Combining DDS and cell therapy generates great interest as it is expected to increase cell engraftment and survival after administration. To date, there are two ways to incorporate cells into DDS: Cells can be encapsulated or adhered to the DDS surface.

Drug Delivery Systems with Myoblasts

The first study combining cell therapy with DDS in an animal MI model was performed by Christman et al. who seeded skeletal myoblasts in a fibrin glue scaffold. The group treated with myoblasts combined with the fibrin glue scaffold presented higher myoblast density within the infarct area and smaller infarct scar size when compared to fibrin glue, cells, and PBS groups 5 weeks after administration (Christman et al., 2004).

Skeletal myoblasts were also seeded and cultured on a biodegradable collagen and Matrigel™ hydrogel by Giraud et al. These authors tested the system's effectiveness in a rat MI model. Four weeks postimplantation they observed that the majority of the cells were washed out from the heart. However, systolic function and neovascularization were improved, presumably due to the cell paracrine effect (Giraud et al., 2008). This group also adhered skeletal myoblasts to polyurethane scaffolds. When implanted in a rat MI model, a delay in functional impairment was observed both in the free myoblasts group and in the scaffold group. Nevertheless, it must be noted that DDS use prolonged the beneficial effect on global heart function. In fact, scaffolds showed vascularization within them, suggesting that they were able to facilitate good nutrient and oxygen cell supply, improving cell viability. However, after 1 year, these authors observed that neither of the therapies prevented progression toward heart failure, so the system failed to produce a long-term effect (Giraud et al., 2010).

In another study, Blumenthal et al. used polyurethane scaffolds seeded with myoblasts, which were previously genetically modified to augment their paracrine activity in order to enhance their possible beneficial effect in a rat MI model. After 6 weeks, angiogenic effects and infarct size reduction were observed, probably due to VEGF, HGF, and SDF released from the cells (Blumenthal et al., 2010).

More recently, von Wattenwyl et al. seeded skeletal myoblasts overexpressing VEGF on polyurethane scaffolds and epicardially implanted them in MI rats. The treatment enhanced angiogenesis although infarction size was not reduced and cardiac function was not improved (von Wattenwyl et al., 2012).

Drug Delivery Systems with Embryonic Stem Cells

Regarding ESC, they were seeded in Matrigel™ and studied in a rat MI model. Interestingly, animals treated with ESC-Matrigel™ showed greater improvements in cardiac function and cardiac remodeling after 2 weeks (Kofidis et al., 2004). One year later, the same group seeded ECSs in a collagen I matrix, and they observed the formation of a stable IM graft into the surrounding infarcted area without distorting myocardial geometry in a rat MI model. This construct was able to prevent wall thinning (Kofidis et al., 2005). The same cell type was also used by the group of Ke et al., who grafted them on poly-glycolic acid scaffolds. Eight weeks after administration in a mice MI model, the system improved left ventricular function and reduced scar size. Interestingly, cells presented a higher survival ratio when attached to the scaffold than when freely administered (Ke et al., 2005).

In another study, ESCs were seeded onto porous fibrin scaffolds and were injected in the peri-infarct region of rat and swine MI models. First, in the rat MI model, cells were detected 1 month postinjection, and a significant improvement in cardiac function was found. In the swine MI model, 4 weeks after injection, infarct size was significantly smaller in the ESC fibrin scaffold group than in controls. Left ventricular contractile function was also improved as well as angiogenesis processes (Xiong et al., 2011).

More recently, a study demonstrated that ESC engraftment via fibrin-based patches represented a promising therapeutic approach to achieve efficient cell implantation in a rat MI model. Authors observed an improvement in global and regional cardiac function (Vallee et al., 2012).

Drug Delivery Systems with Mesenchymal Stem Cells

In the last years, numerous studies including MSCs in DDS have been performed with encouraging results. In a pioneering study conducted by Simpson et al., MSCs were embedded in collagen patches and epicardially applied in a rat MI model. One week after implantation, MSC collagen patch–treated rats showed progenitor cell engraftment increase in all heart regions but more specifically in the epicardium.

At 4 weeks, a significant improvement in full myocardial remodeling and cardiac function was observed. The authors concluded that a marked increase in α-smooth muscle actine positive cell number in patch-treated animals suggests that myofibroblast recruitment and differentiation was promoted (Simpson et al., 2007). The same group also performed a study with collagen patches to compare the effect of human MSC with human ESC-derived mesenchymal cells in a rat MI model. Both cell types incorporated in the patch allowed similar cardiac function and angiogenesis response (Simpson et al., 2012).

Similar results were obtained by Dai et al. in a rat MI model after seeding MSC onto a collagen matrix. They reported an increase in cell retention and survival. A reduction in the relocation of transplanted cells to noninfarcted areas was observed, possibly due to cell adhesion to the matrix interfering with the washout from the infarcted area (Dai et al., 2009).

Jin et al. adhered MSC to poly(lactid-co-ε-caprolactone) (PLCL) scaffolds, an elastic and biodegradable polymer with good cell interaction. The study, performed in a rat MI model, did not show statistical differences in the LVEF compared with the free MSC group. Both groups, MSC-PLCL and MSC, had reduced infarction size compared to the saline group (29% and 18%, respectively). Although in the infarction size there were no statistical differences, the expression of cardiac markers (MHC, α-actin, troponin-1) and GATA-4 was significantly greater in the MSC-PLCL scaffold group with respect to free MSC, indicating that the scaffolds favor higher cardiac differentiation (Jin et al., 2009).

In another study, MSC were encapsulated in RGD-alginate microbeads. The in vitro study demonstrated good cell growth and a satisfactory survival rate. The in vivo study in a rat acute MI model showed that after 10 weeks in MSC-microspheres and non-loaded microspheres groups there was a significant improvement in the cardiac function and arteriole formation enhancement when compared to free MSC and control groups (Yu et al., 2010). In the same year, Lin et al. combined MSC with self-assembling peptide NF. After 28 days of implanting the system in a pig MI model, capillary density increase was observed, accompanied by an increase in cell engraftment and survival. The ability of peptide NF to provide a suitable microenvironment for MSC adherence and the maintenance of their ability to perform normal cellular function might be responsible for the positive effect. These effects allowed a higher MSC differentiation ratio in endothelial and smooth muscle cells although not in cardiomyocytes. The study also demonstrated a synergistic effect between NF and the cells. It is known that MSC significantly increase systolic function whereas self-assembling peptide NF increase diastolic function, so as expected, their combination improved both functions (Lin et al., 2010). Similar results were obtained by Cui et al., who seeded MSC on other self-assembling peptide NF and proved their efficacy in a rat MI model. After 4 weeks, infarction size reduction and cardiac function improvement were observed in animals treated with MSC-NF when compared to free MSC (Cui et al., 2010).

More recently, MSC were seeded on collagen-1 scaffolds and administered in a rat MI model. Histological examination showed that patches were well integrated in the tissue. After 1 month, global cardiac function and infarction size were improved in the MSC-scaffold group when compared with untreated ones. The MSC-scaffold also produced an increase in angiogenesis when compared to controls (Maureira et al., 2012).

Another interesting study was accomplished by Le Visage et al. who studied MSC incorporation into a polysaccharide-based porous scaffold in a rat MI model. After 2 months, engraftment was almost three times higher in the MSC-scaffold group than when the cells were endocardially administered. Left ventricular fractional shortening was improved in the MSC-scaffold group when compared to the rest of the groups, possibly due to a paracrine cell effect (Le Visage et al., 2012).

Drug Delivery Systems with Bone Marrow–Derived Stem Cells

In 2005, Ryu et al. combined BMSCs with a fibrin matrix. This matrix facilitated cell survival until its complete degradation (8 weeks) in a rat MI model. This prolonged cell survival allowed better heart vascularization, producing a significant increase in microvessel density with larger average of internal diameter when compared with the free BMSC group (Ryu et al., 2005).

Two years later, BMSC were seeded in a biodegradable poly-glycolide-co-caprolactone (PGCL) scaffold and tested in a rat MI model by Piao et al. After 4 weeks, both BMSC scaffolds and nonseeded scaffolds showed mechanical properties against progressive left ventricle dilation, suggesting that PGCL acted as a mechanical barrier. However, only BMSC scaffolds showed an effective neovascularization induction. Interestingly, a portion of the BMSC seeded on scaffolds exhibited cardiomyocyte differentiation markers (Piao et al., 2007).

More recently, BMSC were incorporated into self-assembling peptide NF by Guo et al. and studied in a rat MI model. In one of the animal groups, peptide NF was combined with RGD, showing that the BMSC-RGD-NF group had collagen deposition decrease and higher heart function improvement when compared with free BMSC and BMSC-NF. BMSC-RGD-NF also allowed mature muscle fiber and gap junction formation within the myocardium. This higher beneficial effect observed when the NF were combined with RGD was attributed to RGD's ability to give the cells a temporary three-dimensional NF microenvironment, which favors survival and cardiomyogenic differentiation, having a key role in improving stem cell transplantation efficiency (Guo et al., 2010).

Drug Delivery Systems with Cardiac Progenitor Stem Cells

The combination of CSC with DDS has not yet been extensively studied. Tokunaga et al. analyzed the regenerative properties of different cell populations adhered to Puramatrix™ complex, a self-assembling nanopeptide, in a mouse MI model. The cell populations studied were CSC, BMSC, skeletal myoblasts, and ADSC. They observed that the matrix with CSC produced the highest improvement in capillary density, cardiac remodeling, and dysfunction prevention, all of which could be attributed to its angiogenic and antiapoptotic effects. One of the proposed mechanisms by which CSC produced this benefit was by VEGF secretion, highlighting the importance of the paracrine effect. The other cell types combined with the matrix produced a benefit in the infarcted area, but it was not as pronounced as with the CSC. Despite the promising results obtained, the system still requires further improvements as it was shown that most of the cells were eliminated from the treatment area in the first 24 h (Tokunaga et al., 2010).

Drug Delivery Systems with Adipose-Derived Stem Cells (ADSC)

In 2010, Danoviz et al. evaluated the effects of free ADSC or ADSC seeded either into collagen or fibrin scaffolds on cardiac performance in a rat MI model. ADSC on either scaffold, regardless of its composition, retained significantly more cells than the control group 24 hours and 4 weeks after its administration. A significant improvement in cardiac function and cardiac structure was observed 4 weeks post-treatment in the ADSC scaffold groups with respect to controls (Danoviz et al., 2010). In the same year, Zhang et al. isolated rat ADSC and loaded them onto fibrin glue scaffolds, which were then injected in a rat MI model. After 4 weeks, the ADSC scaffold group showed higher cell retention, significant arteriole density increase, and cardiac function improvement compared to free ADSC or to nonloaded scaffold groups. Moreover, animals treated with ADSC scaffold showed infarct size reduction and higher left ventricular thickness (Zhang et al., 2010).

More recently, Araña et al. incorporated ADSC into collagen patches with a different cross-linking degree. In vitro, ADSCs adhered homogenously and showed a similar proliferation ratio in the different collagen patches. However, when collagen patches were tested in vivo, only the non-cross-linked one was able to have a complete, long-lasting adhesion 1 month after its injection in a chronic rat MI model. One week after ADSC non-cross-linked collagen patch administration, 25.3% of the transplanted cells were detected, whereas no cells were found in animals receiving free ADSCs (Araña et al., 2013). Further efficacy studies are needed to confirm the benefits of collagen patches in cardiac repair.

Tissue Engineering

As stated above, the combination of more than one GF is required for mature vessel formation and global cardiac regeneration. This multiple factor effect can be achieved by combining a DDS with cells in order to take advantage of its paracrine effect. Moreover, if GF are incorporated into the DDS they could promote tissue regeneration and/or potentiate the cell regenerative role by increasing cell engraftment, proliferation, and survival. The combination of GFs, cells, and biomaterials is what is known as tissue engineering. At present, only a few studies have assessed the efficacy of tissue engineering strategies for MI treatment. However, preliminary but very promising results have been obtained.

In the study by Fukuhara et al., the authors adhered BMSC into a bFGF-loaded polyglycolic acid scaffold impregnated with collagen I hydrogel and studied them in a rat MI model. Interestingly, the bFGF-BMSC-scaffold group obtained the highest density vessel formation and the best cardiac function, leading to a better improvement with respect to the BMSC-scaffold group, 4 weeks post-treatment. It was thus demonstrated that a further response was obtained when bFGF was present (Fukuhara et al., 2005).

More recently, Kang et al. used a porous collagen scaffold to incorporate VEGF and FGF in combination with MSC, which was tested in a rat MI model. The GFs-MSC-scaffold treated group showed a higher angiogenic effect and better cardiac function compared to the MSC-scaffold group. This higher effect could be related to a higher cell survival in the GF-scaffold (Kang et al., 2012).

Penna et al. encapsulated VEGF in PLGA MP, which were then coated with fibronectin for MSC adhesion, aiming to obtain a good candidate to produce more global heart regeneration. In vitro results showed that the system was able to enhance cell proliferation and survival, but further studies are required (Penna et al., 2013). Díaz-Herráez et al. used PLGA MP for NRG encapsulation. The particles were next coated with collagen and/or poly-D-lysine for ADSC adhesion and studied in vivo in a rat MI model. After 2 weeks, the systems were well integrated in the peri-infarcted area, indicating that they were biocompatible. This work, although preliminary, has yielded favorable results that require further effectiveness studies (Díaz-Herráez et al., 2013).

Finally, there is an ongoing Phase I trial named ALCADIA in which human CSC IM injected are being combined with a gelatin hydrogel sheet incorporating bFGF for its controlled release (ClinicalTrials.gov identifier NCT00981006).

DRUG DELIVERY SYSTEMS IN HEART REGENERATION: LIMITATIONS AND FUTURE PERSPECTIVES

As has been discussed in the previous section, numerous studies involving DDS have been designed to tackle MI. Different materials have been used, from materials naturally present in the heart tissue to synthetic acrylic polymers, as shown in Table 17.4. At the moment, no evidence has been reported demonstrating the supremacy of one over the others. All DDS allow local delivery. Whereas particles, hydrogels, and liposomes can be administered by transendocardial injection, patches and scaffolds need to be attached to the pericardium, so a more invasive administration technique is required. On the other hand, these systems have been proven to be able to contribute more efficiently to the heart mechanical properties.

DDS for delivering GFs and/or cells are showing improvements in infarcted heart regeneration. Nevertheless, there are still many limitations that must be overcome (Figure 17.5 summarizes most of them), and further studies are required in this area.

For instance, one challenge is to obtain systems that can tightly control GF release. Many of the DDS mentioned in the previous section showed a high initial rate of GF delivery, which is known as a burst effect. A strategy to obtain a more sustained release could be to control GF affinity with the biomaterial. For example, as many GFs possess a high affinity with heparin, some in vitro and in vivo studies have incorporated this molecule in the formulation obtaining a delay in GF release (Cai et al., 2005; Huang et al., 2007). Controlling biomaterial porosity and/or biodegradation rate could be another way to control GF release. Alginates, for instance, typically present low and uncontrolled degradation. However, partial alginate oxidation or alginate combination with polymers that possess different molecular weights can provide controlled degradation kinetics, allowing better control of incorporated factor release (Hao et al., 2007).

Cell survival in the tissue has increased with DDS use. However, cell survival rates need to be ameliorated. In this sense, a better interaction between cells and biomaterials could help for this purpose. As previously mentioned, natural polymers can be easily recognized by the cell-surface receptors. On the other hand, synthetic polymers, as they are hydrophobic and lack cell-recognition moieties, are preferably

TABLE 17.4
Biomaterials Under Investigation for Drug Delivery of Proteins and Cells in the Myocardial Infarction Context

Material	DDS	Proteins	Cells
Chitosan	NP	PIGF (Binsalamah et al., 2011)	
	Hydrogel	FGF (Fujita et al., 2005; Wang et al., 2010)	
Alginate	NP	PIGF (Binsalamah et al., 2011)	
	Hydrogel	VEGF + PDGF (Hao et al., 2007) IGF + HGF (Ruvinov et al., 2011)	MSC (Yu et al., 2010)
Hyaluronic acid	Hydrogel	SDF (Purcell et al., 2012)	
Collagen/ gelatin	Hydrogel	FGF (Sakakibara et al., 2003; Fukuhara et al., 2005; Shao et al., 2006)	BMSC (Fukuhara et al., 2005) ESC (Kofidis et al., 2005) Myoblasts (Giraud et al., 2008)
	Scaffold	VEGF (Zhang et al., 2009; Miyagi et al., 2011) VEGF + FGF (Kang et al., 2012)	MSC (Simpson et al., 2007; Dai et al., 2009; Kang et al., 2012; Simpson et al., 2012; Maureira et al., 2012) ADSC (Danoviz et al., 2012; Araña et al., 2013)
	Microsphere	VEGF + IGF (Cittadini et al., 2011)	
Fibrin	Scaffold		ESC (Xiong et al., 2011; Vallee et al., 2012) ADSC (Danoviz et al., 2010; Zhang et al., 2010)
	Hydrogel		Myoblasts (Christman et al., 2004) BMSC (Ryu et al., 2005) MSC (Lisi et al., 2012)
PLGA	MP	VEGF (Formiga et al., 2010; Simón-Yarza et al., 2013; Penna et al., 2013) FGF + NRG (Formiga et al., 2013) NRG (Díaz-Herráez et al., 2013)	ADSC (Díaz-Herráez et al., 2013) MSC (Penna et al., 2013)
Peptide nanofibers	Hydrogel	VEGF (Guo et al., 2012; Lin et al., 2012) PDGF (Hsieh et al., 2006a,b) IGF (Davis et al., 2006; Padin-Iruelas et al., 2009) PDGF + FGF (Kim et al., 2011)	MSC (Lin et al., 2010; Cui et al., 2010) BMSC (Guo et al., 2010) CSC, BMSC, myoblasts, ADSC (Tokunaga et al., 2010)
Acrylic polymers	Hydrogel	FGF (Garben et al., 2011)	
	Scaffold		Myoblast (Giraud et al., 2010; Blumenthal et al., 2010; von Wattenwyl et al., 2012)

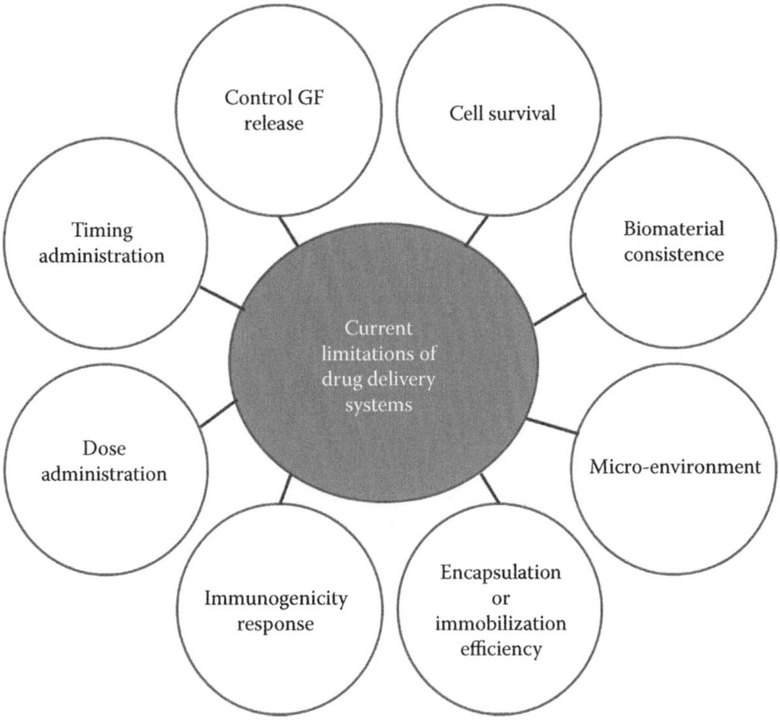

FIGURE 17.5 Current limitations of drug delivery systems used for growth factor and/or cell administration in cardiac regeneration.

used in combination with natural polymers or small peptide sequences in order to promote cell-biomaterial interactions (Ravichandran et al., 2012). Another way to increase cell interactions with synthetic polymers is by covering their surfaces with biomimetic substances, such as collagen (Lu et al., 2007; Hao et al., 2008; Qu et al., 2009; Díaz-Herráez et al., 2013), fibronectin (Garbayo et al., 2011), poly-D-lysine (Lu et al., 2006; Lin et al., 2009; Díaz-Herráez et al., 2013), laminine (Jung et al., 2012), and tenascine (Sahoo et al., 2010; Chen et al., 2012), among others.

Biomaterial consistence is another aspect under investigation. Most of the biomaterials used until now have unmatched mechanical properties with the infarcted myocardium. For example, they are significantly softer than the human cardiac muscle at the end of diastole (Ravichandran et al., 2012). However, this point has generated some controversy between authors since softer biomaterials are more flexible, facilitating normal heart contraction, and harder ones could hinder this function. Thus, biomaterials with strength similar to normal human cardiac muscle seem to be the most appropriate.

Furthermore, biomaterials have to improve the generation of a suitable microenvironment that facilitates cell survival and engraftment and new vessel formation. It has been seen that some hydrogels are formed really fast on the implantation area, forming a consistent structure that does not allow the correct oxygen and nutrient entrance inside the system and the surrounding area while scaffolds with an adequate porosity facilitates it. Self-assembling NFs have also been shown to be able to create NF microenvironments that can promote vascular cell recruitment and cell survival (Davis et al., 2005).

Encapsulation efficiency or immobilization rate are other important aspects that have to be optimized since GFs are expensive. Currently, different manufacturing processes and the affinity between GFs and biomaterial are being studied to reduce protein loss during the production process and consequently minimizing global treatment cost. In addition, by increasing the percentage of GF that is encapsulated or immobilized, the quantity of biomaterial administered can be reduced, lowering the possible immunogenic response. Another way to reduce immunogenicity is by increasing surface hydrophilicity with the incorporation of, for example, PEG chains (Simon-Yarza et al., 2013).

Dose and timing of administration and the choice of the optimal GFs or cells are also under study. At present, VEGF and BMSC are the GF and cells that are receiving most attention, but further research is required to find out more about the real ischemic heart requirements. A deeper knowledge of the processes implicated in cardiac disorders and cardiac repair will help to establish which GFs are most adequate for each situation and at which time and dose they should be administered.

In conclusion, combining DDS with GF and/or cell therapy can be crucial in increasing the beneficial results in MI regeneration. In this regard, it is expected that in the next 10–20 years, these therapies will constitute more than half of the new drugs introduced in the market (Tarun et al., 2011). At the moment, more preclinical studies with consistent results are required in order to proceed to clinical trials.

LIST OF ABBREVIATIONS

ADSC	adipose-derived mesenchimal stem cells
BMSC	bone marrow–derived stem cells
CSC	cardiac progenitor stem cells
CT	clinical trial
CVD	cardiovascular disease
DDS	drug delivery system
DES	drug-eluting stents
EPO	erythropoietin
ESC	embryonic stem cells
FGF	fibroblast growth factor
G-CSF	granulocyte colony stimulating factor
GF	growth factor
HGF	hepatocyte growth factor
IC	intracoronary
IGF	insulin-like growth factor-1
IM	intramyocardial
iPS	induced pluripotent stem cells
IV	intravenous
LVEF	left ventricular ejection fraction

MI	myocardial infarction
MP	microparticle
MSC	mesenchymal stem cells
NF	nanofiber
NP	nanoparticle
NRG	neuregulin
PDGF	platelet-derived growth factor
PIGF	placental growth factor
PLGA	poly lactic co-glycolic acid
PLLA	poly-L-lactid acid
SC	subcutaneous
SDF	stromal cell-derived factor-1
TGF-β	transforming growth factor-β
VEGF	vascular endothelial growth factor

REFERENCES

Achilli, F., Malafronte, C., Lenatti, L., Gentile, F., Dadones, V., Gibelli Mircli, L., Capogrossi, M. C. et al. 2010. Granulocyte colony-stimulating factor attenuates left ventricular remodelling after acute anterior STEMI: Results of the single-blind, randomized, placebo-controlled multicentre Stem cell mobilization in acute myocardial infarction MI (STEM-AMI) trial. *Eur J Heart Fail.* 12: 1111–1121.

Akar, A. R., Durdu, S., Arat, M., Kilickap, M., Kucuk, N. O., Arslan, O., Kuzu, I. et al. 2009. Five-year follow-up after transepicardial implantation of autologous bone marrow mononuclear cells to ungraftable coronary territories for patients with ischaemic cardiomyopathy. *Eur J Cardiothorac Surg.* 36(4): 633–643.

Akbarzadeh, A., Rezaei-Sadabady, R., Davaran, S., Joo, S. W., Zarghami, N., Hanifehpour, Y., Samiei, M. et al. 2013. Liposome: Classification, preparation, and applications. *Nanoscale Res Lett.* 8(1): 102.

Almeida, A. J., and Souto, E. 2007. Solid lipid nanoparticles as a drug delivery system for peptides and proteins. *Adv Drug Deliv.* 59(6): 478–490.

Ang, K. L., Chin, D., Leyva, F., Foley, P., Kubal, C., Chalil, S., Srinivasan, L. et al. 2008. Randomized, controlled trial of intramuscular or intracoronary injection of autologous bone marrow cells into scarred myocardium during CABG versus CABG alone. *Nat Clin Pract Cardiovasc Med.* 5(10): 663–670.

Araña, M., Peña, E., Abizanda, G., Cille, M., Ochoa, I., Gavira, J. J., Espinosa, G. et al. 2013. Preparation and characterization of collagen-based ADSC-carrier sheets for cardiovascular application. *Acta Biomater.* 9(4): 6075–6083.

Assmus, B., Honold, J., Schächinger, V., Britten, M. B., Fischer-Rasokat, U., Lehmann, R., Teupe, C. et al. 2006. Transcoronary transplantation of progenitor cells after myocardial infarction. *N Engl J Med.* 355: 1222–1232.

Beitnes, J. O., Hopp, E., Lunde, K., Solheim, S., Arnesen, H., Brinchmann, J. E., Forfang, K. et al. 2009. Long-term results after intracoronary injection of autologous mononuclear bone marrow cells in acute myocardial infarction: The ASTAMI randomised, controlled study. *Heart.* 95(24): 1983–1989.

Biagini, E., Valgimigli, M., Smits, P. C., Poldermans, D., Schinkel, A. F., Rizzello, V., Onderwater, E. E. et al. 2006. Stress and tissue Doppler echocardiographic evidence of effectiveness of myoblast transplantation in patients with ischaemic heart failure. *Eur J Heart Fail.* 8: 641–648.

Binsalamah, Z. M., Paul, A., Khan, A. A., Prakash, S., and Shum-Tim, D. 2011. Intramyocardial sustained delivery of placental growth factor using nanoparticles as a vehicle for delivery in the rat infarct model. *Int J Nanomedicine*. 6: 2667–2678.

Blumenthal, B., Golsong, P., Poppe, A., Heilmann, C., Schlensak, C., Beyersdorf, F., and Siepe, M. 2010. Polyurethane scaffolds seeded with genetically engineered skeletal myoblasts: A promising tool to regenerate myocardial function. *Artif Organs*. 34(2): E46–E54.

Briguori, C., Reimers, B., Sarais, C., Napodano, M., Pascotto, P., Azzarello, G., Bregni, M. et al. 2006. Direct intramyocardial percutaneous delivery of autologous bone marrow in patients with refractory myocardial angina. *Am Heart J*. 151(3): 674–680.

Britten, M. B., Abolmaali, N. D., Assmus, B., Lehmann, R., Honold, J., Schmitt, J., Vogl, T. J. et al. 2003. Infarct remodeling after intracoronary progenitor cell treatment in patients with acute myocardial infarction (TOPCARE-AMI): Mechanistic insights from serial contrast-enhanced magnetic resonance imaging. *Circulation*. 108: 2212–2218.

Cai, S., Liu, Y., Zheng Shu, X., and Prestwich, G. D. 2005. Injectable glycosaminoglycan hydrogels for controlled release of human basic fibroblast growth factor. *Biomaterials*. 26(30): 6054–6067.

Centers for Disease Control and Prevention (CDC). 2012. CDC Grand Rounds: The Million Hearts Initiative. *MMWR Morb Mortal Wkly Rep*. 61(50): 1017–1021.

Chachques, J. C., Acar, C., Herreros, J., Trainini, J. C., Prosper, F., D'Attellis, N., Fabiani, J. N. et al. 2004. Cellular cardiomyoplasty: Clinical application. *Ann Thorac Surg*. 77: 1121–1130.

Chen, S. L., Fang, W. W., Qian, J., Ye, F., Liu, Y. H., Shan, S. J., Zhang, J. J. et al. 2004. Improvement of cardiac function after transplantation of autologous bone marrow mesenchymal stem cells in patients with acute myocardial infarction. *Chin Med J (Engl)*. 117(10): 1443–1448.

Chen, K., Sahoo, S., He, P., Ng, K. S., Toh, S. L., and Goh, J. C. 2012. A Hybrid Silk/RADA-Based Fibrous Scaffold with Triple Hierarchy for Ligament Regeneration. *Tissue Eng. Part. A*. 18(13–14): 1399–1409.

Christman, K. L., Fok, H. H., Sievers, R. E., Fang, Q., and Lee, R. J. 2004. Fibrin glue alone and skeletal myoblasts in a fibrin scaffold preserve cardiac function after myocardial infarction. *Tissue Eng*. 10(3–4): 403–409.

Chung, H. J., and Park, T. G. 2007. Surface engineered and drug releasing pre-fabricated scaffolds for tissue engineering. *Adv. Drug Delivery Rev*. 59(4–5): 249–269.

Cittadini, A., Monti, M. G., Petrillo, V., Esposito, G., Imparato, G., Luciani, A., Uciuolo, F. et al. 2011. Complementary therapeutic effects of dual delivery of insulin-like growth factor-1 and vascular endothelial growth factor by gelatin microspheres in experimental heart failure. *Eur J Heart Fail*. 13(12): 1264–1274.

Cui, X. J., Xie, H., Wang, H. J., Guo, H. D., Zhang, J. K., Wang, C., and Tan, Y. Z. 2010. Transplantation of mesenchymal stem cells with self-assembling polypeptide scaffolds is conducive to treating myocardial infarction in rats. *Tohoku J Exp Med*. 222(4): 281–289.

Dai, W., Hale, S. L., Kay, G. L., Jyrala, A. J., and Kloner, R. A. 2009. Delivering stem cells to the heart in a collagen matrix reduces relocation of cells to other organs as assessed by nanoparticle technology. *Regen Med*. 4(3): 387–395.

Danoviz, M. E., Nakamuta, J. S., Marques, F. L., dos Santos, L., Alvarenga, E. C., dos Santos, A. A., Antonio, E. L. et al. 2010. Rat adipose tissue-derived stem cells transplantation attenuates cardiac dysfunction post infarction and biopolymers enhance cell retention. *PLoS One*. 5(8): e12077.

Davis, M. E., Motion, J. P., Narmoneva, D. A., Takahashi, T., Hakuno, D., Kamm, R. D., Zhang, S. et al. 2005. Injectable self-assembling peptide nanofibers create intramyocardial microenvironments for endothelial cells. *Circulation*. 111(4): 442–450.

Davis, M. E., Hsieh, P. C., Takahashi, T., Song, Q., Zhang, S., Kamm, R. D., Grodzinsky, A. J. et al. 2006. Local myocardial insulin-like growth factor 1 (IGF-1) delivery with biotinylated peptide nanofibers improves cell therapy for myocardial infarction. *Proc Natl Acad Sci USA*. 103(21): 8155–8160.

de la Fuente, L. M., Stertzer, S. H., Argentieri, J., Peñaloza, E., Miano, J., Koziner, B., Bilos, C. et al. 2007. Transendocardial autologous bone marrow in chronic myocardial infarction using a helical needle catheter: 1-year follow-up in an open-label, nonrandomized, single-center pilot study (the TABMMI study). *Am Heart J*. 154(1): 79.e1–7.

Díaz-Herráez, P., Garbayo, E., Simón-Yarza, T., Formiga, F. R., Prosper, F., and Blanco-Prieto, M. J. 2013. Adipose-derived stem cells combined with Neuregulin-1 delivery systems for heart tissue engineering. *Eur. J. Pharm. Biopharm*. 85: 143–150.

Dib, N., Michler, R. E., Pagani, F. D., Wright, S., Kereiakes, D. J., Lengerich, R., Binkley, P. et al. 2005. Safety and feasibility of autologous myoblast transplantation in patients with ischemic cardiomyopathy: Four-year follow-up. *Circulation*. 112: 1748–1755.

Dib, N., Henry, T., DeMaria, A., Itescu, S., McCarthy, M. M., Jaggar, S. C., Taylor, N. et al. 2009a. The First US Study to Assess the Feasibility and Safety of Endocardial Delivery of Allogenic Mesenchymal Precursor Cells in Patient With Heart Failure: Three-Month Interim Analysis. *Circulation*. 120: S810.

Dib, N., Dinsmore, J., Lababidi, Z., White, B., Moravec, S., Campbell, A., Rosenbaum, A. et al. 2009b. One-year follow-up of feasibility and safety of the first U.S., randomized, controlled study using 3-dimensional guided catheter-based delivery of autologous skeletal myoblasts for ischemic cardiomyopathy. *J Am Coll Cardiol Interv*. 2(1): 9–16.

Duckers, H. J., Houtgraaf, J., Hehrlein, C., Schofer, J., Waltenberger, J., Gershlick, A., Bartunek, J. et al. 2011. Final results of a phase IIa, randomized, open-label trial to evaluate the percutaneous intramyocardial transplantation of autologous skeletal myoblasts in congestive heart failure patients: The SEISMIC trial. *Eurointervention*. 6: 805–812.

Engelmann, M. G., Theiss, H. D., Theiss, C., Henschel, V., Huber, A., Wintersprínger, B. J., Schoenberg, S. O. et al. 2010. G-CSF in patients suffering from late revascularised ST elevation myocardial infarction: Final 1-year-results of the G-CSF-STEMI trial. *Int J Cardiol*. 144: 399–404.

Erbs, S., Linke, A., Adams, V., Lenk, K., Thiele, H., Diederich, K. W., Emmrich, F. et al. 2005. Transplantation of blood-derived progenitor cells after recanalization of chronic coronary artery occlusion: First randomized and placebo-controlled study. *Circ Res*. 97(8): 756–762.

Fernández-Avilés, F., San Román, J. A., García-Frade, J., Fernández, M. E., Peñarrubia, M. J., de la Fuente, L., Gómez-Bueno, M. et al. 2004. Experimental and clinical regenerative capability of human bone marrow cells after myocardial infarction. *Circ Res*. 95(7): 742–748.

Formiga, F. R., Pelacho, B., Garbayo, E., Abizanda, G., Gavira, J. J., Simon-Yarza, T., Mazo, M. et al. 2010. Sustained release of VEGF through PLGA microparticles improves vasculogenesis and tissue remodeling in an acute myocardial ischemia-reperfusion model. *J Control Release*. 147(1): 30–37.

Formiga, F. R., Tamayo, E., Simón-Yarza, T., Pelacho, B., Prosper, F., and Blanco-Prieto, M. J. 2012. Angiogenic therapy for cardiac repair based on protein delivery systems. *Heart Fail Rev*. 17(3): 449–473.

Formiga, F. R., Pelacho, B., Garbayo, E., Imbuluzqueta, I., Díaz-Herráez, P., Abizanda, G., Gavira, J. J. et al. 2014. Controlled delivery of fibroblast growth factor-1 and neuregulin-1 from biodegradable microparticles promotes cardiac repair in a rat myocardial infarction model through activation of endogenous regeneration. *J. Control Release*. 173: 132–139.

Fuchs, S., Kornowski, R., Weisz, G., Satler, L. F., Smits, P. C., Okubagzi, P., Baffour, R. et al. 2006. Safety and feasibility of transendocardial autologous bone marrow cell transplantation in patients with advanced heart disease. *Am J Cardiol.* 97(6): 823–829.

Fujita, M., Ishihara, M., Morimoto, Y., Simizu, M., Simizu, M., Saito, Y., Yura, H. et al. 2005. Efficacy of photocrosslinkable chitosan hydrogel containing fibroblast growth factor-2 in a rabbit model of chronic myocardial infarction. *J Surg Res.* 126(1): 27–33.

Fukuhara, S., Tomita, S., Nakatani, T., Fujisato, T., Ohtsu, Y., Ishida, M., Yutani, C. et al. 2005. Bone marrow cell-seeded biodegradable polymeric scaffold enhances angiogenesis and improves function of the infarcted heart. *Circ J.* 69(7): 850–857.

Gao, R., Zhang, J., Cheng, L., Wu, X., Dong, W., Yang, X., Li, T. et al. 2010. A Phase II, randomized, double-blind, multicenter, based on standard therapy, placebo-controlled study of the efficacy and safety of recombinant human neuregulin-1 in patients with chronic heart failure. *J Am Coll Cardiol.* 55: 1907–1914.

Garbayo, E., Raval, A. P., Curtis, K. M., Della-Morte, D., Gomez, L. A., D'Ippolito, G., Reiner, T. et al. 2011. Neuroprotective properties of marrow-isolated adult multilineage-inducible cells in rat hippocampus following global cerebral ischemia are enhanced when complexed to biomimetic microcarriers. *J Neurochem.* 119(5): 972–988.

Garbern, J. C., Minami, E., Stayton, P. S., and Murry, C. E. 2011. Delivery of basic fibroblast growth factor with a pH-responsive, injectable hydrogel to improve angiogenesis in infarcted myocardium. *Biomaterials.* 32(9): 2407–2416.

Gavira, J. J., Herreros, J., Perez, A., Garcia-Velloso, M. J., Barba, J., Martin-Herrero, F., Cañizo, C. et al. 2006. Autologous skeletal myoblast transplantation in patients with nonacute myocardial infarction: 1-year follow-up. *J Thorac Cardiovasc Surg.* 131: 799–804.

Gibson, C., Laham, R., and Giordano, F. 1999. Magnitude and location of new angiographically apparent coronary collaterals following IV VEGF administration. *J Am Coll Cardiol.* 33(A): 65A.

Giraud, M. N., Ayuni, E., Cook, S., Siepe, M., Carrel, T. P., and Tevaearai, H. T. 2008. Hydrogel-based engineered skeletal muscle grafts normalize heart function early after myocardial infarction. *Artif Organs.* 32(9): 692–700.

Giraud, M. N., Fweckiger, R., Cook, S., Ayuni, E., Siepe, M., Carrel, T., and Tevaearai, H. 2010. Long-term evaluation of myoblast seeded patches implanted on infarcted rat hearts. *Art. Org.* 34(6): E184–E192.

Gnecchi, M., Zhang, Z., Ni, A., and Dzau, V. J. 2008. Paracrine mechanisms in adult stem cell signaling and therapy. *Circ Res.* 103(11): 1204–1219.

Go, A. S., Mozaffarian, D., Roger, V. L., Benjamin, E. J., Berry, J. D., Borden, W. B., Bravata, D. M. et al. 2013. On behalf of the American Heart Association Statistics Committee and Stroke Statistics Subcommittee. Heart disease and stroke statistics—2013 update: A report from the American Heart Association. *Circulation.* 127:e6–e245.

Grundmann, S., van Royen, N., Pasterkamp, G., Gonzalez, N., Tijsma, E. J., Piek, J. J., and Hoefer, I. E. 2007. A new intra-arterial delivery platform for pro-arteriogenic compounds to stimulate collateral artery growth via transforming growth factor-beta1 release. *J Am Coll Cardiol.* 50(4): 351–358.

Guo, H. D., Cui, G. H., Wang, H. J., and Tan, Y. Z. 2010. Transplantation of marrow-derived cardiac stem cells carried in designer self-assembling peptide nanofibers improves cardiac function after myocardial infarction. *Biochem Biophys Res Commun.* 399(1): 42–48.

Guo, H. D., Cui, G. H., Yang, J. J., Wang, C., Zhu, J., Zhang, L. S., Jiang, J. et al. 2012. Sustained delivery of VEGF from designer self-assembling peptides improves cardiac function after myocardial infarction. *Biochem Biophys Res Commun.* 424(1): 105–111.

Gyöngyösi, M., Lang, I., Dettke, M., Beran, G., Graf, S., Sochor, H., Nyolczas, N. et al. 2009. Combined delivery approach of bone marrow mononuclear stem cells early and late after myocardial infarction: The MYSTAR prospective, randomized study. *Nat Clin Pract Cardiovasc Med.* 6(1): 70–81.

Hao, X., Silva, E. A., Mansson-Broberg, A., Grinnemo, K. H., Siddiqui, A. J., Dellgren, G., Wardell, E. et al. 2007. Angiogenic effects of sequential release of VEGF-A165 and PDGF-BB with alginate hydrogels after myocardial infarction. *Cardiovasc Res.* 75(1): 178–185.

Hao, W., Hu, Y. Y., Wei, Y. Y., Pang, L., Lv, R., Bai, J. P., Xiong, Z. et al. 2008. Collagen I gel can facilitate homogenous bone formation of adipose-derived stem cells in PLGA-beta-TCP scaffold. *Cells Tissues Organs.* 187(2): 89–102.

Hare, J. M., Traverse, J. H., Henry, T. D., Dib, N., Strumpf, R. K., Schulman, S. P., Gerstenblith, G. et al. 2009. A randomized, double-blind, placebo-controlled, dose-escalation study of intravenous adult human mesenchymal stem cells (prochymal) after acute myocardial infarction. *J Am Coll Cardiol.* 54(24): 2277–2786.

Heldman, A. W., Cheng, L., Jenkins, G. M., Heller, P. F., Kim, D. W., Ware, M., Jr., Nater, C. et al. 2001. Paclitaxel stent coating inhibits neointimal hyperplasia at 4 weeks in a porcine model of coronary restenosis. *Circulation.* 103(18): 2289–2295.

Hendel, R. C., Henry, T. D., Rocha-Singh, K., Isner, J. M., Kereiakes, D. J., Giordano, F. J., Simons, M. et al. 2000. Effect of intracoronary recombinant human vascular endothelial growth factor on myocardial perfusion: Evidence for a dose-dependent effect. *Circulation.* 121: 118–121.

Hendrikx, M., Hensen, K., Clijsters, C., Jongen, H., Koninckx, R., Bijnens, E., Ingels, M. et al. 2006. Recovery of regional but not global contractile function by the direct intramyocardial autologous bone marrow transplantation: Results from a randomized controlled clinical trial. *Circulation.* 114(1 Suppl): I101–I107.

Henry, T. D., Rocha-Singh, K., and Isner, J. M. 2001. Results of intracoronary recombinant vascular endothelial growth factor (rhVEGF) administration trial. *Am Heart J.* 142: 872–880.

Henry, T. D., Annex, B. H., McKendall, G. R., Azrin, M. A., Lopez, J. J., Giordano, F. J., Shah, P. K. et al. 2003. The VIVA trial: Vascular endothelial growth factor in Ischemia for Vascular Angiogenesis. *Circulation.* 107: 1359–1365.

Herbots, L., D'hooge, J., Eroglu, E., Thijs, D., Ganame, J., Claus, P., Dubois, C. et al. 2009. Improved regional function after autologous bone marrow-derived stem cell transfer in patients with acute myocardial infarction: A randomized, double-blind strain rate imaging study. *Eur Heart J.* 30(6): 662–670.

Hirsch, A., Nijveldt, R., van der Vleuten, P. A., Tijssen, J. G., van der Giessen, W. J., Tio, R. A., Waltenberger, J. et al. 2011. Intracoronary infusion of mononuclear cells from bone marrow or peripheral blood compared with standard therapy in patients after acute myocardial infarction treated by primary percutaneous coronary intervention: Results of the randomized controlled HEBE trial. *Eur Heart J.* 32(14): 1736–1747.

Hsieh, P. C., Davis, M. E., Gannon, J., MacGillivray, C., and Lee, R. T. 2006a. Controlled delivery of PDGF-BB for myocardial protection using injectable self-assembling peptide nanofibers. *J Clin Invest.* 116(1): 237–248.

Hsieh, P. C., Davis, M. E., Gannon, J., MacGillivray, C., Gannon, J., Cruz, F. U., and Lee, R. T. 2006b. Local Controlled Intramyocardial Delivery of Platelet-Derived Growth Factor Improves Postinfarction Ventricular Function Without Pulmonary Toxicity. *Circulation.* 114(7): 637–644.

Huang, M., Vitharana, S. N., Peek, L. J., Coop, T., and Berkland, C. 2007. Polyelectrolyte complexes stabilize and controllably release vascular endothelial growth factor. *Biomacromolecules.* 8(5): 1607–1614.

Huikuri, H. V., Kervinen, K., Niemelä, M., Ylitalo, K., Säily, M., Koistinen, P., Savolainen, E. R. et al. 2008. Effects of intracoronary injection of mononuclear bone marrow cells on left ventricular function, arrhythmia risk profile, and restenosis after thrombolytic therapy of acute myocardial infarction. *Eur Heart J.* 29(22): 2723–2732.

Ince, H., Petzsch, M., Rehders, T. C., Chatterjee, T., and Nienaber, C. A. 2004. Transcatheter transplantation of autologous skeletal myoblasts in postinfarction patients with severe left ventricular dysfunction. *J Endovasc Ther.* 11: 695–704.

Ince, H., Petzsch, M., Kleine, H. D., Schmidt, H., Rehders, T., Körber, T., Schümichen, C. et al. 2005. Preservation from left ventricular remodelin by front-integrated revascularization and stem cell liberation in evolving acute myocardial infarction by use of granulocyte-colony-stimulating factor (FIRSTLINE-AMI). *Circulation.* 112: 3097–3106.

Jabbour, A., Hayward, C. S., Keogh, A. M., Kotlyar, E., McCrohon, J. A., England, J. F., Amor, R. et al. 2011. Parenteral administration of recombinant human neuregulin-1 to patients with stable chronic heart failure produces favourable acute and chronic haemodynamic responses. *Eur J Heart Fail.* 13: 83–92.

Janssens, S., Dubois, C., Bogaert, J., Theunissen, K., Deroose, C., Desmet, W., Kalantzi, M. et al. 2006. Autologous bone marrow-derived stem-cell transfer in patients with ST-segment elevation myocardial infarction: Double-blind, randomised controlled trial. *Lancet.* 367(9505): 113–121.

Jin, J., Jeong, S. I., Shin, Y. M., Lim, K. S., Shin, H. S., Lee, Y. M., Koh, H. C. et al. 2009. Transplantation of mesenchymal stem cells within a poly(lactide-co-epsilon-caprolactone) scaffold improves cardiac function in a rat myocardial infarction model. *Eur J Heart Fail.* 11(2): 147–153.

Jung, S. Y., Kim, J. M., Min, S. K., Kim, O. B., Jang da, H., and Min, B. M. 2012. The potential of laminin-2-biomimetic short peptide to promote cell adhesion, spreading and migration by inducing membrane recruitment and phosphorylation of PKCdelta. *Biomaterials.* 33(15): 3967–3979.

Kang, H. J., Kim, H. S., Zhang, S. Y., Park, K. W., Cho, H. J., Koo, B. K., Kim, Y. J. et al. 2004. Effects of intracoronary infusion of peripheral blood stem-cells mobilised with granulocyte-colony stimulating factor on left ventricular systolic function and restenosis after coronary stenting in myocardial infarction: The MAGIC cell randomised clinical trial. *Lancet.* 363(9411): 751–756.

Kang, K., Sun, L., Xiao, Y., Li, S. H., Wu, J., Guo, J., Jiang, S. L. et al. 2012. Aged human cells rejuvenated by cytokine enhancement of biomaterials for surgical ventricular restoration. *J Am Coll Cardiol.* 60(21): 2237–2249.

Ke, Q., Yang, Y., Rana, J. S., Chen, Y., Morgan, J. P., and Xiao, Y. F. 2005. Embryonic stem cells cultured in biodegradable scaffold repair infarcted myocardium in mice. *Sheng Li Xue Bao.* 57(6): 673–681.

Kharlamov, A. N., Duckers, H. J., van Beusekom, H. M., Smits, P. C., Perin, E. C., and Serruys, P. W. 2012. Do we have a future with transcatheter adventitial delivery of stem cells? *Int J Cardiol.* 165(2): 217–221.

Kim, J. H., Jung, Y., Kin, S. H., Sun, K., Choi, J., Kim, H. C., and Park, Y. 2011. The enhancement of mature vessel formation and cardiac function in infarcted hearts using dual growth factor delivery with self-assembling peptides. *Biomaterials.* 32(26): 6080–6088.

Kofidis, T., de Bruin, J. L., Hoyt, G., Lebl, D. R., Tanaka, M., Yamane, T., Chang, C. P. et al. 2004. Injectable bioartificial myocardial tissue for large-scale intramural cell transfer and functional recovery of injured heart muscle. *J Thorac Cardiovasc Surg.* 128(4): 571–578.

Kofidis, T., de Bruin, J. L., Hoyt, G., Ho, Y., Tanaka, M., Yamane, T., Lebl, D. R. et al. 2005. Myocardial restoration with embryonic stem cell bioartificial tissue transplantation. *J Heart Lung Transplant.* 24(6): 737–744.

Kurrelmeyer, K., Kalra, D., Bozkurt, B., Wang, F., Dibbs, Z., Seta, Y., Baumgarten, G. et al. 1998. Cardiac remodeling as a consequence and cause of progressive heart failure. *Clin Cardiol.* 21: I14–9.

Laham, R. J., Rezaee, M., Post, M., Sellke, F. W., Braeckman, R. A., Hung, D., and Simons, M. 1999. Intracoronary and intravenous administration of basic fibroblast growth factor: Myocardial and tissue distribution. *Drug Metab Dispos.* 27: 821–826.

Laham, R. J., Chronos, N. A., Pike, M., Leimbach, M. E., Udelson, J. E., Pearlman, J. D., Pettigrew, R. I. et al. 2000. Intracoronary basic fibroblast growth factor (FGF-2) in patients with severe ischemic heart disease: Results of a phase I open-label dose escalation study. *J Am Coll Cardiol.* 36: 2132–2139.

Langer, R., and Peppas, N. A. 2003. Advances in biomaterials, drug delivery and bionanotechnology. *AIChE J.* 49(12): 2990–3006.

Le Visage, C., Gournay, O., Benguirat, N., Hamidi, S., Chaussumier, L., Mougenot, N., Flanders, J. A. et al. 2012. Mesenchymal stem cell delivery into rat infarcted myocardium using a porous polysaccharide-based scaffold: A quantitative comparison with endocardial injection. *Tissue Eng Part A.* 18(1–2): 35–44.

Lin, S. P., Kyriakides, T. R., and Chen, J. J. 2009. On-line observation of cell growth in a three-dimensional matrix on surface-modified microelectrode arrays. *Biomaterials.* 30(17): 3110–3117.

Lin, Y. D., Yeh, M. L., Yang, Y. J., Tsai, D. C., Chu, T. Y., Shih, Y. Y., Chang, M. Y. et al. 2010. Intramyocardial peptide nanofiber injection improves postinfarction ventricular remodeling and efficacy of bone marrow cell therapy in pigs. *Circulation.* 122(11): S132–141.

Lin, Y. D., Luo, C. Y., Hu, Y. N., Yeh, M. L., Hsueh, Y. C., Chang, M. Y., Tsai, D. C. et al. 2012. Instructive nanofiber scaffolds with VEGF create a microenvironment for arteriogenesis and cardiac repair. *Sci Transl Med.* 4(146): 146ra109.

Lipsic, E., van der Merr, P., Voors, A. A., Westenbrink, B. D., van den Heuvel, A. F., de Boer, H. C., van Zonneveld, A. J. et al. 2006. A single bolus of a long-acting erythropoietin analogue darbepoetin alfa in patients with acute myocardial infarction: A randomized feasibility and safety study. *Cardiovasc Drugs Ther.* 135: 135–141.

Lu, S., Bansal, A., Soussou, W., Berger, T. W., and Madhukar, A. 2006. Receptor-ligand-based specific cell adhesion on solid surfaces: Hippocampal neuronal cells on bilinker functionalized glass. *Nano Lett.* 6(9): 1977–1981.

Lu, J. T., Lee, C. J., Bent, S. F., Fishman, H. A., and Sabelmal, E. E. 2007. Thin collagen film scaffolds for retinal epithelial cell culture. *Biomaterials.* 28(8): 1486–1494.

Lunde, K., Solheim, S., Aakhus, S., Arnesen, H., Abdelnoor, M., Egeland, T., Endresen, K. et al. 2006. Intracoronary injection of mononuclear bone marrow cells in acute myocardial infarction. *N Engl J Med.* 355(12): 1199–1209.

Martin-Rendon, E., Brunskill, S. J., Hyde, C. J., Stanworth, S. J., Mathur, A., and Watt, S. M. 2008. Autologous bone marrow stem cells to treat acute myocardial infarction: A systematic review. *Eur Heart J.* 29: 1807–1818.

Maureira, P., Marie, P. Y., Yu, F., Poussier, S., Liu, Y., Groubatch, F., Falanga, A. et al. 2012. Repairing chronic myocardial infarction with autologous mesenchymal stem cells engineered tissue in rat promotes angiogenesis and limits ventricular remodeling. *J Biomed Sci.* 19: 93.

Meier, P., Gloekler, S., de Marchi, S. F., Indermuehle, A., Rutz, T., Traupe, T., Steck, H. et al. 2009. Myocardial salvage through coronary collateral growth by granulocyte colony-stimulating factor in chronic coronary artery disease: A controlled randomized trial. *Circulation.* 120: 1355–1363.

Menasche, P., Hagege, A. A., Vilquin, J. T., Desnos, M., Abergel, E., Pouzet, B., Bel, A. et al. 2003. Autologous skeletal myoblast transplantation for severe postinfarction left ventricular dysfunction. *J Am Coll Cardiol.* 41: 1078–1083.

Menasche, P., Alfieri, O., Janssens, S., McKenna, W., Reichenspurner, H., Trinquart, L., Vilquin, J. T. et al. 2008. The Myoblasts Autologous Grafting in Ischemic Cardiomyopathy (MAGIC) trial: First randomized placebo-controlled study of myoblast transplantation. *Circulation*. 117: 1189–1200.

Menasche, P. 2011. Cardiac cell therapy: Lessons from clinical trials. *J Mol Cell Cardiol*. 50(2): 258–265.

Meng, E., and Hoang, T. 2012. Micro- and nano-fabricated implantable drug-delivery systems. *Ther Deliver*. 3(12): 1457–1467.

Meluzín, J., Mayer, J., Groch, L., Janousek, S., Hornácek, I., Hlinomaz, O., Kala, P. et al. 2006. Autologous transplantation of mononuclear bone marrow cells in patients with acute myocardial infarction: The effect of the dose of transplanted cells on myocardial function. *Am Heart J*. 152(5): 975.e9–15.

Meyer, G. P., Wollert, K. C., Lotz, J., Steffens, J., Lippolt, P., Fichtner, S., Hecker, H. et al. 2006. Intracoronary bone marrow cell transfer after myocardial infarction: Eighteen months' follow-up data from the randomized, controlled BOOST (BOne marrOw transfer to enhance ST-elevation infarct regeneration) trial. *Circulation*. 113(10): 1287–1294.

Miyagi, Y., Chiu, L. L., Cimini, M., Weisel, R. D., Radisic, M., and Li, R. K. 2011. Biodegradable collagen patch with covalently immobilized VEGF for myocardial repair. *Biomaterials*. 32(5): 1280–1290.

Mocini, D., Staibano, M., Mele, L., Giannantoni, P., Menichella, G., Colivicchi, F., Sordini, P. et al. 2006. Autologous bone marrow mononuclear cell transplantation in patients undergoing coronary artery bypass grafting. *Am Heart J*. 151(1): 192–197.

Morice, M., Serruys, P. W., Sousa, J. E., Fajadet, J., Hayashi, E. B., Perin, M., Colombo, A. et al. 2002. A randomized comparison of a sirolimus-eluting stent with a standard stent for coronary revascularization. *New Eng J Med*. 346(23): 1773–1780.

Mundargi, R. C., Babu, V. R., Rangaswamy, V., Patel, P., and Aminabhavi, T. M. 2008. Nano/micro technologies for delivering macromolecular therapeutics using poly(D,L-lactide-co-glycolide) and its derivatives. *J Control Release*. 125(3): 193–209.

Oberhoff, M., Herdeg, C., Baumbach, A., and Karsch, K. R. 2002. Stent-based antirestenostic coatings (Sirolimus/Paclitaxel). *Catheter Cardio Int*. 55(3): 404–408.

Onuba, Y., Ormiston, J., and Serruys, P. W. 2011. Bioresorbable scaffold technologies. *Circ J*. 75: 509–520.

Padin-Iruegas, M. E., Misao, Y., Davis, M. E., Segers, V. F., Esposito, G., Tokunou, T., Urbanek, K. et al. 2009. Cardiac progenitor cells and biotinylated insulin-like growth factor-1 nanofibers improve endogenous and exogenous myocardial regeneration after infarction. *Circulation*. 120(10): 876–887.

Patel, N. R., Lee, P. S., Kim, J. H., Weinhouse, G. L., and Koziel, H. 2005. The influence of diagnostic bronchoscopy on clinical outcomes comparing adult autologous and allogeneic bone marrow transplant patients. *Chest*. 127(4): 1388–1396.

Pelacho, B., Mazo, M., Montori, S., Simon-Yarza, A. M., Gavira, J. J., Blanco-Prieto, M. J., and Prósper, F. 2013. Cardiac regeneration with stem cells. In *Regenerative Medicine and Cell Therapy*, ed. H. Baharvand, and N. Aghdami, 65–112. Humana Press.

Penna, C., Perrelli, M. G., Karam, J. P., Angotti, C., Muscari, C., Montero-Menei, C. N., and Pagliaro, P. 2013. Pharmacologically active microcarriers influence VEGF-A effects on mesenchymal stem cell survival. *J Cell Mol Med*. 17(1): 192–204.

Perin, E. C., Dohmann, H. F., Borojevic, R., Silva, S. A., Sousa, A. L., Silva, G. V., Mesquita, C. T. et al. 2004. Improved exercise capacity and ischemia 6 and 12 months after transendocardial injection of autologous bone marrow mononuclear cells for ischemic cardiomyopathy. *Circulation*. 110(11 Suppl 1): II213–II218.

Piao, H., Kwon, J. S., Piao, S., Sohn, J. H., Lee, Y. S., Bae, J. W., Hwang, K. K. et al. 2007. Effects of cardiac patches engineered with bone marrow-derived mononuclear cells and PGCL scaffolds in a rat myocardial infarction model. *Biomaterials*. 28(4): 641–649.

Pisal, D. S., Kosloski, M. P., and Balu-Lyer, S. V. 2010. Delivery of therapeutic proteins. *J Pharm Sci.* 99(6): 2557–2575.

Plewka, M., Krzemińska-Pakuła, M., Lipiec, P., Peruga, J. Z., Jezewski, T., Kidawa, M., Wierzbowska-Drabik, K. et al. 2009. Effect of intracoronary injection of mononuclear bone marrow stem cells on left ventricular function in patients with acute myocardial infarction. *Am J Cardiol.* 104(10): 1336–1342.

Povsic, T. J., O'Connor, C. M., Henry, T., Taussig, A., Kereiakes, D. J., Fortuin, F. D., Niederman, A. et al. 2011. A double-blind, randomized, controlled, multicenter study to assess the safety and cardiovascular effects of skeletal myoblast implantation by catheter delivery in patients with chronic heart failure after myocardial infarction. *Am Heart J.* 162: 654–662.

Purcell, B. P., Elser, J. A., Mu, A., Margulies, K. B., and Burdick, J. A. 2012. Synergistic effects of SDF-1a chemokine and hyaluronic acid release from degradable hydrogels on directing bone marrow derived cell homing to the myocardium. *Biomaterials.* 33(31): 7849–7857.

Qu, C., Xiong, Y., Mahmood, A., Kaplan, D. L., Goussev, A., Ning, R., and Chopp, M. 2009. Treatment of traumatic brain injury in mice with bone marrow stromal cell-impregnated collagen scaffolds. *J Neurosurg.* 111(4): 658–665.

Ravi Kumar, M. N. 2000. Nano and microparticles as controlled drug delivery devices. *J Pharm Pharmaceut Sci.* 3(2): 234–258.

Ravichandran, R., Venugopal, J. R., Sundarrajan, S., Mukherjee, S., and Ramakrishna, S. 2012. Minimally invasive cell-seeded biomaterial systems for injectable/epicardial implantation in ischemic heart disease. *Int J Nanomedicine.* 7: 5969–5994.

Reinecke, H., Minami, E., Zhu, W. Z., and Laflamme, M. A. 2008. Cardiogenic differentiation and transdifferentiation of progenitor cells. *Circ Res.* 103(10): 1058–1071.

Ripa, R. S., Jørgensen, E., Wang, Y., Thune, J. J., Nilsson, J. C., Søndergaard, L., Johnsen, H. E. et al. 2006. Stem cell mobilization induced by subcutaneous granulocyte-colony stimulating factor to improve cardiac regeneration after acute ST-elevation myocardial infarction: Result of the double-blind, randomized, placebo-controlled stem cells in myocardial infarction (STEMMI) trial. *Circulation.* 113: 1983–1992.

Rolfes, C., Howard, S., Goff, R., and Iaizzo, P. A. 2012. Localized drug delivery for cardiothoracic surgery. In *Current Concepts in General Thoracic Surgery*, ed. L. Cagini, 279–304. In Tech.

Ruvinov, E., Leor, J., and Cohen, S. 2011. The promotion of myocardial repair by the sequential delivery of IGF-1 and HGF from an injectable alginate biomaterial in a model of acute myocardial infarction. *Biomaterials.* 32(2): 565–578.

Ryu, J. H., Kim, I. K., Cho, S. W., Cho, M. C., Hwang, K. K., Piao, H., Piao, S. et al. 2005. Implantation of bone marrow mononuclear cells using injectable fibrin matrix enhances neovascularization in infarcted myocardium. *Biomaterials.* 26(3): 319–326.

Sahoo, S., Ang, L. T., Cho-Hong Goh, J., and Toh, S. L. 2010. Bioactive nanofibers for fibroblastic differentiation of mesenchymal precursor cells for ligament/tendon tissue engineering applications. *Differentiation.* 79(2): 102–110.

Sakakibara, Y., Tambara, K., Sakaguchi, G., Lu, F., Ymamoto, M., Nishimura, K., Tabata, Y. et al. 2003. Toward surgical angiogenesis using slow-released basic fibroblast growth factor. *Eur J Cardiothorac Surg.* 24(1): 105–111; discussion 112.

Salimath, A. S., Phelps, E. A., Boopathy, A. V., Che, P. L., Brown, M., Garcia, A. J., and Davis, M. E. 2012. Dual delivery of hepatocyte and vascular endothelial growth factors via a protease-degradable hydrogel improves cardiac function in rats. *PLoS One.* 7(11): e50980.

Schächinger, V., Erbs, S., Elsässer, A., Haberbosch, W., Hambrecht, R., Hölschermann, H., Yu, J. et al. 2006. REPAIR-AMIInvestigators. Intracoronary bone marrow-derived progenitor cells in acute myocardial infarction. *N Engl J Med.* 355(12): 1210–1221.

Schumacher, B., Pecher, P., von Specht, B. U., and Stegmann, T. 1998. Induction of neoangiogenesis in ischemic myocardium by human growth factors: First clinical results of a new treatment of coronary heart disease. *Circulation*. 97: 645–650.

Scott, R. C., Crabbe, D., Krynska, B., Ansari, R., and Kiani, M. F. 2008. Aiming for the heart: Targeted delivery of drugs to diseased cardiac tissue. *Expert Opin Drug Deliv*. 5(4): 459–470.

Scott, R. C., Rosano, J. M., Ivanov, Z., Wang, B., Chong, P. L., Issekutz, A. C., Crabbe, D. L. et al. 2009. Targeting VEGF-encapsulated immunoliposomes to MI heart improves vascularity and cardiac function. *FASEB J*. 23(10): 3361–3367.

Segers, V. F., and Lee, R. T. 2010. Protein therapeutics for cardiac regeneration after myocardial infarction. *J Cardiovasc Transl Res*. 3(5): 469–477.

Segers, V. F. and Lee, R. T. 2011. Biomaterials to enhance stem cell function in the heart. *Circ Res*. 109(8): 910–922.

Seiler, C., Pohl, T., Wustmann, K., Hutter, D., Nicolet, P. A., Windecker, S., Eberli, F. R. et al. 2001. Promotion of collateral growth by granulocyte-macrophage colony-stimulating factor in patients with coronary artery disease: A randomized, double-blind, placebo-controlled study. *Circulation*. 104: 2012–2017.

Shao, Z. Q., Takaji, K., Katayama, Y., Kunitomo, R., Sakaguchi, H., Lai, Z. F., and Kawasuji, M. 2006. Effects of intramyocardial administration of slow-release basic fibroblast growth factor on angiogenesis and ventricular remodeling in a rat infarct model. *Circ J*. 70(4): 471–477.

Silva, A. K., Richard, C., Bessodes, M., Scherman, D., and Merten, O. W. 2009. Growth factor delivery approaches in hydrogels. *Biomacromolecules*. 10(1): 9–18.

Siminiak, T., Kalawski, R., Fiszer, D., Jerzykowska, O., Rzezniczak, J., Rozwadowska, N., and Kurpisz, M. 2004. Autologous skeletal myoblast transplantation for the treatment of postinfarction myocardial injury: Phase I clinical study with 12 months of follow-up. *Am Heart J*. 148: 531–537.

Siminiak, T., Fiszer, D., Jerzykowska, O., Grygielska, B., Rozwadowska, N., Kalmucki, P., and Kurpisz, M. 2005. Percutanous trans-coronary-venous transplantation of autologous skeletal myoblasts in the treatment of post-infarction myocardial contractility impairment: The POZNAN trial. *Eur Heart J*. 26: 1188–1195.

Simon-Yarza, T., Formiga, F. R., Tamayo, E., Pelacho, B., Prosper, F., and Blanco-Prieto, M. J. 2013. PEGylated-PLGA microparticles containing VEGF for long term drug delivery. *Int J Pharm*. 440(1): 13–18.

Simón-Yarza, T., Tamayo, E., Benavides, C., Lana, H., Formiga, F. R., Grama, C. N., Ortiz-de-Solorzano, C. et al. 2013. Functional benefits of PLGA particulates carrying VEGF and CoQ_{10} in an animal of myocardial ischemia. *Int J Pharm*. 454: 784–790.

Simons, M., Annex, B. H., Laham, R. J., Kleiman, N., Henry, T., Dauerman, H., Udelson, J. E. et al. 2002. Pharmacological treatment o coronary artery disease with recombinant fibroblast growth factor-2: Double-blind, randomized controlled clinical trial. *Circulation*. 105: 788–793.

Simpson, D. L., Liu, H., Fan, T. H., Nerem, R., and Dudley, S. C., Jr. 2007. A tissue engineering approach to progenitor cell delivery results in significant cell engraftment and improved myocardial remodeling. *Stem Cells*. 25(9): 2350–2357.

Simpson, D. L., Boyd, N. L., Kaushal, S., Stice, S. L., and Dudley, S. C., Jr. 2012. Use of human embryonic stem cell derived-mesenchymal cells for cardiac repair. *Biotechnol Bioeng*. 109(1): 274–283.

Smits, P. C., van Geuns, R. J., Poldermans, D., Bountioukos, M., Onderwater, E. E., Lee, C. H., Maat, A. P. et al. 2003. Catheter-based intramyocardial injection of autologous skeletal myoblasts as a primary treatment of ischemic heart failure: Clinical experience with six-month follow-up. *J Am Coll Cardiol*. 42: 2063–2069.

Stamm, C., Kleine, H. D., Choi, Y. H., Dunkelmann, S., Lauffs, J. A., Lorenzen, B., David, A. et al. 2007. Intramyocardial delivery of CD133+ bone marrow cells and coronary artery bypass grafting for chronic ischemic heart disease: Safety and efficacy studies. *J Thorac Cardiovasc Surg*. 133(3): 717–725.

Strauer, B. E., Brehm, M., Zeus, T., Köstering, M., Hernandes, A., Sorg, R. V., Kögler, G. et al. 2002. Repair of infarcted myocardium by autologous intracoronary mononuclear bone marrow cell transplantation in humans. *Circulation*. 106: 1913–1918.

Strauer, B. E., Yousef, M., and Schannwell, C. M. 2010. The acute and long-term effects of intracoronary Stem cell Transplantation in 191 patients with chronic heARt failure: The STAR-heart study. *Eur J Heart Fail*. 12(7): 721–729.

Sy, J. C., and Davis, M. E. 2010. Delivering regenerative cues to the heart: Cardiac drug delivery by microspheres and peptide nanofibers. *J Cardiovasc Transl Res*. 3(5): 461–468.

Takahashi, K., and Yamanaka, S. 2006. Induction of pluripotent stem cells from mouse embryonic and adult fibroblast cultures by defined factors. *Cell*. 126(4): 663–676.

Takahashi, K., Tanabe, K., Ohnuki, M., Narita, M., Ichisaka, T., Tomoda, K., and Yamanaka, S. 2007. Induction of pluripotent stem cells from adult human fibroblasts by defined factors. *Cell*. 131(5): 861–872.

Tan, M. L., Choong, P. F., and Dass, C. R. 2010. Recent developments in liposomes, microparticles and nanoparticles for protein and peptide drug delivery. *Peptides*. 31(1): 184–193.

Tang, Y. D., Hasan, F., Giordano, F. J., Pfau, S., Rinder, H. M., and Katz, S. D. 2009. Effects of recombinant human erythropoietin on platelet activation in acute myocardial infarction: Results of a double-blind, placebo-controlled, randomized trial. *Am Heart J*. 158: 941–947.

Tarun, G., Ajay, B., Bhawna, K., Sunil, K., and Arsh, C. 2011. Current status and future directions of new drug delivery technologies. *IRJP*. 2(12): 61–68.

Tendera, M., Wojakowski, W., Ruzyłło, W., Chojnowska, L., Kepka, C., Tracz, W., Musiałek, P. et al. 2009. REGENT Investigators. Intracoronary infusion of bone marrow-derived selected CD34+CXCR4+ cells and non-selected mononuclear cells in patients with acute STEMI and reduced left ventricular ejection fraction: Results of randomized, multicentre Myocardial Regeneration by Intracoronary Infusion of Selected Population of Stem Cells in Acute Myocardial Infarction (REGENT) Trial. *Eur Heart J*. 30(11): 1313–1321.

Theiss, H. D., Brenner, C., Engelmann, M. G., Zaruba, M. M., Huber, B., Henschel, V., Mansmann, U. et al. 2010. Safety and efficacy of SITAgliptin plus Granulocyte-colony-stimulating factor in patients suffering from acute myocardial infarction (SITAGRAMI-trial)-rationale, design and first interim analysis. *Int J Cardiol*. 145: 282–284.

Tokunaga, M., Liu, M. L., Nagai, T., Iwanaga, K., Matsuura, K., Takahashi, T., Kanda, M. et al. 2010. Implantation of cardiac progenitor cells using self-assembling peptide improves cardiac function after myocardial infarction. *J Mol Cell Cardiol*. 49(6): 972–983.

Traverse, J. H., Henry, T. D. Ellis, S. G., Pepine, C. J., Willerson, J. T., Zhao, D. X., Forder, J. R. et al. 2011. Effect of intracoronary delivery of autologous bone marrow mononuclear cells 2 to 3 weeks following acute myocardial infarction on left ventricular function: The Late TIME randomized trial. *J Am Med Assoc*. 306(19): 2110–2119.

Tse, H. F., Thambar, S., Kwong, Y. L., Rowlings, P., Bellamy, G., McCrohon, J., Thomas, P. et al. 2007. Prospective randomized trial of direct endomyocardial implantation of bone marrow cells for treatment of severe coronary artery diseases (PROTECT-CAD trial). *Eur Heart J*. 28(24): 2998–3005.

Udelson, J. E., Dilsizian, V., Laham, R. J., Chronos, N., Vansant, J., Blais, M., Galt, J. R. et al. 2000. Therapeutic angiogenesis with recombinant fibroblast growth factor-2 improves stress and rest myocardial perfusion abnormalities in patients with severe chronic coronary artery disease. *Circulation*. 102: 1605–1610.

Unger, E. F., Goncalves, L., Epstein, S. E., Chew, E. Y., Trapnell, C. B., Cannon, R. O., and Quyyumi, A. A. 2000. Effects of a single intracoronary injection of basic fibroblast growth factor in stable angina pectoris. *Am J Cardiol.* 15: 1414–1419.

Valgimigli, M., Rigolin, G. M., Cittanti, C., Malagutti, P., Curello, S., Percoco, G., Bugli, A. M. et al. 2005. Use of granulocyte-colony stimulating factor during acute myocardial infarction to enhance bone marrow stem cell mobilization in humans: Clinical and angiographic safety profile. *Eur Heart J.* 26: 1838–1845.

Vallee, J. P., Hauwel, M., Lepetit-Coiffe, M., Bei, W., Montet-Abou, K., Meda, P., Gardier, S. et al. 2012. Embryonic stem cell-based cardiopatches improve cardiac function in infarcted rats. *Stem Cells Transl Med.* 1(3): 248–260.

van Ramshorst, J., Bax, J. J., Beeres, S. L., Dibbets-Schneider, P., Roes, S. D., Stokkel, M. P., de Roos, A. et al. 2009. Intramyocardial bone marrow cell injection for chronic myocardial ischemia: A randomized controlled trial. *J Am Med Assoc.* 301(19): 1997–2004.

Verma, R. K., and Garg, S. 2001. Current status of drug delivery technologies and future directions. *Pharm Technol.* 25(2): 1–14.

Viswanathan, C., Davidson, Y., Cooper, K., Tipnis, S., Pujari, G., and Kurian, V. M. 2010. Tansplantation of autologous bone marrow derived mesenchymal stem cells trans-epicardially in patients undergoing coronary bypass surgery. *Indian Heart J.* 62(1): 43–48.

von Wattenwyl, R., Blumenthal, B., Heilmann, C., Golsong, P., Poppe, A., Beyersdorf, F., and Siepe, M. 2012. Scaffold-based transplantation of vascular endothelial growth factor-overexpressing stem cells leads to neovascularization in ischemic myocardium but did not show a functional regenerative effect. *ASAIO J.* 58(3): 268–274.

Voors, A. A., Belonje, A. M., Zijlstra, F., Hillege, H. L., Anker, S. D., Slart, R. H., Tio, R. A. et al. 2010. A single dose of erythropoietin in ST-elevation myocardial infarction. *Eur Heart J.* 31: 2593–2600.

Wang, N., Tong, G., Yang, J., Zhou, Z., Pan, H., Huo, Y., Xu, J. et al. 2009. Effect of hepatocyte growth-promoting factors on myocardial ischemia during exercise in patients with severe coronary artery disease. *Int Heart J.* 50: 291–299.

Wang, H., Zhang, X., Li, Y., Ma, Y., Zhang, Y., Liu, Z., Zhou, J. et al. 2010. Improved myocardial performance in infarcted rat heart by co-injection of basic fibroblast growth factor with temperature-responsive chitosan hydrogel. *J Heart Lung Transplant.* 29(8): 881–887.

World Health Organization. Media Center. Cardiovascular diseases (CVDs). Fact sheet No. 317 http://www.who.int/mediacentre/factsheets/fs317/en/index.html (Updated March 2013).

Wollert, K. C., Meyer, G. P., Lotz, J., Ringes-Lichtenberg, S., Lippolt, P., Breidenbach, C., Fichtner, S. et al. 2004. Intracoronary autologous bone-marrow cell transfer after myocardial infarction: The BOOST randomised controlled clinical trial. *Lancet.* 364(9429): 141–148.

Wu, J., Zeng, F., Huang, X. P., Chung, J. C., Konecny, F., Weisel, R. D., and Li, R. K. 2011. Infarct stabilization and cardiac repair with a VEGF-conjugated, injectable hydrogel. *Biomaterials.* 32(2): 579–586.

Xiong, Q., Hill, K. L., Li, Q., Suntharalingam, P., Mansoor, A., Wang, X., Jameel, M. N. et al. 2011. A fibrin patch-based enhanced delivery of human embryonic stem cell-derived vascular cell transplantation in a porcine model of postinfarction left ventricular remodeling. *Stem Cells.* 29(2): 367–375.

Yancopoulos, G. D., Davis, S., Gale, N. W., Rudge, J. S., Wiegand, S. J., and Holash, J. 2000. Vascular-specific growth factors and blood vessel formation. *Nature.* 407(6801): 242–248.

Yu, J., Du, K. T., Fang, Q., Gu., Y., Mihardja, S. S., Sievers, R. E., Wu, J. C. et al. 2010. The use of human mesenchymal stem cells encapsulated in RGD modified alginate microspheres in the repair of myocardial infarction in the rat. *Biomaterials.* 31(27): 7012–7020.

Zbinden, S., Zbinden, R., Meier, P., Windecker, S., and Seiler, C. 2005. Safety and efficacy of subcutaneous-only granulocyte macrophage colony stimulating factor for collateral growth promotion in patients with coronary artery disease. *J Am Coll Cardiol.* 46: 1636–1642.

Zhang, J., Ding, L., Zhao, Y., Sun, W., Chen, B., Lin, H., Wang, X. et al. 2009. Collagen-targeting vascular endothelial growth factor improves cardiac performance after myocardial infarction. *Circulation.* 119(13): 1776–1784.

Zhang, X., Wang, H., Ma, X., Adila, A., Wang, B., Liu, F., Chen, B. et al. 2010. Preservation of the cardiac function in infarcted rat hearts by the transplantation of adipose-derived stem cells with injectable fibrin scaffolds. *Exp Biol Med (Maywood).* 235(12): 1505–1515.

Zhao, Q., Sun, Y., Xia, L., Chen, A., and Wang, Z. 2008. Randomized study of mononuclear bone marrow cell transplantation in patients with coronary surgery. *Ann Thorac Surg.* 86(6): 1833–1840.

Zohlnhöfer, D., Ott, I., Mehilli, J., Schömig, K., Michalk, F., Ibrahim, T., Meisetschläger, G. et al. 2006. Stem cell mobilization by granulocyte colony-stimulating factor in patients with acute myocardial infarction: A randomized controlled trial. *J Am Med Assoc.* 295: 1003–1010.

18 Current Developments in Nanotherapeutics for Airway Diseases

Indrajit Roy, Ridhima Juneja, Komal Sethi, and Neeraj Vij

CONTENTS

INTRODUCTION

The advent of nanotechnology has transformed several industrial and medical technologies. There has been an extensive use of engineered nanoparticle-based products in myriad aspects of daily human use. In recent years, extensive research on the toxicity and health risks of nanoparticle exposure has raised a concern over the unrestrained use of nano-based products and applications. The airway is one of the primary routes of nanoparticle exposure, and several studies highlight the debilitating effects of acute or chronic nanoparticle exposure. Some of the common outcomes of nanoparticle exposure on the pulmonary system include inflammation, oxidative stress, and DNA damage. Moreover, nanoparticles have been shown to exacerbate chronic lung diseases like asthma and COPD-emphysema. In contrast, nanotechnology has very useful applications in pulmonary nanomedicine as a therapeutic and diagnostic tool. One of the important therapeutic applications of nanoparticles in airway diseases is the targeted delivery of DNA, short interfering RNA, drugs, or peptides to hematopoietic progenitor cells and pulmonary epithelium to control chronic pathophysiology of obstructive (Chronic Obstructive Pulmonary Disease, COPD, and asthma) and conformational disorders (cystic fibrosis, CF). In addition, nanosystems have important applications in imaging technologies used to diagnose various pulmonary complications. However, it is critical that polymers and chemical reagents used for nanoparticle synthesis are nontoxic and biodegradable. Moreover, these nano-based systems need to be fine-tuned for providing sustained drug delivery to the selected cell type to overcome potential toxicity and side effects. We propose that strategies for designing safe nano-based technologies for therapeutic and diagnostic (theranostic) applications in the airway diseases are needed.

COMMON AIRWAY DISEASES AND THERAPEUTIC APPLICATIONS

Common airway disease states include inflammatory (e.g., asthma, bronchitis), obstructive (e.g., COPD, CF, and asthma), autosomal recessive (e.g., CF, alpha-1-trypsin deficiency [Z-mutation], ATD), and pathogenic (e.g., tuberculosis, influenza) conditions and lung cancer, and so on. Obstructive lung diseases, such as COPD and CF, have unique characteristics, such as excessive mucus buildup and inflammatory cells (macrophages and neutrophils), that serve as a challenge for nano-based airway delivery. These conditions are also prone to bacterial and viral infections, resulting in changes in the airway that interfere with the ability to design a safe and effective drug delivery system capable of circumventing multiple physical challenges. Noteworthy, the chronic conditions pose a severe clinical challenge as they not only have increased mortality and morbidity globally but also result in significant increase in health care costs.

Conventional Treatment Options, Drug Types, and Routes of Administration

A number of drug types and therapeutics have been identified for the treatment of airway diseases, but the challenge is to selectively deliver these to specific areas of the lungs or individual cell types. These therapeutics include small organic molecules (e.g., corticosteroids, nonsteroidal anti-inflammatory drugs, NSAIDs), peptides (antimicrobials, WLBU-2, LL-37, etc.), antibiotics (erythromycin, prednisone, etc.), antioxidants (N-acetyl cysteine, NAC, cysteamine, etc.), plasmid DNA, siRNA, and so on that can be encapsulated in nanoparticles for selective delivery. As an example, inflammatory diseases, such as asthma, can be treated with corticosteroids and NSAIDS while antibiotics can be used to treat pathogenic conditions. Gene therapy using plasmid DNA is exploratory but is a viable option for combating autosomal diseases of the airways where nanosystems can play an effective role. Moreover, siRNA treatment is emerging as another promising option for treating viral infections and lung cancer, but it needs an efficient delivery system.

Therapeutics can be targeted to the lungs either directly via intranasal administration (inhaler/nebulizers, nanosystems, etc.) or systemic circulation. The former route is the preferred approach as it enables direct or localized pulmonary deposition of therapeutics with avoidance of, interference of homeostatic mechanisms and therapeutic delivery to nontarget organs. Moreover, the presence of an extensive capillary network with high surface area (about 100 m^2) and extensive vascularization in the deep lungs leads to the rapid absorption of the drugs. Lower amounts of degradative enzymes within the lungs are another advantage of direct delivery. Finally, the minimally invasive nature of inhalation delivery leads to optimal dosing and better patient compliance. The lung-targeted drug delivery via the systemic (e.g., intravenous) route is available but not preferred as drug translocation in the lungs can be limited by RES-mediated drug sequestration and impaired permeation of the drug across the blood–air barrier.

Advantages of Nanodrug Formulations over Conventional Drug Delivery

The drugs in their free form encounter a number of drawbacks related to their formulation, delivery, bioavailability, and efficacy. These drawbacks include poor aqueous solubility, inconsistent size and large size distribution, instability of aqueous or dry powder formulations, impaired permeation across biological barriers, capture and degradation by macrophages, and so on. In order to overcome these drawbacks, it is necessary to formulate them with nanoparticulate carriers, which impart them with properties that ideally suit pulmonary delivery [Ali et al., 2014; Azarami et al., 2008]. Nanocarriers can deliver a wide variety of drugs, help evade them from capture by the immune system and other biological barriers, target them to sites of interest, release them at target sites in a sustained manner, and protect them from degradation and inactivation by the body. They have the capacity to improve drug action and decrease undesirable systemic side effects. Recently, nanoparticles are also being used for advanced therapeutic techniques, such as externally activated drug delivery and real-time monitoring of therapy.

In order for successful drug targeting following inhalation delivery, drug formulations have to be aerosolized with optimal size and aerodynamic properties. These properties, in turn, depend on a number of physical parameters of the micro-nanocarriers, such as their size, shape, porosity, surface charge, density, hygroscopicity, and so on. Thus, for optimal pulmonary drug delivery, it is critical to select appropriate materials and synthesize them with the desired size and other physical parameters. Drug loading and release characteristics of the carriers are also important parameters. Moreover, along with enhanced efficacy, nanodelivery has posed some concurrent health risks. Therefore, it is important to analyze the prospect of nanodelivery to the lungs by carefully analyzing their risk-to-benefit ratio.

Drug formulations are delivered to the lungs in mainly two forms, (a) as colloidal dispersions in aqueous medium via a process called nebulization and (b) as dried powders, using both dry powder inhalers (DPI) and pressurized metered dose inhalers (pMDIs). These formulations are generated from drug carriers, in bulk phase or dispersed in a medium, using techniques such as spray-drying, freeze-drying, ultracentrifugation, ball milling, and so on. The synthetic strategies and advantages or disadvantages of such formulations are reviewed elsewhere [Muralidharan et al., 2015]. In general, the dry powder formulations are favored as a result of their better stability (for both storage and transportation), protection of drugs from leakage and degradation, ease of administration, better aerodynamic properties, and so on.

Extensive research in the past few years has led to the recognition that formulations in the diameter range of 100–500 nm are optimal for absorption and retention by the lungs for desired drug action. While larger particles are trapped by the mucus proteins present in the lungs and are cleared by the mucociliary escalator, smaller particles are often exhaled out or deposited in alveoli, leading to toxicity. These aspects are reviewed elsewhere [Paranjpe and Müller-Goymann, 2014].

NANOPARTICLE TYPES, STRATEGIES OF DRUG INCORPORATION, ROUTES OF ADMINISTRATION

Nanoparticles are composed of inorganic, polymeric, and lipidic materials. Several inorganic materials display unique physical properties at the nanoscale, which are exploited in various diagnostic and sensing applications [Prasad, 2003]. However, most inorganic-based nanoparticles are also known to exert toxic effects in the lungs via either leaking of toxic ions or their reactive surfaces [Prasad, 2012]. Therefore, with the exception of iron oxide nanoparticles, the application of inorganic nanoparticles in the lungs is restricted to in vitro or ex vivo diagnostic assays of pulmonary disorders. On the other hand, most reported nanoparticles used in pulmonary drug delivery are made up of lipid- and polymer-based components, which may be purely lipidic (e.g., liposomes, solid lipid nanoparticles), purely polymeric (e.g., polymeric nanoparticles, block-co-polymeric micelles), and hybrid (e.g., phospholipid-polymer micelles) nanosystems [Paranjpe and Müller-Goymann, 2014; Weber et al., 2014; Ungaro et al., 2012; Mansour et al., 2009; Beck-Broichsitter et al., 2012]. The following diagram (Figure 18.1) presents the various types of such nanoparticles used in pulmonary drug delivery along with their components.

Distinct Nanocarriers Available for Airway Delivery

Liposomes

Liposomes are probably the oldest nanocarriers known and have been used for the last four decades for drug delivery. They are synthesized by spontaneous self-assembly of their components (phospholipids, diglycerides, and cholesterol) in aqueous solution [Sawant and Torchillin, 2012]. These are soft vesicles, which first form large multilamellar vesicles (LMVs), which are subsequently converted to small unilamellar vesicles (SUVs) using extrusion or sonication techniques [Prasad, 2012]. Their phospholipid bilayered composition resembles that of cellular membranes. They can encapsulate either hydrophilic (in their aqueous core) or hydrophobic (within their lipophilic bilayer) drugs as shown in Figure 18.1. Moreover, the use of cationic lipids (diglycerides containing quarternary ammonium groups) as components allow for the fabrication of cationic liposomes, which are used as gene carriers for gene therapy, as also shown in Figure 18.1.

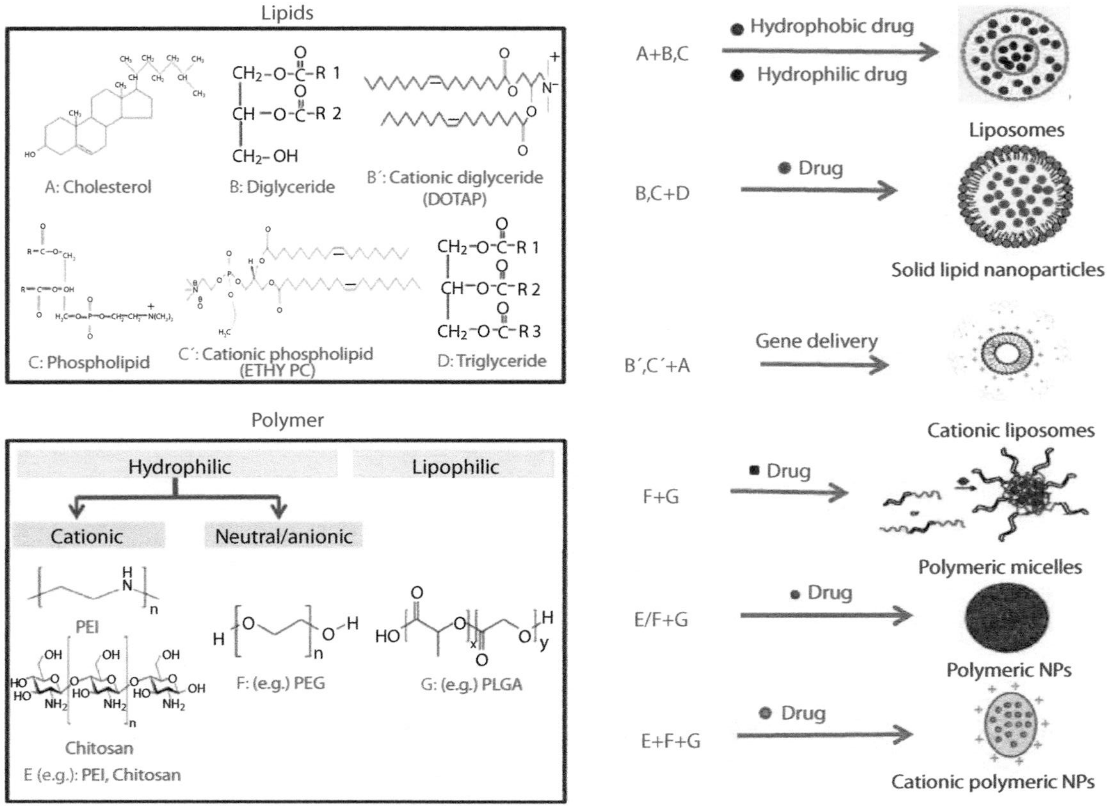

FIGURE 18.1 Types of nanomaterials used in pulmonary delivery.

Liposomes are specially suited for lung applications as phospholipids are natural components of surfactant proteins that are inherent to the lungs. The essential functions of these lung surfactants are maintenance of optimal surface tension and reduction of friction in the lung tissue [Beck-Broichsitter et al., 2011]. Liposomes can be formulated as both liquid aerosols and dry powders although their production with desired diameter and aerodynamic properties for pulmonary delivery can be challenging.

Initially, liposomal formulations for pulmonary delivery were based on liquid aerosols delivered via nebulizers [Schreier et al., 1993]. Alveofact®, the first aerosol-based liposomal product, was introduced in the 1990s to treat acute respiratory distress syndrome (ARDS) after pulmonary instillation [Mansour et al., 2008]. However, these liquid-based formulations were fraught with stability and leakage issues [Taylor et al., 1990]. The focus then shifted to dry powder inhaler (DPI) formulations, which since have been extensively used for delivery of small molecule drugs for treatment of both lung and systemic diseases via the pulmonary route [Joshi et al., 2001].

Solid Lipid Nanoparticles (SLNs)

SLNs are made of a combination of solid, high-melting lipids (e.g., triglycerides) and oil-rich surfactants (e.g., phospholipids). They form nanoparticle suspensions in the aqueous media with a diameter range of 50–500 nm [Weber et al., 2014; Schwartz et al., 1994; Cavalli et al., 1997]. Since SLNs are solid at physiological temperatures, they are structurally stable and can be formulated as inhalable carriers (e.g., dry powders) for delivery to the deep lungs. They can encapsulate lipophilic drugs in their matrix from which the drugs can be released in a sustained manner with a release profile superior to that of polymeric carrier.

Like liposomes, SLNs are also highly suited for lung applications with lung-friendly phospholipids as constituents. In an experiment involving cytokine activation measurements, Nassimi et al. demonstrated the nontoxicity of SLNs using in vitro, ex vivo, and in vivo models of lung. No activation of proinflammatory cytokines (TNF-α and chemokine-KC) were observed when the SLN were administered in mice via nebulization [Nassimi et al., 2010].

Polymeric Nanoparticles (PNPs)

PNPs have been an exciting approach for lung delivery due to their ability to enter intracellular compartments and escape macrophage phagocytosis. Furthermore, they provide the possibility of achieving high drug loading capacity, sustained release, and enhanced drug stability and absorption as well as targeted deposition [Mansour et al., 2009]. As shown in Figure 18.1, polymeric nanoparticles can form from several combinations of hydrophilic and lipophilic polymers. A large number of polymers have been utilized in formulating delivery systems for pulmonary applications [Rytting et al., 2008; Lebhardt et al., 2010]. The selection of an appropriate polymer is mainly based on criteria such as its biocompatibility and degradability [Pilcer and Amighi, 2010]. Aliphatic polyesters like poly(-lactide-co-glycolide) (PLGA) have been most extensively used due to their low toxicity [Anderson and Shive, 1997; Bala et al., 2004]. Other types of biodegradable polymers suitable for pulmonary application are biodegradable poly(anhydride)s and poly(ketal)s [Fiegel et al., 2004; Fiore et al., 2011]. In addition, cationic polymers, such as chitosan and polyethyleneimine (PEI), are useful components of polymeric carriers for gene therapy [Li and Birchall, 2006].

Block Co-Polymeric Micelles

These nanosized micelles result from the spontaneous self-assembly of surfactant-like block co-polymers, comprised of lipophilic and hydrophilic blocks [Cabral and Kataoka, 2014]. They can encapsulate lipophilic drugs. Polymeric micelles have much lower critical micelle concentration (CMC) than surfactant micelles and can retain their structural integrity even at high dilution. However, they do suffer from the drawback of premature and burst drug release. Phospholipid-polymer micelles (or diacyllipid-polymer micelles) are a special type of polymeric micelles in which the hydrophobic block is made up of lipids instead of polymers [Zhaveri and Torchillin, 2014]. They also have very low CMC values, making them efficient drug delivery vehicles for lipophilic blocks.

Candidates for Nano-Based Airway Delivery

Steroids, NSAIDs, Antioxidants

These drugs are commonly used for the treatment of airway inflammatory diseases, such as asthma [Ozbakir et al., 2014]. As discussed before, nanoformulations enhance their delivery and bioavailabilty in the lungs via deep lung deposition, controlled release, and so on. An example in support of this is study by Moritz Beck-Broichsitter et al., who prepared biocompatible polymeric nanoparticles of poly(vinyl sulfonate-co-vinyl alcohol)- graft-poly(D,L-lactide-co-glycolide) (VS(72)-10) loaded with the corticosteroid Salbutamol. After inhalative administration, this formulation demonstrated a sustained pulmonary drug release [Beck-Broichsitter et al., 2010]. This formulation has potential to treat airway inflammatory diseases. Another report shows the development of a novel therapeutic agent for airway inflammatory diseases based on hydroxybenzyl alcohol (HBA)-incorporated polyoxalate (HPOX) [Park et al., 2010; Kim et al., 2011]. HPOX was designed to incorporate antioxidant and anti-inflammatory agent HBA and peroxalate ester linkages capable of reacting with hydrogen peroxide (H_2O_2) in its backbone. When HPOX encapsulated within biodegradable PLGA nanoparticles was administered in asthma mice models, using the intranasal route, a notable decrease in critical proinflammatory cytokines was observed, thus underscoring the promise of this nanoformulation for treatment of airway inflammatory diseases [Yoo et al., 2013].

Solid lipid nanoparticles (SLNs) serve as another category of popular nanocarriers of this category of drugs. The antioxidant and anti-inflammatory drug quercetin was encapsulated in SLNs, which displayed acceptable aerodynamic properties [Silva et al., 2013]. In vitro deposition studies following delivery via nebulization showed predominant deposition in the deep lung areas. Wang et al. developed curcumin-loaded SLNs for treatment of asthma. When this nanoformulation was administered intraperitoneally in an ovalbumin (OVA)-induced allergic rat model of asthma, a decrease in cytokine levels (interleukin-4 and interleukin-13) was observed in comparison to the untreated group, along with suppression of airway hyper-response and inflammatory cell infiltration. These observations suggested the suitability of curcumin-SLN for the treatment of asthma [Wang et al., 2012].

Hoesel and colleagues reported the use of a liposomal formulation containing a cocktail of antioxidants, such as n-acetylcysteine (NAC), vitamin E, and glutathione, for treatment of airway inflammation. In an in vivo study involving experimental rats with a lung injury model, a decrease in proinflammatory cytokine levels was observed in the bronchoalveolar lavage fluid (BAL) fluid after direct pulmonary delivery [Hoesel et al., 2008]. Such antioxidant nanoparticles can prove useful in the therapy for hypoxia and oxidative stress–related injuries of the lungs.

Nanoformulation of anticancer drugs can be used for the treatment of lung cancer. In a study, paclitaxel-loaded PEGylated polymeric micelles were administered in mice using both intratracheal instillation and intravenous administration. The former mode of delivery led to better drug absorption and maximum drug localization in the lung tissue [Gill et al., 2011]. Roa et al. encapsulated doxorubicin-loaded nanoparticles into inhalable effervescent powder formulations and tested the prepared formulations in a tumor-bearing mouse model [Roa et al., 2011]. Animals treated with inhalable effervescent nanoparticle powders showed an improved survival compared to control groups. Moreover, nanoencapsulation of doxorubicin reduced toxic side effects.

Nanoformulation of drugs not only allows better drug efficacy in the lungs, but it also facilitates concurrent bioimaging via the coincorporation of diagnostic agents. For example, Guthi et al. have described a multifunctional polymeric micelle system encoded with a lung cancer–targeting peptide and encapsulated with super paramagnetic iron oxide and doxorubicin, which potentially enables magnetic resonance imaging and target-specific treatment of lung cancer [Guthi et al., 2010].

Antibiotics

Nanoencapsulated antibiotics are promising inhaled formulations for the treatment of bacterial infections of the lung, associated with diseases, such as chronic obstructive pulmonary diseases (COPD) [Hadinoto and Cheow, 2014]. Clinical therapy involves inhalation of antibiotics, such as tobramycin (TOBI®)—a cationic aminoglycoside—which represents the most widely accepted antibiotic in the treatment of chronic lung infection with *P. aeruginosa* [Herrmann et al., 2010]. Even though various approaches have been followed to improve its efficacy [Tre-Hardy et al., 2009; Macleod et al., 2012], the delivery of free-form of antibiotics inevitably suffers from low antibiotic exposures due to their rapid clearance by the mucosal barrier, which, in the long run, promotes emergence of antibiotic-resistant bacteria. Encapsulation of antibiotics into nanoparticle carriers is a promising formulation approach to overcome the mucus barrier and to prolong the antibiotic retention in the lung. Nanoencapsulation of antibiotics also allows their targeted delivery and controlled release at the site of infection [Alhajlan et al., 2013; Serisier et al., 2013]. Besides, nanoencapsulation also facilitates the coincorporation of other antimicrobial agents, such as silver nanoparticles, with the antibiotic.

The antipseudomonal efficacy of liposomal antibiotics has been shown in numerous in vivo studies to be clearly superior to that of the free antibiotics. In the former, the same therapeutic benefit is obtained upon once-daily dosage as that obtained with twice-daily dosage for the free antibiotics. At present, two dry powder–based liposomal drugs, Arikace® (amikacin, Insmed, Monmouth Junction, NJ, USA) and Pulmaquin™ (ciprofloxacin, Aradigm Corp., Hayward, CA, USA), are undergoing advanced clinical trials for the treatment of lung infections [Paranjpe et al., 2014]. A recently concluded Phase II clinical trial involving intranasal delivery of Arikace in CF patients with *P. aeroginosa* infection demonstrated marked reduction in the level of the bacteria in the sputum with general improvement in the lung activity of treated patients in comparison to that of the untreated group [Clancy et al., 2013].

Similarly, ciprofloxacin liposomes were tested for lung infections. In a study performed by Liu et al., ciprofloxacin-loaded liposomes were prepared using phospholipids and cholesterol by the film-hydration method. These liposomes were found to have an average particle size of 350 nm and a high encapsulation efficacy of up to 93%. Furthermore, an in vitro drug release study was performed using simulated lung fluid (SLF) and saline solution as the release medium. The authors observed a higher cumulative release of ciprofloxacin-liposomes in SLF compared to saline solution. In an in vivo experiment performed in rats, they found a higher drug targeting efficiency of ciprofloxacin-liposomes compared to ciprofloxacin solution [Liu et al., 2015].

The potential of PLGA nanoparticles as carriers for lung delivery of antibiotics has been also deeply investigated [Toti et al., 2011; Cheow et al., 2010]. Here, the primary goal is to increase the local concentration of the antibiotic within the macrophages, the host cells for some bacteria, such as Mycobacterium tuberculosis. Although some successful attempts have been made to deliver antibiotics to the lungs via PLGA microparticles, nanoparticles seem to better fit the purpose. When encapsulated into PLGA nanoparticles, the half-life and mean residence time of the entrapped antibiotics are significantly prolonged as compared with the orally administered parent drugs, resulting in an enhanced drug bioavailability.

Tuberculosis (TB) is the leading infectious killer of youth and adults worldwide due to a single infectious agent. In 2010, Saraogi et al. showed that Rifampicin encapsulated natural polymeric gelatin nanoparticles for cytotoxicity study on J-774 macrophage cell lines and in vivo biodistribution and antitubercular studies on a mice model [Saraogi et al., 2010f].

Nucleic Acids

Several lung diseases occur as a result of genetic malfunction or infection by pathogenic genes (via viral invasion). Such diseases can be cured by the delivery of therapeutic nucleic acids (DNA and RNA) [Xu and Anchordoquy, 2011]. However, such anionic nucleic acids cannot be delivered in the free form. Therefore, they require nano-based carriers that would (a) provide a suitable formulation, such as dry powders; (b) protect them from enzymatic degradation; (c) prevent their capture by various biological barriers; (d) deliver them to target sites; and (e) enable their controlled release.

As described in Figure 18.1, various cationic nanocarriers form electrostatic complexes with anionic genetic materials. A number of lipid-based and polymer-based nonviral vectors have been developed to formulate nucleic acids into nanosized particles for pulmonary delivery [Roy and Vij, 2010]. One of the most prominent polymeric gene delivery vectors is poly(ethylene imine) (PEI). There is tremendous potential in targeting genes to the lungs [Birchall, 2007]. Nucleic acids can also be potentially delivered to the lungs via nebulizers, dry powder inhalers (DPIs), or pressurized metered dose inhalers (pMDIs) [Li et al., 2005; Bains et al., 2010; Arulmuthu et al., 2007; Seville et al., 2002]. Nebulization has many advantages, but it is less efficient and less convenient than portable devices. The advantages of nebulizers are associated with DPIs as they are propellant-free, portable, simple to use, have good shelf-life, and need less time for administration. However, there are also some disadvantages associated with the delivery of genes with DPIs, as for example potential problems in dose uniformity, dependency on patient's inspiratory flow rate, and less protection from environmental effects. Genes can also be delivered to the lungs using pressurized metered dose inhalers (pMDIs). However, pMDIs have received considerably less attention than DPIs and nebulizers. The only work discussing gene delivery in hydrofluoroalkane (HFA)-based pMDIs consists of using surfactant-coated DNA particles prepared by reverse microemulsion. pMDIs are simple to use, have high compliance, and are extensively used for drug delivery to the lungs [Bains et al., 2010].

The study by D. S. Conti et al. demonstrates that DNA can be successfully delivered using pMDIs, where chitosan (CS)-DNA nanoparticles (NPs) were prepared by complex coacervation method [Conti et al., 2012]. These polyplexes were successfully encapsulated with high DNA loading efficiency within water-soluble, biodegradable, and HFA-philic co-oligomer shell—up to 90% (w/w). These results suggested that formulating polyplexes in core–shell particles is an efficient approach to deliver genes to the lungs using inexpensive and portable pMDIs to treat medically relevant pulmonary diseases, including asthma, COPD, and cancer.

Pulmonary siRNAs

siRNAs offer a new way to treat various lung diseases by controlling transcript/protein levels of various therapeutic molecular targets. Poly(ethylene imines) (PEIs) serve as promising cationic nanocarriers for siRNA. Different nonviral polycationic nanocarriers have also been tested with promising in vitro properties focused on siRNA delivery to the lungs for their effective in vivo performance in a mouse model [Prasad, 2012; Gunther et al., 2011; Roy and Vij, 2010]. As far as pulmonary siRNA delivery is concerned, mucoadhesive chitosan enjoys great popularity. Matrix systems based on biocompatible and biodegradable polymers, like the Food and Drug Administration (FDA)-approved polymer poly(DL-lactide-co-glycolide acid) (PLGA), are promising for the delivery of small interfering RNA (siRNA) due to favorable safety profiles, sustained release properties, and improved colloidal stability as compared to polyplexes. A dry powder formulation based on cationic lipid-modified PLGA nanoparticles was designed for treatment of severe lung diseases by pulmonary delivery of siRNA.

Spray-dried formulation containing siRNA with characteristics known to be optimal for inhalation therapy without compromising the activity of the siRNA have also been optimized. siRNA delivery to the lungs using nebulizers offers great potential, but to date there has been little research on the aerosol properties of nebulized siRNA. During the process of nebulization, biopharmaceuticals (proteins, peptides, DNA, siRNA, etc.) may be degraded by shear stresses within the nebulizer and effects resulting from adsorption at the liquid–air interface. Hence, in order to improve the stability and aerosolization of biopharmaceuticals from nebulizers, a carrier is often needed. The features of nanoparticles, such as stability at the homeostatic pH of lungs/airways, high encapsulation efficiency, low cytotoxicity, and efficient aerosolization suggest that biodegradable nanoparticles, such as chitosan, can be a suitable siRNA carrier for improving in vivo efficacy.

PERSPECTIVE

As we are gaining more knowledge with respect to pulmonary disease pathophysiology and cellular mechanisms, more specific drugs and nanotherapeutic strategies are being developed. To achieve optimal specificity and potency of therapeutics, novel delivery systems are absolutely required. Nano-based delivery systems have tremendous potential as multifunctional drug carriers; however, several major roadblocks must be overcome before their potential can be realized. Sustained gene, drug, molecular probe release and intracellular entry capability and properties of a nanoscale delivery system need to be carefully controlled to minimize the side effects and allow the treatment of the cause of the disease instead of symptoms.

There is a clear imperative to systematically approach each major roadblock of nanoparticle efficacy in order to rapidly translate nano-based therapeutics from a promising strategy to novel clinical application. The development of novel nontoxic nanosystems for pulmonary gene or drug delivery applications may provide a convenient, noninvasive method for treating specific disease cell types or tissue. Moreover, packaging of imaging modalities, such as molecular probes, allows real time noninvasive quantitative assessment of the disease state and therapeutic efficacy as we recently demonstrated [Vij et al., 2016].

REFERENCES

Alhajlan M, Alhariri M, Omri A. 2013. Efficacy and safety of liposomal clar-ithromycin and its effect on Pseudomonas aeruginosa virulence factors. *Antimicrob. Agents Chemother.* 57, 2694–2704.

Ali ME, McConville JT, Lamprecht A. 2014. Pulmonary delivery of anti-inflammatory agents. *Expert Opin Drug Deliv.* Dec 23, 1–17.

Anderson JM, Shive MS. 1997. Biodegradation and biocompatibility of PLA and PLGA microspheres. *Adv. Drug Deliv. Rev.* 28, 5–24.

Arulmuthu ER, Williams DJ, Baldascini H, Versteeg HK, Hoare M. 2007. Studies on aerosol delivery of plasmid DNA using a mesh nebulizer. *Biotechnol. Bioeng.* 98, 939–955.

Azarmi S, Roa WH, Löbenberg R. 2008. Targeted delivery of nanoparticles for the treatment of lung diseases. *Adv. Drug Deliv. Rev.* 60, 863–875.

Bains BK, Birchall JC, Toon R, Taylor G. 2010. In vitro reporter gene transfection via plasmid DNA delivered by metered dose inhaler. *J Pharm Sci.* 99(7), 3089–3099.

Bala I, Hariharan S, Kumar MNVR. 2004. PLGA nanoparticles in drug delivery: The state of the art. *Crit. Rev. Ther. Drug Carrier Syst.* 21, 387–422.

Beck-Broichsitter M, Gauss J, Gessler T, Seeger W, Kissel T, Schmehl T. 2010. Pulmonary targeting with biodegradable salbutamol-loaded nanoparticles. *J. Aerosol Med.* 23, 47–57.

Beck-Broichsitter M, Ruppert C, Schmehl T, Guenther A, Betz T, Bakowsky U, Seeger W, Kissel T, Gessler T. 2011. Biophysical investigation of pulmonary surfactant surface properties upon contact with polymeric nanoparticles in vitro. *Nanomed. Nanotechnol. Biol. Med.* 7, 341–350.

Beck-Broichsitter M, Merkel OM, Kissel T. 2012. Controlled pulmonary drug and gene delivery using polymeric nano-carriers. *J. Control. Release* 161, 214–224.

Birchall J. 2007. Pulmonary delivery of nucleic acids. *Expert Opin. Drug Deliv.* 4, 575–578.

Cabral H, Kataoka K. 2014. Progress of drug-loaded polymeric micelles into clinical studies. *J. Control. Release* 190, 465–476.

Cavalli R, Caputo O, Carlotti ME, Trotta M, Scarnecchia C, Gasco MR. 1997. Sterilization and freeze-drying of drug-free and drug-loaded solid lipid nanoparticles. *Int. J. Pharm.* 148, 47–54.

Cheow WS, Chang MW, Hadinoto K. 2010. Antibacterial efficacy of inhal-able antibiotic-encapsulated biodegradable polymeric nanoparticles against E. coli biofilm cells. *J. Biomed. Nanotechnol.* 6, 391–403.

Clancy JP, Dupont L, Konstan MW, Billings J, Fustik S, Goss CH, Lymp J, Minic P, Quittner AL, Rubenstein RC. 2013. Phase II studies of nebulised Arikace in CF patients with Pseudomonas aeruginosa infection. *Thorax* 68, 818–825.

Conti DS, Bharatwaj B, Brewer D, da Rocha SR. 2012. Propellant-based inhalers for the non-invasive delivery of genes via oral inhalation. *J. Control. Release* 157, 406–417.

Fiegel J, Fu J, Hanes J. 2004. Poly(ether-anhydride) dry powder aerosols for sustained drug delivery in the lungs. *J. Control. Release* 96, 411–423.

Fiore VF, Lofton MC, Roser-Page S, Yang SC, Roman J, Murthy N, Barker TH. 2011. Polyketal microparticles for therapeutic delivery to the lung. *Biomaterials* 31, 810–817.

Gill KK, Nazzal S, Kaddoumi A. 2011. Paclitaxel loaded PEG5000–DSPE micelles as pulmonary delivery platform: Formulation characterization, tissue distribution, plasma pharmacokinetics, and toxicological evaluation. *Eur. J. Pharm. Biopharm.* 79, 276–284.

Günther M, Lipka J, Malek A, Gutsch D, Kreyling W, Aigner A. 2011. Polyethylenimines for RNAi-mediated gene targeting in vivo and siRNA delivery to the lung. *Eur. J. Pharm. Biopharm.* 77, 438–449.

Guthi JS, Yang SG, Huang G, Li S, Khemtong C, Kessinger CW, Peyton M, Minna JD, Brown KC, Gao J. 2010. MRI-visible micellar nanomedicine for targeted drug delivery to lung cancer cells. *Mol. Pharm.* 7, 32–40

Hadinoto K, Cheow WS. 2014. Nano-antibiotics in chronic lung infection therapy against *Pseudomonas aeruginosa. Colloids Surf. B Biointerfaces.* 116, 772–785.

Herrmann G, Yang LA, Wu H, Song ZJ, Wang HZ, Hoiby N, Ulrich M, Molin S, Riethmuller J, Doring G. 2010. Colistin-tobramycin combinations aresuperior to monotherapy concerning the killing of biofilm *Pseudomonas aeruginosa. J. Infect. Dis.* 202, 1585–1592.

Hoesel LM, Flierl MA, Niederbichler AD, Rittirsch D, McClintock SD, Reuben JS, Pianko MJ, Stone W, Yang H, Smith M. 2008. Ability of antioxidant liposomes to prevent acute and progressive pulmonary injury. *Antioxid. Redox Signal.* 10, 963–972.

Jhaveri AM, Torchilin VP. 2014. Multifunctional polymeric micelles for delivery of drugs and siRNA. *Front. Pharmacol.* 25, 5–77.

Joshi M, Misra AN. 2001. Pulmonary disposition of budesonide from liposomal dry powder inhaler. *Methods Find. Exp. Clin. Pharmacol.* 23, 531–536.

Kim S, Park H, Song Y, Hong D, Kim O, Jo E, Khang G, Lee D. 2011. Reduction of oxidative stress by P-hydroxybenzyl alcohol-containing biodegradable polyoxalate nanoparticulate antioxidant. *Biomaterials* 32, 3021–3029.

Lebhardt T, Roesler S, Beck-Broichsitter M, Kissel T. 2010. Polymeric nanocarriers for drug delivery to the lung. *J. Drug Deliv. Sci. Technol.* 20, 171–180.

Li HY, Birchall JC. 2006. Chitosan-modified dry powder formulations for pulmonary gene delivery. *Pharm. Res.* 23, 941–950.

Li JY, Seville PC, Williamson IJ, Birchall JC. 2005. The use of amino acids to enhance the aerosolisation of spray-dried powders for pulmonary gene therapy. *J. Gene Med.* 7, 343–353.

Liu C, Shi J, Dai Q, Yin X, Zhang X, Zheng A. 2015. In-vitro and in-vivo evaluation of ciprofloxacin liposomes for pulmonary administration. *Drug Dev. Ind. Pharm.* 41, 272–278.

MacLeod DL, Velayudhan J, Kenney TF, Therrien JH, Sutherland JL, Barker LM, Baker WR. 2012. Fosfomycin enhances the active transport of tobramycinin *Pseudomonas aeruginosa. Antimicrob. Agents Chemother.* 56, 1529–1538.

Mansour HM, Rhee YS, Xiao W. 2009. Nanomedicine in pulmonary delivery. *Int. J. Nanomedicine* 4, 299–319.

Muralidharan P, Malapit M, Mallory E, Hayes D Jr, Mansour HM. 2015. Inhalable nanoparticulate powders for respiratory delivery. Invited review. *Nanomedicine*, 4, 1549–9634.

Nassimi M, Schleh C, Lauenstein H, Hussein R, Hoymann H, Koch W, Pohlmann G, Krug N, Sewald K, Rittinghausen S. 2010. A toxicological evaluation of inhaled solid lipid nanoparticles used as a potential drug delivery system for the lung. *Eur. J. Pharm. Biopharm.*, 75, 107–116.

Ozbakir B, Crielaard BJ, Metselaar JM, Storm G, Lammers T. 2014. Liposomal corticosteroids for the treatment of inflammatory disorders and cancer. *J. Control. Release* 190, 624–636.

Paranjpe M, Müller-Goymann CC. 2014. Nanoparticle-mediated pulmonary drug delivery: A Review. *Int. J. Mol. Sci.* 15, 5852–5873.

Park H, Kim S, Song Y, Seung K, Hong D, Khang G, Lee D. 2010. Antioxidant and anti-inflammatory activities of hydroxybenzyl alcohol releasing biodegradable polyoxalate nanoparticles. *Biomacromolecules* 11, 2103–2108.

Pilcer G, Amighi K. 2010. Formulation strategy and use of excipients in pulmonary drug delivery. *Int. J. Pharm.* 392, 1–19.

Prasad PN. 2003. *Introduction to Biophotonics*. New York: Wiley.

Prasad PN. 2012. *Introduction to Nanomedicine and Nanobioengineering*. New York: Wiley.

Roa WH, Azarmi S, Al-Hallak MH, Finlay WH, Magliocco AM, Löbenberg R. 2011. Inhalable nanoparticles, a non-invasive approach to treat lung cancer in a mouse model. *J. Control. Release* 150, 49–55.

Roy I, Vij N. 2010. Nanodelivery in airway diseases: Challenges and therapeutic applications. *Nanomedicine* 6, 237–244.

Rytting E, Nguyen J, Wang X, Kissel T. 2008. Biodegradable polymeric nanocarriers for pulmonary drug delivery. *Expert Opin. Drug Deliv.* 5, 629–639.

Saraogi GK, Gupta P, Gupta UD, Jain NK, Agrawal GP. 2010. Gelatin nanocarriers as potential vectors for effective management of tuberculosis. *Int. J. Pharm.* 385, 143–149.

Sawant RR, Torchilin VP. 2012. Challenges in development of targeted liposomal therapeutics. *AAPS J.* 14, 303–315.

Schreier H, Gonzalez-Rothi RJ, Stecenko AA. 1993. Pulmonary delivery of liposomes. *J Control Release* 24, 209–223.

Schwarz C, Mehnert W, Lucks JS, Müller RH. 1994. Solid lipid nanoparticles (SLN) for controlled drug delivery. I. Production, characterization and sterilization. *J. Control. Release* 30, 83–96.

Serisier DJ, Bilton D, de Soyza A, Thomson PJ, Kolbe J, Greville HW, Cipolla D, Bruinenberg P, Gonda I. 2013. Inhaled, dualrelease liposomal ciprofloxacin in non-cystic fibrosis bronchiectasis (ORBIT-2): A randomized, double-blind, placebo-controlled trial. *Thorax* 68, 812–817.

Seville PC, Kellaway IW, Birchall JC. 2002. Preparation of dry powder dispersions for non-viral gene delivery by freeze-drying and spray-drying. *J. Gene Med.* 4, 428–437.

Silva, LFC, Kasten G, de Campos CEM, Chinelatto AL, Lemos-Senna E. 2013. Preparation and characterization of quercetin-loaded solid lipid microparticles for pulmonary delivery. *Powder Technol.* 239, 183–192.

Taylor KMG, Taylor G, Kellaway IW, Stevens J. 1990. The stability of liposomes to nebulisation. *Int. J. Pharm.* 58, 57–61.

Toti US, Guru BR, Hali M, McPharlin CM, Wykes SM, Panyam J, Whittum-Hudson JA. 2011. Targeted delivery of antibiotics to intracellular chlamydialinfections using PLGA nanoparticles. *Biomaterials* 32, 6606–6613.

Tre-Hardy M, Traore H, Manssouri NE, Vanderbist F, Vaneechoutte M, Devleeschouwer MJ. 2009. Evaluation of long-term co-administration of tobramycinand clarithromycin in a mature biofilm model of cystic fibrosis clinical isolates of *Pseudomonas aeruginosa. Int. J. Antimicrob. Agents* 34, 370–374.

Ungaro F, d'Angelo I, Miro A, La Rotonda MI, Quaglia F. 2012. Engineered PLGA nano- and micro-carriers for pulmonary delivery: Challenges and promises. *J. Pharm. Pharm.* 64, 1217–1235.

Vij N, Min T, Bodas M, Gorde A, Roy I. 2016. Neutrophil targeted nano-drug delivery system for chronic obstructive lung diseases. *Nanomedicine* 12(8), 2415–2427.

Wang W, Zhu R, Xie Q, Li A, Xiao Y, Liu H, Wang S, Cui D. 2012. Enhanced bioavailability and efficiency of curcumin for the treatment of asthma by its formulation in solid lipid nanoparticles. *Int. J. Nanomedicine* 7, 3667–3677.

Weber S, Zimmer A, Pardeike J. 2014. Solid lipid nanoparticles (SLN) and nanostructured lipid carriers (NLC) for pulmonary application: A review of the state of the art. *Eur. J. Pharm. Biopharm.* 86, 7–22.

Xu L, Anchordoquy T. 2011. Drug delivery trends in clinical trials and translational medicine: Challenges and opportunities in the delivery of nucleic acid-based therapeutics. *J. Pharm. Sci.* 100, 38–52.

Yoo D, Guk K, Kim H, Khang G, Wu D, Lee D. 2013. Antioxidant polymeric nanoparticles as novel therapeutics for airway inflammatory diseases. *Int. J. Pharm.* 450, 87–94.

19 Intravitreal Drug Delivery

Omar Saleh, Mark Ihnen, and Shlomit Schaal

CONTENTS

THE CLINICAL SIGNIFICANCE OF INTRAVITREAL DRUG DELIVERY

To achieve an ocular therapeutic effect, it is necessary that the desired drug is delivered to the target tissues in adequate concentrations and for an adequate duration of time. To reach the innermost tissues of the eye, such as the retina or the retinal pigment epithelium, such an objective can be rather challenging. Intrinsic anatomic and physiologic properties of the eye impose qualitative and quantitative limitations to the design of an efficient drug delivery system. The eye is a relatively isolated organ that receives a small share of the cardiac blood flow. It is essentially a fluid-filled cavity engulfed by avascular tissues, and it has multiple blood–ocular barriers. These factors complicate the dynamics of penetration and distribution of drugs inside the eye.

There are multiple routes to drug delivery into the eye. *Topical* application involves the use of eye drops and allows the transportation of the drug into the anterior segment of the eye, albeit with a bioavailability of usually less than 5% and with only negligible bioavailability in the posterior segment [1]. As penetration of most drugs into the eye from the systemic circulation is poor, *systemic* therapy is practical for few eye conditions, such as intraocular inflammation, in which the blood–ocular barrier is interrupted [2]. Furthermore, adverse effects of systemic medications are a major concern when treating solely ocular conditions. For the treatment of common inner-eye conditions, including age-related macular degeneration (AMD) and diabetic macular edema (DME), local therapy is therefore required. This latter route of drug delivery involves the injection of the drug itself or the implantation of a drug-releasing vehicle into the eye (*intravitreal*, *intracameral*) or in the tissues around the eye (*subconjuctival*, *subtenon*, *peribulbar*, *retrobulbar*). By using the intravitreal route, the poor permeability of ocular structures and the restrictions created by the physiologic barriers of the eye are essentially circumvented. In addition, tissues located in the posterior segment, such as the central retina and the vitreous itself, are easily targeted with high concentrations of the drug. This method of drug delivery involves a relatively invasive procedure, which can be inconvenient to the patient and the physician and can potentially cause serious complications, including endophthalmitis and retinal detachment [3,4].

Although the bulk of ophthalmic research has historically studied drug delivery to the anterior segment of the eye, and even though topical eye drop therapy still represents the most commonly used route of drug delivery, current research in ocular drug delivery is focused on innovative designs in local delivery through the posterior segment [5].

This chapter reviews the anatomical and physiological properties associated with limitations to ocular drug delivery. It enlightens the rationale for the use of the intravitreal drug delivery route, discusses the usefulness as well as the shortcomings of intravitreal therapies currently used in ophthalmic practice, and refers to the potential future innovative ideas for drug delivery designs in the context of the unmet clinical and engineering needs for intravitreal delivery systems.

APPLIED ANATOMY AND PHYSIOLOGY: SUPPORT FOR THE RATIONALE OF THE INTRAVITREAL DRUG DELIVERY ROUTE

Topical and systemic administration of drugs represent two convenient methods of drug delivery into the eye. However, using these routes is far from satisfactory in providing or maintaining adequate levels of most medications in the posterior segment of the eye, which is where many of the important eye diseases prevail. Several factors inherent to the structure and function of different ocular tissues challenge our ability to efficiently exploit topical or systemic drug delivery.

Anatomic and Physiologic Limitations of Topical Therapy

Topically applied medications are useful in treating conditions restricted to the anterior tissues of the eye, such as the conjunctiva, the cornea, the anterior sclera, and the anterior uvea. For the drug to enter into the eye in therapeutic concentrations, many obstacles need to be overcome soon after its application topically. The tear film, with its high turnover rate, comprises the first resistance line. Topically applied solutions can be washed away within 15–30 seconds. Blinking, reflex tearing, and the debris-clearing properties of the mucin layer of the tear film are other precorneal factors that further limit the transport of topically applied eye drops [6]. The cornea has three layers that show different polarities. The corneal epithelium represents the main barrier to drug transport across the cornea. Harboring the majority of the corneal cells, the epithelium is lipoid in nature, which can significantly hinder the diffusion of hydrophilic substances [7]. Additionally, the superficial epithelial cells are tied together by desmosomes and surrounded by tight junctional complexes, therefore limiting paracellular influx of drugs [8]. The corneal stroma is a thick, well-hydrated layer that contains regularly arranged collagen bundles. In contrast to the epithelium, the stroma seems to be an important obstacle to the permeation of lipophilic molecules [7]. The endothelium is a monolayer of hexagonal cells that separate the stroma from the aqueous humor. It is important for maintaining the transparency of the cornea, and it has selective carrier-mediated transport and secretory functions [9].

Studied in isolation, the conjunctiva may be more permeable than the cornea [10], but due to the rich supply of blood and lymphatic vessels to the conjuctiva and episclera, a great amount of topically applied drugs may be cleared quickly into systemic circulation. In addition, the conjunctiva is a multilayered epithelial tissue with tight intercellular junctions, which may further limit diffusion [11]. The sclera is the fibrous outer coat of the eye that extends posteriorly from the limbus to the remainder of the globe, thereby offering a much larger surface area than the cornea for drug transport. Scleral permeability is considered comparable to that of the corneal stroma. However, the sclera has been shown to be permeable to macromolecules [12,13]. Some of the factors that may affect the permeability across the sclera include the drug's molecular radius, which is inversely proportional to its permeablity, and its electrical charge with less permeability to positively charged drugs due to their interaction with the negatively charged proteoglycan scleral matrix [14,15]. Although transcorneal permeation represents the traditional route for topical drug delivery, transport of certain substances into the eye, including certain high molecular weight compounds and molecules considered to have low corneal permeability, have been suggested to occur through the noncorneal conjunctival–scleral route, thereby entering specific intraocular tissues and bypassing the anterior chamber [13].

Clinical Drawbacks of Systemic Therapy

In order for oral or intravenous medications to enter into the eye, the drug has to pass across at least one of the blood–ocular barriers: the blood–aqueous barrier in the anterior segment of the eye or the blood–retina barrier in the posterior segment. The former is composed of an epithelial bilayer located at the surface of the ciliary body and the iris with tight intercellular junctional complexes, which prevent diffusion of most substances from the blood into the anterior chamber. The blood–retina barrier is located in the retina and is functional at two levels: The inner barrier is formed by the retinal vascular endothelium, and the outer barrier is formed by the retinal pigment epithelium (RPE). Both cell types are bound together by tight junctions. The retinal endothelium lines the retinal vessels, which travel in the inner retinal layers. The RPE is a monolayer of specialized cells that separates the neurosensory retina from the choroid. Therefore, whether circulating in the intravascular retinal compartment on the inner side of the retina or extravasating from the fenestrated choriocapillaris into the extravascular compartment on the outer side of the retina, most substances are denied entry into the retinal tissue.

Selective conditions affecting the posterior segment have been reported to show satisfactory responses to topical therapy, including cystoid macular edema associated with cataract surgery or with retinitis pigmentosa [16,17] or to systemic therapy, including posterior uveitis or endophthalmitis [2,18,19] although results from other reports were inconsistent [20,21]. Relatively large or frequent doses may need to be administered to ensure adequate penetration of the drug into the posterior segment, therefore increasing the likelihood of adverse events. By using the intravitreal route, in contrast, the therapeutic agent is given in small amounts and is delivered in close proximity to the site of pathology in the retina or posterior vitreous without the need to traverse the blood–ocular barriers.

Unique Structure and Function of the Vitreous Humor

The vitreous humor is a highly hydrated tissue filling the region between the lens and the retina. It is a gel-like material that is formed essentially of intricate networks of extracellular matrix, and it accounts for around 80% of the tissue volume of the eye (about 4 ml in the adult). It's almost acellular except for a few macrophage-like hyalocytes located in the periphery. Water constitutes about 99% of the vitreous with the solid components mainly formed of fibrillar proteins and glycosaminoglycans (GAGs). The main fibrillar protein in the vitreous is collagen type II and the main GAG is hyaluronan. Collagen endows the vitreous with shape, tensile strength, flexibility, and resistance to tractional forces. GAGs are charged macromolecules that attract water and provide swelling pressure to the vitreous, therefore spacing out the thick collagen bundles and resisting compressive forces [22].

While functions of the vitreous are not completely understood, it is clear that the vitreous and the aging changes it undergoes are central to the development of several common eye conditions, including rhegmatogenous retinal detachment, macular hole formation, and proliferative diabetic retinopathy. There is also evidence that the vitreous regulates eye shape and size during development [23]. It also acts as a barrier to migration of cells and diffusion of macromolecules, which can help maintain its transparency [22]. Hyalocytes, which originate from the bone marrow, have been associated with vitreous cavity–associated immune deviation [24]. Low oxygen tensions in the lens and retina are maintained by ascorbate-dependent oxygen consumption in the vitreous. Adequate levels of ascorbate are, in turn, preserved by the gel form of the vitreous. This may explain the tendency to develop nuclear cataract after vitrectomy surgery or vitreous liquefaction [25].

The vitreous can be divided into the central vitreous, the vitreous cortex, and vitreous base. The density and orientation of collagen fibrils differ at each of these regions. The central region forms the bulk of the vitreous and has the lowest density of collagen fibrils. These fibrils are anchored anteriorly to the vitreous base and run across the globe to join the posterior vitreous cortex at the back of the globe. Collagen fibrils at the vitreous base straddle the ora serrata and are firmly attached to the pars plana and peripheral retina. They are densely packed and are inserted perpendicularly at this region, therefore providing the very strong adhesion of the vitreous base. From the vitreous base, these fibrils arc posteriorly toward the optic nerve. The vitreous cortex is a thin layer of densely packed collagen fibrils (0.1–0.3 mm) that surrounds the central vitreous. The anterior cortex courses from the vitreous base anteriorly to the posterior surface of the lens. Its anterior limit is called the anterior hyaloid face. The posterior hyaloid face is where the posterior cortex lines the surface of the retina posterior to the vitreous base. The cortical collagen fibrils are oriented parallel with the inner retinal surface and do not generally insert directly into the internal limiting membrane (ILM). The posterior cortex is, however, adherent to the ILM, especially at the margins of the optic disc and blood vessels [26].

With age, the vitreous humor experiences several changes. Vitreous syneresis is a process by which the vitreous progressively liquefies and loses its gel-like form. It was estimated that by the age of 18 years, about 20% of the vitreous gel is liquid and about half of it is liquid by the age of 90. The liquefaction process is not uniformly distributed and pockets of fluid in the vitreous center seem to enlarge and fuse [27]. Age-related vitreous liquefaction may be caused by gradual aggregation of the collagen fibrils into macroscopic strands, which leads to the formation of collagen-devoid areas that eventually become liquid. It has been suggested that the age-related loss of type IX collagen renders the “sticky” collagen type II exposed, thereby promoting aggregation of collagen bundles and liquefaction of the gel [28].

Weakening of the vitreous adhesion to the post-basal ILM also occurs with age. This is likely due to age-related biochemical changes that loosen the interaction between components on the surface of the vitreous collagen fibrils and macromolecules on the inner surface of the ILM. Both vitreous syneresis and weakening of post-basal vitreoretinal adhesion play a role in yet another age-related physiological change: posterior vitreous detachment (PVD). In this important process, the cortical vitreous gel splits away from the retina as far anteriorly as the posterior border of the vitreous base. The prevalence of PVD increases with age, and it is estimated to occur in more than 60% of people above 70 years. Although the majority of PVD cases occur without complications, sometimes peripheral retinal tears, vitreous hemorrhage, or retinal detachment can develop. Furthermore, if vitreous attachment at the foveal region persists, vitreo-macular adhesion (vitreo-macular traction) syndrome and macular hole may develop [29].

Factors Affecting Drug Distribution and Drug Elimination in the Vitreous

The inherent differences in the organization of vitreous components, the age-related changes that occur in the vitreous, the presence of physiologic barriers, and other factors, may have important effects on the movement and distribution of intravitreally injected particles, especially nanoparticle suspension-based drugs. The following are factors that may affect the kinetics of distribution and elimination of drugs in the vitreous.

Age-Related Vitreous Liquefaction

Although the proportion of solid components in the vitreous humor is very small (1%), the specific geometric arrangement of collagen bundles in different regions of the vitreous cavity may play a role in dictating where injected drug particles would eventually reside. Figure 19.1 shows possible sites of deposition of injected particles in light of arrangement of collagen fibrils in the vitreous. In addition, the combined arrangement of collagen fibers along with GAGs forms a complex network that acts like a molecular barrier to diffusion. It follows that diffusion of particles in the vitreous humor as compared to water would be different. In an experiment where the vitreous was treated with hyaluronidase, the diffusion rate of materials from the mid-vitreous to the choroid was significantly increased [30]. With vitreous liquefaction, convection currents in the eye may become more important. Hydraulic stresses attributed to change in intraocular pressure, blinking, or head movement may have an exaggerated effect on water flux and has been shown to result in complex three-dimensional vortex flow patterns in the eye [31,32]. It has been shown that high molecular weight particles experienced a temporary forward flux in the first few hours after injection and were cleared faster in liquefied vitreous compared to normal vitreous [33].

Status Post Vitrectomy Surgery

A pharmacokinetic effect similar to that observed in liquefied vitreous would be expected to be seen after vitrectomy surgery. Indeed, more rapid clearance has been demonstrated in vitrectomized animal eyes for intravitreally injected substances, including bevacizumab, triamcinolone acetonide, vancomycin, amikacin, amphotericin B, and vascular-endothelial growth factor (VEGF) [34–39]. This was not necessarily true for other therapies, however. For example, reports have shown similar drug levels in the vitreous humor in vitrectomized versus nonvitrectomized rabbit eyes

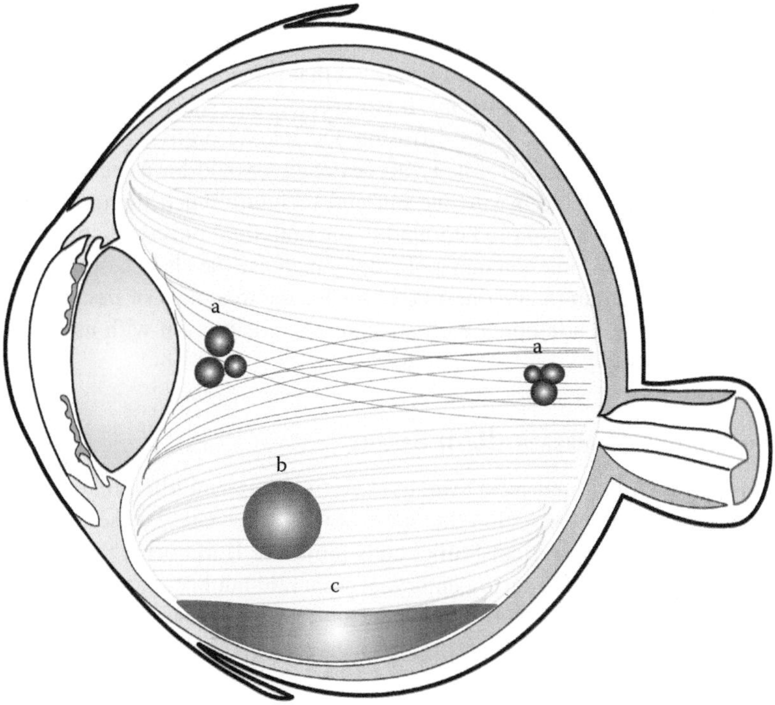

FIGURE 19.1 Illustration of the arrangement of collagen fibers in the vitreous cavity. The potential sites of deposition of injected particles in the vitreous cavity are shown. Some particles injected into the central vitreous remain associated with the back of the lens or near the optic nerve (a). Charged nanoparticles may associate with the collagen fibers (b). Heavy particles settle to the bottom of the eye (c).

after injection of a dexamethasone sustained-release implant [40]. This was supported by the observation of similar clinical responses in vitrecomized and nonvitrectomized eyes of patients who have received this implant [41]. These considerations may be clinically relevant during the management of elderly patients or in vitrectomized eyes with conditions, such as AMD, DME, or retinal vein occlusion (RVO).

Status Post Lens Surgery

It has been also suggested that lens surgery, such as phacoemulsification for cataract extraction, may have an effect on the convection currents in the vitreous and forward clearance of large drug molecules, including anti-VEGF drugs, injected into the vitreous. Because such surgeries may also cause damage to the zonules and compromise the barrier between the anterior and posterior segments, these changes are likely to facilitate drug clearance from the anterior segment [42].

Vitreous Substitutes

In vitreo-retinal surgery, some substances may be injected into the vitreous cavity, usually to provide retinal tamponade. Sulfur hexafluoride and perfluoropropane gas bubbles injected into the vitreous cavity may induce a temporary breakdown of the blood–aqueous barrier [43]. This may alter the pharmacokinetics of intravitreal therapies. Silicone oil is a viscous material that provides long-term tamponade after injection into the vitreous cavity. It is expected that substances injected into silicone oil may experience altered diffusion and release profiles. For example, a drug injected into a silicone oil–filled vitreous cavity would have much less room to disperse if it is insoluble in silicone oil, and therefore much higher than usual drug concentration is expected to be found in the preretinal or retinal compartment [42]. Although this phenomenon may potentially increase the chance of toxicity, the injection of bevacizumab in silicone-filled eyes for the treatment of iris rubeosis or rubeotic glaucoma was attempted with no signs of toxicity even with using double the normal dose [44,45].

Internal Limiting Membrane (ILM) Barrier

The ILM represents the innermost layer of the retina. It is a multilaminar semitransparent basement membrane with a thickness of 0.5–2 μm and is closely associated with the footplates of the retinal Müller cells [46]. The ILM seems to be essential for the support of glial cells during embryogenesis [26] but becomes less important later in life. Indeed, peeling of the ILM may be of benefit in several disorders and is frequently performed as part of the surgical management of macular hole, epiretinal membrane, and DME [47–49].

The ILM may pose a significant barrier to intravitreally injected particles, particularly large charged cationic species, including liposomal and polymeric gene delivery systems [50]. This may also be true for intravitreal Adeno-associated viral (AAV) gene therapy, which has recently shown promise in the potential treatment of certain retinal disorders, including retinitis pigmentosa [51]. Intravitreally injected AAV particles have to bind specific receptors on the ILM and then traverse the ILM in order to infect retinal cells and mediate gene expression. For many AAV serotypes, the ILM acts as a barrier. What's more, it was demonstrated in the laboratory that digestion of the ILM by a nonspecific protease was followed by significantly enhanced transduction of AAV particles from the vitreous, which allowed the virus particles to be expressed in multiple retinal cell types [52]. It seems likely that the ILM can be a staging area for certain intravitreal particles targeting the retina, where movement across the ILM may be mediated by specific active carriers and is preceded by binding to specific ILM receptors. This may be true for bevacizumab, a monoclonal anti-VEGF antibody, widely used for the treatment of choroidal or retinal neovascularization, which was shown to be able to bind and penetrate the ILM and the retina and reach the choroid [53].

Intraocular Inflammation

Ocular inflammation is associated with hyperemia and disruption of the blood–ocular barriers, which may lead to enhanced drug penetration. In animal experiments, it was demonstrated that intravenous injection of bacterial toxin was associated with enhanced penetration of systemic grepafloxacin to the vitreous [54]. A similar effect on fluorescein penetration into the vitreous was observed 1 month after vitrectomy surgery [55], which may be explained by surgically induced trauma or inflammation. Also, endotoxin-induced ocular inflammation resulted in retinal edema and swelling of the Müller cells [56], which may compromise the barrier and transport function of the ILM, thereby facilitating access of intravitreal drugs into the retina.

Transport Molecules

Many types of transport molecules exist in various ocular tissues, including the endothelium of retinal vessels, the RPE, the cornea, the conjunctiva, and the ciliary body. These transporters are usually large protein molecules that control the influx and efflux of particles, thereby regulating the traffic of many substances, including nutrients, solutes, and drugs across ocular barriers. Peptide transporters are a group of proton-coupled transporters that translocate di- and tri-peptide molecules and are expressed on human RPE. They include PepT1, PepT2, and peptide/histidine (PHT1 and PHT2) transporters. β-lactams and angiotensin-converting enzyme and renin inhibitors are known substrates for these transporters [57]. Targeted drug delivery may be achieved by modifying drugs to enhance their recognition by transporters. Such an engagement of the drugs in transporter-mediated mechanisms leads to better tissue specificity and ocular bioavailability. For example, it was reported that higher concentrations of acyclovir in the aqueous humor were attained after systemic administration of two prodrugs (valine-acyclovir or valine-valine-acyclovir) rather than the parent drug due to enhanced transport of these molecules by peptide transporters [58]. In another study, the intravitreal injection of dipeptide monoester prodrugs of ganciclovir, which are substrates for retinal peptide transporters, resulted in the doubling of retinal concentrations of ganciclovir compared to injection of the parent drug [59]. Efflux transporters, on the other hand, function to clear drugs and other compounds from ocular tissues. They constitute a large superfamily of ATP-binding cassette proteins. Blocking these transporters may be another way to exploit transporter-mediated mechanisms to achieve targeted drug delivery and better bioavailability [60].

Effect of Particle Size and Charge

The size of a particle is an important determinant of its diffusion and elimination characteristics in the vitreous. Small molecules with low molecular weight (MW) encounter lower steric hindrance, and therefore, their migration in the vitreous is largely in the form of simple diffusion. Injection via the pars plana into the anterior part of the vitreous cavity allows free diffusion in all directions toward the anterior chamber and retina [42,61]. The movement of larger molecules, however, is also dependent on the intravitreal convection currents, which are generated by pressure and temperature differences between the anterior chamber and the surface of the retina. During and soon after injection, excess pressure is generated by expansion of the vitreous volume, and there is temporary alteration of vitreous integrity. These hydraulic changes may have potential effects on the convection currents in the vitreous. The effect of convection has been proposed to account for approximately

30% of the intravitreal transport of small molecules. For larger molecules, where the diffusion process is limited, it may become the main transport mechanism [62]. In general, the intravitreal half-life of low MW drugs is usually a few hours, but when MW rises above 10 kDa, clearance slows down. For instance, the intravitreal half-lives for dexamethasone (392 Da), vancomycin (1.5 kDa), ranibizumab (48 kDa), and bevacizumab (149 kDa) have been found to be 5.5 hours, 25 hours, 3 days, and 4 days, respectively [63–66].

For nanospheres, the relationship between size and half-life in the vitreous may be more complex. It has been demonstrated, using polystyrene nanospheres tagged with sodium fluorescein, that the elimination half-life from the vitreous increased with decreased particle diameter (approximately 5 days for 2-μm particles, 9 days for 200-nm particles, and 10 days for 50-nm particles). Size also appears to be related to where the particles resided in the eye with larger particles (2 μm) detected in the vitreous and the trabecular meshwork and particles under 200 nm found also in retinal tissues [67]. This relationship between particle size and clearance rate from the vitreous may not hold true, however, for other substances with different surface features. For example, it was demonstrated in a recent study that larger (4 μm) iron oxide particles coated with polystyrene could remain in the vitreous for 5 weeks after injection whereas smaller iron oxide particles (50 nm) coated with dextran could not [68]. It follows that the nanoparticle's surface qualities are important as well for determining its clearance rate. More insight on this may be brought about by further studies that compare elimination rates for nanoparticles with varying sizes but with the same composition and polymer coating.

The charge of the particle is also a significant factor that may affect movement of particles after intravitreal injection. This was studied when anionic and cationic nanoparticles were created from human serum albumin and tagged with a fluorescent dye and then injected into the vitreous cavity. Distribution of the particles was tracked by epifluorescence microscopy performed on thin cross-sections of the vitreous after enucleation. Five hours postinjection, the signal intensity from the cationic nanoparticles in the vitreous remained high because those particles were unable to freely penetrate through the vitreous into other ocular tissues. On the other hand, the signal intensity generated from anionic nanoparticles was much lower as the majority of anionic particles was able to penetrate through the vitreous and was located in the retina by that time [69]. This means that negatively charged anionic nanoparticles, in general, appear to move through the vitreous with little restriction, therefore reaching the ILM and penetrating into the retina. And although it has been generally accepted that a positive surface charge for nanoparticles may promote cellular uptake [70], the barrier that the vitreous humor creates for distribution of positivity charged particles represents a major limitation to their use in the treatment of posterior eye disease.

DRUG DELIVERY TO THE POSTERIOR SEGMENT OF THE EYE

At present, commercially available ocular drug delivery systems are designed to be administered mainly by the intravitreal route. However, many other routes are continually under experimentation and evaluation by both preclinical and clinical studies. Examples include subconjunctival, subtenon's capsule, intrascleral, subretinal, and suprachoroidal routes. In addition, there are various improvements to topical application of drugs including the use of unique fornix devices or punctual placements (Figure 19.2) [71].

The intravitreal injection drug delivery route has surged in popularity in recent years. Intravitreal injections may contain a simple drug solution or more sophisticated drug-loaded vehicles, such as microspheres, nanospheres, and liposomes [71,72]. Intravitreal or trans-scleral sustained-delivery devices may be implanted by injection or by surgery to provide long-term drug release [73].

Direct intravitreal injection delivers a relatively high dose of the drug to the vitreous and retina. Intravitreal injection is an effective route for a wide range of drugs, including low molecular mass drugs as well as macromolecules, such as oligonucleotides and monoclonal antibodies or their fragments. However, because most drugs used in intravitreal injections have a short half-life, repeated injections are needed to sustain therapeutic drug concentrations for long-term treatment. Repeated injections lead to patient discomfort and can be associated with several complications, including serious infection, vitreous hemorrhage, lens injury, and retinal detachment. Furthermore, frequent appointments needed for repeated injections or for evaluation of the response or adverse events may pose significant social and financial burdens. Clearly, a longer half-life for drugs makes them more suitable for intravitreal

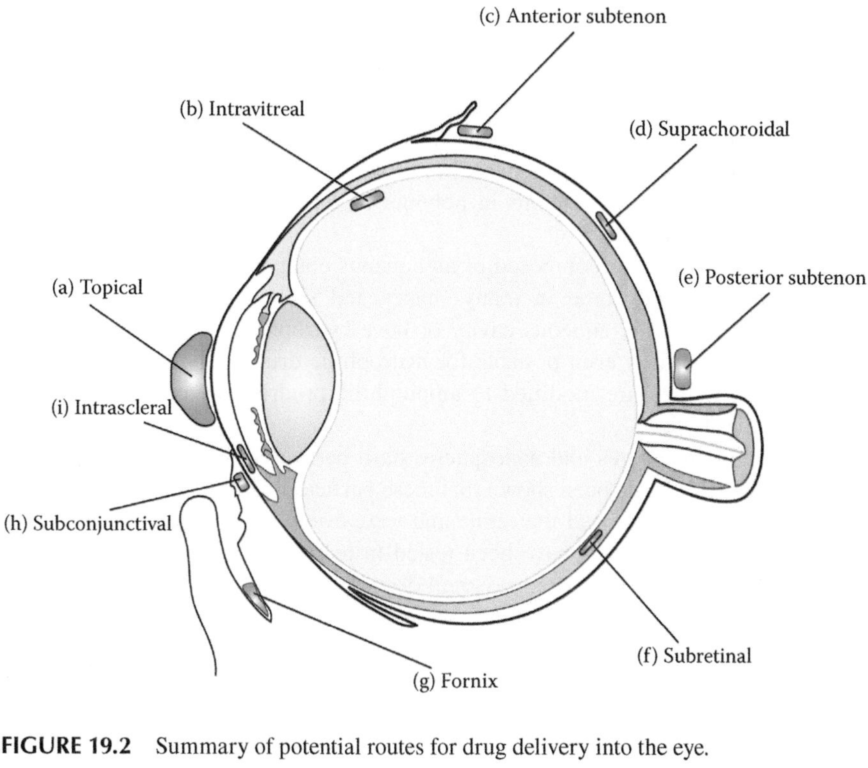

FIGURE 19.2 Summary of potential routes for drug delivery into the eye.

injection. A scientific understanding of the relationship between drug elimination patterns and physicochemical properties of the drug, including molecular weight, lipophilicity/hydrophilicity, and solubility is essential for the improvement of its intravitreal pharmacokinetic properties. Furthermore, alternative approaches to drug delivery and the employment of advanced technologies to ensure safe and long-term intraocular supply of the medication are essential.

Injectable Microparticles

The intravitreal injection of colloid-based vehicles, such as microspheres [74], liposomes [75], and nanospheres [76] provides a longer period of drug release than conventional solutions and potentially reduces drug degradation and toxicity as there is less direct contact between the ocular tissues and the free drug [77,78]. Suspended in a carrier solution to enable ocular injection, these microparticles can be conveniently injected into the vitreous cavity using a fine needle and can achieve therapeutic levels of the drug for extended periods. In microspheres or microcapsules (1–1000 μm in diameter) and in their nano-counterparts (<1 μm), the desired drug is incorporated into biodegradable polymers to form either a matrix system or a reservoir system [79]. In a matrix system, used for micro- and nanospheres, the drug and the polymer matrix are combined. The drug is released through diffusion from the polymer matrix as the polymer undergoes degradation. For micro- and nanocapsules, the reservoir-type system is used, in which drugs are encapsulated within polymeric shells. The choice of the polymer is essential. Commonly used synthetic biodegradable polymers include aliphatic polyesters, such as PLA (poly-lactic acid), PGA (poly-glycolic acid), PLGA (poly-lactide-co-glycolide), and poly-caprolactone. These polymers are suitable for controlled-release applications because they are nontoxic, nonimmunogenic, and degrade through enzymatic reactions and hydrolysis to natural metabolic products over a period of months to years. Drug-release kinetics can be controlled by modifications in polymer molecular weights and copolymer formulations and ratios [80].

Liposomes are vesicles composed of an aqueous compartment bound by a lipid bilayer membrane and come in many shapes and sizes. They can encapsulate hydrophilic drugs in the aqueous cavity or have hydrophobic drugs incorporated into the membrane. It is even possible for hydrophilic drugs to be introduced into the membrane if they are modified to amphiphilic prodrugs by conjugation with other molecules [79].

Polymeric microspheres and nanospheres have been used for targeting drugs to the RPE and retina. It has been shown that these particles, which can be loaded with different substances, accessed the retina and were eventually taken up by the RPE cells [81,82]. Corticosteroids have been tested in micro- and nanospheres for sustained drug delivery [83]. Also, intravitreal drug-delivery vehicles have been introduced using nanoparticles. For example, vehicles called "Trojan particles" permitted slower drug release patterns in vitro and were developed from spray-drying suspensions of dexamethasone-loaded PLGA nanoparticles (230 nm) along with other substances [84]. Several medications, encapsulated in micro- and nanospheres, have been experimented and showed sustained drug release and favorable safety profiles.

Examples include antiviral medications, such as ganciclovir, used for the treatment of CMV retinitis [85]; antiproliferative medications, including 5-fluoruracil and adriamycin, used in proliferative vitreoretinopathy [72,78]; and steorids, such as dexamethasone used to treat uveitis [86]. Due to such qualities as cellular penetration, protection of contents from degradation, and long-term sustained drug release, micro- and nanoparticles have applications as nonviral vectors in gene therapy. Gene therapy involves the delivery of nucleic acids (DNA or RNA) into target cells for the purpose of manipulating transcription and/or translation and eventually expression of certain genes in those cells [58]. Micro- and nanoparticles have shown promise in enabling gene transfer and expression in RPE cells with nontoxic profiles [87]. Nanoparticles have been used also to deliver VEGF antisense oligonucleotide to a human ARPE-19 cell line, therefore inhibiting mRNA expression and VEGF secretion [88].

Intravitreal injection of microparticulates may cause temporary cloudiness of ocular media. Nonetheless, microspheres larger than 2 μm tend to settle at the bottom of the vitreous cavity after injection, similar to triamcinolone acetonide. Also, nanoparticles diffuse rapidly and are internalized by ocular tissues and therefore should not interfere with vision. Another potential problem is a faster clearance rate of microspheres in vitrectomized eyes. One study showed that PLA microspheres remained in the vitreous body for 6 weeks compared to 2 weeks in vitrectomized eyes [89]. Several limitations have been reported with liposomes; there are difficulties in the preparation and storage of liposomes compared with microspheres. Liposomes may burst due to interaction of their membrane components with other proteins, lipids, or cellular components in the eye. This may make drug release from liposomes less predictable. Liposomal instability has been greatly improved, however, with the addition of polyethyleneglycol (PEG). These PEGylated liposomes have much more stable structure and their uptake by the reticulo-endothelial system is minimal [79].

It is worth mentioning that alternative methods for delivering anti-VEGF therapies for the treatment of posterior segment disease, including trans-scleral delivery of PLA or PLGA nano- and microparticles are being evaluated as a feasible and effective method for administrating these drugs. With particle sterilization using γ-radiation proven to be feasible, it is expected that studies of these novel drug-delivery routes will soon include clinical trials [80].

Intravitreal Implantable Device Technology

The concept of implanting an intravitreal device for sustained-release of a therapeutic agent makes sense in many ways. The intraocular structures are relatively easy to access and are almost isolated from the systemic circulation by the inner and outer blood–ocular barriers. This makes local delivery of drugs a favorable approach. Furthermore, the eye benefits from an "immune privilege" particularly observed in the anterior segment and in the subretinal space, which limits the risk of an exaggerated inflammatory reaction to foreign antigens or rejection of cell grafts. Although intravitreal device implantation may be associated with serious complications, several advantages are expected. First, drugs are delivered in close proximity to the target tissue, and when compared to systemic administration of the drug, higher local concentrations are achieved with less amounts of drug. In addition, systemic absorption and undesirable effects on other parts of the body are minimized. Even when local adverse events or unexpected immunological reactions occur, it should be possible to immediately remove the implant and eliminate the problem, a task that may not be as simple with an injected drug, let alone a drug administered systemically. Intravitreal implants are ideal for therapeutic agents whose administration by other routes may be difficult, ineffective, or associated with poor patient compliance. Furthermore, the containment of the medication inside the implant environment may offer protection to medications that may be unstable or exhibit short-half life in vivo [71].

INTRAVITREAL INJECTABLE DRUGS IN CURRENT OPHTHALMIC PRACTICE

Intravitreal injection of drug solutions is an extremely valuable and commonly practiced method for the treatment of various posterior segment conditions, including AMD, DME, RVO, uveitis, vitreo-retinal interface abnormalities, infections, and others. Many formulations may be prepared for intravitreal injection, including anti-VEGF, anti-inflammatory, antimicrobial, and antimetabolite drugs. In addition, enzymes that possess fibrinolytic (tissue plasminogen activator, tPA) or vitreolytic (ocriplasmin) function can be also used. The following is a brief summary of some of these medications.

Anti-VEGF Agents

There are four major anti-VEGF agents that are used in ophthalmic practice: pegaptanib sodium (Macugen®, Eyetech, New York, NY), ranibizumab (Lucentis®, Genentech, Inc., South San Francisco, CA), bevacizumab (Avastin®, Genentech, Inc., South San Francisco, CA), and aflibercept (VEGF Trap-Eye or Eylea®, Regeneron Pharmaceuticals, Inc., Tarrytown, NY, and Bayer Healthcare Pharmaceuticals, Berlin, Germany). The three major eye diseases in which these drugs are being used are wet AMD, DME, and CME secondary to RVO. Nonetheless, these medications are occasionally used in other ocular conditions, such as retinopathy of prematurity, neovascular glaucoma, and radiation retinopathy [90–92].

Macugen® is an oligoribonucleotide aptamer that binds and blocks the activity of the 165 isoform of extracellular VEGF [93]. It was shown in a randomized trial to have a smaller proportion of patients who lost <15 letters of visual acuity compared with sham injection at 1 year although more than half of the treated patients lost >15 letters, and only a third maintained or gained vision [94]. It was approved by the FDA in 2004 for the treatment of all subtypes of wet AMD [95].

Lucentis® is a recombinant, humanized, monoclonal antigen-binding Fab antibody fragment that neutralizes all active forms of VEGF-A. Monthly intravitreal injections of ranibizumab over the course of 24 months were compared with verteporfin and sham injection in large randomized trials and were found to be effective in the treatment of all forms of AMD-related choroidal neovascularization with a breakthrough mean increase in visual acuity of 5.4–10.7 letters in the ranibizumab groups compared with a decrease of 14.9 and 9.8 in the sham-injection and verteporfin groups, respectively [96,97]. Multiple large randomized trials evaluating ranibizumab in the treatment of DME and RVO were also conducted with similarly impressive results [98,99]. Ranibizumab was approved by the FDA in 2006 for the treatment of all subtypes of wet AMD and was approved in 2010 for the treatment of CME associated with RVO [95].

Avastin® is the humanized full-size anti-VEGF antibody that blocks all VEGF-A isoforms. It has shown comparable results to ranibizumab in wet AMD in many uncontrolled clinical trials [100,101]. In addition, a head-to-head comparison in a controlled randomized trial between the two medications in the treatment of wet AMD revealed similar efficacy and safety at 2 years [102]. Moreover, many other studies have demonstrated the usefulness of bevacizumab in CME due to RVO, DME, and several other conditions [103,104]. Although ocular use of bevacizumab is off-label, it was already approved by the FDA for intravenous use in the treatment of metastatic colorectal and other cancers [95]. Due to its substantially lower cost and more widespread availability, bevacizumab accounts for the majority of intravitreal anti-VEGF injections used in ophthalmic practice [93,105].

Eylea® is a fusion protein that consists of VEGF receptors 1 and 2 fused to the crystallizable Fc fragment portion of human immunoglobulin G. It binds both VEGF-A with high affinity and placental growth factor (PlGF). Aflibercept is the most recent anti-VEGF pharmacotherapy introduced into clinical practice and has been demonstrated by randomized controlled trials to be similar to ranibizumab in efficacy and safety in wet AMD [106]. In addition, it has shown outstanding results in DME and RVO as well [107,108]. Aflibercept was approved by the FDA for the treatment of wet AMD in 2011 and for the treatment of CME associated with central RVO in 2012 [95,109]. Figure 19.3 illustrates the structures of anti-VEGF agents used in clinical practice.

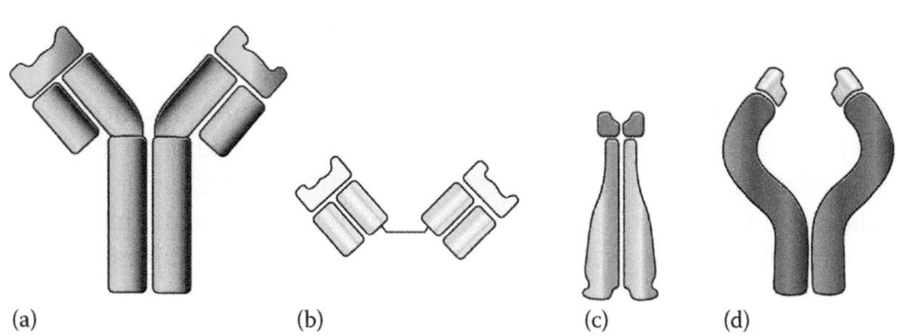

FIGURE 19.3 The structure of anti-VEGF drugs used in clinical practice. Bevacizumab (Avastin®) is a full-size antibody (a). Ranibizumab (Lucentis®) is a Fab antibody fragment (b). Macugen® is an oligoribonucleotide aptamer (c). Aflibercept (Eylea®) is a fusion protein of VEGF receptors and Fc fragment of IgG (d).

Anti-Inflammatory and Immunosuppressive Agents

Triamcinolone acetonide ($C_{24}H_{31}FO_6$, MW 434.5 Da) is a conventional corticosteroid with typical glucocorticoid and mineralocorticoid anti-inflammatory activity [110]. Corticosteroids have anti-inflammatory, antiangiogenic, and antifibrotic properties. They inhibit key processes and mediators that may be important in the pathogenesis of various retinal vascular and inflammatory conditions, including proinflammatory leukocytes, remodeling of extracellular matrix, VEGF expression, and various pro-angiogenic cytokines and inflammatory mediators, including IL-6, phospholipase A2, arachidonic acid, prostaglandins, and leukotrienes. These actions explain the ability of triamcinolone to downregulate VEGF, decrease blood–retinal barrier permeability, and contribute toward the resolution of CME [111,112].

In ophthalmic practice, it is usually available as a 4-mg injectable suspension. Although many commercial preparations exist, one of the most commonly used preparations is *Kenalog-40*® (Bristol-Myers-Squibb, Peapack, NJ), on which a black box warning against intravitreal use exists. A novel, preservative-free proprietary variant of triamcinolone acetonide injectable suspension 40 mg/ml (Triesence®, Alcon Labs, Fort Worth, TX) has been developed and approved by the FDA for intraocular use. It is applied for the treatment of uveitis, sympathetic ophthalmia, temporal arteritis, and other ocular inflammatory conditions unresponsive to topical corticosteroids as well as for visualization during vitrectomy surgery [112].

Dexamethasone ($C_{22}H_{29}FO_5$, MW 392.5 Da) is a synthetic glucocorticoid that has the highest relative strength of any other corticosteroid used in ophthalmic practice and is five times more potent than triamcinolone [113]. However, it has the short half-life of about 5 hours in the vitreous, compared to approximately 18 days for triamcinolone [113,114]. Intravitreal dexamethasone has been shown to suppress VEGF-induced retinal blood–retinal barrier breakdown in rabbits [115]. When administered in pulse injections, it may be less likely to result in glaucoma or cataract progression than other long-acting steroids [112]. Triple therapy using PDT, intravitreal dexamethasone, and anti-VEGF agents is sometimes employed in patients with wet AMD not responding to typical anti-VEGF therapy [116]. Dexamethasone is used in the FDA-approved sustained-release biodegradable implant known as *Ozurdex*® (described later in the chapter).

Methotrexate is a folate analogue that competitively inhibits the enzyme dihydrofolate reductase, thereby blocking purine synthesis and leading to inhibition of rapidly dividing cells. It also inhibits cytokine production and leads to adenosine accumulation at the site of inflammation. Methotrexate thus exhibits antiangiogenesis, anti-inflammatory, and humoral and cellular immunosuppressive properties [117,118]. Methotrexate is mainly used systemically in ophthalmic practice to treat noninfectious posterior uveitis. Nonetheless, intravitreal methotrexate injections were successfully used in the treatment of intraocular lymphoma, some types of uveitis, and relapsing retinoblastoma [119–122]. Typically, intravitreal therapy is initially administered twice weekly and then is reduced in frequency. Injections are generally tolerated with the main adverse event being transient corneal toxicity [120].

Antimicrobial Agents

A large number of antibiotics, antiviral, and antifungal medications are available for intravitreal injections for the treatment of infectious endophthalmitis. A few examples include cephalosporins, such as ceftazidime; aminoglycosides, such as amikacin; and vancomycin (antibiotics); ganciclovir (antiviral); and amphotericin B and voriconazole (antifungal) [123–125].

Enzymes

Tissue plasminogen activator (tPA) is a naturally occurring polypeptide enzyme found on the vascular endothelium and containing 527 amino acid residues with a MW of 72 kDa. It is a serine protease that mediates clot-specific fibrinolysis by converting plasminogen to plasmin [126]. The fibrinolytic effect and enhanced clearance rate of blood clots achieved relatively safely with intravitreal tPA led to its application in cases of subretinal macular hemorrhage, particularly in association with wet AMD [127]. A large number of uncontrolled case series report variable results for the use of tPA, usually in combination with pneumatic retinopexy, for submacular hemorrhage, whether injected intravitreally as an outpatient procedure or delivered surgically into the subretinal space [128–130].

Ocriplasmin (Jetrea®, Thrombogenics NV, Leuven, Belgium) is a 27 kDa recombinant truncated form of plasmin, a human serine protease. It has proteolytic activity against fibronectin and laminin, which are two major components of the biochemical proteoglycan glue that contributes to adhesion forces at the vitreoretinal interface [131]. Vitreomacular adhesion (VMA) follows anomalous PVD and may result in the development of VMA syndrome, a condition highlighted by persistent vitreomacular attachment. It is characterized by symptoms such as metamorphopsia and decreased central visual function and could be complicated by foveal distortion, CME, and macular hole formation. Furthermore, VMA has also been implicated in the pathogenesis and progression of exudative AMD and proliferative diabetic retinopathy [132].

Pharmacological or enzymatic vitreolysis has been attempted in animal studies using various molecules, including hyalouronidase, plasmin, chondroitinase, and dispase [132,133]. Some of these enzymes showed limited efficacy or unacceptable complications [134,135]. However, the experience with others was more favorable, and there were recommendations for use of these enzymes as adjuncts in vitreoretinal surgery [133]. Ocriplasmin was approved by the FDA for use in symptomatic VMA in October 2012 [136].

INTRAVITREAL IMPLANTS IN CURRENT OPHTHALMIC PRACTICE

Several intravitreal implants can be inserted into the vitreous cavity for long-term treatment of important chronic eye conditions, including noninfectious uveitis, cytomegalovirus (CMV) retinitis, DME, and RVO [137–140]. Whether or not implants are degraded into nontoxic products and excreted from the body depends largely on the types of polymers used in the implant. Accordingly, they can be classified into biodegradable and nonbiodegradable implants. Polymers commonly used for nonbiodegradable implants are polyvinyl alcohol (PVA), ethylene vinyl acetate (EVA) and silicone. For biodegradable implants, a wider variety of polymers can be used, including PLA, PGA, PLGA, polycaprolactones, polyanhydrides, and polyorthoesters [141]. Nonbiodegradable implants offer more accurate control of drug release and longer release periods compared to biodegradable implants. In the latter, drug release may occur in different phases, and its kinetics may be complex, especially during the phase where the drug release is coupled with continuous erosion of the polymer. Therefore, many factors, including the size, shape, surface area, and the characteristics of the polymers used in the manufacturing of the implant, need to be considered to avoid drug bursts and keep drug concentrations under control [79,142]. Although insertion of either type of implant may be considered invasive, a major difference is that nonbiodegradable implants require surgical implantation, and after a certain amount of time, may require surgical removal. This can be associated with complication risks and poor patient compliance [141].

Nonbiodegradable Implants

Vitrasert® (Chiron Vision Inc., Irvine, CA) was the first implantable ganciclovir delivery device developed in 1992 for the treatment of cytomegalovirus (CMV) retinitis. Several animal and later human studies demonstrated long-term release of the drug (80 days) and control of the retinitis [143,144]. Subsequently, the device was approved by the FDA in 1996 for clinical use in CMV retinitis. It is a reservoir-based device composed of the drug and polymeric coats of PVA and EVA. It is relatively large and requires a 4–5 mm sclerotomy at the pars plana for surgical implantation [71]. It offered a convenient and less expensive way to control CMV retinitis without the systemic complications of the drug. However, it was associated with risks of endophthalmitis and retinal detachment [142]. Additionally, it didn't protect against nonocular CMV disease and CMV retinitis in the contralateral eye [145]. The disease is more commonly treated nowadays with by oral valganciclovir, intravenous ganciclovir, or weekly intravitreal ganciclovir injections [146].

Retisert® (Bausch & Lomb Inc., Rochester, NY) is a reservoir-based fluocinolone acetonide-loaded implant designed to provide drug release over a period of about 3 years. The implant is about 5 × 3 × 2 mm and is composed of silicone laminate and PVA polymer and contains 0.59 mg of the steroid. A drug tablet is contained in a cup-like drug core affixed by a silicone adhesive to a 0.2-mm-thick platform, the suture strut [147,148]. Feasibility and safety of the implant were demonstrated by animal experiments, and then effective control of posterior noninfectious uveitis for up to 3 years was shown in a human clinical trial [137,149,150]. In a prospective randomized clinical trial, the implant was found to be noninferior to systemic steroids and immunosuppression therapy for posterior noninfectious uveitis [2]. Significant complications, nonetheless, have been observed with this implant. More than 90% of phakic patients needed cataract extraction surgery, and 40% of patients needed glaucoma surgery at 3 years [150]. In addition, complications related to implantation or removal surgery or related to long-term retention of the implant were reported [71,147]. Although Retisert was evaluated for the treatment of other conditions,

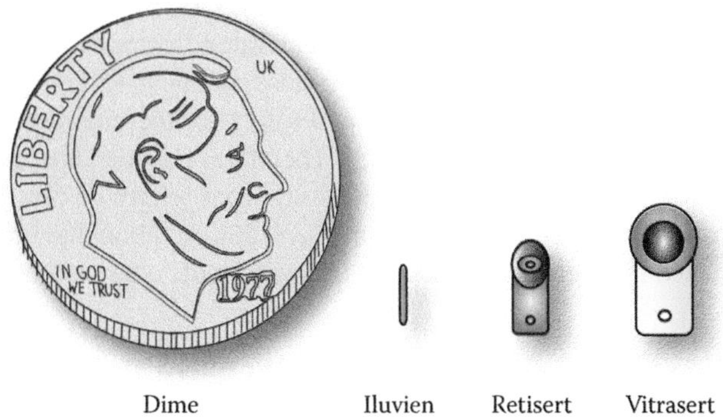

FIGURE 19.4 Comparative sizes of different nonbiodegradable implants.

including central RVO and DME, it has received FDA approval (in 2005) only for the treatment of noninfectious posterior uveitis [151,152].

Iluvien® is also a nonbiodegradable silicone-PVA implant containing fluocinolone acetonide (Alimera Sciences Inc., Alpharetta, GA). However, being much smaller (3.5 mm length × 0.37 mm diameter) than Retisert, the rod-shaped implant can be injected into the vitreous cavity through the pars plana using a 25-gauge needle in an outpatient or office setting. As expected, it will be freely floating in the vitreous compartment after its administration, in contrast to Retisert and Vitrasert [58]. Iluvien has been evaluated for the treatment of DME in randomized clinical trials. It was demonstrated that visual gain was significantly increased up to 36 months in patients who received the implant compared to those who received sham therapy. Almost all phakic patients needed cataract extraction, but the implant enjoyed a more favorable ocular hypertensive profile, compared to Retisert, with only 5%–8% of patients needing incisional glaucoma surgery [153]. Although approved in several European countries, the FDA has not yet approved Iluvien for DME and has requested two additional clinical trials to demonstrate its safety and efficacy. Currently, fluocinolone implants are being investigated in Phase II trials for the use in wet AMD as an adjunct to ranibizumab, in dry AMD, and in RVO [58]. Figure 19.4 shows the comparative sizes of Vitrasert, Retisert, and Iluvien nonbiodegradable implants.

Biodegradable Implants

Ozurdex® (Allergan Inc., Irvine, CA), formerly known as Posurdex, is a 6.5 mm × 0.45 mm rod-shaped drug pellet containing 0.7 mg of dexamethasone contained in a PLGA copolymer matrix (Novadur™ technology, Allergan, Inc.). The implant is injected into the vitreous cavity through the pars plana using a single-use 22-gauge microinjector in an outpatient setting [154]. It releases the drug by diffusion in a biphasic fashion with a peak drug level maintained for up to 60 days, followed by a rapid decline between days 60 and 90 and then a steady lower therapeutic level up to 6 months after injection. Randomized, sham-controlled clinical trials have demonstrated efficacy of Ozurdex in improving visual acuity and resolving CME in RVO.

The safety concerns were much less compared to Retisert with complications including cataract formation in about 30% of patients and elevated intraocular pressure, which was mainly manageable by hypotensive medications, in about 15% of patients [139]. In another controlled clinical trial, efficacy and safety for the treatment of posterior noninfectious uveitis was demonstrated [155]. Therefore, Ozurdex has received FDA approval in 2009 for the treatment of CME arising from branch or central RVO and for the treatment of noninfectious posterior uveitis [156]. Additionally, Phase III trials are being conducted to determine efficacy of Ozurdex in the treatment of DME [58].

NOVEL INTRAVITREAL AND SCLERAL IMPLANTS

Many other intraocular devices have been designed and developed for the use in various eye diseases, including those that can be implanted in the anterior segment for the treatment of conditions, such as corneal graft rejection, postoperative inflammation, glaucoma, and dry eye syndrome [154]. Research and development related to intravitreal implants for posterior segment diseases currently occupy yet a larger area in the field of ocular drug delivery. Most of these novel devices are currently investigational and are subject to ongoing development and clinical trials. The following is a summary of a few examples of delivery systems that target the posterior segment.

Encapsulated Cell Technology (ECT)

This comprises a nonbiodegradable semipermeable hollow fiber polymeric membrane supported by a polyethylene terephthalate scaffold encompassing genetically modified cells (ARPE-19 line) that synthesizes a desired protein, such as ciliary neurotrophic factor (CNTF) or other growth factors. The polymeric membrane in the device is permeable to oxygen and nutrients that are vital for the survival of the cell line but is impermeable to white blood cells, which prevents immunogenic host response to the encapsulated cells. This implant is stitched to the sclera in the vitreous cavity by the implant's suture loop to makes it easily retrievable for dose adjustments or therapy discontinuation. It has been demonstrated in Phase II clinical trials that the NT-501 product by Neurotech (Lincoln, RI), designed for the treatment of geographic atrophy in AMD and retinitis pigmentosa, was well-tolerated by patients with no increased IOP, retinal detachment, infection, or serious inflammation up to 18 months postimplantation. Photoreceptors in retinitis pigmentosa were significantly preserved over 24 months in patients who received the implant. There exist controversies, however, about ECT, including the potential production of other substances by these cells and their biological effects [58,71].

Nonbiodegradable and Biodegradable Injectable Systems

I-vation™ (SurModics Ltd., Eden Prairie, MN) is a 0.5 × 0.21 mm nonbiodegradable helical nonferrous alloy coil with an eluting polymer containing 925 μg triamcinolone acetonide. It is implanted through a 25G needle-stick and is self-anchoring within the sclera. It was designed to provide intravitreal triamcinolone release for up to 2 years. The evaluation of this interesting technology for the treatment of DME by a Phase II randomized clinical trial was unfortunately terminated early due to unstable pharmacokinetics and rapid cataract progression in nearly all treated eyes [58,71,112].

Verisome™ (Icon Bioscience Inc., Sunnyvale, CA) is a biodegradable nonpolymer-based drug delivery system that can deliver peptides, nucleic acids, small molecules, and monoclonal antibodies for up to a year in either the anterior segment or posterior segment of the eye. Verisome can be formulated as a solid, a gel, or a liquid and is injected using a 30-gauge needle into the target site with stability up to 2 years. IBI-20089/Verisome is a gel with triamcinolone as the active ingredient. Phase I/II clinical trials evaluating its use in CME secondary to RVO have been completed [58].

Scleral Plugs and Intrascleral Implants

These comprise drug-loaded biodegradable polymers. They have various dimensions and can be implanted at the pars plana to gradually release effective doses of drugs into the vitreous over several months. One such plug (8.5 g in weight, 5 mm in length) is prepared from PLA or PLGA and contains various quantities of ganciclovir. The implantable scleral plug may be useful in diseases such as CMV retinitis and proliferative vitreoretinopathy. Other device forms have been developed including a nonerodible, refillable reservoir device and a coated coil matrix device (Figure 19.5). The devices can be implanted at the pars plana through a scleral

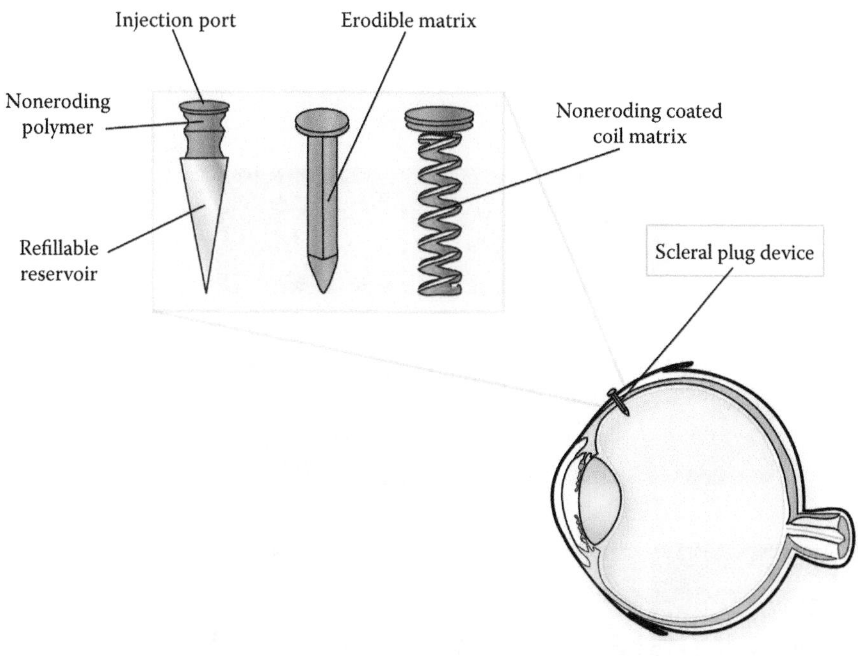

FIGURE 19.5 Illustration of different scleral plugs. These biodegradable devices may be implanted through a scleral incision without suturing and may not need removal once their drug-load is depleted.

incision without the need of a suture. Since they are biodegradable or have refillable reservoirs, they don't need to be removed once the drug load is depleted. Scleral plug implants may have disadvantages, including unpredictable burst phases during drug release. Scientists have tried to address these undesirable drug release kinetics by modifying the geometric properties of the scleral implants and developed other devices, including discoid or doughnut-shaped intrascleral devices. A discoid intrascleral PVA/EVA device (4 mg in mass, 1 mm thick, and 4 mm in diameter) containing betamethasone was evaluated in rabbits and showed sustained drug release into the vitreous for 4 weeks with no burst effects [157]. Another scleral disc utilizing polymethylidene malonate (PMM2.1.2) as the polymer/matrix was shown to be biocompatible in rabbits and released triamcinolone into the vitreous for 5 weeks [158]. Unlike in implantable scleral plugs and devices, a sclerotomy isn't required in intrascleral devices, and therefore complications associated with ocular perforation may be avoided. However, the duration of drug release in these relatively noninvasive devices is shorter [71].

UNCONVENTIONAL ROUTES OF DRUG DELIVERY TO THE VITREOUS AND THE POSTERIOR SEGMENT OF THE EYE

There are many other active research programs that may utilize novel or unconventional routes or methods to effectively deliver prolonged therapeutic concentrations of drugs to the posterior segment. Other programs work on refining existing methods in ways that result in more effective therapy or extended duration of action or less invasive approach. Figure 19.6 is flowchart highlighting the main drug delivery routes to the vitreous.

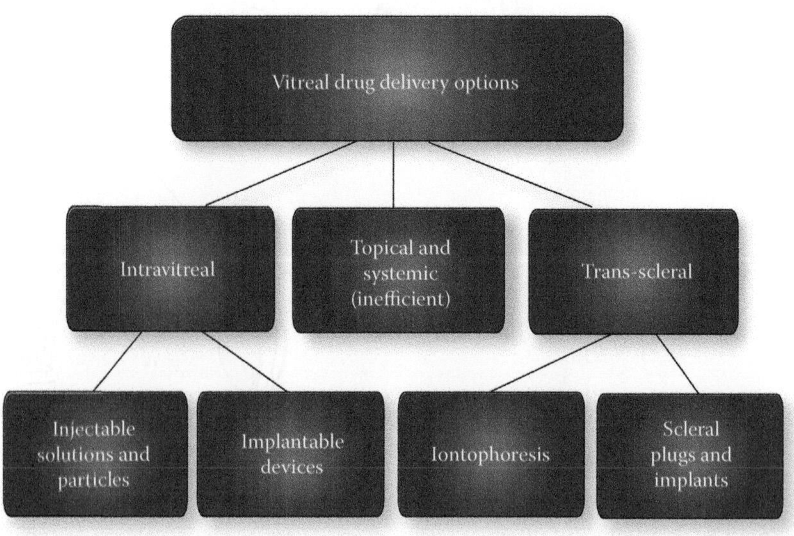

FIGURE 19.6 Summary of options for drug delivery to the vitreous.

Trans-Scleral Iontophoresis

Mainly described in the field of dermatology, this delivery system is a promising non-invasive technique for drug delivery to the posterior segment of the eye. In summary, charged drug molecules act as a conductor of a low electrical current through ocular tissues. A donor electrode with the same charge as the drug is placed on the scleral surface, and a return electrode with an opposite charge is placed on another body surface [141]. Several processes in iontophoresis may contribute to drug penetration into the eye. Electrophoresis is the movement of the charged drug particles into the eye in response to electrical current. Electroporation is an enhancement of drug penetration because of increased intrinsic tissue permeability to the drug due to the electric field. Electro-osmosis is the transport of both neutral and charged species by an electric field–induced convective flow observed in the solvent [159]. The process of ocular iontophoresis typically lasts minutes to tens of minutes [160]. Before the iontophoresis device is used, the drug solution can be loaded into a 5–10 mm eye cup that is applied to the eye with gentle suction. Alternatively, the drug can be loaded into hydrogels made of hydrophilic polymers. These have attracted increasing attention in recent years in view of their swelling behavior, biocompatibility, and stability. Furthermore, hydrogels allow modulation of drug release kinetics and offer target tissue specificity [141,161]. Many medications, including antibiotics, antivirals, antimetabolites, and steroids, in addition to oligonucleotides and genes and charged nanoparticles have been successfully delivered to the vitreous of animals using trans-scleral iontophoresis [141,162–165]. Several investigators conducted clinical studies using trans-scleral iontophoresis of methylprednisolone. In a Phase II clinical trial, the technique was found to be safe, well tolerated, and easily applied for the treatment of severe ocular inflammation, thereby reducing the need for systemic corticosteroids [141]. Saline iontophoresis on healthy volunteers using the OcuPhor™ (Iomed, Inc., Salt Lake City, Utah, USA) applicator demonstrated that the procedure was well tolerated [166]. Although iontophoresis enjoys the advantages of introducing high doses of drug into the eye, avoiding systemic side effects and circumventing the use of intraocular injections, adverse events may occur. Several factors play a role in these side reactions, including the density of the current, the site of application, and the duration of treatment. Conjuctival injection and a burning sensation are common. With higher currents or multiple applications, burns affecting the scleral, corneal, and chorioretinal tissues, retinal edema, hemorrhagic necrosis of chorioretinal tissue, fibrosis, and RPE hyperplasia at the site of iontophoresis have been reported [79,141].

Ultrasound-Mediated Microbubble Drug Delivery

Ultrasound has long been used for diagnostic imaging, but recently there has been a focus on its therapeutic applications in drug delivery and gene transfection. Due to their efficient acoustic reflectivity, gas-filled microbubbles (1–8 μm diameter) with stable shell coatings containing phospholipids, surfactant, denatured serum albumin, or synthetic polymer are being used as contrast agents for the enhancement of ultrasound images [167]. It has been shown that ultrasonic waves targeting tissues that harbor these microbubbles result in the destruction of the bubbles and release of their contents as well as enhancement of the permeability of the target tissue [168]. Drugs and genes can be incorporated inside the microbubble or in its shell. Drug-loaded bubbles can then be delivered to the target tissue using various routes, including intravenous and intravitreal injections. A novel controlled-release delivery system for the posterior segment utilized mathematically modeled acoustic signals to induce drug or gene release from subconjuctivally injected polymeric nano- and microbubbles by fracturing the polymeric shell and increasing scleral permeability for drug transfer into the vitreous [80]. Microbubble targeting is mediated by the intrinsic binding properties of the microbubble shells and can be further enhanced by site-specific ligands. Exposure to a carefully controlled ultrasound field with varying powers and frequencies mediates transport, permeation into tissues, and site-specific destruction of the bubbles with the release of their contents [168]. Experiments have also demonstrated that exposure to ultrasound increased drug release up to 20-fold from biodegradable polymeric implants and up to tenfold from nonbiodegradable implants in a reversible ultrasound intensity-dependent fashion [169]. Ultrasound-mediated delivery has been tested in animals and resulted in successful delivery of drugs, proteins, genes, and gene-silencing therapies to various organ systems [170].

Thermoresponsive Hydrogels

Hydrogels are polymeric networks that absorb large amounts of water while remaining insoluble in aqueous solutions. They allow for the manipulation of permeation and diffusion kinetics, thus allowing optimized drug delivery. They also prolong the drug residence in the vitreous, which could be important in vitrectomized eyes. Compared to hydrophobic polymers such as PLA or PLGA, hydrogels don't have the hydrophobic interactions that normally denature biomolecules. This makes them excellent for encapsulating macromolecules, such as proteins and DNA. In addition, the formation of hydrogels usually occurs at ambient temperatures, and organic solvents are rarely needed. Hydrogels can be made from natural or synthetic polymers. Natural polymers provide increased biocompatibility and biodegradability. However, they largely lack the mechanical properties that synthetic polymers possess, and they may carry pathogens and evoke inflammatory responses within the body [171]. Certain types of hydrogels exhibit rapid reversible change in physical state in response to external stimuli, such as temperature, pH, glucose, or light. For example, poly N-isopropylacrylamide hydrogel is a thermosensitive material that occurs as a swollen gel below a critical solution temperature and collapses above that temperature. These properties have introduced hydrogels as a useful tool in nanodrug delivery and have stimulated research in the application of hydrogels in the field of sustained-release delivery of various substances, including anti-VEGF drugs. For instance, a recent experiment involved the encapsulation of a thermosenstive hydrogel (PNIPAAm–PEG-diacrylate) with various proteins, including bovine albumin, IgG, bevacizumab, and ranibizumab, and then injection of the hydrogel as a liquid to the juxtascleral region or in the vitreous cavity via a small-gauge needle. Once it was exposed to body temperature, the hydrogel rapidly became a solid gel that started releasing the anti-VEGF with an initial burst of release within 2 days followed by a steady-state level of drug, which was maintained for 3 weeks [80].

Electromagnetically Steerable Intravitreal Inserts

Microrobotic devices represent an emerging tool for localized drug delivery using minimally invasive surgery. The use of electromagnetically controlled microrobots that act as intravitreal inserts with drug reservoirs that may contain substances, such as anti-VEGF drugs for the treatment of AMD has been suggested. The ability to move these devices in a controlled manner allows for their positioning and removal in the eye, potentially without the need for vitrectomy [172]. Microrobotic devices are nonbiodegradable, but they can be made biocompatible using various coatings [173]. The microrobots may have a shape similar to that of the Iluvien implant. The outer diameter is less than 0.5 mm, and they can fit in a 23-gauge needle. Their length (reservoir) can be adjusted to carry larger payloads for higher dosage or extended durations. They are inserted into the vitreous cavity through the pars plana, and with the eye located within the field of action of an electromagnetic control system, the microrobots are wirelessly controlled to the macula where they release their payload. They can be placed in an area along the lower vessel arcade without significant effects on vision until their reservoirs are depleted, at which time they are controlled back toward the entry site and are removed by a magnetic tool. The eye is illuminated trans-sclerally, and images are captured by a camera mounted on a microscope during the implantation or removal process. Successful ex vivo experiments on porcine eyes were conducted and demonstrated feasibility of inserting microrobotic devices and steering them to the target site without the need for vitrectomy [172].

Vascular Targeted Photodynamic Therapy

The only compound approved by the FDA for the use in ocular photodynamic therapy (PDT) is verteporfin (Visudyne®, Novartis Pharmaceuticals, East Hanover, NJ). Verteporfin is a lipophilic photosensitizer prepared in a liposome formulation. The mechanism of action for PDT involves radiating the retina with nonthermal laser after the intravenous infusion of the photosensitizer. The photosensitizer in the target cell (endothelium of the neovascular membrane) is then activated and leads to the generation of cytotoxic free radicals, thereby occluding the targeted blood vessels. Studies evaluating this therapy have revealed some adverse events that may occur with verteporfin-PDT, including damage to the RPE and photoreceptor cells. Stakel® (Steba Biotech, Luxembourg, Germany), a modified palladium-substituted bacteriochlorophyll compound, is also a photosensitizer that has very high vascular affinity with minimal migration into the surrounding ocular tissues. Studies in rabbits demonstrated that Stakel, unlike Visudyne, does not destroy retinal or RPE cell layer. Phase II clinical trials to assess the safety and preliminary efficacy of vascular targeted PDT using Stakel in patients with wet AMD are currently underway. It seems the need for multiple PDT treatments observed with verteporfin and for anti-VEGF therapy may be both reduced with Stakel-PDT [58].

CLINICALLY UNMET NEEDS

A dramatic improvement in our understanding and in our ability to treat various ocular diseases has recently occurred. The clinical outcomes for previously devastating ocular conditions have been upgraded with the emergence of new therapeutic agents and novel drug delivery methods. Better understanding of the basic underlying mechanism of ocular diseases, more effective screening methods, and the ability to accurately identify the high-risk patient population have all contributed to the emergence of new concepts and paradigm shifts in the management of many common and blinding eye conditions, such as AMD, DME, posterior uveitis, and RVO.

Anti-VEGF drugs and steroids delivered to the posterior segment by intravitreal injection, sometimes on a monthly basis, have become the standard of care for most of patients with these conditions. Although it may be a temporarily effective method, simple intravitreal injection of the drug solution is far from optimal [93]. First, the invasiveness of the intravitreal injection procedure is an important consideration. It is inconvenient compared to topical or systemic therapy and may be an important cause of poor patient compliance. Second, adverse events associated with an intravitreal injection include not only minor complications, such as eye pain or conjunctival bleeding, but also sight-threatening complications, such as endophthalmitis, vitreous hemorrhage, lens injury, and retinal detachment. In addition, drug molecules injected into the vitreous cavity are allowed to diffuse to areas other than their target tissues and may cause local or systemic complications. Examples include the frequent development of cataract and glaucoma with steroid injections. The relatively short half-life of drugs in the vitreous, which may be even shorter in vitrectomized eyes, is also a problem because it creates a need for repetitive injections. Considering the chronicity of many ocular diseases, frequent injections in these patients for years to come would not qualify as a safe or convenient management plan. Furthermore, frequent injections pose a significant cost on the health care system and may require logistical preparations that may be dramatic to patients and physicians. It is therefore clear that development of new routes of drug delivery to the posterior segment or revision and refinement of existing routes have become necessary. The development of new therapeutic agents and their evaluation in clinical trials should be paralleled by research and development in drug delivery. The optimal drug delivery method would be minimally invasive and convenient and would offer efficient drug penetration, extended bioavailability, excellent biocompatibility, nontoxicity, target-selectivity, and cost-effectiveness.

The concept of a drug delivery system, as compared to simple injection, is gaining more traction and acceptance across many medical and pharmaceutical communities. Biodegradable polymer-based drug delivery systems show considerable promise in tailoring drug release and providing a sustained-release platform. In addition, drugs that may be ineffective by conventional routes may become useful when incorporated into these systems.

Trans-scleral iontophoresis represented a relatively noninvasive method for drug delivery and enhanced penetration through otherwise nonpermeable barriers. However, practical and safety issues in this system are still to be assessed.

Several implantable devices provide controlled and extended zero-order drug release but require invasive procedures or surgery for implantation or removal and may have substantial complication profiles. Particulate drug delivery systems can be administered by different routes without the need for surgery. Furthermore, engineering the size and composition of these particles allows for a controllable slow release of the encapsulated drugs for extended durations along with the potential for specific cell or tissue targeting. Another plus is the possibility to develop thermo or light labile particles that allows for time and site control of drug release and the ability to respond to external stimuli or to certain manifestations of the disease.

Because the epidemiology of such disease as AMD or DME creates a great impact on public health, it is likely that successful patient management will require a drug delivery system or a combination of systems. One possible approach would utilize combinations of drugs and drug delivery devices to counteract multiple pathophysiological disease processes, for example, an antineovascularization drug plus an anti-inflammatory drug delivered by two or more devices or systems. Better yet, development of a "standard" biocompatible drug delivery system to the posterior segment that can be safely administered or implanted around the eye to treat different diseases may not be far from reality. It may be designed to simultaneously store different types of drug-loaded tissue-targeting nanoparticles and offer a drug release profile that is titrated by specific disease events or external cues. In addition, an electronic shut down mechanism could be incorporated in the system to mediate a wirelessly controlled "override" if significant adverse events are encountered. Currently, no single device or technology meets the wide range of ever-increasing needs, and a combination of approaches with multidisciplinary integration is demanded to optimize drug delivery. Indeed, the scope of active research and development efforts that the drug delivery field is now experiencing predicts a bright future for ocular drug therapy. It is quite reasonable to envision several novel designs and methods for drug delivery systems to the posterior segment of the eye over the next decade.

REFERENCES

1. Urtti, A., Challenges and obstacles of ocular pharmacokinetics and drug delivery. *Adv Drug Deliv Rev*, 2006. 58(11): p. 1131–5.
2. Multicenter Uveitis Steroid Treatment Trial Research Group et al., Randomized comparison of systemic anti-inflammatory therapy versus fluocinolone acetonide implant for intermediate, posterior, and panuveitis: The multicenter uveitis steroid treatment trial. *Ophthalmology*, 2011. 118(10): p. 1916–26.
3. Sampat, K. M. and S. J. Garg, Complications of intravitreal injections. *Curr Opin Ophthalmol*, 2010. 21(3): p. 178–83.
4. Rifkin, L. and S. Schaal, Factors affecting patients' pain intensity during in office intravitreal injection procedure. *Retina*, 2012. 32(4): p. 696–700.
5. Velez, G. and S. M. Whitcup, New developments in sustained release drug delivery for the treatment of intraocular disease. *Br J Ophthalmol*, 1999. 83(11): p. 1225–9.
6. Gaudana, R. et al., Ocular drug delivery. *AAPS J*, 2010. 12(3): p. 348–60.
7. Klyce, S. D. and C. E. Crosson, Transport processes across the rabbit corneal epithelium: A review. *Curr Eye Res*, 1985. 4(4): p. 323–31.

8. Prausnitz, M. R. and J. S. Noonan, Permeability of cornea, sclera, and conjunctiva: A literature analysis for drug delivery to the eye. *J Pharm Sci*, 1998. 87(12): p. 1479–88.
9. Barar, J., A. R. Javadzadeh, and Y. Omidi, Ocular novel drug delivery: Impacts of membranes and barriers. *Expert Opin Drug Deliv*, 2008. 5(5): p. 567–81.
10. Wang, W. et al., Lipophilicity influence on conjunctival drug penetration in the pigmented rabbit: A comparison with corneal penetration. *Curr Eye Res*, 1991. 10(6): p. 571–9.
11. Saha, P., K. J. Kim, and V. H. Lee, A primary culture model of rabbit conjunctival epithelial cells exhibiting tight barrier properties. *Curr Eye Res*, 1996. 15(12): p. 1163–9.
12. Raghava, S., M. Hammond, and U.B. Kompella, Periocular routes for retinal drug delivery. *Expert Opin Drug Deliv*, 2004. 1(1): p. 99–114.
13. Ahmed, I. and T. F. Patton, Importance of the noncorneal absorption route in topical ophthalmic drug delivery. *Invest Ophthalmol Vis Sci*, 1985. 26(4): p. 584–7.
14. Geroski, D. H. and H. F. Edelhauser, Transscleral drug delivery for posterior segment disease. *Adv Drug Deliv Rev*, 2001. 52(1): p. 37–48.
15. Kim, S. H. et al., Transport barriers in transscleral drug delivery for retinal diseases. *Ophthalmic Res*, 2007. 39(5): p. 244–54.
16. Chalam, K., V. Khetpal, and C. J. Patel, Spectral domain optical coherence tomography documented rapid resolution of pseudophakic cystoid macular edema with topical difluprednate. *Clin Ophthalmol*, 2012. 6: p. 155–8.
17. Ikeda, Y. et al., The clinical efficacy of a topical dorzolamide in the management of cystoid macular edema in patients with retinitis pigmentosa. *Graefes Arch Clin Exp Ophthalmol*, 2012. 250(6): p. 809–14.
18. Breit, S. M. et al., Management of endogenous fungal endophthalmitis with voriconazole and caspofungin. *Am J Ophthalmol*, 2005. 139(1): p. 135–40.
19. George, J. M. et al., Aqueous and vitreous penetration of linezolid and levofloxacin after oral administration. *J Ocul Pharmacol Ther*, 2010. 26(6): p. 579–86.
20. Verbraeken, H. et al., Penetration of gentamicin and ofloxacin in human vitreous after systemic administration. *Graefes Arch Clin Exp Ophthalmol*, 1996. 234 Suppl 1: p. S59–65.
21. Smith, A. et al., Fluoroquinolones: Place in ocular therapy. *Drugs*, 2001. 61(6): p. 747–61.
22. Le Goff, M. M. and P.N. Bishop, Adult vitreous structure and postnatal changes. *Eye (Lond)*, 2008. 22(10): p. 1214–22.
23. Halfter, W. et al., Regulation of eye size by the retinal basement membrane and vitreous body. *Invest Ophthalmol Vis Sci*, 2006. 47(8): p. 3586–94.
24. Sonoda, K. H. et al., The analysis of systemic tolerance elicited by antigen inoculation into the vitreous cavity: Vitreous cavity-associated immune deviation. *Immunology*, 2005. 116(3): p. 390–9.
25. Shui, Y. B. et al., The gel state of the vitreous and ascorbate-dependent oxygen consumption: Relationship to the etiology of nuclear cataracts. *Arch Ophthalmol*, 2009. 127(4): p. 475–82.
26. Mains, J. and C. G. Wilson, The Vitreous Humor As a Barrier to Nanoparticle Distribution. *J Ocul Pharmacol Ther*, 2012.
27. Sebag, J., Ageing of the vitreous. *Eye (Lond)*, 1987. 1 (Pt 2): p. 254–62.
28. Bishop, P. N. et al., Age-related changes on the surface of vitreous collagen fibrils. *Invest Ophthalmol Vis Sci*, 2004. 45(4): p. 1041–6.
29. Regillo, C. D., *Basic and Clinical Science Course Section 12 2009–2010: Retina and Vitreous*. 2009: American Academy of Ophthalmology.
30. Foulds, W. S. et al., Effect of intravitreal hyaluronidase on the clearance of tritiated water from the vitreous to the choroid. *Br J Ophthalmol*, 1985. 69(7): p. 529–32.

31. Missel, P. J., Hydraulic flow and vascular clearance influences on intravitreal drug delivery. *Pharm Res*, 2002. 19(11): p. 1636–47.
32. Stocchino, A., R. Repetto, and C. Cafferata, Eye rotation induced dynamics of a Newtonian fluid within the vitreous cavity: The effect of the chamber shape. *Phys Med Biol*, 2007. 52(7): p. 2021–34.
33. Tan, L. E. et al., Effects of vitreous liquefaction on the intravitreal distribution of sodium fluorescein, fluorescein dextran, and fluorescent microparticles. *Invest Ophthalmol Vis Sci*, 2011. 52(2): p. 1111–8.
34. Kakinoki, M. et al., Effect of vitrectomy on aqueous VEGF concentration and pharmacokinetics of bevacizumab in macaque monkeys. *Invest Ophthalmol Vis Sci*, 2012. 53(9): p. 5877–80.
35. Pflugfelder, S. C. et al., Intravitreal vancomycin. Retinal toxicity, clearance, and interaction with gentamicin. *Arch Ophthalmol*, 1987. 105(6): p. 831–7.
36. Mandell, B. A. et al., Effects of inflammation and surgery on amikacin levels in the vitreous cavity. *Am J Ophthalmol*, 1993. 115(6): p. 770–4.
37. Doft, B. H. et al., Amphotericin clearance in vitrectomized versus nonvitrectomized eyes. *Ophthalmology*, 1985. 92(11): p. 1601–5.
38. Lee, S. S. et al., Vitreous VEGF clearance is increased after vitrectomy. *Invest Ophthalmol Vis Sci*, 2010. 51(4): p. 2135–8.
39. Chin, H. S. et al., Difference in clearance of intravitreal triamcinolone acetonide between vitrectomized and nonvitrectomized eyes. *Retina*, 2005. 25(5): p. 556–60.
40. Chang-Lin, J. E. et al., Pharmacokinetics of a sustained-release dexamethasone intravitreal implant in vitrectomized and nonvitrectomized eyes. *Invest Ophthalmol Vis Sci*, 2011. 52(7): p. 4605–9.
41. Shaikh, A. H. et al., Comparative effectiveness of the dexamethasone intravitreal implant in vitrectomized and non-vitrectomized eyes with macular edema secondary to central retinal vein occlusion. *Ophthalmic Surg Lasers Imaging*, 2012: p. 1–6.
42. Laude, A. et al., Intravitreal therapy for neovascular age-related macular degeneration and inter-individual variations in vitreous pharmacokinetics. *Prog Retin Eye Res*, 2010. 29(6): p. 466–75.
43. Ogura, Y. et al., Integrity of the blood-ocular barrier after intravitreal gas injection. *Retina*, 1989. 9(3): p. 199–202.
44. Falavarjani, K. G., M. Modarres, and H. Nazari, Therapeutic effect of bevacizumab injected into the silicone oil in eyes with neovascular glaucoma after vitrectomy for advanced diabetic retinopathy. *Eye (Lond)*, 2010. 24(4): p. 717–9.
45. Salman, A. G., Intrasilicone bevacizumab injection for iris neovascularization after vitrectomy for proliferative diabetic retinopathy. *Ophthalmic Res*, 2013. 49(1): p. 20–4.
46. Kalvoda, J. et al., Morphometry of surgically removed internal limiting membrane during vitrectomy in diabetic macular edema. *Graefes Arch Clin Exp Ophthalmol*, 2009. 247(10): p. 1307–14.
47. Chang, S., Controversies regarding internal limiting membrane peeling in idiopathic epiretinal membrane and macular hole. *Retina*, 2012. 32 Suppl 2: p. S200–3; discussion S203–4.
48. Lois, N. et al., Internal limiting membrane peeling versus no peeling for idiopathic full-thickness macular hole: A pragmatic randomized controlled trial. *Invest Ophthalmol Vis Sci*, 2011. 52(3): p. 1586–92.
49. Yamakoshi, T. et al., Triamcinolone-assisted removal of internal limiting membrane enhances the effect of vitrectomy for diabetic macular edema. *Ophthalmic Res*, 2009. 41(4): p. 203–9.
50. Pitkanen, L. et al., Neural retina limits the nonviral gene transfer to retinal pigment epithelium in an in vitro bovine eye model. *AAPS J*, 2004. 6(3): p. e25.

51. Koch, S. et al., Gene therapy restores vision and delays degeneration in the CNGB1(-/-) mouse model of retinitis pigmentosa. *Hum Mol Genet*, 2012. 21(20): p. 4486–96.
52. Dalkara, D. et al., Inner limiting membrane barriers to AAV-mediated retinal transduction from the vitreous. *Mol Ther*, 2009. 17(12): p. 2096–102.
53. Heiduschka, P. et al., Penetration of bevacizumab through the retina after intravitreal injection in the monkey. *Invest Ophthalmol Vis Sci*, 2007. 48(6): p. 2814–23.
54. Perez-Olivan, S. et al., Grepafloxacin concentration in ocular tissues after intravenous infusion in rabbits with intraocular inflammation. *Ophthalmic Res*, 2005. 37(6): p. 335–40.
55. Knudsen, L. L. et al., Ocular fluorescein kinetics before and after vitrectomy on swine. *Graefes Arch Clin Exp Ophthalmol*, 2001. 239(11): p. 832–9.
56. Pannicke, T. et al., Ocular inflammation alters swelling and membrane characteristics of rat Muller glial cells. *J Neuroimmunol*, 2005. 161(1–2): p. 145–54.
57. Gaudana, R. et al., Recent perspectives in ocular drug delivery. *Pharm Res*, 2009. 26(5): p. 1197–216.
58. Rawas-Qalaji, M. and C. A. Williams, Advances in ocular drug delivery. *Curr Eye Res*, 2012. 37(5): p. 345–56.
59. Majumdar, S., V. Kansara, and A. K. Mitra, Vitreal pharmacokinetics of dipeptide monoester prodrugs of ganciclovir. *J Ocul Pharmacol Ther*, 2006. 22(4): p. 231–41.
60. Karla, P. K. et al., Molecular evidence and functional expression of a novel drug efflux pump (ABCC2) in human corneal epithelium and rabbit cornea and its role in ocular drug efflux. *Int J Pharm*, 2007. 336(1): p. 12–21.
61. Park, J. et al., Evaluation of coupled convective-diffusive transport of drugs administered by intravitreal injection and controlled release implant. *J Control Release*, 2005. 105(3): p. 279–95.
62. Xu, J. et al., Permeability and diffusion in vitreous humor: Implications for drug delivery. *Pharm Res*, 2000. 17(6): p. 664–9.
63. Gan, I. M. et al., Effect of intravitreal dexamethasone on vitreous vancomycin concentrations in patients with suspected postoperative bacterial endophthalmitis. *Graefes Arch Clin Exp Ophthalmol*, 2005. 243(11): p. 1186–9.
64. Aguilar, H. E. et al., Vancomycin levels after intravitreal injection. Effects of inflammation and surgery. *Retina*, 1995. 15(5): p. 428–32.
65. Bakri, S. J. et al., Pharmacokinetics of intravitreal bevacizumab (Avastin). *Ophthalmology*, 2007. 114(5): p. 855–9.
66. Bakri, S. J. et al., Pharmacokinetics of intravitreal ranibizumab (Lucentis). *Ophthalmology*, 2007. 114(12): p. 2179–82.
67. Sakurai, E. et al., Effect of particle size of polymeric nanospheres on intravitreal kinetics. *Ophthalmic Res*, 2001. 33(1): p. 31–6.
68. Raju, H. B. et al., Investigation of nanoparticles using magnetic resonance imaging after intravitreal injection. *Clin Experiment Ophthalmol*, 2012. 40(1): p. 100–7.
69. Kim, H., S. B. Robinson, and K. G. Csaky, Investigating the movement of intravitreal human serum albumin nanoparticles in the vitreous and retina. *Pharm Res*, 2009. 26(2): p. 329–37.
70. Verma, A. and F. Stellacci, Effect of surface properties on nanoparticle-cell interactions. *Small*, 2010. 6(1): p. 12–21.
71. Choonara, Y. E. et al., A review of implantable intravitreal drug delivery technologies for the treatment of posterior segment eye diseases. *J Pharm Sci*, 2010. 99(5): p. 2219–39.
72. Moritera, T. et al., Microspheres of biodegradable polymers as a drug-delivery system in the vitreous. *Invest Ophthalmol Vis Sci*, 1991. 32(6): p. 1785–90.
73. Ambati, J. et al., Transscleral delivery of bioactive protein to the choroid and retina. *Invest Ophthalmol Vis Sci*, 2000. 41(5): p. 1186–91.

74. Herrero-Vanrell, R. et al., Biodegradable PLGA microspheres loaded with ganciclovir for intraocular administration. Encapsulation technique, in vitro release profiles, and sterilization process. *Pharm Res*, 2000. 17(10): p. 1323–8.
75. Cheng, L. et al., Intravitreal toxicology and duration of efficacy of a novel antiviral lipid prodrug of ganciclovir in liposome formulation. *Invest Ophthalmol Vis Sci*, 2000. 41(6): p. 1523–32.
76. Merodio, M. et al., Ocular disposition and tolerance of ganciclovir-loaded albumin nanoparticles after intravitreal injection in rats. *Biomaterials*, 2002. 23(7): p. 1587–94.
77. Bochot, A., P. Couvreur, and E. Fattal, Intravitreal administration of antisense oligonucleotides: Potential of liposomal delivery. *Prog Retin Eye Res*, 2000. 19(2): p. 131–47.
78. Moritera, T. et al., Biodegradable microspheres containing adriamycin in the treatment of proliferative vitreoretinopathy. *Invest Ophthalmol Vis Sci*, 1992. 33(11): p. 3125–30.
79. Yasukawa, T. et al., Drug delivery systems for vitreoretinal diseases. *Prog Retin Eye Res*, 2004. 23(3): p. 253–81.
80. Shah, S. S. et al., Drug delivery to the posterior segment of the eye for pharmacologic therapy. *Expert Rev Ophthalmol*, 2010. 5(1): p. 75–93.
81. Bourges, J. L. et al., Ocular drug delivery targeting the retina and retinal pigment epithelium using polylactide nanoparticles. *Invest Ophthalmol Vis Sci*, 2003. 44(8): p. 3562–9.
82. Moritera, T. et al., Feasibility of drug targeting to the retinal pigment epithelium with biodegradable microspheres. *Curr Eye Res*, 1994. 13(3): p. 171–6.
83. Kompella, U. B., N. Bandi, and S. P. Ayalasomayajula, Subconjunctival nano- and microparticles sustain retinal delivery of budesonide, a corticosteroid capable of inhibiting VEGF expression. *Invest Ophthalmol Vis Sci*, 2003. 44(3): p. 1192–201.
84. Gomez-Gaete, C. et al., Dexamethasone acetate encapsulation into Trojan particles. *J Control Release*, 2008. 128(1): p. 41–9.
85. Veloso, A. A., Jr. et al., Ganciclovir-loaded polymer microspheres in rabbit eyes inoculated with human cytomegalovirus. *Invest Ophthalmol Vis Sci*, 1997. 38(3): p. 665–75.
86. Barcia, E. et al., Downregulation of endotoxin-induced uveitis by intravitreal injection of polylactic-glycolic acid (PLGA) microspheres loaded with dexamethasone. *Exp Eye Res*, 2009. 89(2): p. 238–45.
87. Bejjani, R. A. et al., Nanoparticles for gene delivery to retinal pigment epithelial cells. *Mol Vis*, 2005. 11: p. 124–32.
88. Aukunuru, J. V., S. P. Ayalasomayajula, and U. B. Kompella, Nanoparticle formulation enhances the delivery and activity of a vascular endothelial growth factor antisense oligonucleotide in human retinal pigment epithelial cells. *J Pharm Pharmacol*, 2003. 55(9): p. 1199–206.
89. Hsu, J., Drug delivery methods for posterior segment disease. *Curr Opin Ophthalmol*, 2007. 18(3): p. 235–9.
90. Wu, W. C. et al., An updated study of the use of bevacizumab in the treatment of patients with prethreshold retinopathy of prematurity in taiwan. *Am J Ophthalmol*, 2013. 155(1): p. 150–8 e1.
91. Park, S. C., D. Su, and C. Tello, Anti-VEGF therapy for the treatment of glaucoma: A focus on ranibizumab and bevacizumab. *Expert Opin Biol Ther*, 2012. 12(12): p. 1641–7.
92. Finger, P. T. and S. K. Mukkamala, Intravitreal anti-VEGF bevacizumab (Avastin) for external beam related radiation retinopathy. *Eur J Ophthalmol*, 2011. 21(4): p. 446–51.
93. Yoreh Barak, M. A. I., Shlomit Schaal, Anti-vascular Endothelial Growth Factor Pharmacotherapy in the Treatment of Subretinal Choroidal Neovascularization, in *US Ophthalmic Review*, 2012. 5(2): p. 107–10.
94. Gragoudas, E. S. et al., Pegaptanib for neovascular age-related macular degeneration. *N Engl J Med*, 2004. 351(27): p. 2805–16.

95. Ho, A. C. et al., Anti-vascular endothelial growth factor pharmacotherapy for diabetic macular edema: A report by the American Academy of Ophthalmology. *Ophthalmology*, 2012. 119(10): p. 2179–88.
96. Rosenfeld, P. J. et al., Ranibizumab for neovascular age-related macular degeneration. *N Engl J Med*, 2006. 355(14): p. 1419–31.
97. Brown, D. M. et al., Ranibizumab versus verteporfin photodynamic therapy for neovascular age-related macular degeneration: Two-year results of the ANCHOR study. *Ophthalmology*, 2009. 116(1): p. 57–65 e5.
98. Brown, D. M. et al., Ranibizumab for macular edema following central retinal vein occlusion: Six-month primary end point results of a phase III study. *Ophthalmology*, 2010. 117(6): p. 1124–33 e1.
99. Nguyen, Q. D. et al., Ranibizumab for diabetic macular edema: Results from 2 phase III randomized trials: RISE and RIDE. *Ophthalmology*, 2012. 119(4): p. 789–801.
100. Arevalo, J. F. et al., Intravitreal bevacizumab for subfoveal choroidal neovascularization in age-related macular degeneration at twenty-four months: The Pan-American Collaborative Retina Study. *Ophthalmology*, 2010. 117(10): p. 1974–81, 1981 e1.
101. Bashshur, Z. F. et al., Intravitreal bevacizumab for treatment of neovascular age-related macular degeneration: The second year of a prospective study. *Am J Ophthalmol*, 2009. 148(1): p. 59–65 e1.
102. Comparison of Age-related Macular Degeneration Treatments Trials Research Group et al., Ranibizumab and bevacizumab for treatment of neovascular age-related macular degeneration: Two-year results. *Ophthalmology*, 2012. 119(7): p. 1388–98.
103. Hung, K. H. et al., Intravitreal bevacizumab (avastin) in the treatment of macular edema associated with perfused retinal vein occlusion. *J Ocul Pharmacol Ther*, 2010. 26(1): p. 85–90.
104. Arevalo, J. F. et al., Intravitreal bevacizumab plus grid laser photocoagulation or intravitreal bevacizumab or grid laser photocoagulation for diffuse diabetic macular edema: Results of the Pan-American Collaborative Retina Study Group at 24 Months. *Retina*, 2013. 33(2): p. 403–13.
105. American Society of Retina Specialists (ASRS), P.a.T. American Society of Retina Specialists (ASRS), Preferences and Trends 2013 1/12/2013]; Available from: http://www.asrs.org/asrs-community/pat-survey/pat-survey-archive.
106. Heier, J. S. et al., Intravitreal aflibercept (VEGF trap-eye) in wet age-related macular degeneration. *Ophthalmology*, 2012. 119(12): p. 2537–48.
107. Do, D. V. et al., One-year outcomes of the DA VINCI Study of VEGF Trap-Eye in eyes with diabetic macular edema. *Ophthalmology*, 2012. 119(8): p. 1658–65.
108. Brown, D. M. et al., Intravitreal Aflibercept Injection for Macular Edema Secondary to Central Retinal Vein Occlusion: 1-Year Results From the Phase 3 COPERNICUS Study. *Am J Ophthalmol*, 2012.
109. Regeneron Pharmaceuticals Inc. Regeneron Announces FDA Approval of EYLEA® (aflibercept) Injection For Macular Edema Following Central Retinal Vein Occlusion. 2012 [cited 2013 2/11/2013]; Available from: http://investor.regeneron.com/release detail.cfm?releaseid=708835.
110. Jermak, C. M. et al., Triamcinolone acetonide in ocular therapeutics. *Surv Ophthalmol*, 2007. 52(5): p. 503–22.
111. McAllister, I. L. et al., Effect of triamcinolone acetonide on vascular endothelial growth factor and occludin levels in branch retinal vein occlusion. *Am J Ophthalmol*, 2009. 147(5): p. 838–46, 846 e1–2.
112. Kiernan, D. F. and W. F. Mieler, Intraocular corticosteroids for posterior segment disease: 2012 update. *Expert Opin Pharmacother*, 2012. 13(12): p. 1679–94.
113. Morse, L. S., S. Modjjtahedi, and Z. Smit-McBride, Use of intravitreal steroids in the clinic. *Retina Today*, 2010 (May/June Supplement).

114. Chang-Lin, J. E. et al., Pharmacokinetics and pharmacodynamics of a sustained-release dexamethasone intravitreal implant. *Invest Ophthalmol Vis Sci*, 2011. 52(1): p. 80–6.
115. Edelman, J. L., D. Lutz, and M. R. Castro, Corticosteroids inhibit VEGF-induced vascular leakage in a rabbit model of blood-retinal and blood-aqueous barrier breakdown. *Exp Eye Res*, 2005. 80(2): p. 249–58.
116. Bakri, S. J. et al., Same-day triple therapy with photodynamic therapy, intravitreal dexamethasone, and bevacizumab in wet age-related macular degeneration. *Retina*, 2009. 29(5): p. 573–8.
117. Saleh, O., A. Kagan Do, Y. Barak, and H. J. Kaplan, Immunomodulatory therapy in noninfectious posterior uveitis. *Retinal Physician*, 2012. 9(September): p. 17–20.
118. Durrani, K. et al., Systemic therapy with conventional and novel immunomodulatory agents for ocular inflammatory disease. *Surv Ophthalmol*, 2011. 56(6): p. 474–510.
119. Taylor, S. R. et al., Intravitreal methotrexate in uveitis. *Ophthalmology*, 2012. 119(4): p. 878–9.
120. Frenkel, S. et al., Intravitreal methotrexate for treating vitreoretinal lymphoma: 10 years of experience. *Br J Ophthalmol*, 2008. 92(3): p. 383–8.
121. Bae, J. H. and S. C. Lee, Effect of intravitreal methotrexate and aqueous humor cytokine levels in refractory retinal vasculitis in Behcet disease. *Retina*, 2012. 32(7): p. 1395–402.
122. Kivela, T., S. Eskelin, and M. Paloheimo, Intravitreal methotrexate for retinoblastoma. *Ophthalmology*, 2011. 118(8): p. 1689, 1689 e1–6.
123. Teoh, S. C., X. Ou, and T. H. Lim, Intravitreal ganciclovir maintenance injection for cytomegalovirus retinitis: Efficacy of a low-volume, intermediate-dose regimen. *Ophthalmology*, 2012. 119(3): p. 588–95.
124. Riddell, J. t., G. M. Comer, and C. A. Kauffman, Treatment of endogenous fungal endophthalmitis: Focus on new antifungal agents. *Clin Infect Dis*, 2011. 52(5): p. 648–53.
125. Group, E. V. S., Results of the Endophthalmitis Vitrectomy Study. A randomized trial of immediate vitrectomy and of intravenous antibiotics for the treatment of postoperative bacterial endophthalmitis. Endophthalmitis Vitrectomy Study Group. *Arch Ophthalmol*, 1995. 113(12): p. 1479–96.
126. Manosroi, J. et al., Secretion of active recombinant human tissue plasminogen activator derivatives in Escherichia coli. *Appl Environ Microbiol*, 2001. 67(6): p. 2657–64.
127. Lewis, H. et al., Tissue plasminogen activator treatment of experimental subretinal hemorrhage. *Am J Ophthalmol*, 1991. 111(2): p. 197–204.
128. Hesse, L. et al., Quantitative effect of intravitreally injected tissue plasminogen activator and gas on subretinal hemorrhage. *Retina*, 2000. 20(5): p. 500–5.
129. Sandhu, S. S., S. Manvikar, and D. H. Steel, Displacement of submacular hemorrhage associated with age-related macular degeneration using vitrectomy and submacular tPA injection followed by intravitreal ranibizumab. *Clin Ophthalmol*, 2010. 4: p. 637–42.
130. Tennant, M. T., J. L. Borrillo, and C. D. Regillo, Management of submacular hemorrhage. *Ophthalmol Clin North Am*, 2002. 15(4): p. 445–52, vi.
131. Goldenberg, M. M., Pharmaceutical approval update. P T, 2012. 37(12): p. 668–708.
132. Sebag, J., Pharmacologic vitreolysis—Premise and promise of the first decade. *Retina*, 2009. 29(7): p. 871–4.
133. Tezel, T. H., L. V. Del Priore, and H. J. Kaplan, Posterior vitreous detachment with dispase. *Retina*, 1998. 18(1): p. 7–15.
134. Stalmans, P. et al., Enzymatic vitreolysis with ocriplasmin for vitreomacular traction and macular holes. *N Engl J Med*, 2012. 367(7): p. 606–15.
135. Hesse, L. et al., Induction of posterior vitreous detachment in rabbits by intravitreal injection of tissue plasminogen activator following cryopexy. *Exp Eye Res*, 2000. 70(1): p. 31–9.

136. (FDA), U.S.F.a.D.A. FDA approves Jetrea for symptomatic vitreomacular adhesion in the eyes. 2012 2/12/13]; Available from: http://www.fda.gov/NewsEvents/Newsroom/PressAnnouncements/ucm324369.htm.
137. Jaffe, G. J. et al., Fluocinolone acetonide implant (Retisert) for noninfectious posterior uveitis: Thirty-four-week results of a multicenter randomized clinical study. *Ophthalmology*, 2006. 113(6): p. 1020–7.
138. Marx, J. L. et al., Use of the ganciclovir implant in the treatment of recurrent cytomegalovirus retinitis. *Arch Ophthalmol*, 1996. 114(7): p. 815–20.
139. Haller, J. A. et al., Dexamethasone intravitreal implant in patients with macular edema related to branch or central retinal vein occlusion twelve-month study results. *Ophthalmology*, 2011. 118(12): p. 2453–60.
140. Kane, F. E. et al., Iluvien: A new sustained delivery technology for posterior eye disease. *Expert Opin Drug Deliv*, 2008. 5(9): p. 1039–46.
141. Eljarrat-Binstock, E., J. Pe'er, and A. J. Domb, New techniques for drug delivery to the posterior eye segment. *Pharm Res*, 2010. 27(4): p. 530–43.
142. Bourges, J. L. et al., Intraocular implants for extended drug delivery: Therapeutic applications. *Adv Drug Deliv Rev*, 2006. 58(11): p. 1182–202.
143. Smith, T. J. et al., Intravitreal sustained-release ganciclovir. *Arch Ophthalmol*, 1992. 110(2): p. 255–8.
144. Anand, R. et al., Control of cytomegalovirus retinitis using sustained release of intraocular ganciclovir. *Arch Ophthalmol*, 1993. 111(2): p. 223–7.
145. Musch, D. C. et al., Treatment of cytomegalovirus retinitis with a sustained-release ganciclovir implant. The Ganciclovir Implant Study Group. *N Engl J Med*, 1997. 337(2): p. 83–90.
146. Sandler, S. F. and J. B. Rosenberg, Ganciclovir for cytomegalovirus retinitis. *Ophthalmology*, 2012. 119(11): p. 2418–9; author reply 2419.
147. Nicholson, B. P. et al., Evaluation of fluocinolone acetonide sustained release implant (Retisert) dissociation during implant removal and exchange surgery. *Am J Ophthalmol*, 2012. 154(6): p. 969–73 e1.
148. Hudson, H. L., Retisert: A step forward in treating chronic noninfectious posterior uveitis. *Retinal Physician*, 2005 (July/August Issue).
149. Jaffe, G. J. et al., Safety and pharmacokinetics of an intraocular fluocinolone acetonide sustained delivery device. *Invest Ophthalmol Vis Sci*, 2000. 41(11): p. 3569–75.
150. Callanan, D. G. et al., Treatment of posterior uveitis with a fluocinolone acetonide implant: Three-year clinical trial results. *Arch Ophthalmol*, 2008. 126(9): p. 1191–201.
151. Ramchandran, R. S. et al., Fluocinolone acetonide sustained drug delivery device for chronic central retinal vein occlusion: 12-month results. *Am J Ophthalmol*, 2008. 146(2): p. 285–91.
152. Schwartz, S. G. and H. W. Flynn, Jr., Fluocinolone acetonide implantable device for diabetic retinopathy. *Curr Pharm Biotechnol*, 2011. 12(3): p. 347–51.
153. Campochiaro, P. A. et al., Sustained delivery fluocinolone acetonide vitreous inserts provide benefit for at least 3 years in patients with diabetic macular edema. *Ophthalmology*, 2012. 119(10): p. 2125–32.
154. Lee, S. S. et al., Biodegradable implants for sustained drug release in the eye. *Pharm Res*, 2010. 27(10): p. 2043–53.
155. Lowder, C. et al., Dexamethasone intravitreal implant for noninfectious intermediate or posterior uveitis. *Arch Ophthalmol*, 2011. 129(5): p. 545–53.
156. Arcinue, C. A., O. M. Ceron, and C. S. Foster, A Comparison Between the Fluocinolone Acetonide (Retisert) and Dexamethasone (Ozurdex) Intravitreal Implants in Uveitis. *J Ocul Pharmacol Ther*, 2013.

157. Okabe, K. et al., Intraocular tissue distribution of betamethasone after intrascleral administration using a non-biodegradable sustained drug delivery device. *Invest Ophthalmol Vis Sci*, 2003. 44(6): p. 2702–7.
158. Felt-Baeyens, O. et al., Biodegradable scleral implants as new triamcinolone acetonide delivery systems. *Int J Pharm*, 2006. 322(1–2): p. 6–12.
159. Eljarrat-Binstock, E. and A. J. Domb, Iontophoresis: A non-invasive ocular drug delivery. *J Control Release*, 2006. 110(3): p. 479–89.
160. Behar-Cohen, F., Current-mediated ocular drug delivery: Iontophoresis and electroporation as drug-delivery systems. *Retinal Physician*, 2012. 9(July/August): p. 52–6.
161. Peppas, N. A. et al., Hydrogels in pharmaceutical formulations. *Eur J Pharm Biopharm*, 2000. 50(1): p. 27–46.
162. Asahara, T. et al., Induction of gene into the rabbit eye by iontophoresis: Preliminary report. *Jpn J Ophthalmol*, 2001. 45(1): p. 31–9.
163. Eljarrat-Binstock, E. et al., Charged nanoparticles delivery to the eye using hydrogel iontophoresis. *J Control Release*, 2008. 126(2): p. 156–61.
164. Yoshizumi, M. O. et al., Experimental transscleral iontophoresis of ciprofloxacin. *J Ocul Pharmacol*, 1991. 7(2): p. 163–7.
165. Lam, T. T. et al., Intravitreal delivery of ganciclovir in rabbits by transscleral iontophoresis. *J Ocul Pharmacol*, 1994. 10(3): p. 571–5.
166. Parkinson, T. M. et al., Tolerance of ocular iontophoresis in healthy volunteers. *J Ocul Pharmacol Ther*, 2003. 19(2): p. 145–51.
167. Tinkov, S. et al., Microbubbles as ultrasound triggered drug carriers. *J Pharm Sci*, 2009. 98(6): p. 1935–61.
168. Price, R. J. and S. Kaul, Contrast ultrasound targeted drug and gene delivery: An update on a new therapeutic modality. *J Cardiovasc Pharmacol Ther*, 2002. 7(3): p. 171–80.
169. Kost, J., K. Leong, and R. Langer, Ultrasound-enhanced polymer degradation and release of incorporated substances. *Proc Natl Acad Sci U S A*, 1989. 86(20): p. 7663–6.
170. Mayer, C. R. et al., Ultrasound targeted microbubble destruction for drug and gene delivery. *Expert Opin Drug Deliv*, 2008. 5(10): p. 1121–38.
171. Lin, C. C. and A. T. Metters, Hydrogels in controlled release formulations: Network design and mathematical modeling. *Adv Drug Deliv Rev*, 2006. 58(12–13): p. 1379–408.
172. Bergeles, C. et al., Steerable intravitreal inserts for drug delivery: In vitro and ex vivo mobility experiments. *Med Image Comput Comput Assist Interv*, 2011. 14(Pt 1): p. 33–40.
173. Sivaraman, K. M. et al., Tailoring the drug loading capacity of polypyrrole films for use in intraocular biomicrorobots. *Conf Proc IEEE Eng Med Biol Soc*, 2010. 2010: p. 4359–62.

20 Drug Delivery in Obstetrics and Gynecology

David Shveiky, Yael Hants, and Sarit Helman

CONTENTS

INTRODUCTION

The field of obstetrics and gynecology is dedicated to women's health. We treat medical and surgical conditions throughout a woman's lifetime. In addition to assisting in the creation of new lives through infertility treatment and obstetrics, we treat serious conditions, such as infections and tumors of the female reproductive tract. Also, attention is being turned into improving women's quality of life. As a population ages, we understand that our role as physicians continues through life in treating these conditions.

In this chapter we discuss different mechanisms of drug delivery in several clinical conditions in obstetrics and gynecology. We chose to present it on a time axis of a modern woman's lifetime. In early reproductive years, many women try to postpone childbirth; drugs and devices used for contraception are discussed. While most women conceive spontaneously, some will need assistance with infertility treatment. Here also, different medications are being used. We will discuss drug delivery in the special interface connecting the fetus and its mother during pregnancy: the placenta. Later in life, usually after childbearing age, other clinical conditions may interfere with quality of life, such as menopausal symptoms and overactive bladder. We will discuss different drug delivery mechanisms in treating these conditions.

TRYING TO POSTPONE CHILDBIRTH

CONTRACEPTION

Decreased fertility is a known characteristic of affluent western societies. This is mainly due to effective family planning measures and a desire to postpone childbearing. Despite that, it was estimated that about 54% of all pregnancies and up to 78% of teenage pregnancies in the United States are unintended.[1] The most common family planning measures include periodic abstinence; withdrawal; barrier methods, such as condom or diaphragm use; spermacides; oral contraceptives ("the pill"); and intrauterine devices (IUDs) as well as male or female permanent sterilization. Hormonal contraceptives depend on adherence to the regimen; despite high theoretical effectiveness of hormonal methods, typical use has less favorable results.[2] The wide gap between theoretical and actual effectiveness is attributed to human factors. Repetitive and correct use by the woman is critical for successful use of the combined oral contraceptives (COCs), progestin-only pills, the patch, the vaginal ring, and injectable contraceptives. In contrast, the effectiveness of other hormonal contraceptives, including the levonorgestrel intrauterine system and subdermal delivery systems, depend less on the patient's compliance.

An "ideal" contraceptive would be characterized by easy use, minimal side effects, excellent tolerability, and high continuation rates.

The search for such a contraceptive led to the introduction of low-dose pills and combined injectables as well as new contraceptive delivery systems, such as the skin patch, hormone-releasing intrauterine system, and intravaginal ring.

Clinical Problems with COCs

- Gastrointestinal malabsorption: Occasionally, a situation may be encountered when an alternative to oral administration of contraceptive pills is required, for example, in the case of simple gastroenteritis or, less commonly, patients receiving chemotherapy (significant nausea and vomiting or mucositis), both of which would prevent oral drug administration. The low-dose oral contraceptives can be administered vaginally.[3]
- Drug interactions: There are many anecdotal reports of patients who have conceived on oral contraceptives while taking antibiotics. There is little evidence, however, that antibiotics that reduce the bacterial flora of the gastrointestinal tract affect oral contraceptive efficacy. Studies indicate that while antibiotics can alter the excretion of contraceptive steroids, plasma levels are unchanged, and there is no evidence of ovulation.[4]
- Liver metabolism: Drugs that stimulate the liver's metabolic capacity, for example, antiepileptic drugs, can affect oral contraceptive efficacy.

  To be cautious, patients on medications that affect liver metabolism should choose an alternative contraceptive.

Intrauterine Device (IUD)

An intrauterine device (IUD) is one of the most effective methods to prevent unwanted pregnancy. It lacks the systemic metabolic effects associated with oral contraceptives, and it provides long-term protection. In Western European countries, 15%–30% of married couples use IUDs as compared to less than 1% in the United States.[2] According to a frequently told urban legend, the first IUD users were desert caravan drivers who used intrauterine stones to protect their female camels from pregnancy.[3] This story, despite being not well documented, is a demonstration of an early use of biomaterials as a contraceptive method. In 1909, Richter reported his experience with a silkworm catgut ring with coils of nickel and bronze. This preliminary IUD was the base of the 1930s Grafenberg ring made of coiled silver and gold.

Modern IUDs include copper IUD and progesterone (or levonorgestrel LNG) eluding IUDs (Mirena™).

The Copper IUD is made of a plastic stem and arm, covered with coiled copper.

The TCu380A IUD (Paragard™) currently approved by the Food and Drug Administration is widely used in the United States. This IUD creates a copper surface area of 300 mm^2 in the vertical arm and 40 mm^2 on each of the transverse arms. The lifespan of this IUD is at least 10 years with reported efficacy even after 12 years of use.

Mechanism of action: The contraceptive action of all IUDs is mainly in the uterine cavity. Ovulation is not affected.

It is currently believed that the mechanism of action for IUDs is the production of an intrauterine environment that is spermicidal. Nonmedicated IUDs depend for contraception on the general reaction of the uterus to a foreign body. It is believed that this reaction, a sterile inflammatory response, produces tissue injury of a minor degree but sufficient enough to be spermicidal.

The copper IUD releases free copper ions and copper salts that have both a biochemical and morphologic impact on the endometrium and also produce alterations in cervical mucus and endometrial secretions.

Copper has many specific actions, including the enhancement of prostaglandin production and the inhibition of various endometrial enzymes. The endometrium becomes decidualized with atrophy of the glands.

The LNG-releasing IUD (Mirena) was approved by the FDA in 2000. This T-shaped device contains a reservoir of LNG on its vertical arm. LNG is a progestin (a synthetic derivative of testosterone that activates progesterone receptors) that is being released at a rate of 20 micrograms per 24 hours by this intrauterine system. It acts directly on the endometrium, interfering with endometrial maturation required for implantation. In addition, it has an inhibitory effect on ovulation as well as an effect on thickening the cervical mucous. The inhibitory effect on endometrial maturation is responsible for a significant reduction in menstrual blood flow and dysmenorrhea (pain with menstruation). Indeed, Mirena was approved by the FDA in 2009 for the indication of heavy menstrual bleeding. It reduces menstrual blood loss by 90% 1 year after insertion.

Efficacy: Both copper IUDs and LNG-releasing IUDs have excellent efficacy with a 5-year pregnancy rate of only 1.4% for the TCu380A IUD and 0.7% for the Mirena.

When comparing efficacy of contraceptive devices, one must take into consideration that there is a difference between "typical failure rate" and "perfect failure rates." For example, if a couple is relying on condoms for contraception, the typical failure rate will be higher than the perfect rate because couples tend, too often, to forget to use the condom. In the case of IUD, the typical failure rate almost equals the perfect failure rate.

Adverse effects of IUD include the risk for an infection and pelvic inflammatory disease, especially around insertion, heavy menstrual bleeding (with the copper IUD) and menstrual abnormalities, uterine perforation at insertion, and septic abortion in the case of pregnancy in the presence of IUD. Despite that, IUD remains a safe and effective contraception method, utilizing biomaterials to increase women's liberty and choice.

Implantable Devices

Norplant is a levonorgestrel (LNG) subdermal implant. It is implanted under the skin in a simple office procedure under local anesthesia and provides contraceptive protection for 5 years. It releases LNG to the bloodstream at a rate of 80 mg/day in the first year, then 30–35 mg/day for another 4 years. The blood levels of this progestin remain stable at 0.25–0.35 ng/dl, sufficient for its contraceptive activity. LNG blocks the LH surge required for ovulation. It also thickens the cervical mucous to prevent transport of sperm to the uterus.

Norplant is a very effective contraceptive agent with only 1% pregnancy over 5 years. It consists of six rods measuring 34 × 2.4 mm; each contains 36 mg of LNG.

It is inserted under the skin at the upper arm, using a special trocar and is removed after 5 years of use.[5]

Spermicides

A spermicidal agent is a material introduced into the vagina before intercourse that immobilizes or kills sperm cells. Spermicides typically contain a surfactant, Nonoxynol 9, that is spermicidal and also provides a mechanical barrier that blocks sperm transfer into the cervical canal.

Spermicides are available in the form of foam, cream, and suppositories. A contraceptive sponge made of polyurethane that contains 1 mg of Nonoxynol 9 was available in the United States until 1994 and is still available in some European countries. The advantage of this device is that it remains effective for 24 hours after insertion and does not need to be inserted right before intercourse.

In addition to its contraceptive activity, Nonoxynol 9 is known to reduce the risk of vaginal infections, such as bacterial vaginosis and other sexually transmitted diseases, including HIV.

Although in vitro studies have demonstrated that spermicides kill or inactivate most STI pathogens, including HIV, it cannot be said that spermicides provide protection against sexually transmitted infections. Spermicides have been reported to prevent HIV serocon-version as well as to have no effect; therefore, spermicides by themselves cannot be counted on for protection against HIV.[3]

Being toxic to some of the normal flora of the vagina, spermicides may increase the risk for colonization of pathogenic bacteria, such as E. coli, thus increasing the risk of urinary tract infection.

Although older studies raised concerns about potential teratogenicity of Nonoxynol 9, several large studies found no greater risk of congenital malformations in embryos conceived despite using this contraceptive agent.

Finally, spermicides are much more effective when used along with mechanical barriers, such as a condom or a diaphragm.[5]

Permanent Tubal Sterilization

Essure®, Conceptus, Inc. After completion of the family, many women seek permanent measure of contraception. Until recently, the most popular permanent contraception was tubal ligation. This operative procedure, usually done laparoscopically, requires general anesthesia and a short hospital stay. New emerging technology, first approved by the FDA in 2002, has revolutionized permanent sterilization. Essure is a transcervical contraceptive device that offers women seeking permanent contraception a nonsurgical, nonhormonal solution. In this office procedure, flexible inserts are inserted into the fallopian tube through the cervix and the uterus via hysteroscopy. The inserts are made of inner polyethylene terephthalate (PET) fibers to inducea tissue fibrotic reaction and are held in place bya flexible stainless steel inner coil and a dynamic outer nickel–titanium alloy coil. PET fibers are used because of their ability to induce tissue ingrowth into medical devices in other procedures, such as arterial grafts. The physician is performing hysteroscopy, identifying the fallopian tube ostia and inserting these coils. During the next 3 months, there is an inflammatory response caused by the invasion of macrophages, fibroblasts, giant cells, and plasma cells, resulting in fibrosis in the fallopian tube around the insert. This natural "plug" prevents sperm from reaching the eggs. After 3 months, hysterosalpingogram is performed with injecting dye through the cervix to ensure complete blockade of both fallopian tubes. A follow-up study of 5 years reported excellent results with zero pregnancies and 99.74% success rate. Failure in this study was due to inability to insert or expulsion of the device. The risks include pain and cramping, uterine perforation, inability to insert, allergic reaction to the materials or vasovagal response (fainting) during insertion. In the first 3 months, there is risk of failure as well as ectopic pregnancy and therefore complementary contraceptive method is recommended.[6]

Adiana® Hologic, Inc. This permanent sterilization method is a combination of controlled thermal damage to the lining of the fallopian tube followed by insertion of a nonabsorbable biocompatible silicone elastomer matrix into the tubal lumen. This procedure is done under hysteroscopic guidance as well. A catheter is inserted into the tubal ostium and delivers radiofrequency (RF) energy for 1 minute, causing a lesion in the fallopian tube lumen. Then, a 3.5-mm silicone matrix is placed in the injured area. During the next few weeks, tubal occlusion is achieved by fibroblast ingrowth into the matrix, which serves as permanent scaffolding and allows for "space-filling." As with the Essure device, tubal occlusion is assessed 3 months after device placement. Adiana matrix is not visible by X-ray but can be seen by ultrasound.[7,8]

TRYING TO CONCEIVE

Delivery of Drugs and Biomaterial Used for Prevention and Treatment of Infertility

Infertility is generally defined as 1 year of unprotected intercourse without conception. This is a common condition, which affects 10%–15% of couples and has important psychological and medical as well as economic and demographic implications. During the last three decades, there was no change in the prevalence of infertility, but the demand for infertility treatment has grown substantially. During this period, new emerging technologies, mainly assisted reproductive technologies (ART), have inflicted a dramatic change in the field of infertility treatments and improved the prognosis for many infertile couples.

In vitro fertilization requires that ovulation occurs in a controlled manner, which facilitates retrieval of the mature eggs. In order to prevent uncontrolled or premature ovulation, drugs are used to "switch off" (downregulate) the pituitary gland. Drugs commonly used for this purpose are gonadotrophin-releasing hormone agonists (GNRHa). These drugs mimic the action of naturally produced gonadotrophin-releasing hormone but are more powerful. GNRHa causes a temporary rapid increase in the production of two other hormones (luteinizing hormone [LH] and follicle-stimulating hormone [FSH]), but after this brief surge, the pituitary gland stops production and ovulation is prevented. Controlled ovulation is then stimulated by use of synthetic gonadotrophins. One of the most common side effects of fertility drugs is ovarian hyperstimulation syndrome (OHSS), which can cause the ovaries to become swollen and painful.

There are several options for GnRHa use. Long courses of GnRHa can be given either as daily low-dose injections or using a single higher-dose longer-acting injection (depot version).

The review of 16 randomized controlled trials found no evidence that depot versus daily GnRHa injections produce different rates of live birth/ongoing pregnancy, clinical pregnancy, or ovarian hyperstimulation syndrome (OHSS). However, substantial differences could not be ruled out.[9,10]

Pelvic Adhesions

About 60% of infertility cases of are attributed to the female factor. One of the most common identifiable female causes of infertility is the presence of pelvic adhesions causing tubal blockage. This factor constitutes up to 23% of female causes. Pelvic adhesions occur in 60%–90% of women following major gynecologic surgery. They cause infertility by preventing the normal transport of the oocyte, sperm, or the fertilized egg through the fallopian tube. Apart from preventing conception, adhesions can cause considerable acute or chronic pelvic and abdominal pain and small bowel obstruction. They may also complicate future surgeries by causing difficulties in access and dissection, prolongation of operative time, increase in blood loss, and predisposition to injury to the bowel or urinary system.[11–13]

Adhesions usually result from the normal peritoneal inflammatory wound-healing response and develop in the first 5 to 7 days after surgery.[14] They are composed of fibrous tissue but also contain blood vessels, fat, and nerves. Several factors involved in mechanisms of adhesion formation include peritoneal injury, the attendant inflammation, imbalance in the plasmin system, and the proximity of injured surfaces.[11]

Hence, preventive strategies have been designed in order to target these steps individually or in combination. Limiting of the injured area, a vital aspect of prophylaxis, is largely a surgical endeavor achieved by meticulous attention to operative technique and tissue handling as well as by using minimally invasive techniques when possible.

However, since injury can only be minimized but not completely abolished, adjuncts to injury limitation techniques are necessary to reduce the risk of adhesions.[11]

Barriers agents are one of the methods traditionally employed for this purpose. These agents represent a direct drug delivery mechanism, where the biomaterial is directly applied over the injured target tissue. Barriers may be either liquid or solid, and the latter can be absorbable or nonabsorbable. Several synthetic barriers with different characteristics are commercially available, but the evidence for the use of these products is not adequate for definite conclusions to be drawn, and further research in this field is warranted.

The following biomaterials are examples of products being used for adhesion prevention.[12,13]

Interceed®, ETHICON Women's Health & Urology, Somerville, NJ, USA

Interceed is an oxidized regenerated cellulose. It was the first degradable barrier used in clinical practice to cover traumatized peritoneum in the pelvis. Interceed can be cut as necessary, requires no suturing, and is completely absorbable. It is applied over raw tissue surfaces at the end of surgery after hemostasis has been achieved. It forms a gelatinous protective coat within 8 hours of application and is broken down into its monosaccharide constituents and absorbed within 2 weeks. In order to evaluate the efficacy of Interceed in the prevention of the development of postsurgical adhesions, many studies have been carried out. A meta-analysis of 11 randomized controlled trials has shown that the barrier is safe and significantly reduces the incidence of the-novo adhesions as well as the reformation of adhesions that were previously lysed as compared with no treatment in laparoscopy. Rather than acting systemically, this product is site-specific. Therefore, its efficacy is limited to surgical situations where raw surfaces can be completely covered with the product, and its benefit is limited to the site of barrier placement. The main disadvantage of this product is that it is not effective unless the entire area is completely hemostatic. The presence of small amounts of blood in the peritoneal cavity or postoperative bleeding results in blood permeating the mesh, fibrin deposition, and, finally, adhesion formation. Therefore, there is no substitute for meticulous hemostasis and good surgical technique and tissue handling to maximize the benefit from this product.

Intercoat®, ETHICON Women's Health & Urology, Somerville, NJ, USA

INTERCOAT is an absorbable adhesion barrier gel used to prevent adhesion formation in women. Its gel formulation makes it easy to apply on surgical areas with precision. It is an effective adjunct to peritoneal surgery and is intended to reduce the incidence, extent, and severity of postoperative adhesions at the surgical site. This barrier is composed of a combination of polyethylene oxide (PEO) and sodium carboxymethyl cellulose (CMC), which is stabilized with calcium and made isotonic through the use of sodium chloride. As oppose to the solid alternative, Intercoat is injected into the peritoneal cavity with a syringe that is provided with the product instead of being placed directly over the exposed area. It allows for application in one single layer to the traumatized tissue, thus creating a temporary barrier during the healing process.

The effectiveness of INTERCOAT was proved in two clinical trials. Using the American Fertility Society (AFS) adnexal score as a measure of the severity of pelvic adhesions, it was shown that application of INTERCOAT improved or did not worsen in 91% of cases as opposed to the 63% in the control group.[15,16]

Seprafilm®, Genzyme, Cambridge, Massachusetts, USA

Seprafilm is an adhesion barrier composed of hyaluronic acid and carboxymethylcellulose. It is a membrane applied to the traumatized tissue during surgery and is absorbed from the peritoneal cavity within 7 days.

Seprafilm is a site-specific agent and acts as a mechanical barrier, preventing opposite tissue surfaces from sticking to each other. Its function lasts for 7 days, and it is completely excreted from the body within 28 days. It is a brittle film that has a tendency to fracture when bent, thus making it hard to use in laparoscopic surgery. In a blind prospective, randomized, multicenter study, the treatment of patients after myomectomy (resection of uterine fibroids) with Seprafilm significantly reduced the extent and area of postoperative adhesions. Potential side effects include induced foreign body reaction, higher incidence of pulmonary emboli and intraperitoneal abscess formation, but these findings were not statistically significant in the relevant trials. High cost is another limitation because, for an effective protection from intestinal obstruction, a mean of 4.5 sheets per patient is required. Seprafilm has been approved by the FDA for use in open surgery in the USA in 2006 (10,11,13).[12,13]

Fallopian Tube Blockage

There are instances where fallopian tube blockage is desired. Hydrosalpinx is a condition when the fallopian tube is dilated and filled with fluid. This condition may be secondary to pelvic inflammatory disease or surgery of the reproductive system and results in a dilated, nonfunctional fallopian tube. Hydrosalpinx appears as an irregular cystic mass in the pelvis, and it may cause no symptoms, but in some instances, it may get infected and cause tubo-ovarian abscess. In cases of severe infertility requiring assisted reproductive technologies, in vitro fertilization (IVF) is commonly performed. During this treatment, after ovarian hyperstimulation with hormones (gonadotropins), eggs are retrieved from the ovaries. These eggs are fertilized in vitro with the male partner's sperm to create embryos. These embryos are then transferred into the uterus for implantation of pregnancy. In the past 2 decades, studies have shown lower implantation rates in women with hydrosalpinx. Further studies demonstrated that the fluid in these dilated fallopian tubes is toxic to the embryos. In addition, this fluid may mechanically wash out the recently transferred embryos from the uterus. Therefore, disconnection of the fallopian tubes from the uterus is desired in these cases. While traditionally performed surgically by tubal ligation or resection of the fallopian tubes, this can be now achieved by using the Essure or Adiana® procedure, previously discussed in detail.[6,7] Thus, using the biomaterials originally designed for contraception, we are able to assist reproduction.

"A TIME TO BE BORN" (ECCLESIASTES 3:2)

Drug Delivery during Pregnancy, Labor, and Delivery

Drug Delivery in Pregnancy

Major adaptations in maternal anatomy, physiology, and metabolism are required for a successful pregnancy. Hormonal changes, initiated before conception, significantly alter maternal physiology and persist through both pregnancy and the initial postpartum period. These adaptations are profound and affect nearly every organ system.[17]

These may alter the exposure to xenobiotics between pregnant and nonpregnant women who receive similar doses with implications for different susceptibility to environmental pollutants or therapeutic agents.[18] Physiological changes occurring during pregnancy can alter exposure to drugs. Examples include increased gastric pH, volume of distribution, glomerular filtration and cardiac output, decreased protein binding, and alteration of cytochrome P450 activity.[19]

Many medical conditions during pregnancy and lactation are best treated initially with nonpharmacologic remedies. Before a drug is administered in pregnancy, the indications should be clear, and the risk-to-benefit ratio should justify drug use.

The evaluation of the risk-to-benefit ratio of drug administration during pregnancy often constitutes a challenge. The deleterious effects of a drug on the fetus depend on 1) the chemical and physical nature of the drug; 2) the extent of fetal exposure based on its pharmacokinetics and primarily placental transfer and drug disposition in the fetus; and 3) most importantly, on the developmental stage at the time of exposure.[20]

Patients should be educated about avenues other than the use of drugs to cope with tension, aches, and pains and viral illnesses during pregnancy. Drugs should be used only when necessary. The risk-to-benefit ratio should justify the use of a particular drug, and the minimal effective dose should be employed. Because long-term effects of drug exposure in utero may not be revealed for many years, caution with regard to the use of any drug in pregnancy is warranted.

A unique topic for pregnancy is the treatment of fetal diseases through the mother; this could be done either by oral treatment or directly through use of intra-amniotic instillation of different drugs.

For example,

- Persistent fetal AF/SVT could cause fetal heart failure. Therefore, drug treatment is offered to most mothers who present with frequent or persistent fetal AF/SVT. Digoxin is the most often used first-line antiarrhythmic drug. Numerous retrospective studies have demonstrated that transplacental therapy with digoxinand other drugs is useful in terminating fetal tachyarrhythmias[21]
- Fetal anemia

  During the last 50 years, intrauterine red cell transfusion (IUT), first via the intraperitoneal route and later directly to fetal circulation, is the standard practice in most centers, with survival rates that exceed 90%, particularly if anemia is diagnosed early and treated in a timely manner[22]
- Lung maturation

  There are a few reports on the use of intra-amniotic instillation of surfactant for women at risk of preterm birth. According to the Cochrane analysis, the use of intra-amniotic surfactant should be limited to randomized controlled trials[23]
- Treatment of fetal hypothyroidism by intra-amniotic injection of levothyroxine (LT4) was reported successful[24–26]

Most medications taken by the mother appear in the milk, but the calculated doses consumed by the nursing infant range from 0.001% to 5% of the standard therapeutic doses and are tolerated by infants without toxicity.

Drug Delivery during Labor and Delivery

Labor and delivery is a natural process that we strive to keep natural. Nevertheless, in the developed world, it is usually done under medical supervision in order to be able to provide medical assistance and to respond promptly to complications during or after labor. As a natural process with minimal intervention, very few biomaterials are used during labor. In this chapter, we present a biomaterial used for induction of labor.

Induction of labor is a medical intervention meant to initiate the process of labor in order to deliver the baby earlier than expected. Indications for induction may include high-risk conditions in pregnancy, such as post-term, gestational hypertensive disorders and preeclampsia, diabetes, and more. Nonmedical and sometimes controversial indications may include planned delivery for patient or doctor's reasons.

Parturition or the initiation of labor is a complex process involving both maternal and fetal signals that are not fully understood. It does include a local secretion of prostaglandins, mainly prostaglandin E2 (PGE2), in the cervix in a process called cervical ripening. Cervical ripening includes softening, some shortening, and initial dilatation of the cervix preparing for labor. Prostaglandins also increase the concentration of receptors to the hormone oxytocin in the uterine muscle to enable effective contractions.

Administration of PG results in dissolution of collagen bundles and an increase in submucosal water content of the cervix. These changes in cervical connective tissue at term are similar to those observed in early labor. PGs are endogenous compounds found in the myometrium, deciduas, and fetal membranes during pregnancy. The chemical precursor is arachidonic acid. PG formulations have been used since they were first synthesized in the laboratory in 1968. Prostaglandin analogs were originally given by intravenous and oral routes. Later, local administration of prostaglandins in the vagina or the endocervix became the route of choice because of fewer side effects and acceptable clinical response. Side effects of all PG formulations and routes may include fever, chills, vomiting, and diarrhea.

Prostaglandins can be given directly into the cervix or vagina. The various administration vehicles (tablet, gel, and timed-release pessary) appear to be equally efficacious. The optimal route, frequency, and dose of prostaglandins of all types and formulations for cervical ripening and labor induction have not been determined. Also, prostaglandin formulations of any kind should be avoided in women with a prior uterine scar, such as a prior cesarean delivery or myomectomy, because their use appears to increase the risk for uterine rupture.

Both prostaglandin E (PGE) 1 and 2 have been found to be effective agents for labor induction.[27]

Dinoprostone, a synthetic PGE2 analog, is currently available in several formulations in the United States and the EU, such as a cervical gel, vaginal tablet, or vaginal insert. The products are administered locally to the reproductive tract: Prepidil® (Pfizer, NY, USA) is a gel formulation that is introduced directly into the cervix; Prostin E2® (Pfizer) gel or tablet is administered intravaginally; Cervidil® (Forest Laboratories, NY, USA)/Propess® (Ferring Controlled Therapeutics, Scotland, UK) are controlled-release formulations that have a retrieval tape, allowing removal of the drug quickly and easily in case of excessive uterine stimulation.[28,29]

There appears to be no difference in clinical outcomes when comparing intravaginal or intracervical PGE2 preparations, and for ease of administration and patient satisfaction, vaginal administration is recommended.

Multiple studies suggest that misoprostol tablets placed vaginally are either superior to or equivalent in efficacy compared with intracervical PGE2 gel.[17]

Misoprostol is a synthetic PGE1 analog and is U.S. FDA-approved in its oral form, Cytotec® (Pfizer), for use as a gastric protectant in patients treated with NSAIDs. However, the oral tablets have been used off-label vaginally, orally, and sublingually since the 1980s for cervical ripening and labor induction. A meta-analysis of 62 studies, completed by Hofmeyr et al., found that a 25-µg tablet placed vaginally every 4 h had similar efficacy to intravaginal or intracervical dinoprostone (PGE2) with regards to delivery time.

Oxytocin is a polypeptide hormone produced in the hypothalamus and secreted from the posterior lobe of the pituitary gland in a pulsatile fashion. It is identical to its synthetic analog, which is among the most potent uterotonic agents known.

Synthetic oxytocin is an effective means of labor induction although oxytocin is more effective in augmenting labor than in inducing labor and even less successful as a cervical ripening agent.

Oxytocin is most often given intravenously. It cannot be given orally because the polypeptide is degraded to small, inactive forms by gastrointestinal enzymes. The plasma half-life is short, estimated at 3 to 6 minutes, and steady-state concentrations are reached within 30 to 40 minutes of initiation or dose change.[17]

Postpartum hemorrhage is an obstetrical emergency; it is a major cause of maternal morbidity and mortality. Uterotonic medications represent the mainstay of drug therapy for postpartum hemorrhage secondary to uterine atony.

Oxytocin is usually given as a first-line agent. Intravenous therapy is the preferred route of administration, but intramuscular and intrauterine dosing is possible.

When oxytocin fails to produce adequate uterine tone, second-line therapy must be initiated. Currently, a variety of other uterotonic agents are available for use.

Misoprostol (Cytotec) is attractive as a second-line agent in that it has multiple administration routes that can be combined; it is a safe, inexpensive, and efficacious uterotonic medication.[30]

Traditionally, it has been used rectally, but the sublingual route allows for lower dosing with higher bioavailability.

Methylergonovine (Methergine) has limited usefulness in the acute postpartum hemorrhage because of its relatively long half-life and its potential for worsening hypertension in patients with preexisting disease.

Prostaglandins are highly effective uterotonic agents. Both natural and synthetic prostaglandin formulations are available. Intramuscular and intrauterine administration of prostaglandin F2α (Hemabate) can be used for control of uterine atony.

IMPROVING QUALITY OF LIFE

The Use of Drugs and Biomaterials in the Treatment of Benign Gynecologic Conditions

Uterine Artery Embolization

Uterine fibroids (leiomyomas, myomas) are the most common tumors of the female genital tract. According to recent studies, the lifetime risk of fibroids in a woman over the age of 45 years is more than 60% with incidence higher in blacks than in whites. Although most fibroids cause no symptoms, fibroid uterus remains a leading cause for hysterectomy. Fibroid tumors are regulated by many factors, mainly ovarian steroids: estrogen and progesterone, growth factors, and angiogenic factors. Black race, nulliparity, obesity, polycystic ovary syndrome, hypertension, and diabetes are associated with increased risk of fibroids. The genetic basis of uterine fibroids has not been elucidated yet; however, recent studies demonstrated the role of key genes in the pathogesesis of these tumors, including genes related to alcohol metabolism and apoptosis. Additionally, a few familial syndromes of uterine fibroids were described, raising the possible role of the gene coding to the protein fumarate hydratase, a Krebs cycle enzyme.

Until recently, the mainstay of treatment of uterine fibroids was hysterectomy. In the past two decades, minimally invasive techniques are being utilized to improve symptoms of fibroids without hysterectomy. One of the most effective uterine sparing methods is uterine fibroid embolization (UFE). This is another example of a direct biomaterial delivery mechanism. Embolization is a minimally invasive means of blocking the arteries that supply blood to the fibroids. In this procedure, a catheter is introduced into the uterine arteries using angiographic techniques. Then, small particles of polyvinyl alcohol (PVA) are injected into the arteries, which results in their blockage. This procedure was first used to reduce blood loss during resection of fibroids (myomectomy). Surprisingly, patients who were treated with UFE prior to myomectomy showed reduction in their fibroid size and improvement of symptoms while awaiting surgery. Recent studies have shown that UFE is a safe and effective uterine sparing treatment for uterine fibroids.

The same technique is being used to treat severe bleeding after childbirth. Despite modern medicine, bleeding remains a leading cause of mortality during labor. When possible to transfer a bleeding patient to the interventional radiology suite, this treatment may save the patient's life without the need for hysterectomy. In conclusion, UFE, with the injection of PVA particles into the uterine arteries is a minimally invasive uterine sparing treatment for fibroids that may also be utilized as a lifesaving measure (21–24).[31–33]

Endometriosis

Endometriosis is a common disease that causes pain symptoms and/or infertility in women in their reproductive years. The disease is characterized by the presence of endometrium-like tissue—glands and stroma—outside the uterine cavity.

The treatment of endometriosis depends on the women's age, desire for pregnancy, the degree of pain, and the impact on the work capacity and the quality of life.

Different treatment options exist for endometriosis, including medical and surgical treatments or a combination of the two approaches.

The most commonly used medications are nonsteroidal anti-inflammatory drugs; GnRH agonists; androgen derivatives, such as danazol; combined oral contraceptive pills; progestogens; and more recently, the levonorgestrel intrauterine system.

Most currently used medical treatments aim at suppressing the stimulatory effect of sex steroids on endometriotic lesions, leading to quiescence and regression of active lesions. Hormonal treatments used in endometriosis achieve their effect either by suppressing the hypothalamo-pituitary-ovarian axis and/or by acting directly on the steroid receptors of the lesions themselves.

All currently used hormonally active treatments have been shown equally effective in the treatment of endometriosis-related pain symptoms, and the choice of treatment depends on the long-term safety and adverse effect profiles.[34]

GnRH Agonists

GnRH agonists exert a continuous, very potent action on the GnRH receptor, leading to an initial short stimulatory—flare-up—effect on the gonadotrophin secretion, followed by a deep suppression of the gonadotrophin secretion. The ovarian function is suppressed in a pseudomenopausal state, resulting in an absence of follicular growth, ovulation, and therefore very low local and circulating estrogen levels. The weaning from the stimulatory effect of estrogens leads to a quiescence of endometriotic lesions during the time of the treatment. The effect is only suppressive and not curative.

The profound hypo-estrogenism related to the use of GHRH agonist leads to frequent adverse effects, such as hot flashes, headaches, vaginal dryness, and so on.

Moreover, a prolonged use has been associated with a loss of bone mineral density.[35]

In the last decade, the option of giving an add-back therapy during the use of GnRH agonist has emerged. Surprisingly, giving a hormonal treatment to normalize estrogen levels (add-back therapy) does not reduce the efficacy of GnRH on pain symptoms while reducing adverse effects.

Progestogens

Progestogens have a therapeutic action in women with endometriosis.

A wide variety of oral and injectable progestogens have been used for the treatment of endometriosis, such as medroxyprogesterone acetate (MPA), desogestrel, dienogest, cyproterone acetate, and so on, as a sole therapy or in combination with estrogens.

Dienogest

A new synthetic oral progestogen for the indication of endometriosis-related pain, dienogest is highly selective for the progesterone receptor and exerts in vivo a strong progestational effect and a moderate antigonadotropic effect. Dienogest does not seem to affect bone mineral density.[36]

Levonorgestrel Intrauterine System

The levonorgestrel intrauterine system (LNG-IUS) releases 20 μg/24 h of levonorgestrel (LNG) for 5 years, resulting in mean plasma concentrations between 100 and 200 pg/ml.[37]

The exact mechanism by which LNG-IUS decreases endometriosis-related symptoms is not known. Since LNG-IUS do not inhibit ovulation in most women and do not induce a hypo-estrogenic state, a direct action of LNG on endometriotic lesions can be hypothesized.

Androgens

Danazol, a synthetic androgen that acts by inducing atrophy of ectopic endometriotic implants and by its antigonadotropic effect, has been widely used for treating endometriosis-related pain symptoms in the 1970s and1980s. The use of this treatment declined thereafter with the introduction of GnRH agonists. Other hormonal treatments with less adverse effects are now available, and danazol is scarcely prescribed nowadays because of the many adverse effects experienced by patients, such as weight gain, lipid profile alterations, acne, hirsutism, alopecia, etc.

IMPROVING QUALITY OF LIFE LATER IN LIFE

The menopausal transition, most commonly occurring around the age of 50, may be associated with symptoms that interfere with women's quality of life. These include hot flashes, mood swings, decreased libido, skin changes, and more. Controversy exists regarding hormone therapy for postmenopausal women. This discussion is beyond the scope of this chapter, and the benefits of this treatment should be weighed against its risks.

Hormone therapy (HT) is used for controlling menopausal symptoms.

HT includes either estrogen alone (estrogen-only HT) or estrogen combined with a progestogen (combined HT). It is used in a variety of formulations and doses, which can be taken orally, vaginally, intranasally, or as an implant, skin patch, cream, or gel. Clinical effects vary according to the type of HT and the duration of its use.[38]

Overactive Bladder

Overactive bladder (OAB) is a collection of symptoms consisting of urinary urgency (the sudden compelling desire to void that is difficult to defer), frequency and nocturia (usually), and incontinence (sometimes).[39]

Approximately 16% of the general population is affected by OAB. There is an age-related increase in the prevalence of OAB, which is more pronounced in women, particularly after the age of 40.

OAB is highly prevalent in the community and is likely significantly underreported and untreated. OAB has a significant effect on quality of life (QOL), particularly if associated with incontinence.[40]

The mainstay of medical therapy for OAB management has been anticholinergic or antimuscarinic medications administered orally.

One of the first anticholinergic medications used for OAB was immediate release (IR) oral oxybutynin (OXY-IR). Although it has the drawbacks of multiple daily dosing and bothersome side effects, it is still being used today.

Subsequent numerous anticholinergic formulations have been developed to improve compliance by reducing the required dosing frequency and minimizing the side effect profile. More recent developments include the use of mirabegron, an oral β-3 adrenergic receptor (β3-AR) agonist, and the injection of botulinum toxin into the bladder walls. These agents avoid anticholinergic side effects by their alternative mechanism of action.[40]

CONCLUSION

In this chapter, we described several drug delivery mechanisms in commonly used medical interventions in obstetrics and gynecology. We demonstrated their use earlier in life, when pregnancy is not desired, in fertility treatment, during pregnancy and delivery, and in the treatment of common gynecologic problems later in life. Knowledge of the different mechanisms to deliver a drug or a biomaterial to its target is essential in improving the ability to tailor the best treatment for the patient.

REFERENCES

1. Henshaw SK. Unintended pregnancy in the United States. *Fam Plan Perspect* 1998;30:24.
2. Halpern V, Lopez LM, Grimes DA, Gallo MF. Strategies to improve adherence and acceptability of hormonal methods of contraception. *Cochrane Database Syst Rev* 2011 Apr;13;(4).
3. Speroff L. Oral Contraception in Speroff L et al. Eds. *Clinical Gynecologic Endocrinology and Infertility*. 8th Edition. Lippincott, Williams and Wilkins.
4. Helms SE BD, Zajic J, Jarjoura D, Brodell RT, Krishnarao I. Oral contraceptive failure rates and oral antibiotics. *J Am Acad Dermatol* 1997;36:705.
5. Stubblefield PG C-ES, Kapp N., ed. *Berek and Novak's Gynecology*, 14th edition. Lippincott, Williams and Wilkins.
6. www.essure.com.
7. www.adiana.com.
8. Palmer SN, Greenberg JA. Transcervical Sterilization: A Comparison of Essure® Permanent Birth Control System and Adiana® Permanent Contraception System. *Rev Obstet Gynecol* 2009;2(2):84–92.
9. Albuquerque LE, Tso LO, Saconato H, Albuquerque MC, Macedo CR. Depot versus daily administration of gonadotrophin-releasing hormone agonist protocols for pituitary down regulation in assisted reproduction cycles. *Cochrane Database Syst Rev* 2013 Jan;31.
10. Farquhar C, Rishworth JR, Brown J, Nelen WL, Marjoribanks J. Assisted reproductive technology: An overview of Cochrane Reviews. *Cochrane Database Syst Rev* 2013.
11. Kumar S, Wong PF, Leaper DJ. Intra-peritoneal prophylactic agents for preventing adhesions and adhesive intestinal obstruction after non-gynaecological abdominal surgery. *Cochrane Database Syst Rev* 2009.
12. Ahmad G, O'Flynn H, Hindocha A, Watson A. Barrier agents for adhesion prevention after gynaecological surgery. *Cochrane Database Syst Rev* 2015;30:4.
13. Pados G, Venetis CA, Almaloglou K, Tarlatzis BC. Prevention of intra-peritoneal adhesions in gynaecological surgery: Theory and evidence. *Reprod Biomed Online*. 2010;21(3):290–303.
14. DeCherney AH, Kumar S. Postoperative peritoneal adhesions in adults and their prevention. https://www.uptodate.com/contents/postoperative-peritoneal-adhesions-in-adults-and-their-prevention. Oct, 2016.
15. Lundorf P, Donnez J, Korell M, Audeburt AJM, Block K, diZerega GS. Clinical evaluation of a viscoelastic gel for reduction of adhesions following a gynaecological surgery by laparoscopy in Europe. *Human Reproduction* 2005;20:514–20.
16. Young P, Johns A, Templeman C, Witz C, Webster B, Ferland R, Diamond M, Block K, diZerega GS. Reduction of postoperative adhesions after laparoscopic gynaecological surgery with Oxiplex/AP Gel: A Pilot Study. *Fertility and Sterility* 2005;845:1450–6.

17. Gabbe SG, ed. *Obstetrics: Normal and problem pregnancies*, 6th edition. Saunders, an imprint of Elsevier Inc.; 2012.
18. Abduljalil K, Furness P, Johnson TN, Rostami-Hodjegan A, Soltani H. Anatomical, physiological and metabolic changes with gestational age during normal pregnancy: A database for parameters required in physiologically based pharmacokinetic modelling. *Clin Pharmacokinet* 2012;51(6):365–96.
19. Colbers A, Greupink R, Burger D. Pharmacological considerations on the use of antiretrovirals in pregnancy. *Curr Opin Infect Dis* 2013 Dec;26(6):575–88.
20. Jacqz-Aigrain E, Koren G. Effects of drugs on the fetus. *Semin Fetal Neonatal Med* 2005 Apr;10(2):139–47.
21. Jaeggi ET, Carvalho JS, De Groot E, Api O, Clur SA, Rammeloo L, McCrindle BW, Ryan G, Manlhiot C, Blom NA. Comparison of transplacental treatment of fetal supraventricular tachyarrhythmias with digoxin, flecainide, and sotalol: Results of a nonrandomized multicenter study. *Circulation* Oct 18, 2011;124(16):1747–54.
22. Papantoniou N, Sifakis S, Antsaklis A. Therapeutic management of fetal anemia: Review of standard practice and alternative treatment options. *A J Perinat Med* 2013 Jan;41(1):71–82.
23. Abdel-Latif ME, Osborn DA, Challis D. Intra-amniotic surfactant for women at risk of preterm birth for preventing respiratory distress in newborn. *Cochrane Database Syst Rev* Jan 20, 2010.
24. Grüner C, Kollert A, Wildt L, Dörr HG, Beinder E, Lang N. Intrauterine treatment of fetal goitrous hypothyroidism controlled by determination of thyroid-stimulating hormone in fetal serum. A case report and review of the literature. *Fetal Diagn Ther* 2001.
25. Yanai N, Shveiky D. Fetal hydrops, associated with maternal propylthiouracil exposure, reversed by intrauterine therapy. *Ultrasound Obstet Gynecol* 2004 Feb;23(2):198–20.
26. Matsumoto T, Miyakoshi K, Saisho Y, Ishii T, Ikenoue S, Kasuga Y, Kadohira I, Sato S, Momotani N, Minegishi K, Yoshimura Y. Antenatal management of recurrent fetal goitrous hyperthyroidism associated with fetal cardiac failure in a pregnant woman with persistent high levels of thyroid-stimulating hormone receptor antibody after ablativetherapy. *Endocr J* 2013;60(12):1281–7.
27. Rayburn WF, Powers BL, Plasse TF, Carr D, Spirito MD. Pharmacokinetics of a controlled-release misoprostol vaginal insert at term. *J Soc Gynecol Investig* 2006;13:112–7.
28. Powers BL, Wing DA, Carr D, Ewer K, Spirito MD. Pharmacokinetic profiles of controlled-release hydrogel polymer vaginal inserts containing misoprostol. *J Clin Pharmacol* 2008;48:26–34.
29. Stephenson ML, Hawkins JS, Powers BL, Wing DA. Misoprostol vaginal insert for induction of labor: A delivery system with accurate dosing and rapid discontinuation. *Womens Health* 2014 Jan;10(1):29–36.
30. Hofmeyr GJ, Gülmezoglu AM, Novikova N, Linder V, Ferreira S, Piaggio G. Misoprostol to prevent and treat postpartum haemorrhage: A systematic review and meta-analysis of maternal deaths and dose-related effects. *Bull World Health Org* 87:666, 2009.
31. Shveiky D, Shushan A, Ben Bassat H, Klein BY, Ben Meir A, Levitzky R, Rojansky N. Acetaldehyde differentially affects the growth of uterine leiomyomata and myometrial cells in tissue cultures. *Fertil Steril* 2009 91:575–9.
32. Goodwin SC, Spies JB. Uterine fibroid embolization. *N Engl J Med* 2009 361:690–7.
33. Bloom AI, Vestandig A, Gielchinsky Y, Nadiari M, Elchalal U. Arterial embolisation for persistent primary postpartum haemorrhage: Before or after hysterectomy? *BJOG* 2004;111:880–4.
34. Streuli I, de Ziegler D, Santulli P, Marcellin L, Borghese B, Batteux F, Chapron C. An update on the pharmacological management of endometriosis. *Expert Opin Pharmacother* 2013 Feb.

35. Sagsveen M, Farmer JE, Prentice A et al. Gonadotrophin-releasing hormone analogues for endometriosis: Bone mineral density. *Cochrane Database Syst Rev* 2003.
36. McCormack PL. Dienogest: A review of its use in the treatment of endometriosis. *Drugs* 2010;70:2073–88.
37. Luukkainen T, Lähteenmäki P, Toivonen J. Levonorgestrel-releasing intrauterine device. *Ann Med* 1990;22:85–90.
38. Marjoribanks J, Farquhar C, Roberts H, Lethaby A. Long term hormone therapy for perimenopausal and postmenopausal women. *Cochrane Database Syst Rev* 2012 Jul 11.
39. Abrams P, Cardozo L, Fall M, Griffiths D, Rosier P, Ulmsten U, van Kerrebroeck P, Victor A, Wein A. Standardization Sub-Committee of the International Continence Society. The standardization of terminology in lower urinary tract function: Report from the standardization sub-committee of the International Continence Society. *Urology* 2003;61(1):37–49.
40. Jayarajan J, Radomski SB. Pharmacotherapy of overactive bladder in adults: A review of efficacy, tolerability, and quality of life. *Res Rep Urol* 2013 Dec 6;6:1–16.

21 Drug Delivery Systems
A Regulatory Perspective

Pablo Gurman, Noel M. Elman, and Yitzhak Rosen

CONTENTS

The views and conclusions expressed in this work are those of the authors and do not necessarily represent those of or imply endorsement from the Food and Drug Administration.

INTRODUCTION

During the last decades, a vast number of drugs have entered the market, producing revolutionary changes in health care, improving the quality of life of millions of people worldwide. It was realized that as important as having the appropriate drug for a specific application was to administer the drug effectively. For example, many drugs cannot be administered by the oral route because they are enzymatically degraded in the gastro-intestinal tract, or they are too insoluble in water to be administered intravenously. In addition, because many drugs suffer from broad biodistribution inside the human body and the fact that most drug receptors are located in more than one tissue, unspecific interaction of drugs with healthy tissues is a common event, resulting in unwanted side effects. Therefore, in order to circumvent these issues and achieve the desired clinical effect with a particular selected drug, there is a critical need for a system capable of protecting the drug against the harsh environment of the human body, controlling drug distribution across the tissues, transporting the drug to the biophase, and achieving selective binding of the drug molecules to their receptors, which ultimately will result in a pharmacologic response. The "magic bullet" concept, adopted by Paul Erlich 200 years ago is becoming a reality with the help of technological advances in the fields of pharmaceutical technology, computer-aided rational drug design, molecular biology, genetic engineering, and in the last years, micro- and nanotechnology. All these advances led to the development of new field known as drug delivery systems (DDS) [1].

What Are Drug Delivery Systems? Why Drug Delivery Systems?

According to Jain [2], a drug delivery system (DDS) is defined as a "formulation or a device that enables the introduction of a therapeutic substance in the human body and improves its efficacy and safety by controlling the rate, time, and place of release of drugs in the body."

There are a number of reasons why the drug delivery field has attracted so much attention from both academia and the industry in recent years, specifically:

1. Drug delivery systems could diversify the portfolio of a company more easily than developing a new drug. This is because, whereas for a new

molecular entity there is only a potential single product, for a DDS multiple combinations can be developed between the DDS and different drugs.
2. Proteins and peptides are among the fastest growing markets in the pharmaceutical industry; however, they require administration for routes other than oral because of the enzymatic and the acidic environment existing in the gut, leading to their degradation. DDS could provide an attractive solution by allowing administration of peptides and proteins by the oral route, protecting them against degradation.
3. Drug delivery systems using new technologies, such as nanotechnology, could extend the time of patent exclusivity. This is because "new nanoformulations" of existing old drugs might be patentable [3].
4. Drug delivery systems may allow the use of drugs otherwise prohibitive because their potential toxicity, for example, by transporting the drug to specific sites of the human body, thus avoiding the interaction of the drug with healthy tissues that could otherwise lead to toxic side effects in that tissue (recycled drugs) [2].

Several different types of DDS have been developed, varying substantially according to the route of administration, site of implantation (for implantable DDS), the characteristics of the drug being used (therapeutic index, drug solubility in water, etc.) mechanism of release (pulsatile vs. continuous or both), materials utilized in their construction (polymer, ceramic, metal, or a combination of them), size (macro implants vs. micro implants, microparticles vs. nanoparticles), geometry (spherical, tubular, hexagonal), architecture (unimodular vs. multimodular, mobile parts vs. no mobile parts), and whether they are biodegradable or not, among other critical features.

As stated above, due to the enormous number of DDS being developed, their complexity and heterogeneity makes it impossible to overview all existing DDS in a single chapter. Instead, a brief description of the routes of administration and some of the DDS used for each route are described. This description is followed by an introduction to the Food and Drug Administration, the main federal agency responsible for the regulation of DDS in the United Staes. The chapter describes the FDA's origin and its organization, followed by a description of some of the standards that have been either adopted or developed to address critical technical issues in DDS. The chapter continues with an overview of the FDA regulatory pathways involved in the regulation of DDS and a brief overview on micro- and nanotechnologiesm which are predicted to play a critical role in the future of DDS. Finally, the ethical implications involved in FDA regulation are briefly discussed.

DRUG DELIVERY SYSTEMS: ROUTES OF ADMINISTRATION

One of the most important issues in drug therapy is the route of administration that determines the onset of action of the drug and some side effects that are specifically related to each route. Several routes of administration are available in the human body with an amazing repertoire of DDS developed for each one of them. Every route of administration has unique requirements that are reflected in the design of the DDS, including form factor, materials, and controlled release mechanisms. A brief description of the main routes of administration is detailed below.

Oral Route

Ninety percent of all medicines use the oral route. The oral route is preferred by the patients, since it is easy, painless, and does not require any training by the patient. However, because of the anatomical and physiological barriers existing in the gastrointestinal tract, it becomes difficult for some drugs to arrive to the site of action intact (the biophase). To address this issue, a number of DDS have been developed.

A first classification of DDS is based on the different timing/rate of release, dividing oral DDS into immediate-release and modified-release DDS. Among modified-release DDS, there are extended-release products (such as osmotic DDS, known as gastrointestinal therapeutic systems [GITS]), delayed-released products (such as enteric coated tablets), targeted-release products, and orally disintegrating tablets. In addition to modifying the release kinetics profile, improving the dissolution and absorption rate in the intestine have been key issues in DDS developers. In this regard, micro- and nanosizing techniques, such as wet milling and high-pressure homogenization, are some of the tools developed to improve drug dissolution and absorption. Ultimately, all these DDS technologies are designed to overcome the anatomical and physiological barriers presented by the gastrointestinal tract (GI), including acidity (Ph), GI motility, mucus, and bubbles, and to allow an optimal dissolution, diffusion, and absorption needed for the drug to reach the site of action [4]. In relation to the latter, the drug has to be absorbed in the right place, at the right time, and to the right extent. Because failure to accomplish these objectives could pose a risk for the patient, regulations exist to comply with standards for DDS developed for the oral route. One of the important parameters to evaluate the safety of DDS for the oral route is bioavailability. Bioavailability refers to the percentage of administered drug that reaches the systemic circulation and is used by regulatory agencies to compare two different products using the same active principle (chemically equivalent). When two different formulations containing the same active principle have the same bioavailability, the products are said to be bioequivalent. This is an important issue for generic drug manufacturers. It is also critical for DDS manufacturers that want to avoid regulatory delays by taking advantage of existing FDA-approved drugs [5].

Parenteral Route

The parenteral route is the fastest route to achieve therapeutic concentrations of a drug and thus is the favorite in the management of emergencies. In addition, the parenteral route allows the administration of a drug to unconscious patients and the use of drugs that are poorly absorbed in the GI tract (low bioavailability). On the other hand, the parenteral route could also present serious risks associated with its use since the drug immediately reaches systemic circulation. The parenteral route includes intravenous, intramuscular, and subcutaneous [6].

Existing DDS for the parenteral route includes catheters, prefilled syringes, auto injectors with cartridges, and syringes with ampules. Pen injectors and prefilled syringes became a very popular DDS for the parenteral route due to their ease of use, self-administration, safety, and portability. Prefilled devices have reached many disease areas, including diabetes management, migraine, multiple sclerosis, rheumatoid arthritis, and infertility, among other clinical conditions. These DDS need to be highly regulated in terms of many of their features, including drug shelf-life inside the injector (for prefilled devices), biocompatibility of the container, and performance of the material, among others [2,7].

Transdermal Route

Transdermal drug delivery is a growing segment of the DDS market. The transdermal route allows the avoidance of first-pass metabolism by the liver and is a convenient route for the patient. Transdermal DDD have evolved rapidly as they incorporated new mechanisms to enhance permeation across the skin. Among these permeation enhancers, it is worth mentioning iontoporetic and sonophoretic enhancers. Furthermore, microfabrication technologies allowed the incorporation of microneedle array patches that penetrate the skin in a painless manner. The degree in which the drug penetrates the skin or mucosa determines the amount of drug that is absorbed into general circulation. Some of the issues that have called for regulation of transdermal patches are the amount of drug present following the intended use, since it could pose a danger for children who may be in contact with the product [2,8].

Pulmonary Route

Pulmonary drug delivery systems involve the use of the inhalation route of substances for the treatment of a variety of diseases involving the respiratory tract, lungs, or for systemic diseases where the pulmonary route could provide an advantage over other routes of administration. Examples of pharmacotherapies using pulmonary delivery systems include the use of beta adrenergic drugs and corticoids for the management of asthma/chronic obstructive pulmonary disease (COPD), vaccines for influenza management, chemotherapeutic drugs for lung cancer treatment, and immunosuppressive agents for lung transplantation. For the pulmonary route, several DDS have been developed, including dry powder inhalers (DPI) where the drug in powder form is aerosolized by means passive (patient inhalation) or active (compressed gas, loaded spring, electric energy provided by a battery). It is important to notice that in many of these devices the innovation relies both in the drug formulation and the device itself [2,9].

Devices for pulmonary delivery are subject to several standards and regulatory assessment. Some examples include a full description of the mechanism of actuation used to create the aerosol (pneumatic, ultrasonic), description of the components of the device, in vitro and in vivo testing, characterization of the aerosol plume, including particle size distribution, among others.

Nasal Route

The nasal route could be used for topical administration of drugs, including decongestants, saline, and corticoids for the treatment of some of the most common disorders, such as chronic rinosinusitis. The nasal cavity and nasal mucosae also provide a high surface area for absorption, allowing the drug to get access to the systemic circulation for the treatment of systemic diseases. In addition, the existence of the olfactory epithelia in the nasal cavity allows the use of delivery systems for the management of brain diseases.

Spray pumps are a class of nasal delivery systems. These devices are regulated in terms of spray weight, plume geometry (allowing comparison of the same spray product among different manufacturers or a change on an existing spray product), and particle size distribution among other critical parameters. Another interesting nasal delivery system is the recently developed bidirectional delivery device, where the delivery occurs during exhalation avoiding the entrance of the drug to the lungs [2,10].

Intraosseous Route

Intraoseus delivery constitutes an alternative to the intravenous route, and it is used when peripheral access is not available for administration of drugs during emergency situations. From a regulatory standpoint, some of the information on the product that should be submitted for regulatory approval include, but is not limited to: device design, type of needle, site of injection, force or pressure needed, and depth of needle insertion. An example of DDS developed for this route is the "injection gun" [11].

Ocular Route

The ocular route favors the local administration of drugs for the treatment of eye disorders, such as glaucoma, macular degeneration, diabetic retinopathy, and others. Several types of delivery devices have been developed to be implanted in different regions of the eyeball to address diseases of the anterior chamber or posterior chamber of the eye. Examples of DDS developed for the eye route include eye droplets, such as the drug timolol for the treatment of glaucoma; passive implants for the posterior chamber containing corticoids for the management of uveitis; and an active implant under investigation consisting of an electrochemically driven micropump implanted trans-sclerally for the management of various eye disorders [12].

Intravaginal Route

The intravaginal route allows for the treatment of local diseases, such as fungal and bacterial infections, and the use of contraceptive drugs to prevent conception. In addition, because of the large surface area and rich blood supply provided by the vaginal mucosa, a number of DDS for the treatment of systemic disorders have been developed. Examples of local DDS include contraceptive DDS containing the spermicide Nonoxynol 9. In the case of systemic diseases, a remarkable example is the formulation of antiretroviral drugs in gel form for the management of HIV infection. Intravaginal delivery systems have been developed in a variety of formulations, including gels, creams, intravaginal rings, pessaries, suppositories, and tablets. Novel approaches in DDS for the vagina have incorporated mucoadhesive molecules to increase the residence time of the drug in the vagina. The particular use of one delivery system over another would depend on different issues, including drug properties, clinical application, and user acceptance. Due to the enormous implications of HIV in public health, regulatory guidelines for the development of vaginal microbicides for the prevention of HIV infection have been developed [13–15].

Central Nervous System (CNS) Route

The brain is one of the organs that are highly protected from the entrance of foreign substances, including drugs, by the blood–brain barrier (BBB). In order to circumvent the BBB, several approaches have been investigated, including intracerebroventricular delivery systems and intrathecal delivery systems. In these DDS, the drug is delivered into the cerebrospinal fluid by passing the blood–brain barrier. Another approach to overcome the BBB is direct implantation of a DDS in the brain. An example of the latter is a DDS available in the market containing the chemotherapeutic drug carmustine for the treatment of glioblastoma, an aggressive type of brain cancer. From a technical standpoint, both approaches differ significantly; while intrathecal catheter DDS utilize a micropump to control the infusion rate of the drug, the brain implant consists of a polymer implant that passively releases the drug at constant rate. In addition to measuring drug plasma concentrations, monitoring drug concentration in the cerebrospinal fluid represents an additional regulatory requirement for this route [16].

FDA APPROACHES FOR REGULATION OF DDS

FDA: An Overview

The Food and Drug Administration is responsible for regulation of medical products, including DDS, in the United States. In the following, a description of the FDA history and organization will be provided.

Brief History of FDA

The Food and Drug Administration (FDA) is a federal agency with the mission of "ensuring the safety, efficacy, and security of human and veterinary drugs, biological products, medical devices, food supply, cosmetics, and products that emit radiation" (www.fda.gov). The history of the FDA dates back to the Food and Drug Act that was launched in 1906 to monitor counterfeiting of food and medicines. In 1938, after a tragic accident where more than 100 patients died as a result of the presence of diethylenglycol in a sulfonamide product, a comprehensive law called the Federal Food and Drug Cosmetic Act was passed to enforce the safety of foods, drugs, and cosmetics. With the tragedy of thalidomide in Europe (in the United States the drug had not been approved, and therefore, no cases were reported) in 1962, which caused many pregnant women to give birth to newborns with deformities (such as absence of arms and heart defects), a new law known as the Kefauver-Harris Drug Amendments Act was approved to strengthen the power of the FDA to monitor drug safety in United States. In 1976 the Medical Device Amendment Act became the first medical device regulation in the United States. This amendment called for quality control procedures and registering of manufacturers of medical devices with the FDA. In 1990, the safe Medical Device Act required post-marketing surveillance of medical devices. In 1997, the Food and Drug Administration Act was approved, strengthening the FDA commitment to protect public health. In 2002, the Medical Device User Fee and Modernization and the Office of Combination Products (OCP) were created [17–19].

FDA Organization

The FDA is divided in several centers: the Center for Biological Research (CBR), the Center for Drugs and Evaluation Research (CDER), the Center for Food Safety and Applied Nutrition (CFSAN), the Center for Tobacco Products (CTP), the Center for Veterinary Medicine (CVM), the Center for Medical Devices and Radiological Health (CDRH), the National Center for Toxicological Research (NCTR), the Office of Regulatory Affairs (ORA), and the Office of the Commissioner. A brief description of each center is detailed below:

1. Center for Biologics and Evaluation Research (CBER) is responsible for the regulation of products, such as gene therapy, blood and blood components, vaccines, tissues (such as biological heart valves), and tissue engineering products among others. FDA supervises product and manufacturing establishment inspections, licensing, and safety of blood supplies (blood and blood components), and post-marketing surveillance of biological products.
2. Center for Drugs and Evaluation Research (CDER) is in charge of assessing the safety and effectiveness of drugs.
3. Center for Food Safety and Applied Nutrition (CFSAN) takes regulatory action on the labeling and safety of food and cosmetics.
4. Center for Tobacco Products (CTP) is responsible for surveillance of tobacco products and their manufacturing.
5. Center for Veterinary Medicine (CVM) assesses the safety and effectiveness of animal food, drugs, and devices.
6. Center for Medical Devices and Radiological Health (CDRH) supervises medical devices, including premarket approval of new devices, manufacturing and performance standards, tracking reports of device malfunctioning, and serious adverse reactions.
7. National Center for Toxicological Research (NCTR) plays a critical role in assessing the safety of new products.
8. Office of Regulatory Affairs (ORA): Among other relevant tasks, the ORA is responsible for FDA inspections of manufacturer's facilities and products and the control of imported products.
9. Office of the Commissioner is responsible for ensuring the FDA's mission [17,18].

FDA AND STANDARDS

Voluntary Standards

A standard could be defined as "a document that provides requirements, specifications, guidelines, or characteristics that can be used consistently to ensure that materials, products, processes, and services are fit for their purpose." Standards are redacted by experts on the field through voluntary standard organizations. Two main standard organizations are the International Standard Organization (ISO) and ASTM international (formerly known as The American Society for Testing and Materials). Voluntary standard organizations are important because (a) setting standards for every product becomes prohibitively expensive for federal agencies and (b) they allow the industry to adopt the standard that better fulfills its needs. Because they exhibit a competitive advantage, standards are many times adopted by industry. In some cases, standards are adopted by regulatory agencies and become mandatory. In some other cases, standards are submitted by the manufacturer as a replacement for other requisitions that would otherwise increase the costs and delay of the regulatory process. Because of the hazards that might accompany the malfunctioning of a DDS, several standards covering materials performance, device performance, and biocompatibility have been developed to ensure the safety and effectiveness of DDS.

International Standard Organization (ISO)

The International Standard Organization (ISO) was founded in 1947. To date the ISO has written more than 19,500 standards. The ISO is divided into several committees, each of them dedicated to writing guidance documents in a specific field, which become standards after being approved by a majority of the members of that committee. Some examples of ISO committees focused on issues related to DDS are ISOTC194 (which focuses on the biological evaluation of medical devices) and the ISOTC229 WG3 (nanotechnologies in health). Standards related to DDS currently in use are the ISO10993, for the evaluation of biocompatibility of medical devices, and ISO 13485, a quality standard for medical devices. Other standards related to DDS are listed in Table 21.1 [20].

ASTM

ASTM international (formerly known as the American Society for Testing and Materials) develops standards for procedures related to classification and testing of materials. The ASTM has developed several standard specifications and standard terminology for a wide variety of materials used for DDS, which were later adopted by the FDA. A list describing some of the ASTM standards used for DDS are listed in Table 21.1 [21].

TABLE 21.1
ISO and ASTM Standards Related to DDS

Standard	Organization	Comments	References
ASTM D4775/ D4775M-09	ASTM	Standard Specification for Identification and Configuration of Prefilled Syringes and Delivery Systems for Drugs	[21]
ISO11608/2000	ISO	Pen injectors for medical use	[20]
ISO 10993	ISO	A number of battery test to evaluate biocompatibility on medical implants (e.g., implantable micropumps, implantable microchips)	[20]
ISO 21649/2006	ISO	A standard related to Needle free injectors for medical use	[20]
ISO 20072-2009	ISO	Aerosol drug delivery design verification and requirement test and methods	[20]
ISO [12417:2011	ISO	This standard was developed in the assessment of combinatory products where one component is a catheter or guidewire and the other component is drug that coats the catheter. Delivery pumps or delivery catheters are not covered in this standard	[20]
ISO 27427/2010	ISO	A standard developed to assess Anesthetic and respiratory equipment	[20]

MANDATORY STANDARDS

The FDA enforces the compliance with regulations set forth in the Code of Federal Regulations (CFR). The CFR is a list with the rules compiled by all the federal agencies of the U.S. government. In some cases, the FDA could enforce compliance with standards developed by voluntary organizations. In this case these standards become "mandatory." For this purpose, the FDA has created the Standard Management Staff (SMS) within the CDRH. The SMS is responsible for the recognition of standards related to medical devices developed by the voluntary standard organizations. The SMS has developed a database with the FDA-recognized standards that assist manufacturers to keep FDA compliance. Of particular interest in medical products are a set of standards known as Good Manufacturing Practices (GMP), Good Laboratory Practices (GLP), and Good Clinical Practices (GCP). GMP, GLP, and GCP comprise a set of regulations agreed by the International Conferences on Harmonization (ICH), between Europe, Japan, and the United States to define guidelines for conducting biomedical research to ensure the quality, integrity, and ethical behavior during the development, laboratory testing, and clinical evaluation of medical products [22,23].

Good manufacturing practices (GMP) are a production and testing practice to ensure product quality. The FDA has adopted GMP to ensure that medical product manufacturing is safe. In order to enforce compliance with GMP, the FDA conducts inspections at the manufacturer site where several features of the manufacturing process are reviewed, including manufacturing processes, records, and personnel training, among other requirements. Should a violation of GMP be detected, the FDA can detain the production of the medical product for up to 30 days. For DDS (most of them are a combination between a drug and a device), specific GMPc regulation applies for each component. For drugs, FDA enforces compliance with GMPc whereas for devices FDA enforces compliance with the Quality System Regulation (QSReg). If the drug and device are manufactured separately, the drug should comply with GMPc while the device should comply with QSReg. If the drug and device are manufactured as a single entity or copackaged, both sets of regulations (GMP and QSReg) should apply for the product. This is because, although GMP and QSReg share in common many features, (management organization, record keeping) there are specific requirements that apply for each one.

Good Laboratory Practices (GLP) are standards developed to ensure the validation of the data generated during preclinical studies (in vitro studies, animal testing) of medical products. FDA-GLP inspections within a laboratory will supervise organization and personnel, facilities, equipment, records and reports, and protocols for conducting a nonclinical laboratory study.

Good Clinical Practices (GCP) ensure that the scientific procedures, organization, and ethical principles governing the development of a clinical trial are followed according to the highest standards set forth by the International Conference on Harmonization (ICH). GCP contains a number of topics, including ethical considerations and technical issues, such as how a clinical protocol must be written; responsibilities of the principal investigator during a clinical study; quality assurance of the clinical study; and monitoring the clinical study among other important issues. The interested reader is referred to the references [18,24] for more information about GMP, GLP, and GCP.

FDA: REGULATORY PATHWAYS FOR DDS

Combination Products

Because DDS systems are made of more than one component, including a drug, a device, or a biologic, they enter into the category of combination products. Combination products could be defined as "therapeutic and diagnostic products that combine drugs, devices, and/or biological products" and are first reviewed by the Office of Combination Products (OCP). The OCP was created in 2002 as a stipulation of the Medical Device User Fee and Modernization Act of 2002 (MDUFMA). The office addresses the regulatory gap existing for the increasing number of products made of more than one technology, such as drug-eluting stents, drug-delivery polymer scaffolds, antibiotic bone cements, and others. The OCP has a jurisdictional and classification authority to determine which center will be responsible for reviewing a combination product. This is accomplished by defining which is the primary mode of action of the product. The primary mode of action of a combination product is the one in which the product exerts its intended therapeutic effect. It is, however, the OCP that dictates the jurisdictional authority over a combination product. It is also possible that a manufacturer of a DDS presents a request for designation (RFD). A RFD involves the submission of a document from a manufacturer to the OCP to identify which is the primary mode of action of the DDS and select a center for review accordingly. The decision process takes 60 days, after which the manufacturer is notified of which office center will be responsible for the evaluation of the product. Most DDS depend on the drug to produce the intended therapeutic effect and thus fall under the jurisdiction of the CDER. However, some DDS fall under the category of devices (e.g., a drug-eluting stent) and are therefore designated for review to the CDRH [25].

FDA: CLINICAL DEVELOPMENT

IND AND IDE

Once the OCP has established which office will have jurisdictional authority on the DDS, the manufacturer of a DDS is ready to submit either an Investigational New Drug (IND) through the CDER (if the OCP determines that the primary mode of action depends on the drug or a biologic) or an Investigational Device Exemption (IDE) through the CDRH (if the OCP determines that the primary mode of action is based on the device) in order to start the clinical investigation of the DDS. An IND is a document that contains information on animal pharmacology and toxicology, manufacturing information, and the clinical protocol for the proposed clinical trial. The IDE is required in most cases for high-risk devices. Some of the requirements for an IDE application include report of prior investigations (laboratory, animal, clinical), the investigational plan, information on the manufacturing, packaging, storage, and labeling of the devices, and informed consent forms, among others.

DRUGS AND MEDICAL DEVICES CLINICAL TRIALS

The clinical investigation of a medical product, such as a DDS, involves a controlled experiment in a small population of human subjects that represents the entire population (a "clinical trial") to assess whether the medical product is safe and effective to be commercialized. Clinical trials are required when the data collected through preclinical studies and laboratory studies do not conform to the level of safety and effectiveness required by the FDA to approve the marketing and commercialization of a medical product. FDA guidelines assist manufacturers in classifying which medical products will require further clinical studies. Furthermore, the manufacturer is advised to consult to the FDA in the early stages of development for which regulatory pathways and requirements apply for the medical product.

As described above, clinical development starts soon after an IND or IDE has been approved. Clinical trials involve a number of phases in which the safety and effectiveness of a medical product is evaluated in humans. For DDS considered devices, the clinical development includes a biocompatibility phase (analogue to Phase I in drug clinical trials), a feasibility phase trial (equivalent to Phase II drug trials), and a larger trial known as pivotal studies (usually multicenter studies) to assess the safety and effectiveness of the device against the current standard. A premarket approval (PMA) or premarket notification (known as 510K) should be submitted in order to obtain FDA clearance for commercialization. After the medical devices have obtained clearance for commercialization, post-marketing surveillance should be conducted to assess the safety of the device in the general population. Post-marketing surveillance involves the detection of potential adverse effects, failures, or threats that could recall the device or even necessitate its withdrawal from the market. In addition, post-marketing surveillance studies and post-approval studies might be required by the FDA from the manufacturer.

For DDS considered drugs, clinical development includes Phase I (pharmacokinetic studies), Phase IIA and IIB (effectiveness studies), and Phase III (comparative efficacy studies), followed by premarket approval (known as New Drug Application or NDA) and post-market surveillance (Phase IV).

Many manufacturers take advantage of existing drugs for development of new DDS in order to shorten the time for regulatory approval ("generics"). A brief description of the concepts of bioavailability and bioequivalence is provided below [26–28].

Pharmacokinetics: Bioavailability and Bioequivalence

Before a drug can exert its biological effect, it has to reach the site of action (biophase) where it binds to its target (receptor), inducing a biological response. This is achieved after the drug has been administered, absorbed, and distributed throughout the body. After the drug has reached the target (and sometimes even before it does), it suffers from metabolic transformation by several mechanisms (the most important occurs in the liver by a family of enzymes known as CYP450) to a product that is then easier to remove from the body by renal excretion or other routes of elimination. This sequence of processes is known as absorption, distribution, metabolism, and excretion (ADME) and defines the pharmacokinetic profile of a drug. Since DDS control the time, rate, and place of delivery, they can modify the pharmacokinetic profile of a drug. Because the pharmacokinetic profile has direct implications on the clinical effect (pharmacodynamics) of the drug, regulation of DDS pharmacokinetics becomes critical to ensure the effectiveness and safety of DDS intended to enter the market. From a regulatory standpoint, one of the forms to study the pharmacokinetic profile of a drug is by measuring its bioavailability. The term bioavailability (BA) was coined to define the extent and rate at which a drug product reaches the site of action while bioequivalence (BE) could be defined as the lack of significant difference in bioavailability between two different drug formulations (e.g., two different DDS using the same drug). FDA guidelines for industry in bioequivalence and bioavailability describe a number of studies (clinical, but in some cases, in vitro studies are sufficient) to characterize the pharmacokinetic profile of a drug or a drug contained in a DDS. Some of these studies include the systemic exposure profile, which is a measurement of the concentration of the active principle obtained from a clinical sample as a function of time (e.g., taking blood samples at different times). These studies provide relevant information because it is possible to determine if the drug levels are below a reference (lack of efficacy) or above the reference (toxicity). Potential recommendations provided by the FDA arising from these studies range from changing the formulation (or delivery system) and repeating the pharmacokinetic study, to changing the manufacturing process (Box 21.1).

BOX 21.1 QUALITY OF LIFE AND PHARMACOKINETICS

One common side effect of patients suffering from cancer undergoing chemotherapy is emesis. In addition, some chemotherapeutic agents produce adverse effects in the mouth, such as oral inflammation (stomatitis). Because some patients suffer from both emesis and stomatitis, which impede the patient from taking oral pills, an oral spray version of an antiemetic drug was developed to overcome this issue. The FDA requested bioequivalence studies to demonstrate that the bioavailability of the oral pill containing the antiemetic drug was similar to the oral spray in order to ensure that any potential bioavailability change would not produce drug concentrations above or below the therapeutic range, both cases resulting in serious risks for the patient [29].

PREMARKET ASSESSMENT OF DDS

After the clinical development of a DDS has been completed, the manufacturer is required to submit all the information to the FDA as an NDA application (if the OCP has dictated that the DDS should be regulated as a drug) or PMA or 510k application (if the OCP has determined that the DDS should be regulated as a device).

CASE #1: THE DDS IS CLASSIFIED AS A DRUG

FDA Premarket Approval of Drugs

Many DDS have drugs as their primary mode of action and thereby will be evaluated as drugs in order to obtain FDA clearance for commercialization. New drugs (new molecular entities) or drugs that are copies of new drugs (generics) that are intended to enter the market must pass a stringent evaluation process by FDA. The office in charge of such evaluation is the Center for Drug Evaluation and Research (CDER). The document that must be filed and presented to CDER in order to obtain clearance for commercialization is known as NDA or new drug approval. An NDA should contain, in detail, the entire history of the drug, including manufacturing, in vitro testing, preclinical and clinical studies, quality systems, and all the relevant information needed to ensure the safety and effectiveness of the drug. There are several types of NDA:

1. An NDA for a new molecular entity where the manufacturer presents all the information concerning the safety and efficacy of the new drug and where all the studies have been performed by the manufacturer
2. An NDA where the manufacturer presents all the information about the safety and efficacy of the new drug but where one or more studies were conducted by another organization other than the manufacturer (e.g., a contract research organization)
3. An NDA for a copy of an existing drug, called a generic drug (also called an abbreviated new drug application or ANDA) [30].

CASE #2: THE DDS IS CLASSIFIED AS A MEDICAL DEVICE

FDA Premarket Approval of Medical Devices

According to the FDA, a medical device is the following:

> An instrument, apparatus, implement, machine, contrivance, implant, in vitro reagent, which is recognized in the United States Pharmacopoeia, intended for use in the diagnosis of disease or other conditions, or in the cure, treatment, or prevention of disease, or does not achieve its primary intended purposes through chemical action within the body and which is not dependent upon being metabolized for the achievement of any of its primary intended purposes. [16].

There are a variety of medical devices in the market used for either monitoring (glucose monitoring devices), laboratory diagnostics (HIV diagnostic kits), clinical diagnostics (stethoscopes) or therapeutic purposes (heart valves, pacemakers).

Medical Device Regulation

According to the CDRH, there are three categories of medical devices based on their risk: Class I, Class II, and Class III. Class I devices are considered low-risk devices and therefore require low control levels. An example of a Class I device is examination gloves. Class II devices are of intermediate risk and have more control levels than Class I devices. Examples of Class II devices are CT scanners. Finally, Class III devices are high-risk devices, because their malfunction could result in life-threatening adverse effects, and therefore Class III devices require high control levels. Examples of Class III devices include defibrillators and pacemakers. For each category, there are specific requirements and standards that must be followed.

Investigational Device Exemption (IDE)

An IDE should be submitted to the FDA by the manufacturer when a device is intended to be used for the first time in a human subject as an investigational device. An IDE should also be submitted when the sponsor wants to submit a new use for an existing device [31,32].

Humanitarian Device Exemption (HDE)

The HDE constitutes a regulatory pathway that applies for devices which are intended to be used in less than 4,000 patients per year in the United States. This pathway benefits device manufacturers that develop devices that are targeting low prevalent diseases where the economic incentive is low. Manufacturers applying for HDE are benefited through FDA waiver of effectiveness data. Therefore, manufacturers must submit only safety data and confirm that the benefits from using the device outweigh the risks, when comparing with current standard-of-care devices.

Premarket Notification (510k)

Premarket notification (also known as 510k) is a premarket application where the manufacturer claims equivalence of the device with a device already in the market (known as "the predicate device"). The level of equivalence with the predicate devices is established based on the following:

1. Has the device the same intended use as the predicate device and has the same technological characteristics or
2. Has the device the same intended use as the predicate device and has different technological characteristics and the information submitted to FDA
    a. Does not raise new questions of safety and effectiveness
    b. Demonstrates that the device is at least as safe and effective as the legally marketed device

The rationale for this assessment is that if enough similarity exists with an existing device in the market, it will be expected that the new device will perform similarly in terms of safety and effectiveness to the predicate device. If the device does not meet FDA criteria for equivalence to an existing device, a premarket approval (PMA) is required. Class I and Class II devices could be exempted from a 510k if they are pre-amendment devices, which means they have existed in the market before 1976 and have not significantly changed since then or they are exempted by regulation.

Premarket Approval (PMA)

Premarket approval (PMA) applies for high-risk devices (Class III devices). A PMA is required when it is not possible to prove substantial equivalence to an existing device (510k). In addition to bench and preclinical data, PMA usually requires additional clinical data to demonstrate the safety and effectiveness of the device.

FDA: POST-MARKET ASSESSMENT OF MEDICAL PRODUCTS

Post-market requirements for medical products involve a number of regulatory controls after the medical products have been cleared for commercialization. Among these, there are surveillance activities, such as reporting adverse events related to the medical product either by the patient, physician, or manufacturer. To accomplish this task, the FDA has created the Medical Device Reporting system (MDR) where manufacturers must report adverse events associated with a medical device. In addition, Med Watch is a medical report system that can be used by patients and professionals who could report to the FDA any potential adverse event that might be related to a medical product [33]. Manufacturers could also be required to conduct post-marketing surveillance studies. The rationale for post-market surveillance studies is that during the clinical development phase, a very small proportion of the population is tested with the medical product, thereby not reflecting the adverse effects that would be seen in a large population of patients once the medical product is in the market. This could be due to the low prevalence of the problem associated with the medical product, making the odds of detection during clinical trials very low (e.g., allergy to titanium) or because the problem was found in a specific lot of the product that differs from the one used during clinical trials. It is also possible that even if an adverse event is not detected in a patient, a manufacturer might detect a problem or a correction that needs to be made in a medical product. In this case, it is the obligation of the manufacturer to report the problem to the FDA by performing a recall. A recall is an action taken (in most cases by the manufacturer) when a medical product violates FDA law. According to the Code of Federal Regulations CFR Title 21 Volume 7, "A Recall means a firm's removal or correction of a marketed product that the FDA considers being in violation of the laws under its jurisdiction and against which the agency would initiate legal actions." Recalls are classified as Class I, Class II, and Class III according to the severity they represent for public health. Class I recalls represent a serious threat whereas Class III represents almost negligible risk. A market withdrawal involves those cases in which a manufacturer withdraws a product from the market even if no FDA legal action is expected against the product.

Recalls to DDS are based on different issues that range from mechanical problems to electronic or material issues. A problem that has been frequently reported over the last years are infusion pumps. Problems with drug infusion systems, such as corrosion of the motor stall of the pump, incorrect use of the pump by incorporating drugs other than those approved for use with that pump, or a touchscreen unresponsive to user input, resulting in delayed delivery of drugs, are examples of recalls. Another example was described when a pressure switch that was designed to control the drug supply and drug reservoir failed to alert when the reservoir was empty, putting the patient at risk. Problems with drug overdosing were also reported when the alarm that controls the door that opens and releases the drug was not working properly, generating a free flow of drug that would result in drug overdose [34].

FDA AND NEW TECHNOLOGIES FOR DDS: MICRO- AND NANOTECHNOLOGIES

Microtechnologies refer to technologies that enable manipulation of matter in the scale of 1 μm–100 μm (a hair is 80 μm in thickness). Examples include microelectromechanical systems (MEMS). Nanotechnologies are technologies that enable manipulation of matter at the nanoscale level (between 1 and 100 nm; a virus is 50 nm in diameter). Examples include nanoparticles. Nanotechnologies can be further divided into bottom-up and top-down technologies. Bottom-up technologies take advantage of chemical methods of synthesis to produce nanostructures, ranging from atomic clusters up to nanoparticles or thin films. Nanoparticles are structures that range in size between 1 and 100 nm. Because of their nanosize scale, nanoparticles are capable of crossing biological barriers, gaining access to hard-to-reach sites of the human body (blood–brain barrier, retina–blood barrier). In addition, due to their ability to accommodate hydrophobic drugs in their core and their capacity to be functionalized with specific ligands, such as monoclonal antibodies, nanoparticles became an attractive option as drug delivery systems. For example, nanoparticles could greatly benefit cancer therapies by improving the access of anticancer drugs to the tumors and improving the specificity of anticancer drugs. The latter can be achieved by combining molecular moieties to the surface of the nanoparticles that bind to tumor cells selectively. Some of these nanoparticles have been in the market for many years, while others are still at the early stage of development.

What makes nanoparticles as attractive as drug delivery systems is also a matter of concern. The high surface area–to–volume ratio of nanoparticles increases their reactivity and has been cited as a one of the potential causes of their toxicity. The small size of nanoparticles would potentially allow them to penetrate anatomical barriers, such as the skin, and gain access to the systemic circulation. In addition, nanoparticles have been shown to improve antigenicity of some antigens and act as adjuvants to promote an immune response. Some nanoparticles present a high length-to-width ratio and are known as nanofibers. A particular type of nanofibers are carbon nanotubes (CNTs). CNTs have been extensively studied due to their potential lung toxicity. Other nanoparticles, known as semiconductor nanocrystals or quantum dots, which have attracted much attention due to their unique optical properties, have raised concerns due to the presence of cadmium in their core. The possibility of cadmium to be released if the coating of the particle is degraded could result in the potential accumulation of cadmium in the human body. Based on the aforementioned, nanoparticle systems became a focus of debate in terms of their toxicological potential. As a result, several initiatives have been developed. Examples include the Woodrow Wilson Center for Nanotechnologies, which oversees the impact of nanotechnologies in health. Among the federal agencies, the Environmental Protection Agency (EPA), and the National Institutes for Occupational Safety and Health (NIOSH) have created special programs or redacted guidelines concerning the potential risk of nanoparticle exposure in the environment and at the occupational setting. The FDA, as a federal agency controlling the safety of medical products, has created the FDA Nanotechnology Task Force. The Nanotechnology Task Force is in charge of finding regulatory gaps in nanotechnology regulation, addressing these gaps by creating regulatory approaches for nanotechnology products that would result in safer and more effective products entering the market. Several FDA offices are affiliated to the task force. These offices include CDER, CBER, CDRH, CFSAN, CVM, NCTR, the Center of the Commissioner, and the office of Regulatory Affairs.

In addition to specific areas of research in which each office is involved, a center to accelerate the clinical development of innovative nanotechnology products for cancer treatment was developed. This center is known as the Nanotechnology Characterization Laboratory (NCL), which is a joint effort between the FDA, the National Cancer Institute (NCI), and the National Institute for Standards (NIST). The NCL aims at accelerating the transition between fundamental nanoscale sciences into clinical development of anticancer nanoscale systems by providing critical infrastructure to manufacturers interested in bringing their product to the clinical phase. Therefore, the NCL mission is to perform the complete characterization of nanoparticles that are developed for cancer therapies. The characterization includes preclinical toxicology and pharmacology of nanopharmaceutical systems. An example of the work performed at NCL was the characterization of dendrimers as carriers of gadolinium for their use as contrast agents for MRI. The characterization included in vitro studies, such as cytotoxicity and immunotoxicity, physicochemical characterization, including hydrodynamic size distribution by dynamic light scattering, molecular weight measurements by mass spectrometry, and MRI relaxivity measurements [35–44].

Top-down technologies are based on microfabrication technologies, and comprise a number of technologies originally developed by the microelectronic industry, including photolithography, thin-film deposition, doping, dry etching, wet etching, and electroplating among others. These techniques have been used for more than 40 years by the microelectronic industry and are now achieving an astonishing level of resolution that goes well below 100 nm (nanofabrication). More recently, these techniques were adopted to develop micro- and nanoelectromechanical systems (MEMS/NEMS), also known as micromachines, or microsystems. MEMS/NEMS are now being explored to develop DDS. Advantages of MEMS include control over drug release kinetics, multiple pharmacotherapies on a single device, batch fabrication with high reproducibility at low cost, allowing low interbatch variability, active control via integration with microelectronics ("smart pills"), accuracy in the drug payload, and precise control over the geometry, such as asymmetrical microparticles, increasing versatility of the DDS. All these advantages have generated great interest among the academic and industry sectors working in the drug delivery field. Examples of MEMS drug delivery devices being developed or already commercialized include micropumps, microneedles, microchips, and microparticles. Some of these technologies are already in the market (Table 21.2) while others are in the FDA pipeline (Table 21.2) [44,45] (Box 21.2).

TABLE 21.2
FDA Milestones in DDS Approved by FDA

Product Brand Name	Description	Manufacturer	Comment
Exhubera	Inhalatory insulin	Pfizer	One of the first inhalated insulins DDS FDA approved (2006) The DDS was withdrawn from the market one year later
Ambisome	Amphotericin loaded in liposomes	Nexstar	One of the First antilesihmanial drugs approved by FDA
MicroCHIPS	MEMS drug delivery system	MicroCHIPS Inc.	First microchip DDS. IND approved (2012)
Fluzone	Intradermal Flue microneedle vaccine	Sanofi	One of the first microneedle arrays FDA approved
Transdermal Sc	Scopolamine trandermal patch	Novartis	First transdermal patches FDA approved (1979)
ProAir Respiclick	First breath actuated powder inhaler containing albuterol sulphate	Teva	First FDA approved inhalation devices breath actuated for asthma treatment (2014)
EVZIO	Naloxone autoinjector	Kaleo	First autioinjector FDA fast track approved for the management of opioid overdose (2014)

BOX 21.2 INNOVATIVE DDS

Hearing loss represents an important public health issue. More than 28 million Americans suffer from hearing loss. In addition, military personnel exposed to blast-induced cochlear damage, young people using headphones, and newborns with hearing deficiencies at birth (1:3,000) represent groups of the population where there is an urgent need for improving hearing loss. Cochlear prosthesis emerged as a powerful tool for restoring hearing to people where the cochlea is damaged. A recent approach to increase the efficiency of cochlear implants was to incorporate a DDS into the cochlear implant. In spite of the regulatory issues that such an innovative approach might entail, this technological improvement has a number of advantages from a regulatory standpoint including the following:

1. Utilizes the same surgical procedures as current cochlear implants already FDA-approved (there is a precedent that supports its use).
2. The technology complexity is of similar grade to existing cochlear implants without drug delivery capabilities.
3. Integration with current cochlear implants does not compromise implant functionality.
4. A local delivery system decreases the risk of adverse drug reactions as improves efficacy.

This represents an example of how it is possible to address regulatory requirements for novel devices by a strategic design from the early stages of development [46].

ETHICAL CONSIDERATIONS IN FDA REGULATION

Recent publications have called attention to increasing concerns regarding conflict of interest within FDA committees, particularly in the pharmaceutical industry [47,48]. These papers warned about a potential conflict of interest among members of FDA committees, claiming that several members of those committees had ties with the biomedical industry, and that information was not disclosed by the FDA. The consequences of such influences not only could jeopardize the trust in federal agencies and ultimately in the government, but also could weaken the regulatory barriers allowing products of unclear quality enter the market. A recent meta-analysis reported about this issue by analyzing several premarket approvals submitted to the FDA between 2000 and 2007. The study accounted for the lack of the minimum methodological requirements among clinical studies submitted within the PMAs to be considered reliable [49]. This issue of potential conflict of interest within the FDA has raised concerns about how medical products should be regulated. As a result of this controversy, independent committee assessment groups have been created. These committees would collaborate with FDA experts by performing critical reviews of clinical studies in order to ensure the quality of the evidence that is presented for review to the FDA. Some of these groups include the Institute of Medicine (IOM), Medicare, professional associations, and the California Technology Assessment Forum (CATF) [50].

Another subject of increasing concern is the approval times for medical products submitted to the FDA. This is particularly true when approval times are compared with the European Union where some medical devices receive regulatory approval for commercialization long before they do in the United States. For example, the drug-eluting stent was available in Europe a year earlier than in the United States and 75% of cardiovascular devices were tested for the first time outside the United States, while a novel device (artificial retina) developed to restore the vision to people blinded by retinitis picmentosa was launched in Europe almost 1 year before receiving approval by FDA [51,52]. While some political groups and the public opinion entrust the FDA with the task of ensuring that any product entering the market will be safe for the population, other advocate groups (cancer, neurodegenerative disorders, patient advocates) and in particular the biomedical industry, lobby for treatments to be available as soon as possible. For these reasons, the FDA has launched the critical path initiative to accelerate the regulatory process for medical products. The Critical Path Initiative (CPI) addresses critical areas where the FDA pipeline demands urgent solutions for unmet clinical needs in public health. Some of these areas are related to medical devices, including modernization of clinical trials to improve the manner in which medical device trials are designed. Since many DDS are considered medical devices from a regulatory standpoint, it can be thought that DDS regulations will be affected by the CPI if medical device regulations are modified. Lastly, the CPI is bringing together different sectors, including academia, regulatory experts, and industry conforming a multidisciplinary, multitask group, providing outstanding capabilities for the forthcoming challenges that the interdisciplinary field of DDS will present to the FDA [53,54].

ACKNOWLEDGMENT

To Marina Gorgoschidse for her assistance during the review of this manuscript.

REFERENCES

1. Tan, S.Y. and Grimes, S. 2010. Paul Ehrlich (1854–1915): Man with the magic bullet. *Singapore Med J* 51(11): 842.
2. Jain, K.K. 2008. Drug delivery systems: An overview. *Methods Mol Biol* 437: 1–50.
3. Bawa, R. 2008. Nanoparticle therapeutics in humans: A survey. *Nanotechnol Law Business*. 5 (2).
4. Gabor, F., Fillafer, C., Neutsch, L., Ratzinger, G., and Wirth, M. 2010. Improving oral delivery. In *Drug Delivery Systems*. M. Schäfer-Korting (Ed.), Springer: Berlin.
5. Shargel, L., Wu-Pong, S., and Yu, A.B.C. 2005. Drug product performance in vivo: Bioavailability and bioequivalence. In *Applied Biopharmaceutics and Pharmacokinetics*. McGraw Hill: New York.
6. Gulati, N. and Gupta, H. 2011. Parenteral drug delivery: A review. *Recent Pat Drug Deliv Formul*. 5(2): 133–145.

7. U.S. Department of Health and Human Services Food and Drug Administration Center for Devices and Radiological Health, Center for Drug Evaluation Research, Center for Biologics Evaluation and Research, and Office of Combination Products in the Office of the Commissioner Guidance for Industry and FDA Staff: Technical Considerations for Pen, Jet, and Related Injectors Intended for Use with Drugs and Biological Products FDA Guidelines on Injectors. 2013.
8. Huy, R.G. 2010. Transdermal drug delivery. In *Drug Delivery Systems.* M. Schäfer-Korting (Ed.), Springer: Berlin.
9. Henning, A., Hein, S., Schneider, M., Bur, M., and Lehr, C.M. 2010. Pulmonary drug delivery: Medicines for inhalation. In *Drug Delivery Systems.* M. Schäfer-Korting (Ed.), Springer: Berlin.
10. Albu, S. 2012. Novel drug delivery systems for patients with rhinosinusitis. *Drug Des Dev Ther* 6125–6132.
11. Tobias, J.D. and Ross, A.K. 2010. Intraosseous infusions: A review for the anesthesiologist with a focus on pediatric use. *Anesth Analg* 110(2): 391–401.
12. Kompella, U.B., Kadam, R.S., and Lee, V.H.L. 2010. Recent advances in ophthalmic drug delivery. *Ther Deliv* 1(3): 435–456.
13. Woolfson, A.D., Malcolm, R.K., and Gallagher, R. 2000. Drug delivery by the intravaginal route. *Crit Rev Ther Drug Carrier Syst* 17(5): 509–555.
14. Ferguson, L.M. and Cencia Rohan, L. 2011. The importance of the vaginal delivery route for antiretrovirals in HIV prevention. *Ther Deliv* 2(12): 1535–1550.
15. Baloglu, E., Senyigit, Z.A., Karavana, S.Y., and Bernkop-Schnürch, A. 2009. Strategies to prolong the intravaginal residence time of drug delivery systems. *J Pharm Pharm Sci* 12(3): 312–336.
16. Potschk, H. 2010. Targeting the brain—Surmounting or bypassing the blood-brain barrier. In *Drug Delivery Systems.* M. Schäfer-Korting (Ed.), Springer: Berlin.
17. FDA website, available at www.fda.gov (accessed May 2013).
18. *United States FDA Medical Devices Control and Regulation Handbook.* 2010. Vol. 1: Strategic and Practical Information, 4th ed. International Publisher Publications, Washington.
19. Annas, G.J. and Elias, S. 1999. Thalidomide and the Titanic: Reconstructing the technology tragedies of the twentieth century. *Am J Public Health* 89: 98–101.
20. ISO website, available at http://www.iso.org (accessed May 2013).
21. ASTM website, available at http://www.astm.org (accessed May 2013).
22. Code of Federal Regulations website, available at http://www.gpoaccess.gov/cfr/
23. International Conferences on Harmonization website, available at http://www.ich.org (accessed May 2013).
24. FDA website, available at http://www.fda.gov/RegulatoryInformation/Guidances/ucm126198.htm (accessed May 2013).
25. Siegel, E.B. 2008. *Development and Approval of Combination Products.* Wiley: New Jersey.
26. Kaplan, A.V. et al. 2004 Medical Device Regulation: From Prototype to Regulatory Approval. *Circulation* 109: 3068–3072.
27. Mehta, S.S. 2008. *Commercializing Successful Biomedical Technologies.* Cambridge University Press, New York.
28. Lawrence, M.F., Furberg, C.D., and De Mets, D.L. 2010. *Fundamentals of Clinical Trials*, 4th ed. Springer, New York, pp. 1–5.
29. Shargel, L. and Yu, A.B.C. (Eds.). 2012. Drug product performance, in vivo: Bioavailability and bioequivalence. In *Applied Biopharmaceutics and Pharmacokinetics.* McGraw Hill: New York.
30. FDA website, available at http://www.fda.gov/Drugs/DevelopmentApprovalProcess/HowDrugsareDevelopedandApproved/ApprovalApplications/NewDrugApplicationNDA/default.htm (accessed May 2013).

31. Felten, R.P. et al. 2005. Food and drug administration medical device review process: Clearance of a cot retriever for use in ischemic stroke. *Stroke* 34: 404–406.
32. FDA website, available at http://www.fda.gov/MedicalDevices/DeviceRegulationand Guidance/Overview/default.htm (accessed June 2013).
33. FDA website, available at http://www.fda.gov/MedicalDevices/Safety/ReportaProblem /default.htm (accessed May 2013).
34. Brown, S.L., Bright, R.A., and Travis, D.R. 2004. Medical device epidemiology and surveillance: Patient safety is the bottom line. *Expert Rev Med Dev* 1 (1): 1–2.
35. National Nanotechnology Initiative website, available at http://www.nano.gov/html /facts/whatIsNano.html (accessed December 2010).
36. Ferrari, M. 2005. Cancer nanotechnology: Opportunities and challenges. *Nat Rev Cancer* 5(3): 161–71.
37. Vauthier, C. and Couvreur, P. 2007. Nanomedicines: A new approach for the treatment of serious diseases. *J Biomed Nanotechnol* 3: 1–12.
38. Woodrow Wilson Center. Project on Emerging Nanotechnologies website, available at http://www.nanotechproject.org/ (accessed December 2010).
39. NISOH website, available at http://www.cdc.gov/niosh/docs/2009-125/
40. EPA website, available at http://www.epa.gov/nanoscience/
41. Oberdoster, E. and Oberdoster, J. 2005. Nanotoxicology: An emerging discipline evolving from studies of ultrafine particles. *Environ Health Perspect* 113: 823–839.
42. Drobvolskaia, M.A. and McNeil, S. 2007. Immunological properties of nanoscale materials. *Nat Nanotechnol* 2: 469–478.
43. Saho, L., Gao, Y., and Yan, F. 2011. Semiconductor quantum dots for biomedical applications. *Sensors*. 11: 11736–11751.
44. Nanotechnology: A report of the Food and Drug Administration Nanotechnology Task Force 2007. Available at http://www.fda.gov/ScienceResearch/SpecialTopics /Nanotechnology/Nanotechnology Task Force/default.html
45. Staples, M. et al. Application of micro- and nano-electromechanical devices to drug delivery. *Pharm Res* 23(5): 847–863.
46. Borenstein. J.T. 2011. Intracochlear drug delivery systems. *Expert Opin Drug Deliv* 8(9): 1161–1174.
47. Lenzer, J., and Epstein, K. 2012. US advisory panelists on drug's safety had ties to manufacturers. *BMJ* 10: 344.
48. Bitter Pill: Why Medical Bills Are Killing Us. *Time Magazine*, February 2013.
49. Dhruva, S.S., Bero, L.A., and Redberg, R.F. 2009. Strength of study evidence examined by the FDA in premarket approval of cardiovascular devices. *JAMA* 302 (24): 2679–2685.
50. Feldman, M.D. et al. 2008. Who is responsible for evaluating the safety and effectiveness of medical devices? The role of independent technology assessment. *J Gen Intern Med* 23(Suppl. 1): 57–63.
51. Kaplan, A.V. et al. 2004. Medical device regulation: From prototype to regulatory approval. *Circulation* 109: 3068–3072.
52. Second Sight website, available at http://2-sight.eu/en/home-en (accessed June 2013).
53. Critical Path Initiative website, available at http://www.fda.gov/ScienceResearch /special Topics/Critical Path Initiative/
54. Avorn, J. 2007. Keeping science on top of drug evaluation. *N Engl J Med* 357(7): 633–663.

Index

Page numbers followed by f and t indicate figures and tables, respectively.

B

E

H

J

K

L

N

Q

Printed and bound by CPI Group (UK) Ltd, Croydon, CR0 4YY
01/11/2024
01782622-0017